SEMICONDUCTOR LASERS AND HETEROJUNCTION LEDs

QUANTUM ELECTRONICS — PRINCIPLES AND APPLICATIONS

A Series of Monographs

EDITED BY
YOH-HAN PAO
Case Western Reserve University
Cleveland, Ohio

N. S. *Kapany and J. J. Burke.* OPTICAL WAVEGUIDES, 1972

Dietrich Marcuse. THEORY OF DIELECTRIC OPTICAL WAVEGUIDES, 1974

Benjamin Chu. LASER LIGHT SCATTERING, 1974

Bruno Crosignani, Paolo Di Porto, and Mario Bertolotti. STATISTICAL PROPERTIES OF SCATTERED LIGHT, 1975

John D. Anderson, Jr. GASDYNAMIC LASERS: AN INTRODUCTION, 1976

W. W. Duley. CO_2 LASERS: EFFECTS AND APPLICATIONS, 1976

Henry Kressel and J. K. Butler. SEMICONDUCTOR LASERS AND HETEROJUNCTION LEDs, 1977

In preparation

H. C. *Casey and M. B. Panish.* HETEROSTRUCTURE LASERS

SEMICONDUCTOR LASERS AND HETEROJUNCTION LEDs

HENRY KRESSEL
RCA Laboratories
Princeton, New Jersey

J. K. BUTLER
Department of Electrical Engineering
Southern Methodist University
Dallas, Texas

ACADEMIC PRESS   New York   San Francisco   London   1977

A Subsidiary of Harcourt Brace Jovanovich, Publishers

ACADEMIC PRESS, INC.
111 Fifth Avenue, New York, New York 10003

United Kingdom Edition published by
ACADEMIC PRESS, INC. (LONDON) LTD.
24/28 Oval Road, London NW1

Library of Congress Cataloging in Publication Data

Kressel, Henry.
    Semiconductor lasers and heterojunction LEDs

    (Quantum electronics—principles and applications)
    Includes bibliographies.
    1.   Semiconductor lasers.   2.   Light emitting diodes.
I.   Butler, Jerome K., joint author.   II.   Title.
TA1700.K73   621.36'61   76-42974
ISBN 0–12–426250–3

To
Bertha Kressel
and
Virginia M. Butler

Contents

Preface   xiii

Introduction

I.1   Background   1
I.2   Outline   5
      References   7

Chapter 1   Résumé of Relevant Concepts in Solid State Physics

1.1   Crystal Structure   9
1.2   Bonding and Band Structure   11
1.3   Dopants   16
1.4   Electron Distribution and Density of States   21
1.5   Electron–Hole Pair Formation and Recombination   26
1.6   Minority Carrier Diffusion   33
1.7   Radiative Recombination Processes Other than Band-to-Band   35
1.8   Nonradiative Recombination Processes   44
      References   47

Chapter 2   p–n Junctions and Heterojunctions

2.1   Current–Voltage Characteristics   51
2.2   Junction Capacitance   60
2.3   Heterojunctions   61
2.4   Light–Current Relationships in Spontaneous Emission   70

2.5 Diode Frequency Response as Limited by Carrier Lifetime   73
     References   75

Chapter 3 Stimulated Emission and Gain

3.1 Introduction   77
3.2 Optical Gain in the Two-Level Atomic System   82
3.3 Optical Gain in a Direct Bandgap Semiconductor   84
3.4 The Fabry–Perot Cavity and Threshold Condition   95
3.5 Laser Transitions   103
     References   115

Chapter 4 Relevant Concepts in Electromagnetic Field Theory

4.1 Introduction   117
4.2 Maxwell's Equations   119
4.3 Complex Dielectric Constant   120
4.4 Boundary Conditions   122
4.5 Poynting's Theorem   123
4.6 Vector Wave Equation   125
4.7 Plane Waves   127
4.8 Plane Wave Reflection and Transmission at Plane Boundaries   131
     References   136

Chapter 5 Modes in Laser Structures: Mainly Theory

5.1 Laser Topology and Modes   137
5.2 Waveguide Equations   143
5.3 Wave Definitions   145
5.4 Slab Waveguides   146
5.5 Slab Waveguide Mode Characteristics   155
5.6 Propagation in a Dissipative/Gain Medium   162
5.7 Three-Dimensional Modes in Practical Structures   165
5.8 Five-Layer Slab Waveguide Modes   172
5.9 Modal Facet Reflectivity   174
5.10 Mode Selection in Laser Structures   180
     References   183

Chapter 6 Laser Radiation Fields

6.1 Introduction   185
6.2 Radiation from Slab Waveguides   186
6.3 Boundary Solution of the Radiation Fields   191
6.4 Modal Radiation Patterns from Slab Waveguides   195
6.5 Radiation of Three-Layer Slab Modes   198
6.6 Radiation from Two-Dimensional Waveguides   198
     References   202

Chapter 7   Modes in Laser Structures: Mainly Experimental

7.1   Introduction   205
7.2   Double-Heterojunction Lasers   206
7.3   Four-Heterojunction Lasers   222
7.4   Asymmetrical Structures—Single-Heterojunction (Close-Confinement)
        Lasers   228
7.5   Large Optical Cavity Lasers—Symmetrical and Asymmetrical Structures   230
7.6   Experimental/Theoretical Radiation Patterns (Transverse Modes)   234
7.7   Lateral "*s*" Modes   238
7.8   Summary   244
        References   247

Chapter 8   Relation between Electrical and Optical Properties of Laser Diodes

8.1   Carrier Confinement and Injected Carrier Utilization   249
8.2   Threshold Current Density and Differential Quantum Efficiency   261
8.3   Temperature Dependence of J_{th} 275
8.4   Optical Anomalies and Radiation Confinement Loss in Asymmetrical
        Heterojunction Lasers   280
        References   285

Chapter 9   Epitaxial Technology

9.1   Liquid Phase Epitaxy   287
9.2   Vapor Phase Epitaxy   294
9.3   Molecular Beam Epitaxy   296
9.4   Lattice Mismatch Effects   298
9.5   Substrate Considerations   318
        References   322

Chapter 10   Binary III–V Compounds

10.1   Gallium Arsenide   327
10.2   Gallium Phosphide   346
10.3   Gallium Antimonide   351
10.4   Indium Arsenide   352
10.5   Indium Phosphide   352
10.6   Aluminum Arsenide and Aluminum Phosphide   353
        References   353

Chapter 11   Ternary and Quaternary III–V Compounds

11.1   General Considerations   357
11.2   Phase Diagrams—Introduction   363
11.3   Principal Ternary Alloys   369

11.4   Quaternary Compounds   389
       References   393

Chapter 12   **Diode Fabrication and Related Topics**

12.1   Junction Formation and Layer Characterization   399
12.2   Some Key Properties of $Al_xGa_{1-x}As$ Relevant to Device Design   413
12.3   Active Junction Area Definition   420
12.4   Thermal Dissipation of Laser Diodes   428
       References   434

Chapter 13   **Heterojunction Devices of Alloys Other than GaAs–AlAs**

13.1   Introduction   437
13.2   IV–VI Compound Lasers   439
13.3   III–V Compound Lasers   446
13.4   Summary   452
       References   453

Chapter 14   **Devices for Special Applications**

14.1   High Peak Power, Pulsed Operation Laser Diodes   455
14.2   Fiber Concepts Relevant to Optical Communications   465
14.3   Near-Infrared CW Laser Diodes of (AlGa)As   473
14.4   High Radiance Light-Emitting Diodes   485
14.5   Visible Emission Laser Diodes   500
14.6   General Purpose Heterojunction LEDs   510
       References   518

Chapter 15   **Distributed-Feedback Lasers**

15.1   Introduction   523
15.2   Coupled Mode Analysis   523
15.3   Solution of Coupled Modes   526
15.4   GaAs–(AlGa)As DFB Lasers   527
       References   531

Chapter 16   **Device Reliability**

16.1   Facet (Catastrophic) Degradation   533
16.2   Internal Damage Mechanisms   538
16.3   Technology of Reliable Devices   549
       References   553

Chapter 17 **Transient Effects in Laser Diodes**

17.1	Introduction	555
17.2	Turn-On Effects	556
17.3	Continuous Oscillations	566
17.4	Oscillations Related to Nonuniform Population Inversion	573
17.5	Diode Modulation	575
17.6	Summary	578
	References	579

Appendix A **Physical Constants** 581

Appendix B **Gain in Strong Fields and Lateral Multimoding**

B.1	Introduction	585
B.2	Spatial Modulation of the Gain and Multimoding	585
B.3	Optically Induced Saturation of Transition Probabilities	586
B.4	Spontaneous Power in the Lasing Region	588
B.5	Summary	589

Appendix C **Pressure Effects on Heterojunction Laser Diodes**

C.1	Uniaxial Stress	591
C.2	Hydrostatic Stress	592

Appendix D **Atmosphere Attenuation of GaAs Laser Emission** 597

Appendix E **Single Mode Emission Line Width** 599

Index 603

Preface

After more than a decade of research, the semiconductor laser has emerged as an important component in optoelectronic systems. Perhaps the most important emerging application is in the field of optical communications using fibers. Parallel advances in laser diodes and LEDs, as well as fibers, promise to make optical systems viable and cost-effective communication channels.

The purpose of this book is to present an introduction to the subject of semiconductor lasers and heterojunction LEDs, the latter being primarily high radiance devices not generally intended for applications where visibility is important. Although it is not possible to fully do justice to the vast amount of published information concerning these devices, we have selected those areas in theory, material growth, fabrication, and application that we feel are most relevant to practical devices.

Some aspects of the field have reached a reasonable level of maturity, while others are in the process of rapid development—epitaxial technology, for example. Wherever possible we emphasize basic principles in order to provide a useful framework for understanding ongoing trends in device development. The first few chapters review relevant basic solid-state and electromagnetic principles. These introductory chapters are intended to make this book reasonably self-sufficient.

We are indebted to Drs. H. S. Sommers, Jr., J. P. Wittke, M. D. Miller, and D. Redfield for their critical reading and comments on sections of the manuscript. We are pleased to acknowledge useful discussions with M. Ettenberg, F. Hawrylo, I. Ladany, H. F. Lockwood, C. J. Nuese, G. H. Olsen, J. I. Pankove, and J. J. Tietjien. Finally, we are indebted to the management of RCA Laboratories for their continued support of laser and materials research.

Introduction

I.1 Background

The semiconductor laser diode blends the basic p–n junction common to many semiconductor devices with the quantum electronic concepts common to all lasers. Compared to gas or solid state lasers of the HeNe- or Nd-doped YAG types, respectively, the semiconductor laser diode offers considerably smaller size, potentially lower cost, and the unique ability to modulate the optical output up to gigahertz rates by simply changing the current through the device. The unique properties of the laser diode make it an essential component of the emerging field of optical communications using glass fibers.

The laser diode is also related to the low power visible light-emitting diode (LED), but the LED has a broader spectral emission, its emission is less directional, and its modulation capability is limited. In addition, only certain types of semiconductors can be used for lasers ("direct bandgap" ones), and the laser diode must incorporate a narrow region designed for effective mode guiding (radiation confinement) and electron–hole recombination (carrier confinement). These requirements in modern lasers are met with the incorporation of one or more heterojunctions which introduce dielectric steps as well as potential barriers confining minority carriers.

Figure I.1 shows a basic laser diode chip which consists of two cleaved parallel facets and two sawed (roughened) sides. The cleaved facets define the Fabry–Perot cavity. As described in detail in Chapter 12, many lasers are now made in the stripe-contact configuration where the active diode area is defined by the contact area, and therefore roughening of the sides of the laser is not necessary. The emitting width of the laser is varied from about 1 μm to over 1000 μm by changing the diode geometry. Considering a typical diode

1

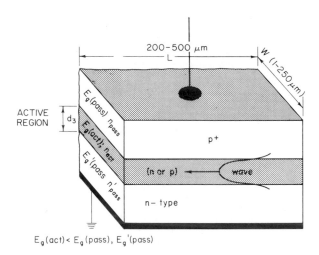

$E_g(act) < E_g(pass), E_g'(pass)$

FIG. I.1 Schematic of a basic laser diode chip formed by cleaving two parallel edges and roughening two sides. The active region of width d_3 is shown.

length of 300 μm, the laser diode's active area of 10^{-5}–10^{-4} cm^2 is small indeed compared to other types of lasers.

The internal laser diode configuration consists basically of a thin (order of 1 μm) *active* planar waveguide provided with injecting surfaces for minority carriers. The internal waveguide plays an essential role in confining the radiation to the region of electron–hole recombination in which light amplification occurs. In the *homojunction* lasers, small differences in doping provide small refractive index steps for this radiation guiding effect. In the *heterojunction* lasers the layer index steps are controlled by the difference in the bandgap energy of the adjoining regions, as shown in Fig. I.1 for the double-heterojunction laser (which is only one of several possible configurations as discussed in Chapter 5).

The width d_3 of the active region (i.e., region of electron–hole recombination) is also controlled in heterojunction lasers by the bandgap energy steps which provide potential barriers sufficient to confine the minority carriers. The term "close confinement lasers" was originally applied to heterojunction laser diodes specifically designed to provide for the first time effective carrier and radiation confinement to a well-defined active region. With the wide acceptance of the heterojunction concepts, the term "heterojunction lasers" denotes devices which incorporate the required control concepts, although poorly designed heterojunction lasers may perform worse than homojunction lasers. At this time, the field of semiconductor lasers is dominated by heterojunction devices and these, therefore, are mainly discussed in this book. However, mention of earlier results dealing with homojunction lasers is included whenever the internal structure is believed not to be relevant to the results discussed.

In this book we also discuss nonlasing heterojunction diodes (LEDs). The technology is similar to that of laser diodes; these are of particular interest as sources for optical communications using fibers because of the high radiance achievable with these structures as well as the ability to modulate their output at high frequencies. Although their operating frequencies are not as high as those achievable with laser diodes, they do meet the needs of many communications systems and are thus finding ever widening use.

The history of the laser diode is traced from the first demonstration in 1962 of stimulated emission in homojunction (diffused) GaAs diodes operating at cryogenic temperatures [1–3]. This work was followed by worldwide research aimed at improving understanding of the theory of stimulated emission in semiconductors, and the expansion of the lasing wavelength into the visible and the infrared spectrum by exploring many III–V and IV–VI compounds. In addition, investigations were made of lasing by electron beam pumping using platelets of II–VI compounds (where p–n junctions could not be formed). By 1968, lasing had been obtained in a spectral range from ∼ 20 to ∼ 0.5 μm, although room temperature operations were achieved with only some materials, the most important being GaAs emitting at ∼ 9000 Å.

The problems facing practical applications of the GaAs lasers were still very serious: (1) The threshold current density was generally in excess of 50, 000 A/cm² at room temperature, thus limiting the duty cycle to a small fraction of 1% because of excessive power dissipation, and (2) the reliability of the lasers was erratic, with operating lifetimes ranging from minutes to perhaps a few hundred hours at best. Thus, laser diodes could not be considered for serious applications when operation at ambient temperature was desired (as it most often is).

The problem of laser diode degradation was particularly troublesome because of the unhappy prior experience with GaAs tunnel diodes which, despite intense effort to remedy their poor lifetimes, failed to ever perform as required for practical use. The nagging question remained whether the laser diode, which also operated at high current densities, was doomed to a similar fate because of ill-understood but nevertheless fundamental reasons. The first hopeful indication that perhaps the degradation process was *not* fundamental came from the identification of the two basic failure causes—facet damage, which was shown related to the optical flux density [4, 5], and internal defect formation, which was shown to be related both to the initial metallurgical quality of the device and to the operating current density (actually the rate of electron–hole recombination in the active region) [6]. From these studies, it became evident that substantial reliability improvements could be made by carefully delineating the safe operating conditions and devising means of increasing the material perfection of the devices, particularly the elimination of dislocations [6].

The improvement in the basic GaAs laser performance, however, could not be brought about by an evolutionary development process. Fortunately, at the same time the degradation process became better defined, came the realization of heterojunction lasers using lattice-matched AlAs–GaAs alloys which dramatically reduced the threshold current density and increased the overall device efficiency. The realization of the heterojunction laser is the achievement of three laboratories working independently. The first room temperature operation heterojunction lasers incorporated a single heterojunction [7, 8] (with threshold current densities of 8000–10,000 A/cm²), followed by the lower threshold (∼ 4000 A/cm²) double-heterojunction devices [9–11] (Fig. I.2).

Note that the double-heterojunction concept was proposed [12] as early as 1963, simply as a means of improving the carrier injection efficiency into the active region compared to a homojunction. However, the construction of a heterojunction laser providing measurable benefits awaited suitable semiconductors and epitaxial technology. This came about with (AlGa)As alloys [13] since they have the nearly unique property that the bandgap energy can be changed over a wide range with negligible lattice parameter change, making low defect heterojunction structures possible.

Progress has continued since 1970 in laser diode technology and reliability,

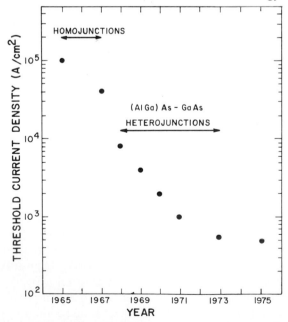

FIG. I.2   State-of-the art GaAs laser diode threshold current density.

and in theoretical understanding. In particular, the clear definition of the role of radiation guiding and a well-defined recombination region have permitted a detailed analysis of the modal properties of the laser diode which can be accurately compared to theory.

With the threshold current density routinely reduced to <4000 A/cm^2 at room temperature, the diodes can be conveniently operated continous wave (CW), or modulated at rates reaching the gigahertz region. In addition to its use in communications, the laser diode provides an interesting replacement for low power gas lasers in applications in which the near-infrared spectral emission is not a drawback. Furthermore, although interest in CW devices has grown, the use of pulsed operation, high power laser diodes (primarily single-heterojunction lasers and specially designed "large optical cavity" (LOC) [14] structures with varying four-heterojunction modifications [15]) has also grown. Thus, both branches of the laser diode family based on (AlGa)As–GaAs heterojunctions have continued to expand their practical applications as their operating lifetimes have increased into the order of years.

The success of these devices had prompted interest in expanding the heterojunction laser concept to other materials in order to obtain lasers in a spectral range beyond that achieved with the AlAs–GaAs alloys. Figure I.3 shows the range of wavelengths now achieved with heterojunction lasers.

I.2   Outline

The purpose of this book is to present a comprehensive treatment of the major aspects of the principles common to all devices irrespective of the semiconductor used. Extensive technological information is also provided on major devices and materials. Whenever possible, we illustrate key theoretical

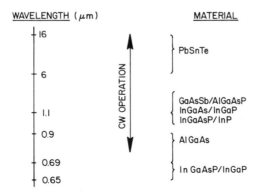

FIG. I.3   Spectral emission range and materials used to fabricate heterojunction laser diodes.

results with experiment and indicate areas in which discrepancies exist or further refinements are called for.

We have included tutorial material which we hope will prove useful to readers as a convenient summary of widely used equations and concepts. For example, Chapter 1 presents a summary of semiconductor concepts, particularly luminescent phenomena relevant to the operation of our devices; Chapter 4 presents a tutorial introduction to Maxwell's equations as relevant to the mode guiding problem.

Chapter 2 is concerned with a review of relevant p–n junction and heterojunction concepts. Chapter 3 introduces a discussion of stimulated emission in general, using the simple two-level atom system, and progresses into stimulated emission in semiconductors with specific application to GaAs.

Following a review of basic electromagnetic theory in Chapter 4, we follow in Chapter 5 with the analysis of the modes in laser diodes with due consideration of the vertical and horizontal geometry. Chapter 6 then adds the analysis of the radiation patterns in the *far field* and their relationship to the internal laser structure. The material in Chapters 4–6 is mainly theoretical, and it is therefore the objective of Chapter 7 to provide experimental comparisons to the theory and describe the major observations in state-of-the-art lasers.

Chapter 8 focuses on the relationship between the electrical and the optical properties of the lasers, including key aspects of the threshold temperature dependence, the role of interfacial recombination, and carrier leakage from the recombination region.

Chapters 9, 10, and 11 discuss basic semiconductor properties and epitaxial synthesis methods of interest in the operation and construction of laser diodes and LEDs covering a broad spectral range. Particular emphasis is placed on liquid phase epitaxy since it has been most widely used for heterojunction diode construction using III–V compounds.

Chapter 12 contains mainly technological information, much of it relevant to the construction of diodes using III–V compounds, including the various methods of preparing stripe-contact diodes.

In Chapter 13 we focus on devices fabricated with IV–VI compounds as well as on III–V compound diodes other than (AlGa)As devices.

The purpose of Chapter 14 is to highlight major diode classes for important applications. Particular emphasis is placed on diodes for fiber optical communications, and a brief review of fiber concepts relevant to diode needs is presented.

Chapter 15 is devoted to the newest addition to the laser diode family, the distributed-feedback laser which uses internal corrugations to produce single longitudinal mode emission.

Diode reliability and relevant models are discussed at length in Chapter 16.

Finally, in Chapter 17 the transient phenomena are discussed. The basic rate equations are developed and used to provide a unifying theme.

The appendixes discuss various topics which do not conveniently fit in any of the chapters.

We have used both the cgs and the MKS unit systems, depending on the material under discussion and what we feel to be most commonly used. The chapters concerned with electromagnetic theory, for example, use MKS units.

The symbols used include, of necessity, some duplications, but every attempt has been made to identify all but the most common symbols within each chapter. Major symbols are listed in Appendix A.

REFERENCES

1. R. N. Hall, G. E. Fenner, J. D. Kinglsey, T. J. Soltys, and R. O. Carlson, *Phys. Rev. Lett.* **9**, 366 (1962).
2. M. I. Nathan, W. P. Dumke, G. Burns, F. H. Dill, Jr., and G. Lasher, *Appl. Phys. Lett.* **1**, 63 (1962).
3. T. M. Quist, R. H. Rediker, R. J. Keyes, W. E. Krag, B. Lax, A. L. McWhorter, and H. J. Ziegler, *Appl. Phys. Lett.* **1**, 91 (1962).
4. C. D. Dobson and F. S. Keeble, *Proc. Int. Symp. GaAs, Reading, England.* Inst. Phys. and the Phys. Soc., 1967.
5. H. Kressel and H. P. Mierop, *J. Appl. Phys.* **38**, 5419 (1967).
6. H. Kressel and N. E. Byer, *Proc. IEEE* **38**, 25 (1969);
   H. Kressel *et al., Met. Trans.* **1**, 635 (1970).
7. H. Kressel and H. Nelson, *RCA Rev.* **30**, 106 (1969).
8. I. Hayashi, M. B. Panish, and P. W. Foy, *IEEE J. Quantum Electron.* **5**, 211 (1969).
9. Zh. I. Alferov, V. M. Andreev, E. L. Portnoi, and M. K. Trukan, *Fiz. Tekh. Poluprov.* **3**, 1328 (1969) [*English transl.: Sov. Phys. Semicond.* **3**, 1107 (1970)].
10. I. Hayashi, M. B. Panish, P. W. Foy, and S. Sumski, *Appl. Phys. Lett.* **17**, 109 (1970).
11. H. Kressel and F. Z. Hawrylo, *Appl. Phys, Lett.* **17**, 169 (1970).
12. H. Kroemer, *Proc. IEEE* **51**, 1782 (1963).
13. H. Rupprecht, J. M. Woodall, and D. G. Pettit, *Appl. Phys. Lett.* **11**, 81 (1967).
14. H. F. Lockwood, H. Kressel, H. S. Sommers, Jr., and F. Z. Hawrylo, *Appl. Phys. Lett.* **17**, 499 (1970).
15. G. H. B. Thompson and P. A. Kirkby, *IEEE J. Quantum Electron.* **9**, 311 (1973).

Chapter 1

Résumé of Relevant Concepts in Solid State Physics

1.1 Crystal Structure

The semiconductor materials used for electronic devices are said to be crystalline in that they consist of a periodic arrangement of atoms with the lattice constant a_0 (also called the lattice parameter) being the measure of the unit cell. The basic concepts concerning the behavior of electrons in solids start with the isolated atom in which a positively charged nucleus is surrounded by a sufficient number of electrons to form a neutral entity. Although a classical particle would have an infinite number of possible orbits, the fact that the electron behaves as a constrained wave rather than a particle results in only a definite number of possible orbits and hence energy levels. The transfer of electrons from one orbit to the next requires a quantum of energy which is either absorbed or emitted by the atom depending on whether it moves into a lower or higher energy orbit.

The crystal structure of Ge and Si, the most widely studied semiconductors, is of the diamond lattice form in which each atom lies in the center of a tetrahedron formed by the four nearest neighbors. The binary compounds of greatest importance for luminescent devices, such as GaAs and GaP, are of the zinc-blende structure similar to the diamond lattice except that two nearest neighbor atomic sites are occupied by different elements, e.g., Ga and As, or Ga and P. One of the elements can be partially replaced by a suitable substitute, for example, P for As, to form a ternary compound, Ga(AsP).

9

Similarly, Al can be substituted for Ga to form (AlGa)As, with the basic lattice structure remaining unchanged, and even more substitutions are possible for more complex compounds. It is generally assumed that these partial element substitutions are random in nature.

Figure 1.1.1 shows the GaAs lattice as viewed in the [111] direction; the lines PQ and RS indicate the difference observed by cutting the crystal through different planes. A surface cut through RS requires three broken bonds per atom, an unfavorable situation which results in the preferred cut being either through the plane PQ or above PQ; in both cases the number of broken bonds per atom is minimized. If the plane is formed by cutting through PQ, then the plane is referred to as the (111) plane and the A atoms (Ga) are exposed. The cut above PQ is a ($\bar{1}\bar{1}\bar{1}$) plane, with the B (As) atoms exposed. The chemical properties of these surfaces differ considerably, particularly in their reaction to etchants [1].

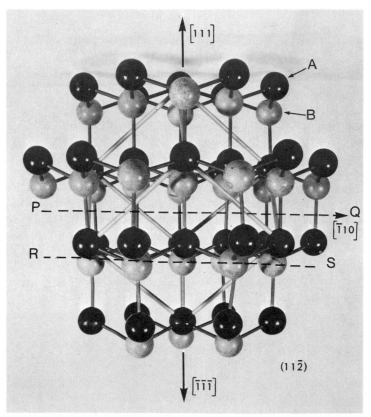

FIG. 1.1.1 View of a zinc-blende compound, consisting of atoms of elements A and B (e.g., Ga = A, As = B) [1].

1.2 Bonding and Band Structure

The bonding of atoms within a solid uses concepts familiar in the area of molecular bonding. In the semiconductors of interest here the binding is basically of the covalent type, with polar contributions for the zinc-blende structures. For the simple elements such as Ge and Si, two atoms contribute electrons of opposite spin to the common space so that each electron contributes to the binding of the two atoms. Since there are four valence electrons for Si and Ge, each electron is shared with a nearest neighbor. Thus, because each of the valence electrons is bound, there are no free electrons in the ideal case at 0 K. However, by absorbing the bandgap energy E_g, electrons can be excited to higher energy levels (i.e., into the conduction band) in which they are free to move through the crystal, leaving behind a *hole* in the valence band. Under application of an electric field, the electron and hole move in opposite directions and at different velocities which depend on the details of the crystal structure which influences their effective mass m_c^*, m_v^*. Figure 1.2.1 shows the schematic band diagram for an intrinsic semiconductor which has equal electron and hole density. The intrinsic carrier concentration is $\propto \exp(-E_g/2kT)$, where k is the Boltzmann constant and T the temperature.

In the zinc-blende compounds, the nearest neighbor atoms have unequal numbers of valence electrons, but the sum of these electrons is always 8. Therefore, each atom, on the average, has four valence electrons for forming the bonds, and the basic covalent bonding process of the diamond lattice is effective here as well, as long as the electron sharing process occurs. However, the differences in the atomic core charges in the zinc-blende compounds also yield an additional ionic bonding contribution because the electron wave function distribution may, on the average, be preferentially skewed in favor of the atom with the higher electronegativity. For example, in GaAs the As atom with its charge of 5 (electronegativity value of 2.0) is preferred to the Ga atom with its charge of 3 (electronegativity value of 1.6).* Thus, the electrons

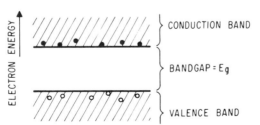

FIG. 1.2.1 Conduction electrons ($\cdot$) and holes ($\bigcirc$) in an intrinsic semiconductor for $T > 0$ K.

*The "electronegativity" of an element is its power to attract an electron to itself when part of a compound. Comparative values are shown in Table 1.2.1.

tend to be preferentially located in the vicinity of the As atom. This gives rise to a net charge difference between the As and Ga atoms which contributes to the atomic bonding. The ionic bonding contribution evidently varies greatly with the nature of the compound, but generally the higher bandgap III–V materials tend to have a larger ionic bonding contribution than the lower bandgap materials.

It is convenient to assign a covalent radius, following the definitions of Pauling [2], to each atom of the compound such that the sum of the two radii in a binary compound provides a reasonable indication of the lattice parameter. Table 1.2.1 presents a list of these covalent radii useful in determining the possibility of substituting one element for another in the formation of alloys or the introduction of dopants. In general, the closer the covalent radius values, the easier it is to substitute elements in a lattice with minimal lattice strain. This concept is one which will be referred to in the discussion of useful compounds and dopants.

We now turn our attention to the band structure of the semiconductor, by which we mean the dependence of the electron energy on momentum. This is obtained from a solution of the Schrödinger equation with an appropriate periodic electronic potential. Many such energy relationships are possible, depending on the electrons with which we are dealing. The electrons closest to

TABLE 1.2.1

Covalent Radii and Electronegativity of Selected Atoms[a]

Element	Covalent radius (Å)	Electronegativity
B	0.88	2.0
C	0.77	2.5
N	0.70	3.0
Al	1.26	1.5
Si	1.17	1.8
P	1.10	2.1
Ga	1.26	1.6
Ge	1.22	1.7
As	1.18	2.0
In	1.44	1.6
Sn	1.40	1.7
Sb	1.36	1.9
Pb	1.46	2.2
Te	1.32	2.1
O	0.66	3.5
S	1.04	2.5
Se	1.14	2.4
Zn	1.31	1.6
Cd	1.48	1.7

[a] L. Pauling, *The Nature of the Chemical Bond.* Cornell Univ. Press, Ithaca, New York, 1948.

the atomic core are clearly the least affected by the incorporation of the atom in the solid. Therefore, these electrons have a narrow energy distribution. The valence electrons, on the other hand, are the most affected, and these can approach the broad continuum of energy levels of nearly free electrons. Of course, the electrons excited into the conduction band are similarly relatively unconstrained. Our interest focuses here on those relatively mobile electrons which contribute to the optical and transport properties of the device of interest. In fact, the carriers in the material can be characterized by properties in many ways comparable to those of free electrons under vacuum, with the exception that their mass is now an *effective mass,* which takes into account the averaged interaction of the carrier with the periodic lattice potential.

A simplifying assumption in the theory used to calculate the energy bands in solids is that the actual crystal can be represented by a perfectly periodic lattice, neglecting defects and lattice vibrations. It is further assumed that the electron moves independently of other electrons in a static potential $V(\mathbf{r})$ having the periodicity of the lattice. The one-electron model appears rather daring, but in fact it has served well in predicting the major properties of materials. In the model, the electrons in the solid are characterized by Bloch functions of the form

$$\Psi_k(\mathbf{r}) = u_k(\mathbf{r}) \exp(i\mathbf{k} \cdot \mathbf{r}) \qquad (1.2.1)$$

where $\mathbf{k}$ is the *wave vector* which characterizes the wave function and $u_k(\mathbf{r})$ is a function with the periodicity of the lattice. The Bloch functions are seen to be plane waves $\exp(i\mathbf{k}\cdot\mathbf{r})$ modulated by $\mathbf{u}_k(\mathbf{r})$, which is related to the potential $V(\mathbf{r})$. The wave vector is related to the momentum $\mathbf{p}$ and wavelength λ of the electron in the solid by

$$k - p/2\pi h, \qquad k = 2\pi/\lambda, \qquad p - h/\lambda \qquad (1.2.2)$$

The periodic lattice is described by a set of vectors $\mathbf{R}_i$ such that a translation by $\mathbf{R}_i$ reproduces the potential at the origin

$$\mathbf{R}_i = M_{i1}\mathbf{a}_1 + M_{i2}\mathbf{a}_2 + M_{i3}\mathbf{a}_3$$

where $\mathbf{a}_1$, $\mathbf{a}_2$, and $\mathbf{a}_3$ are the shortest possible independent periodic translations of the lattice and the M_i are integers.

Another set of vectors $\mathbf{K}_j$ is defined such that

$$\mathbf{K}_j \cdot \mathbf{R}_i = 2\pi n_{ij}$$

where n_{ij} is an integer. The vectors $\mathbf{K}_j$ define a set of points called the *reciprocal lattice,* in terms of elementary translations,

$$\mathbf{K}_j = N_{j1}\mathbf{b}_1 + N_{j2}\mathbf{b}_2 + N_{j3}\mathbf{b}_3$$

These elementary translations in the *reciprocal* lattice are related to those in the *direct* lattice by

$$\mathbf{b}_1 = 2\pi \frac{\mathbf{a}_2 \times \mathbf{a}_3}{\mathbf{a}_1 \cdot \mathbf{a}_2 \times \mathbf{a}_3}, \qquad \mathbf{b}_2 = 2\pi \frac{\mathbf{a}_3 \times \mathbf{a}_1}{\mathbf{a}_1 \cdot \mathbf{a}_2 \times \mathbf{a}_3}, \qquad \mathbf{b}_3 = 2\pi \frac{\mathbf{a}_1 \times \mathbf{a}_2}{\mathbf{a}_1 \cdot \mathbf{a}_2 \times \mathbf{a}_3}$$

$$(1.2.3)$$

Therefore,

$$\mathbf{b}_j \cdot \mathbf{a}_i = 2\pi \, \delta_{ij}$$

where δ_{ij} is the Kronecker delta (i.e., $\mathbf{b}_1 \cdot \mathbf{a}_1 = 2\pi$, $\mathbf{b}_1 \cdot \mathbf{a}_2 = 0$, . . .).

The unit cell of the reciprocal lattice, the *Brillouin zone,* is constructed by drawing the planes which bisect the vectors from the origin to all points of the reciprocal lattice. The reciprocal lattice can be shown to be invariant under the same point group as the real lattice. The utility of the reciprocal lattice formalism arises from the fact that $E(\mathbf{k})$ is periodic in the reciprocal lattice,

$$E(\mathbf{k}) = E(\mathbf{k} + \mathbf{K}_j)$$

Therefore, to define the electron energy dependence on momentum uniquely it suffices to use the $\mathbf{k}$ values within the unit cell of the reciprocal lattice, i.e., the first Brillouin zone. Figure 1.2.2 shows the Brillouin zone for the zinc-blende lattice with the important symmetry points and lines indicated. The center of the zone is denoted Γ; the intersection of the $\langle 111 \rangle$ axes with the zone edge is L; the intersection of the $\langle 100 \rangle$ axes with the zone edge is X; the intersection of the $\langle 110 \rangle$ axes with the zone edge is K. Note that there are several such

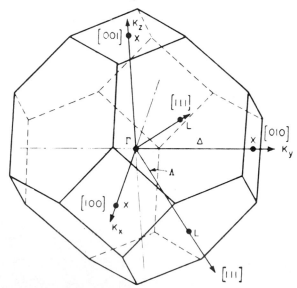

FIG. 1.2.2   First Brillouin zone of the diamond and zinc-blende lattices, with the most important symmetry points and lines indicated. The equivalence of some points are evident. For example, there are six equivalent X points [3].

zone intersection points, and therefore corresponding important equivalent band structure features.

The band structure determination is performed by computer solutions of the Schrödinger equation with appropriate lattice symmetry and potential functions. (An excellent introductory treatment is given by Long [3].) Figure 1.2.3 shows the results of such band structure calculations for GaAs and GaP which illustrate the major features [4]. (These have been largely confirmed by experiment.) The forbidden energy ranges are indicated as well as the variation of the electron energy with direction. Gallium arsenide is an example of a *direct bandgap* semiconductor in which the lowest energy separation E_g between the conduction and the valence band occurs at the center of the zone ($\mathbf{k} - 0$), at Γ.

Gallium phosphide is an example of an *indirect bandgap* semiconductor in which the conduction band minima occur at X, thus away from the valence band maximum at $\mathbf{k} = 0$. The difference between direct and indirect bandgap materials is vital in affecting the optical properties of the semiconductors, as discussed is Section 1.5. Note that there are other direct bandgap semiconductors in which the band extrema are at $\mathbf{k} \neq 0$, for example in PbSe (Chapter 13).

It is important to note that the mixture of miscible direct and indirect bandgap materials provides a means of smoothly altering the band structure between endpoints. As described in Chapter 11, the mixture of GaAs and GaP, for example, results in an increased bandgap energy at Γ. A point is reached, however, as P is substituted for As, at which the X and Γ conduction band minima* are equal in magnitude. Beyond that point the X minima are lower than the Γ minimum.

Finally, we note that the effective mass of the carriers in the various bands

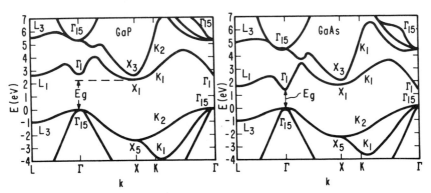

FIG. 1.2.3 Calculated band structure of GaP and GaAs with the major symmetry features indicated. The separation E_g denotes the bandgap energy [4].

*The symbols Γ, X refer to the conduction band minima of interest here, (Γ_1) and (X_1).

is a function of the curvature of the band. Thus,

$$m_v^* \quad \text{or} \quad m_c^* = \frac{h^2}{4\pi^2} \left(\frac{\partial^2 E}{\partial k^2}\right)^{-1}$$

Therefore, the steeper the $E(\mathbf{k})$ vs. $\mathbf{k}$ curve, the lower is the effective carrier mass. Some of the bands near the extremal points can be well approximated by parabolic functions of E vs. k which simplifies calculations. This is the case, for example, for the conduction and valence bands in GaAs.

1.3   Dopants

1.3.1   Low Concentrations

The introduction of dopants into a semiconductor can change the carrier density. The band diagram with donors or acceptors present (extrinsic semiconductors) is shown in Fig. 1.3.1. For simplicity, consider first Si or Ge. If the number of valence electrons of the dopant exceeds four, we have more electrons than needed for covalent bonding to its nearest neighbors. The excess electron is relatively weakly bound to the impurity, and the energy needed to free the electron (the ionization energy) is therefore much less than the bandgap energy. A *donor* is introduced if the number of valence electrons exceeds four in Ge or Si, whereas an *acceptor* is introduced if less than four valence electrons are present.

The concept of donor and acceptor formation in the compound materials is similar, except that the site of the substituted impurity as well as its number of valence electrons is relevant. For example, in the III–V compounds, Zn (group II) placed on Ga sites (group III) provides an acceptor, whereas Te (group VI) placed on an As site (group V) provides a donor. The group IV dopants, such as Ge and Si, may be on either Ga or As sites; when substituting for Ga, they provide a donor, whereas they provide an acceptor when placed on As sites. Thus, they are amphoteric dopants. The preferred location of Ge and Si in the lattice depends on the compound, the method of material synthesis, and the covalent radius relative to the host atoms (Chapter 10). In general, the atom will tend to prefer to substitute for a native atom as close as possible to its covalent radius, since this minimizes the lattice strain and hence the free energy of the crystal.

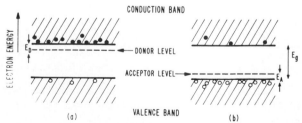

FIG. 1.3.1   Energy levels of doped semiconductors at $T > 0$ K: (a) n-type, (b) p-type.

A conventional estimate of the ionization energy of the typical "shallow" donors and acceptors is obtained by treating the impurity as a hydrogen atom with the modification that the binding of the electron to the impurity is reduced by the host lattice because of its high static dielectric constant ε compared to free space. In addition, it is assumed that the force is acting on a carrier having the effective mass of those in the crystal (m_c^* for an electron and m_v^* for a hole). Therefore, the calculation of the energy E_D needed to ionize a donor, for example, reduces to the hydrogen atom problem calculation with the static dielectric constant of the crystal and the relevant electron effective mass m_c^*. The resultant ground state energy is given by

$$|E_D| = 13.5\,(m_c^*/m_0)(\varepsilon_0/\varepsilon)^2 \quad (\text{eV}) \tag{1.3.1}$$

where ε_0 is the permittivity of free space; E_D is measured relative to the conduction band edge. A similar computation for an acceptor yields the energy level E_A above the valence band.

Following along the hydrogenic model approximation, one may estimate the extent of the wave function of electrons (or holes) bound to impurity centers from the first Bohr radius r_b,

$$r_b = 0.53\,(m_0/m_c^*)\,(\varepsilon/\varepsilon_0) \quad (\text{Å}) \tag{1.3.2}$$

and similarly for holes. The wave function extends over many lattice spacings. For example, $r_b = 86$ Å in GaAs with $\varepsilon = 11\varepsilon_0$ and $m_c^* = 0.068m_0$; therefore, the Bohr radius is considerably in excess of the lattice parameter $a_0 \cong 6$ Å. In fact, the extent of the wave function is used as justification for considering the electron–impurity interaction as involving general properties of the host crystal such as the static dielectric constant and the effective mass.

The concept of the Bohr radius is useful in the first-order analysis of numerous problems in semiconductors, and its value is often approximated by working backward from the known ionization energy E_i of a center to avoid the need to involve the effective mass. Combining (1.3.1) and (1.3.2),

$$E_i = |e^2/2\varepsilon r_b| \quad \text{or} \quad r_b = (7.16/E_i)(\varepsilon_0/\varepsilon) \quad (\text{Å}) \tag{1.3.3}$$

Donor and acceptor levels can also be introduced by intrinsic lattice defects such as vacant atomic sites (vacancies) or interstitially located atoms (interstitials). However, in the majority of cases it is difficult to establish a priori whether a Ga vacancy in GaAs, for example, leads to the formation of an acceptor or a donor since complex bonding arrangements can occur in the vicinity of the vacant site.

The prediction of the ionization energy of a recombination center introduced by doping (or defects) is still an imprecise science because of the complexity of the problem, particularly for centers with large ionization energies such as those due to transition metals.

The ionization energies of donors is typically $\sim$ 5–6 meV in GaAs, and that of the widely used acceptors is ~ 30 meV (Chapter 10). Since at room temperature the thermal energy is 26 meV, the donors and acceptors are ionized, which means that the extra electron is no longer bound to the donor impurity, whereas the acceptor impurity has captured an electron. The free carrier concentration is then equal to the impurity concentration.

When both donors and acceptors are present, the crystal is said to be *compensated*. If donors (hence electrons) predominate, the crystal is n-type while it is p-type when acceptors (holes) predominate. Of course, even in n-type crsytals, holes are present because some electrons acquire energy E_g and thus move upward from the valence band into the conduction band, leaving a hole behind. Similarly, in p-type material, electrons are present in thermal equilibrium. As will be shown in Section 1.4, the product of the electrons and holes in a nondegenerate crystal in thermal equilibrium is a constant at a given temperature, as determined by the intrinsic carrier concentration N_i,

$$P_n N_n = N_i^2 \quad \text{(n-type material)}, \qquad P_p N_p = N_i^2 \quad \text{(p-type material)} \quad (1.3.4)$$

We find it convenient in some cases to use the nomenclature P_n and N_n to denote the hole and electron concentrations in n-type material. In general, however, whenever the meaning is obvious, we will denote the hole concentration P and the electron concentration N. The intrinsic carrier concentration, for parabolic conduction and valence bands, is given by

$$N_i^2 = 4(2\pi k T/h^2)^3 \, (m_c^* m_v^*)^{3/2} \, \exp(-E_g/kT) \qquad (1.3.5)$$

where m_c^* and m_v^* are the "density of states effective masses" in the conduction and valence bands, respectively.

1.3.2 High Concentrations

The impurity ionization energy disappears when the concentration becomes sufficiently high. With increasing concentration, two major effects reduce the ionization energy: the impurity potential is screened by free electrons and the wave functions overlap. We recall that in the hydrogenlike treatment of the impurity atom, we assumed a potential of the form

$$V(r) = e/\varepsilon r \qquad (1.3.6)$$

If the free carrier concentration is significant, we need to consider the reduction of $V(r)$ to a "screened" potential of the form

$$V(r) = (e/r)\exp(-r/L_D) \qquad (1.3.7)$$

where L_D is a screening length, which in a classical (but very limited approximation is a Debye screening length, $L_D = (kT\varepsilon/4\pi Ne^2)$, where N is the electron concentration.

The overlap of wave functions when the Bohr radius is comparable to the interimpurity spacing results in the formation of bands of impurity energy states. At high enough concentrations, these "impurity bands" merge with the nearest band edge.

Since the Bohr radius is an inverse function of ionization energy [Eq. (1.3.3)], the shallow centers are affected at relatively low impurity concentrations. For example, in GaAs with $E_D = 5$ meV ($r_b \cong 130$ Å), wave overlap effects are pronounced for $N_D > 10^{16}$ cm^{-3}. On the other hand, for shallow acceptors in GaAs ($E_A \cong 30$ meV, $r_b \cong 22$ Å) a concentration of $\sim 10^{17}$ cm^{-3} is accommodated before overlap effects reduce E_A.

In many cases, one finds that the ionization energy of the deeper recombination centers (typically acceptors in the III–V compounds) follows an empirical expression of the form

$$E_i = E_i^0 - A N_t^{1/3} \tag{1.3.8}$$

where E_i^0 is the ionization energy for infinite dilution, A a constant on the order of 10^{-8} cm^3-eV, and N_t the concentration of the dopant, assumed here much in excess of compensating dopants. However, at this time insufficient data exist to determine the range of validity of such an expression.

Finally, we note that a high *injected* carrier density will also affect the behavior of the impurities, since screening effects are produced which, via (1.3.7), will reduce the potential $V(r)$. In fact, the considerations of Section 1.7.2 relative to the existence of excitons in the presence of a high free carrier concentration are applicable to determine the carrier concentrations needed to affect the binding energy.

1.3.3 Bandtail States

A consequence of the introduction of a high impurity concentration in crystals is the formation of conduction and valence "bandtail" states. Typically, bandtail effects become significant with impurity concentrations well in excess of 10^{18} cm^{-3} in materials such as GaAs, and compensation increases these effects.

The nature of the states and their extent into the gap have comprised a thoroughly studied subject both theoretically and experimentally. The randomly distributed charged defect centers (when the centers are ionized) produce strong local electrical fields in the crystal [8–10]. A qualitative view of the variation of the potential induced by the random distribution of ionized donors in the lattice is shown in Fig. 1.3.2a. The energy E_c here denotes the conduction band edge energy as a function of position in the crystal. Averaging of the electron energy density of states over the crystal volume results in the distribution shown in Fig. 1.3.2b for the conduction bandtail states. The resultant bandtail states reduce the separation between the valence and conduction band edges.

Similar bandtail effects occur in the valence band when acceptor states are

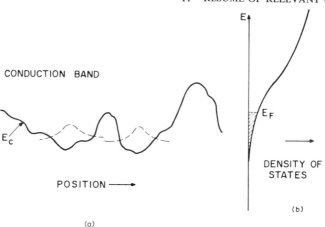

POSITION ⟶

(a)

DENSITY OF
STATES

(b)

FIG. 1.3.2 (a) Spatial variation of the random potential as seen in the conduction band edge E_c (heavy line). Dashed lines indicate wave functions of localized states. (b) Spatial average of the density of states; E_F illustrates the Fermi energy in the bandtail [10].

introduced, although both conduction and valence band edges are perturbed when charged (i.e., ionized) impurities exist in the crystal.

The bandtails affect the mission and absorption properties because a significant fraction of the optical transitions occur at energies less than the bandgap energy of the pure crystal. Figure 1.3.3 illustrates the two-band consequence of bandtails, in a situation in which the crystal contains relatively deep centers at energy E_i below the conduction band. The effect on the average density of states is shown in Fig. 1.3.3b. An important result of the condition presented pictorially in Fig. 1.3.3 is that the electrons will tend to be concentrated in the low lying conduction band valleys of the crystal, whereas the holes will be found preferentially in the spatially distinct, high energy regions of the valence band. Thus, there is only partial overlap of the electron and hole wave functions which extend into the forbidden gap, as shown, and the matrix elements connecting the electrons and holes are altered seriously. An important consequence of the *deep* bandtail states, such as those introduced by doping GaAs with Si under certain conditions, is that the recombination probability of deep bandtail state transitions is reduced compared to bandgap transitions, leading to long carrier lifetimes [11], and hence to long diode recovery times (Section 14.6.2).

Numerical estimates of the density of states in the bandtails for various dopant concentrations have been made. A commonly used (but imprecise) dependence of the density of states is the exponential one of the form

$$\rho(E) \propto \exp(E/E_0) \tag{1.3.9}$$

where E_0 (8–15 meV in GaAs on the basis of absorption measurements) [12]

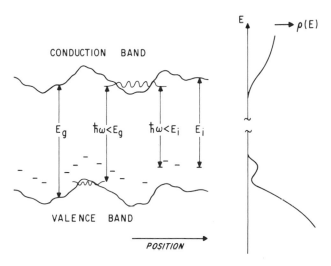

FIG. 1.3.3   Perturbations of the conduction and valence band edges and the consequent formation of bandtail states associated with both bands. Note the displacement of the conduction band minima and the valence band maxima, giving rise to an effective spatial separation of conduction electrons and holes in the crystal. $\rho(E)$ denotes the averaged density of states [10].

is a term which varies with temperature and dopant concentration. The extensive theory of Halperin and Lax [13] provides values for a range of impurity concentrations which were used for optical gain calculations (of the type described in Chapter 3) in highly doped GaAs. The effect of a high dopant concentration in effectively reducing the bandgap energy is discussed in Section 1.4.

1.4   Electron Distribution and Density of States

Section 1.2 called attention to the complexity of the band structure of semiconductors due to differences in their lattice structure and atomic constituents. The parabolic density of states distribution for the conduction and valence bands, although an approximation of varying accuracy in different materials, provides a good estimate in GaAs and other III–V compounds of interest here with appropriate effective mass values. In this section, we summarize the major formulations of interest in this regard.

For the conduction band, if the energy is measured from the edge E_c, the density of states per unit energy interval between E and $E + dE$ is

$$\rho_c(E)\, dE = \frac{4\pi (2m_c{}^*)^{3/2}(E - E_c)^{1/2}}{h^3}\, dE \qquad (1.4.1)$$

For holes in the valence band, energy is measured from the edge of the valence band E_V,

$$\rho_V(E)\,dE = \frac{4\pi(2m_v{}^*)^{3/2}(E_v - E)^{1/2}}{h^3}\,dE \qquad (1.4.2)$$

In GaAs and similar materials, the value taken for the hole mass $m_v{}^*$ includes the contributions from the two valence bands, one of which has a heavy hole mass m_{vh}^* and the other a light hole mass, m_{vl}^* and

$$(m_v{}^*)^{3/2} = (m_{vh}^*)^{3/2} + (m_{vl}^*)^{3/2}$$

In GaAs, $m_{vh}^* = 0.68m_0$, $m_{vl}^* = 0.12m_0$, and hence $m_v{}^* = 0.47m_0$ ($m_v{}^* = 0.5\,m_0$ is generally used).

Both expressions for the density of states include a factor of 2 for spin degeneracy. When these density of states functions are used in the form of a product in integration, a factor of 2 is removed because the spin of the electron is unchanged in a band-to-band transition.

The probability of a state being occupied by an electron is given by the Fermi–Dirac statistics

$$f(E) = \{\exp[(E - E_F)/kT] + 1\}^{-1} \qquad (1.4.3)$$

where E_F is the Fermi level determined from the condition that the free electron density N be given by

$$\int_{E_c}^{\infty} \rho_c(E)f(E)\,dE = N \qquad (1.4.4a)$$

while the total hole density is given by

$$\int_{-\infty}^{E_V} \rho_V(E)[1 - f(E)]\,dE = P \qquad (1.4.4b)$$

Using the density of states functions (1.4.1) and (1.4.2), the density of electrons in the conduction band is

$$N = \left(\frac{4\pi}{h^3}\right)(2m_c{}^*)^{3/2} \int_{E_c}^{\infty} \frac{(E - E_c)^{1/2}\,dE}{\exp[(E - E_F)/kT] + 1} \qquad (1.4.5)$$

Similarly, for the holes in the valence band,

$$P = \left(\frac{4\pi}{h^3}\right)(2m_c{}^*)^{3/2} \int_{-\infty}^{E_V} \frac{(E_v - E)^{1/2}\,dE}{\exp[(E_F - E)/kT] + 1} \qquad (1.4.6)$$

These integrals have been tabulated and E_F calculated for known N or P values. Figure 1.4.1 shows the convenient nomograph of Pankove and Annavedder [14] for calculating the Fermi level separation from the band edges.

The determination of the Fermi level is simple in relatively lightly doped material where the Fermi level is outside the band (i.e., *nondegenerate* carrier population). If E_F is at least 3–4 kT below the conduction band edge in n-type

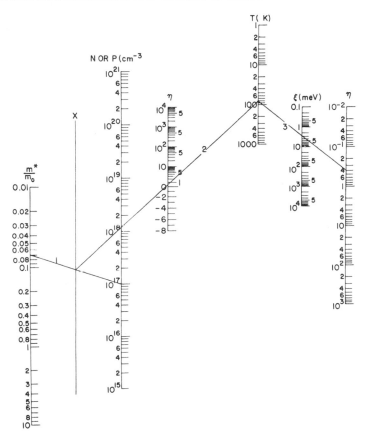

FIG. 1.4.1 Nomograph of the temperature dependence of the Fermi level in a degenerate parabolic band. ξ is the position of the Fermi level with respect to the band edge (corresponding to δ_e and δ_h in the nomenclature used elsewhere in the text), and $\eta = \xi/kT$. The nomograph permits a graphical determination of any parameter N, m^*, ξ, or T when any three of them are known. For example, if N and m^*/m_0 are known, they are joined by a straight line. From the intercept of this straight line with the X axis one draws a straight line to the desired T to find a value η on the left-hand η scale. Transferring this value to the right-hand η scale, one strikes another straight line to T to find ξ. If η is negative, ξ lies outside the parabolic band (i.e., inside the energy gap) [14].

material (or 3–$4kT$ above the valence band edge in p-type material), then the exponential term in the denominators of (1.4.5) and (1.4.6) is large with respect to unity, and the integrals can be greatly simplified as follows.

Using the transformation $x = (E - E_c)/kT$ in (1.4.5), we obtain, with appropriate change in the limits of integration,

$$N = \left(\frac{4\pi}{h^3}\right)(2m_c^*)^{3/2}(kT)^{3/2} \exp\left(\frac{E_F - E_c}{kT}\right)\int_0^\infty x^{1/2}(\exp x)\,dx$$

Since the value of the integral is $\frac{1}{2}\sqrt{\pi}$,

$$N = 2(2\pi m_c^* kT/h^2)^{3/2} \exp[(E_F - E_c)/kT] \tag{1.4.7}$$

which can be rewritten

$$N = N_c \exp[(E_F - E_c)/kT] \tag{1.4.8}$$

Similarly, from (1.4.6),

$$P = N_v \exp[(E_v - E_F)/kT] \tag{1.4.9}$$

Here, N_c and N_v are called the "effective density of states" values in the conduction and valence bands,

$$\begin{aligned} N_c &= 2[2\pi m_c^* kT/h^2]^{3/2} = 4.83 \times 10^{15}(m_c^*/m_0)^{3/2} T^{3/2} \quad (\text{cm}^{-3}) \\ N_v &= 2[2\pi m_v^* kT/h^2]^{3/2} = 4.83 \times 10^{15}(m_v^*/m_0)^{3/2} T^{3/2} \quad (\text{cm}^{-3}) \end{aligned} \tag{1.4.10}$$

In GaAs at 300 K,

$$N_c = 4.26 \times 10^{17} \text{ cm}^{-3}, \qquad N_v = 8.87 \times 10^{18} \text{ cm}^{-3} \tag{1.4.11}$$

The meaning of N_c and N_v is as follows. When the Fermi level is well *within* the gap (i.e., when Boltzmann statistics can be used to describe the carrier distribution in the band), then the conduction band may be treated as a single level at E_c with degeneracy N_c. Similarly, N_v represents the degeneracy of a single level at E_v, the edge of the valence band. In this approximation, the intrinsic electron concentration is related to the Fermi level E_{Fi} by

$$N_i = N_c \exp[(E_{Fi} - E_c)/kT], \qquad P_i = N_i = N_v \exp[(E_v - E_{Fi})/kT] \tag{1.4.12}$$

Hence,

$$N_i^2 = N_c N_v \exp[-(E_c - E_v)/kT] = N_c N_v \exp[-(E_g/kT)] \tag{1.4.13}$$

The Fermi level is in the gap removed from either the conduction or valence band edge by the following energy values. For electrons. (see Fig. 1.4.2),

$$\delta_e = E_c - E_F = kT \ln(N_c/N_n) \tag{1.4.14}$$

and for holes,

$$\delta_h = E_F - E_v = kT \ln(N_v/P_p)$$

For intrinsic material, it is easily seen from this that the Fermi level E_{Fi} is at midgap when $N_c = N_v$. If the densities of states are unequal, then there is a shift toward either band from midgap given by

$$\Delta = \tfrac{1}{2}kT \ln(N_c/N_v) = \tfrac{3}{4}kT \ln(m_c^*/m_v^*) \tag{1.4.15}$$

A useful relationship follows from (1.4.8) and (1.4.9) with regard to the product of electrons and holes in a material with a nondegenerate carrier population,

$$NP = N_c N_v \exp[-(E_c - E_v)/kT] = N_c N_v \exp[-(E_g/kT)] \tag{1.4.16}$$

Hence from (1.4.13), $NP = N_i^2$, a relationship which holds strictly only for nondegenerate materials.

A graphic summary of the electron and hole distribution under various conditions is presented in Fig. 1.4.2: Part a shows an intrinsic material (i.e., containing neither donors nor acceptors) in which electron and hole densities are equal. Figure 1.4.2b shows an n-type material in which the Fermi level is close to the conduction band as a result of the ionization of the donors. However, some holes exist due to the thermal ionization of valence electrons. Figure 1.4.2c shows a p-type material in which the Fermi level is close to the valence band due to the capture of electrons by the acceptors leaving holes behind in the valence band. In addition, free electrons in the conduction band result from thermal ionization from the valence band.

As mentioned in Section 1.3, a high density of impurities changes the density of states at the conduction and valence band edges. In effect, the bandgap energy can be considered to be reduced because the states introduced by the impurities merge with the bands. Figure 1.4.3 shows the calculated density of states in GaAs containing a high concentration of both shallow donors and shallow acceptors [15]. The tail states are seen to extend to a depth in excess of 0.1 eV from the valence band edge, and about 0.05 eV from the conduction band edge. Experimentally, the presence of tail states is reflected in an increase in the absorption coefficient for values of photon energy much below the

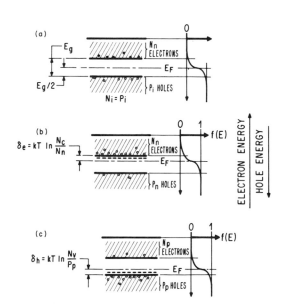

FIG. 1.4.2   Carrier distribution and Fermi–Dirac distribution function $f(E)$ for (a) an intrinsic semiconductor for $T > 0$ K; (b) an n-type semiconductor; (c) a p-type semiconductor.

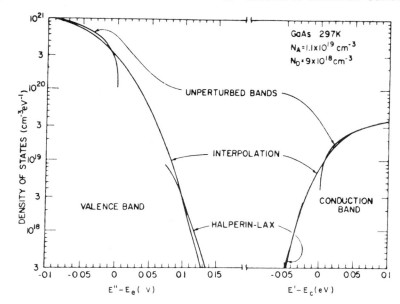

FIG. 1.4.3 Densities of states in the conduction and valence bands for GaAs with $N_A -$ $N_D = 2 \times 10^{18}$ cm^{-3}. The upper curves show the densities of states in the unperturbed bands, the lower curves show the densities of states in the bandtail as calculated from the theory of Halperin and Lax [15].

$E_g = 1.424$ eV value of pure GaAs, as well as a shift in the peak (and broadening) of the luminescence emitted from such crystals, including a reduction in the lasing peak energy as discussed in Chapter 3. An effective bandgap energy has been experimentally defined in terms of the hole concentration P in p-type GaAs of the form [15]

$$E_g = 1.424 - 1.6 \times 10^{-8} P^{1/3} \quad \text{(eV)} \qquad (1.4.17)$$

Thus, for example, for $P = 10^{18}$ cm^{-3}, the effective bandgap energy is 16 meV lower than the value in pure GaAs, and for 3×10^{19} cm^{-3} (near the highest hole concentration commonly used in GaAs), the bandgap energy is effectively reduced by about 50 meV, with the ionization energy of the shallow acceptors being ≈ 0.

The high acceptor concentration also affects the radiative recombination parameters as discussed in Section 1.5.

1.5 Electron–Hole Pair Formation and Recombination

1.5.1 Direct and Indirect Bandgap Materials and Internal Quantum Efficiency

An excess of electrons and holes is created in a semiconductor by several processes which include the absorption of a photon with sufficient energy to move an electron from the valence to the conduction band (or from an impurity center into the conduction band), the incidence of energetic (i.e., with energy substantially in excess of the bandgap energy) particles on the semiconductor which ionize the lattice, or by injection at contacts. The process of *photoluminescence* refers to the radiative recombination of electron–hole pairs generated by shining high energy light on a crystal. *Cathodoluminescence* refers to the radiative processes following energetic (usually several kiloelectronvolts) electron bombardment of the material, and *injection luminescence* refers to radiative processes occurring in structures containing injecting contacts, such as p–n junctions.

A crucial distinction exists between semiconductors in which the lower energy conduction to valence band electron transition occurs without phonon participation and those in which phonon participation is required. In the simplest conditions of a parabolic band in a III–V direct bandgap material, the energy bands are spherical in shape with the extrema occurring at $k = 0$ (as previously noted and shown in Fig. 1.5.1a in detail), and the transition of an electron across the gap at E_g does not involve a change in its momentum. (The small momentum of the emitted or absorbed photon, h/λ, can be neglected for λ in the ~ 1 μm range.) As far as is currently known, direct bandgap materials are essential for laser diode operation.

In other semiconductors, such as Si, Ge, and GaP, where the minima in the energy of the conduction band are located at $k \neq 0$, as shown in Fig. 1.5.1b, electrons will tend to dwell in that band whereas holes will be preferentially at $k = 0$ where their energy is minimal. Hence, when an electron at $k = 0$ recombines with a hole at $k \neq 0$, there is a momentum change. Because momentum must be conserved in a band-to-band electron–hole recombination or pair formation process, these "indirect transitions" require the

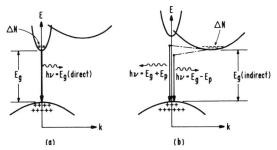

(a)   (b)

FIG. 1.5.1   Electron–hole recombination in the band-to-band process in (a) a direct and (b) an indirect bandgap semiconductor. Because of the need for momentum conservation, the energy of the photon emitted in the indirect bandgap material electron–hole recombination process is either smaller or larger than the bandgap energy by E_p, the energy of the participating phonon.

generation or absorption of a phonon with energy E_p with appropriate momentum. The required simultaneous interaction of a photon and a phonon reduces the probability of such an event compared to the direct transition described earlier. Assuming no competing processes for the disappearance of the electron in the conduction band, it will dwell for a relatively long term in the indirect valley (compared to the dwell time in the direct valley). Unfortunately, competing nonradiative recombination processes involving defects and impurities exist which allow the electron and hole to recombine in a relatively short time interval in most materials. Therefore, the probability of a radiative band-to-band electron–hole recombination process in indirect bandgap materials is considerably lower than that in the direct bandgap materials.

Under continuous injection or carrier generation by optical excitation, a steady state is established in which an excess carrier density exists in the crystal. Since the carriers are formed and recombine in pairs, the excess density of electrons ΔN and holes ΔP is equal, a requirement which also follows from the need for charge neutrality in the crystal. When the injection of carriers ceases, their density must return to the equilibrium value. Most commonly, the excess carrier density decays exponentially with time $\sim\exp(-t/\tau)$, where the time constant τ is the carrier lifetime. As described herein, this lifetime (which can vary from milliseconds to fractions of a nanosecond) is very sensitive to both fundamental parameters and defects, and is of central importance in the operation of optoelectronic devices.

In addition to recombining within the bulk of the crystal, minority carriers can also recombine at the surface of the material and, in thin samples, the surface recombination process can be more important than the bulk recombination process.

The excess carrier population can decrease via *radiative* or *nonradiative* electron–hole recombination. In *nonradiative* recombination, the energy released in the recombination process is dissipated in the form of lattice vibrations (heat) whereas in a radiative recombination a photon is created. In band-to-band *radiative* recombination, the photon energy released is approximately the bandgap energy. If the recombination process proceeds via impurity states, the emitted photon energy is below the bandgap energy.

The quantum efficiency (i.e., the fraction of radiative electron–hole recombinations) is determined by the ratio of radiative lifetime τ_r to the nonradiative lifetime τ_{nr} (with $1/\tau = 1/\tau_r + 1/\tau_{nr}$). Consider a material in which the electron–hole recombination processes are either radiative or nonradiative. The radiative recombination rate per unit volume is R_r and the nonradiative recombination rate is R_{nr}. The total recombination rate $R_{sp} = R_r + R_{nr}$. The ratio of the radiative recombination rate to the total recombination rate is the internal quantum efficiency,

$$\eta_i = R_r/(R_r + R_{nr}) \qquad (1.5.1)$$

Assuming an exponential decay process, the lifetime for radiative recombination is $\tau_r = \Delta N/R_r$, and for nonradiative recombination $\tau_{nr} = \Delta N/R_{nr}$. Hence, the internal quantum efficiency is

$$\eta_i = \tau_r^{-1}/(\tau_r^{-1} + \tau_{nr}^{-1}) = (1 + \tau_r/\tau_{nr})^{-1} \tag{1.5.2}$$

It is evidently desirable to keep τ_r/τ_{nr} as small as possible for high internal quantum efficiency. Since the noradiative lifetime depends on the density of defects, there has been much research connected with defects of all kinds. In addition, the nonradiative lifetime can be influenced by the density of majority carriers (irrespective of defects) because of the possibility of recombination via an Auger process whereby an electron and a hole recombine to release the energy to a third carrier which then becomes "hot" and dissipates its energy to the lattice (Section 1.8).

1.5.2 Carrier Lifetime Limited by Band-to-Band Recombination

As will become clear from the analysis of spontaneous and stimulated transitions in Chapter 3, the absorption and radiative processes are related by means of the principle of detailed balance. It is thus possible to use the measured absorption coefficient to calculate the radiative carrier lifetime, as limited by band-to-band recombination, when the material is not degenerately doped.

As will be shown in Section 3.3, the band-to-band spontaneous recombination rate R_{sp}, under conditions in which monemtum conservation for the band-to-band process is not required, takes on the simple form

$$R_{sp} = B_r NP \tag{1.5.3}$$

where $B_r(cm^3/s)$ is a parameter characteristic of the material. Under conditions of thermal equilibrium, the hole concentration is P_0 and the electron concentration is N_0 with $N_0 P_0 = N_i^2$. Under nonequilibrium conditions, additional carriers $\Delta N = \Delta P$ are introduced into the material. Therefore, the total recombination rate is

$$R_{sp} = B_r(N_0 + \Delta N)(P_0 + \Delta P) \tag{1.5.4}$$

The radiative carrier lifetime is defined in terms of the excess carrier pair density ΔN and τ_r as*

$$R_{sp}^{exc} = \Delta N/\tau_r \tag{1.5.5}$$

where R_{sp}^{exc} is the recombination rate of the injected excess carriers.[†] Thus,

$$R_{sp} = R_{sp}^0 + R_{sp}^{exc} \tag{1.5.6}$$

---

*This implies $\Delta N = (\Delta N)_0 \exp(-t/\tau)$.

[†]In practice, $R_{sp}^e \ll R_{sp}^{exc}$, and R_{sp} adequately accounts for the injected carrier recombination rate.

where R_{sp}^0 is the spontaneous recombination rate in thermal equilibrium. Hence,

$$R_{sp} = B_r [N_0 P_0 + \Delta N(P_0 + N_0) + (\Delta N)^2] \qquad (1.5.7)$$

Since

$$R_{sp}^0 = B_r N_0 P_0 = B_r N_i^2, \qquad R_{sp}^{exc} = R_{sp} - R_{sp}^0,$$
$$R_{sp}^{exc} = B_r \Delta N(P_0 + N_0 + \Delta N) \qquad (1.5.8)$$

Using (1.5.5),

$$\tau_r = [B_r(P_0 + N_0 + \Delta N)]^{-1}$$

We can distinguish two limits for the lifetime depending on the injected carrier density relative to the initial (background) concentration. At high injection levels, where the excess carrier density substantially exceeds the background concentration, $\Delta N > P_0 + N_0$ and τ_r is now a function of the injected carrier density,

$$\tau_r \cong [B_r(\Delta N)]^{-1} \qquad (1.5.9)$$

This is commonly denoted the *bimolecular* recombination region where the lifetime value continually changes as the carrier concentration decays back to its equilibrium value. The term denotes the average carrier decay time starting from a given excess carrier concentration.

At the other extreme is the region in which the injected carrier density is low relative to the background concentration. There, the excess carriers decay exponentially with time with a constant lifetime τ_r determined by the background carrier concentration:

$$\tau_r \cong [B_r(N_0 + P_0)]^{-1} \qquad (1.5.10)$$

Therefore, in p-type material, the hole concentration ($P_0 \gg N_0$) will determine the lifetime, and in n-type material the electron concentration ($N_0 \gg P_0$) will be the relevant quantity. Finally, the longest possible lifetime is calculated in intrinsic material at very low excitation level:

$$\tau_r(max) = (2B_r N_i)^{-1} \qquad (1.5.11)$$

The value of B_r depends on the band structure of the material, with the direct bandgap semiconductors having much larger B_r values than indirect bandgap semiconductors. From the measured values of the absorption coefficient, a semiempirical determination of B_r is possible. Table 1.5.1 shows the values so calculated by Varshni [16] for several semiconductors of interest here. Note that these semiempirical calculated values are more useful as order of magnitude estimates for comparing materials than as absolute quantities for lifetime prediction. The reason is the uncertainty in some of the absorption data used (particularly for high absorption coefficient values most important in determining B_r) and the approximations used in the calculation.

TABLE 1.5.1

Calculated Recombination Coefficient for Representative Direct and Indirect Bandgap Semiconductors[a]

Material	Energy bandgap type	Recombination coefficient, B_r (cm^3/s)
Si	Indirect	1.79×10^{-15}
Ge	Indirect	5.25×10^{-14}
GaP	Indirect	5.37×10^{-14}
GaAs[b]	Direct	7.21×10^{-10}
GaSb	Direct	2.39×10^{-10}
InAs	Direct	8.5×10^{-11}
InSb	Direct	4.58×10^{-11}

[a]Y. P. Varshni, *Phys. Status Solidi* **19**, 353 (1964).
[b]Experimental values are $\sim 10^{-10}$ cm^3/s (see text).

To illustrate the problems in correlating the calculated B_r values with experiment, consider GaAs where numerous attempts have been made to deduce its experimental value. Using absorption data covering a wide range of doping levels, B_r was estimated [15] to vary from 3.8×10^{-10} cm^3/s for $P = 1.2 \times 10^{18}$ cm^{-3}, to 1.7×10^{-10} cm^3/s at $P = 1.6 \times 10^{19}$ cm^{-3}. From other measurements, such as carrier lifetime, B_r values of 1.3 to 0.6×10^{-10} cm^3/s have been deduced in p-type GaAs ($\sim 10^{17}$–10^{19} cm^{-3}) [17–19]. Thus, it appears that a value in the vicinity of 10^{-10} cm^3/s is appropriate for p-type GaAs at room temperature, but it is uncertain within a factor of about 2. A method of deducing B_r in double-heterojunction lasers is described in Section 8.1.

1.5.3 Recombination via Centers in the Forbidden Energy Gap

Energy levels introduced into the forbidden energy gap by impurities or lattice defects may greatly increase the electron–hole recombination rate, and thus reduce the carrier lifetime below the values calculated on the basis of Section 1.5.2. The recombination process via such centers may be either radiative or nonradiative, depending on the nature of the centers. In this section we summarize the results of the simple kinetic theory for the recombination process via intermediate centers as originally worked out by Hall [20], Shockley and Read [21], and Sah *et al.* [22].

Consider a level in the gap at energy E_i as shown in Fig. 1.5.2. Four processes can occur: (a) The center captures an electron from the conduction band; (b) the electron is emitted from the center into the conduction band; (c) the electron recombines with a hole in the valence band, thus completing the band-to-band electron–hole recombination process; (d) the center is occupied by an energetic electron from the valence band.

It is intuitively obvious that processes (b) and (d) will be more likely for shallow centers than for deep ones; therefore, the most likely condition for

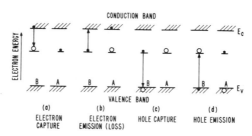

FIG. 1.5.2   Basic processes involving the carrier traffic through a level within the band-gap. B = before process, A = after process, $\bigcirc$ = hole, $\cdot$ = electron.

the band-to-band recombination process to be completed is if the center's energy is at midgap, $E_i \approx E_g/2$. The analysis of the various possibilities, taking into account different capture cross sections for electron and holes, σ_e and σ_h, respectively, yields the trap-determined recombination rate R_{trap}, [22],

$$R_{\text{trap}} = \frac{\sigma_e \sigma_h v_{\text{th}} N_t (PN - N_i{}^2)}{\sigma_e \left[N + N_i \exp\left(\dfrac{E_i - E_{\text{Fi}}}{kT}\right) \right] + \sigma_h \left[P + N_i \exp\left(\dfrac{E_i - E_{\text{Fi}}}{kT}\right) \right]}$$

$$(\text{cm}^{-3}\, s^{-1}) \tag{1.5.12}$$

where v_{th} is the thermal velocity of the carriers, N_t the density of recombination centers, and E_{Fi} the intrinsic Fermi level at termperature T (i.e., the Fermi level for equal electron and hole concentrations, typically $E_{\text{Fi}} \cong E_g/2$); $P = P_0 + \Delta N$ and $N = N_0 + \Delta N$ are the majority and minority carrier densities.

The capture cross section of a center is an indication of how close a carrier has to come to the center for the capture to be effected, and is a function of the carrier effective mass among other more complex factors. The thermal carrier velocity in (1.5.12) is calculated using the free electron mass m_0, $v_{\text{th}} = (3kT/m_0)^{1/2} \approx 10^7$ cm/s at room temperature. Note that the capture cross section may be temperature dependent, as is discussed with respect to certain nonradiative centers in Section 1.8.1.

Equation (1.5.12) can be simplified under conditions of *low carrier injection* (i.e., $\Delta N \ll N_0$ or $\Delta P \ll p_0$) into material in which the ionization energy of the centers is comparatively deep relative to kT. In n-type material, for example,

$$N_0 \gg P_0 \gg N_i \exp[(E_i - E_{\text{Fi}})/kT] \tag{1.5.13}$$

and

$$R_{\text{trap}} \cong \sigma_h N_t v_{\text{th}} \, \Delta N \tag{1.5.14a}$$

Similarly, for p-type material,

$$R_{\text{trap}} = \sigma_e N_t v_{\text{th}} \Delta N \qquad (1.5.14b)$$

From the definition of the minority carrier lifetime as the ratio of the excess carrier density ΔN to net recombination rate, the trap-limited lifetime in n-type material is

$$\tau \cong (\sigma_h v_{\text{th}} N_t)^{-1} \qquad (1.5.15a)$$

and in p-type material,

$$\tau \cong (\sigma_e v_{\text{th}} N_t)^{-1} \qquad (1.5.15b)$$

Under these conditions, where the Fermi level is assumed so placed that the majority carrier density is always sufficient to keep the centers filled, the rate-limiting step for the electron–hole recombination process is the capture of minority carriers by the centers. As indicated by (1.5.15), the lifetime is therefore independent of the minority carrier density and becomes a function of the center's capture cross section (for minority carriers), trap density, and carrier thermal velocity.

The impact of electron–hole recombination via intermediate centers is particularly pronounced in indirect bandgap materials because the competing direct band-to-band recombination process is so slow. It is instructive to consider a simple example for illustration of the internal quantum efficiency comparing GaAs and Si, assuming that the recombination via the deep centers is nonradiative in both cases. With an assumed majority carrier density of 10^{17} cm^{-3}, B_r from, Table 1.5.1 yields an approximate band-to-band recombination carrier lifetime of 6×10^{-3} s for Si, but only 1.4×10^{-8} s for GaAs. Assuming a nonradiative center density of 10^{15} cm^{-3} (a relatively low value), and a reasonable capture cross section of 10^{-15} cm^2, the nonradiative lifetime in both materials is 10^{-7} s. It is clear, therefore, that under conditions of low carrier injection the recombination process in Si is dominated by the centers, whereas in GaAs the band-to-band radiative process is dominant since that lifetime is so much shorter. The internal quantum efficiency is appropriately affected in the two materials. From (1.5.1), the estimated internal quantum efficiency in Si is 1.7×10^{-5} whereas it is 0.88 in GaAs. Although this conclusion must be reconsidered for specific conditions, it is evident that a high internal quantum efficiency is more easily achieved in a direct bandgap material with its short band-to-band radiative lifetime, than in an indirect bandgap material.

1.6   Minority Carrier Diffusion

The carriers which are formed locally, or injected, will diffuse away from their initial position because of the random thermal motion of the carriers. If we consider a given direction x, the flow of excess elections ΔN is proportional to the density gradient $\partial(\Delta N)/\partial x$ and a constant D_e, the electron diffusion constant. Hence, in the absence of an applied electric field, the number of electrons passing through a unit area per second is $D_e \, \partial(\Delta N)/\partial x$ cm^{-2} s^{-1}. Similarly, the number of holes passing through per unit area is $-D_h \, \partial(\Delta P)/\partial x$, where the hole diffusion coefficient is D_h.

The directed flow of electrons or holes gives rise to an electric current which for electrons is given by $eD_e \, \partial(\Delta N)/\partial x$ since each electron carries a charge e. This current flows even in the absence of an electric field applied to the sample solely as a result of the nonuniform carrier distribution. The diffusion coefficient and the carrier mobility are related by the Einstein relation

$$D_e = (kT/e)\mu_e, \qquad D_h = (kT/e)\mu_h \tag{1.6.1}$$

Since we are dealing with the flow of minority carriers, the mobility value used (μ_e or μ_h) is that of the minority carrier, i.e., electrons in p-type material and holes in n-type material. The mobility is a function of the majority carrier density and the charged impurity concentrations as well as the temperature. Since the carriers diffuse along a decreasing gradient, some disappear by recombination. On the average, they move a distance L_e or L_h, for electrons and holes, respectively, which is determined by the diffusion coefficient and the lifetime in the material,

$$L_e = (D_e \tau)^{1/2}, \qquad L_h = (D_h \tau)^{1/2} \tag{1.6.2}$$

An important limiting case is the proximity of a surface which is an infinite sink for minority carriers or which is provided with other means of removing minority carriers as quickly as they appear. If the distance between the source of excess carriers and the infinite sink is $d \ll L_e$, then the excess electron distribution is

$$\Delta N \cong (\Delta N)_0 \left[(d - x)/d\right] \tag{1.6.3}$$

indicating an essentially constant gradient. The important case of a contact with a limited recombination velocity is discussed in Chapter 8 where heterojunction structures are described.

The theoretical maximum diffusion length values can be computed using (1.6.2) with τ and minority carrier mobility values and lifetimes appropriate to the doping level of the material. The mobility is usually estimated on the basis of the mobility of the carrier *if* it was the majority carrier. For example, in p-type material with $p = 10^{17}$ cm^{-3}, the electron's mobility would be estimated as if it were in n-type material with that carrier concentration. Mobility values are given in Chapters 10 and 11 for some materials of current interest.

1.7   Radiative Recombination Processes Other than Band-to-Band [23]

The four major electron–hole recombination processes are summarized in Fig. 1.7.1: (a) band-to-band, as discussed herein; (b) band-to-impurity center; (c) donor-to-acceptor; (d) recombination involving isoelectronic impurities, or nearest neighbor pairs which constitute a neutral complex center. In addition, excitonic effects may be observed in pure materials at low temperatures.

Of these processes, only (a) and (b) constitute important lasing transitions, whereas processes (c) and (d) are particularly important spontaneous recombination processes in indirect bandgap materials such as GaP, and are only very briefly mentioned here.

1.7.1   Free-to-Bound Carrier Recombination

In this section we present a summary of the observations commonly seen when a carrier in a band recombines radiatively with one bound to an impurity. Because of the complications introduced by self-absorption within diodes, the radiative emission is frequently distorted, making it difficult to determine the nature of the process giving rise to the observed emission. The example chosen here, therefore, concerns a sample in which the excess electron–hole pair population is generated by excitation using an external laser source. In this case, the emission (photoluminescence) is generated close to the surface and the observed emission is therefore free from absorption effects within the sample.

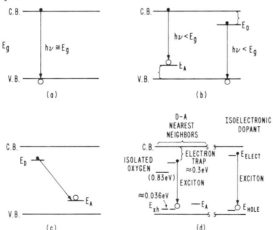

FIG. 1.7.1   Radiative recombination processes: (a) Conduction band-to-valence band transition; (b) conduction band-to-acceptor, or donor-to-valence band transition; (c) donor-to-acceptor transition; (d) left, bound exciton recombination involving nearest neighbor donor O and acceptor Zn (GaP); right, recombination of exciton bound to isoelectronic center.

Consider the recombination of a free carrier, in a sample at temperature T, with a carrier bound to an impurity having an ionization energy E_i. The radiative emission is peaked at a photon energy [24]

$$h\nu_p = E_g - E_i + \tfrac{1}{2}kT \qquad (1.7.1)$$

where the $\tfrac{1}{2}kT$ term accounts for the energy of the free carrier. To illustrate this process, consider an example of recombination of free electrons with holes on acceptors in $In_{0.5}Ga_{0.5}P$, a direct bandgap material [25]. Here, the Cd ionization energy is found to decrease with doping following the empirical relationship (1.3.8):

$$E_A = E_A^{\,\circ} - 2 \times 10^{-8}(N_A - N_D)^{1/3} \quad (eV) \qquad (1.7.2)$$

where $E_A^{\,\circ} = 59$ meV. In the samples studied, as described below, the acceptor concentration was $\sim 10^{18}$ cm^{-3}, resulting in some (~ 20 meV) reduction in the ionization energy of the Cd centers. A shallow donor ($E_D \cong 7$ meV) was also present in low concentration relative to the Cd centers.

Because the centers ionize with increasing temperature, the most interesting effects regarding impurity-related recombination in direct bandgap materials are generally seen at low temperatures. The effect of changing the temperature of the sample is seen in Fig. 1.7.2. The emitted bands, denoted by letters have been identified by studies of variously doped samples. Band A_1 is the band-to-band (intrinsic) recombination emission; A_2 involves the recombination of an electron on the shallow donor with a free hole; and B_1 is due to free electron recombination with a hole on the Cd acceptor. As the temperature of the sample is increased, one notices the disappearance of band A_2 because the shallow donors are becoming ionized thermally. In fact, at 45 K ($kT \cong 4$ meV) so many of the donors are ionized that band A_2 is essentially replaced by the free–free process represented by band A_1. Band B_1, which involves Cd undergoes similar reduction, but only at much higher temperature, and remains significant up to about 140 K. In any case the important conclusion from this example is that the radiative processes at room temperature are not dominated by transitions involving impurities in the concentrations indicated for the present samples. In a direct bandgap material, the intrinsic processes remain the most important ones unless the dopant concentrations become large. Figure 1.7.3 illustrates, as a summary, the shift of the emission peak energy with temperature, and the highest temperature for which the main processes are observable. The downward shift of the intrinsic band peak energy follows that of the bandgap energy with temperature.

It is also important to note that these photoluminescence experiments were conducted under conditions in which the excess carrier density was orders of magnitude below the equilibrium carrier concentration. However, under conditions of high injection, the impurity effects would be much less significant than indicated here. In fact, the competition between the free-to-bound and

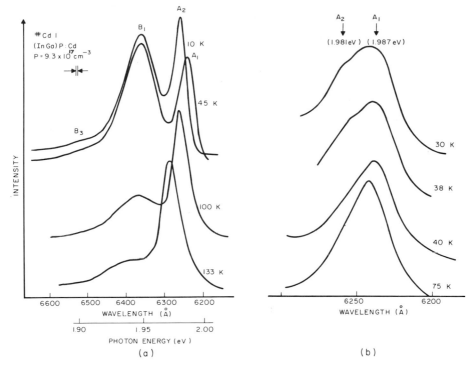

FIG. 1.7.2 Photoluminescence of a Cd-doped sample with $P = 9.3 \times 10^{17}$ cm^{-3} at 10, 45, 100, and 133 K showing the gradual evolution of the various bands. (a) At 10 K, band A$_2$ (donor-to-valence band) dominates the near-bandgap emission, but at high temperatures the intrinsic band A$_1$ is dominant. (b) The evolution of A$_1$ and A$_2$ between 30 and 75 K [25].

intrinsic recombination processes can be characterized by their respective lifetimes. The lifetime for the intrinsic rediative process is obtained as indicated in Section 1.5.2. For the impurity-related radiative recombination, the capture cross section of the center, its ionization energy, and occupancy probability need to be known (Section 1.5.3). For a condition of high injection relative to the impurity concentration, the role of the impurities is reduced relative to the band-to-band recombination process. This is indeed the case under lasing conditions in many materials. For GaAs, a calculation by Moss *et al.* [26] has been performed to predict what dopant concentration is needed to compete with the band-to-band recombination process (i.e., produce a luminescent band equal in intensity to the intrinsic one). They estimate that at 300 K, a shallow acceptor ($E_A = 30$ meV) concentration of 4.8×10^{18} cm^{-3} is needed; at 77 K, because of the higher fraction of unionized centers, only 4.2×10^{15} cm^{-3} acceptors are needed.

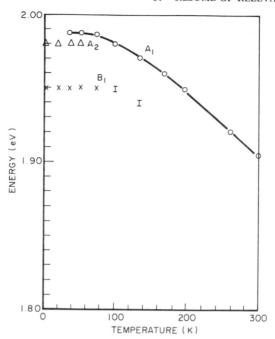

FIG. 1.7.3 Temperature dependence of the various emission bands seen in sample Cd-1 ($P = 9.3 \times 10^{17}$ cm^{-3}) between 4.2 and 300 K. Band B_1 is not resolvable above about 150 K. Thus, the room temperature luminescence is basically intrinsic and does not involve the Cd acceptor levels; $\bigcirc = A_1$ (intrinsic) $\triangle = A_2(D - B)$, $\times = B_1(B - A)$ [25].

1.7.2 Excitonic Effects

Excitons are electron–hole pairs held together by their mutual (screened) Coulomb interaction. One generally speaks of *free* excitions, or excitons *bound* to impurity centers. For the *free exciton*, the energy level scheme is taken as comparable to the hydrogen atom, with the proton being replaced by the heavy hole. The energy needed to dissociate the electron–hole pair is the ionization energy which is calculated from (1.3.1) for the lowest orbit, with the effective mass being given by $m_c^* m_v^* / (m_c^* + m_v^*)$.

When the electron and the hole forming the exciton recombine, a photon is emitted with energy

$$h\nu_p = E_g - E_{exc} \pm KE_p \tag{1.7.3}$$

where KE_p denotes the emission or absorption of K lattice phonons with energy E_p. The value of E_{exc} is a few millielectronvolts in III–V compounds; the most recent value in GaAs is $E_{exc} = 4.2 \pm 0.1$ meV [27].

The exciton localized in the vicinity of a donor, acceptor, or neutral atom is called a *bound exciton*. Because the bound exciton lacks kinetic energy, its emission band upon annihilation is generally narrower than that of the free exciton. If the binding energy of the exciton to the impurity is E_{bx}, the peak of the emitted radiation (neglecting phonon interactions) is

$$h\nu_p = E_g - E_{bx} - E_{exc} \qquad (1.7.4)$$

The value of E_{bx} is a function of the material and the ionization energy E_i of the center to which the exciton is bound. An empirical rule is [28] $E_{bx} \cong E_i/10$. Therefore, the bound exciton energy is a few millielectronvolts. As a result, neither free nor bound excitons play a significant role in the operation of practical direct bandgap devices at room temperature where the thermal energy is far in excess of the exciton binding energies. However, in materials in which isoelectronic impurity effects are important, in particular GaP (described shortly), excitonic effects are important in enhancing the radiative efficiency of the material.

In addition to thermal ionization which reduces the effect of excitons, there is another consideration at low temperatures involving free carriers which screen the exciton–hole attraction of the exciton and reduce their binding energy. Casella [29] suggested a criterion that no bound states exist when the Debye screening length due to the free electrons L_D is less than the Bohr radius of the exciton r_b; hence,

$$r_b = e^2/2\varepsilon E_{exc} < (kT\varepsilon/4\pi Ne^2)^{1/2} \qquad (1.7.5)$$

In GaAs at 77 K, with $E_{exc} = 4.2$ meV, $r_b \cong 150$ A; the free electron concentration must therefore be less than 2×10^{16} cm^{-3} for a significant free exciton density. At elevated temperatures the carrier density limitation is, of course, even more stringent. It is evident, therefore, that the effect of excitons is negligible under high temperature conditions of laser operation because the injected carrier density largely exceeds 10^{16} cm^{-3}. However, as discussed in Section 3.5.1, stimulated emission involving excitons is observed at very low temperatures where the injected carrier densities are low.

1.7.3 Isoelectronic Impurity Effects on Luminescence

Isoelectronic impurities play a key role in the improved efficiency of GaP (indirect gap) LEDs, and are also significant in alloys such as Ga(AsP) and (InGa)P in the indirect bandgap composition ranges. Isoelectronic impurities have the same number of valence electrons as the host but different covalent radius and, most important, electronegativity. The best known and most useful example is nitrogen in GaP which substitutes for P in the lattice. Other known examples are listed in Table 1.7.1.

The isoelectronic substitution is believed to create a *short-range* "potential well" whose magnitude depends on the covalent radius of the substituted atom compared to the replaced atom, and on their difference in electronegativity.

TABLE 1.7.1
Known Examples of Isoelectronic Substitutions

Compound	Isoelectronic center	Replaces	Ref.
GaP	N, Bi	P	a
ZnTe	O	Te	b
CdS	Te	S	c

[a] D. G. Thomas and J. J. Hopefield, *Phys. Rev.* **150**, 680 (1966).
[b] D. G. Thomas, J. J. Hopefield, and R. T. Lynch, *Phys. Rev. Lett.* **17**, 312 (1966).
[c] A. C. Aten, J. H. Haanstra, and H. DeVries, *Phillips Res. Rep.* **20**, 395 (1965).

If the substituted atom has a *lower* electronegativity than the host, then a hole may be trapped at the center. On the other hand, the impurity binds an electron if it has a *higher* electronegativity than the atom it replaces. In GaP, N traps an electron while Bi traps a hole. It is postulated that once a carrier is trapped, the center becomes charged and its long-distance Coulomb potential attracts an oppositely charged carrier. The resultant pair forms a bound exciton with a binding energy which depends on the center. For N in GaP, the exciton binding energy is 11 meV, wheres it is 107 meV for Bi [30–32].

In GaP:N the collapse of the exciton bound to the isolated N center produces the "A line" which at 300 K is centered at 2.24 eV, or about 20 meV below the indirect bandgap energy of 2.26 eV. In addition, recombination involving more complex groupings of nitrogen atoms can occur, particularly at high nitrogen doping levels. These produce lower energy bands, the more important of which is the "NN" line involving a nitrogen atom pair recombination site.

The importance of the nitrogen doping in GaP arises from the fact that the bound exciton process competes relatively efficiently* with the many nonradiative processes which account for the decay of the excess carriers, the intrinsic effects being so slow in the indirect bandgap materials. The benefit of the nitrogen doping is further enhanced by the fact that the isoelectronic impurity introduces no free carriers which could otherwise promote nonradiative Auger recombination (Section 1.8). Hence, very high nitrogen doping (order 10^{19} cm^{-3}) is possible with maximum effect on the radiative efficiency. However, note that even under the most favorable doping conditions, the internal quantum efficiency in GaP:N is between 0.2 and ~1%, values very low compared to the efficiencies of 50–100% achieved with direct bandgap materials such as GaAs [34, 35].

Bound exciton effects similar in their enhancement of radiative efficiency have also been identified in GaP as resulting from the recombination of electron–hole pairs trapped at a neutral complex formed by two atoms on adjoin-

*The N center in GaP has very unusual properties causing its presence to be felt in absorption at temperatures far above those expected on the basis of the rather low ionization energy. It has been suggested by Wolfe *et al.* [33] that this results from a weak coupling between the lattice and N, producing a repulsive potential for the normal phonons of the crystal, and thus extending the lifetime of the electron trapped at the center.

ing sites [36, 37]. The most important of these is the Zn–O pair which has been extensively studied in GaP because it is responsible for the efficient red luminescence ($\sim$1.79 eV) at room temperature. The combination of the Zn acceptor ($E_A = 0.06$ eV) and the deep donor O ($E_D = 0.86$ eV) forms a complex which can bind an electron with an ionization energy of 0.3 eV (Fig. 1.7.1d). A hole is subsequently captured, forming a bound exciton which upon its collapse emits a photon. The emitted band is considerably broadened because of strong lattice interaction (i.e., phonon participation) which produces variation in the photon energy emitted.

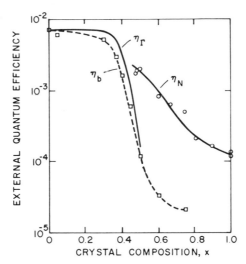

FIG. 1.7.1   GaAs$_{1-x}$P$_x$ electroluminescence quantum efficiency (300 K) versus crystal composition x. The solid curve labeled η_Γ is the calculated contribution to the efficiency resulting from electron–hole recombination external to the N isoelectronic trap. The calculated contribution to the efficiency from excitons bound to N traps, η_N, has been fitted to experimental data by varying the N concentration. For reference the dashed curve ($\square$) shows measured quantum efficiencies η_b on LEDs with no N doping [39].

The addition of nitrogen to (InGa)P and Ga(AsP) can also result in major improvements in the spontaneous emission radiative efficiency in the indirect bandgap composition region (38–40). Figure 1.7.4 shows the improvement in the diode external efficiency obtained by adding N to GaAs$_{1-x}$P$_x$ in the range $x \gtrsim 0.45$, i.e., the composition at which the material is indirect (Chapter 11). A similar improvement is theoretically expected in (InGa)P [41]. However, the emission wavelength with the addition of N may be substantially below the bandgap energy in the alloy. This is shown in Fig. 1.7.5 for Ga(AsP) and calculated in Fig. 1.7.6 for (InGa)P. The reason is that the complex recombination process may dominate over the individual isoelectronic recombination center process (A line) in the alloys.

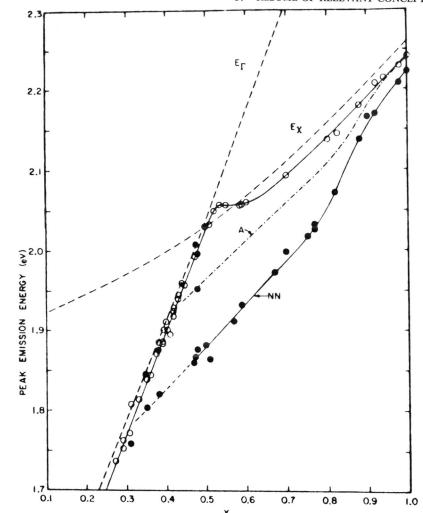

FIG. 1.7.5 Peak emission energy versus alloy composition for $GaAs_{1-x}P_x$ diodes with (•) and without (○) nitrogen doping at 300 K. The diode current is 5 mA (5 A/cm²) [38].

With regard to *stimulated emission*, there is evidence reported in the literature that the presence of N in Ga(AsP) is detectable in the emission spectrum [42].

1.7.4 Donor–Acceptor Pair Radiation

Donor-to-acceptor electron transitions may be observed when the density of donors and acceptors is substantial (typically in excess of 10^{16} cm^{-3}). If the ionization energy of the isolated donor is E_D and that of the acceptor is

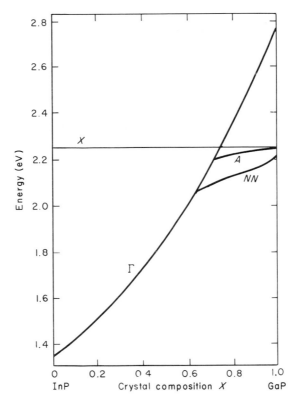

FIG. 1.7.6   Calculated energies (300 K) of the transitions associated with the N isoelectronic trap in $In_{1-x}Ga_xP$ plotted as a function of crystal composition x [39].

E_A, and the pair separation is r, an electron on the donor may recombine with the hole on the acceptor, emitting a photon with energy

$$h\nu_p = E_g - (E_D + E_A) + e^2/\varepsilon r \qquad (1.7.6)$$

where ε is the static dielectric constant. If varying values of the separation r exist, then one can expect to see rather sharp emission lines corresponding to these values [43]. However, commonly one observes a single broad band resulting from donor-acceptor pair recombination, with the peak energy value determined by the average distance r between donors and acceptors.

A characteristic feature of donor–acceptor recombination is the relatively long decay time needed to complete the recombination of excess electron–hole pairs at the end of the excitation. The reason is that the electron–hole interaction is controlled by their wave function overlap [44] which decreases with distance, $\propto \exp(-2r/r_b)$, where r_b is the larger of the two Bohr radii. Because of the slow decay time, competing processes can empty the donors and fill acceptors and lead to recombination by processes other than the donor–acceptor transition process. Thermal ionization of the centers is particularly effective at temperatures at which E_A or E_D approaches kT. Thus, the pair process is rarely seen at room temperature except for very deep recombination centers, a condition not found in the majority of the widely used LED materials. Finally, we note that this process plays no role in laser diodes, although lasing transitions involving tail states resulting from donors and acceptors can occur in very heavily doped materials (Section 3.5.2).

1.8 Nonradiative Recombination Processes

1.8.1 Multiphonon Emission

It has long been recognized that impurity or lattice defect centers exist which produce nonradiative electron–hole recombination. In the case of the important III–V compounds, such as GaAs, deep centers formed by vacancies or metals such as Fe or Cu have long been suspected of being nonradiative, particularly at room tempeature. A model [45, 46] proposed to explain such special centers relates the ionization energy of the center to its position relative to its neighbors in the lattice. In a crystal which has an ionic contribution to binding, the relative positions of an atom and of its immediate neighbors depend on its charge. When the center undergoes a change in charge state (with the capture or release of an electron) the atom is assumed to "rock" momentarily. This rocking, which vibrates the lattice, produces a string of phonons which either partially or totally absorb the energy released by the electron–hole recombination process at the center prior to its relaxation into an equilibrium position. The effect can be expected to be temperature dependent, the higher the temperature of the lattice, the greater is the probability of the nonradiative energy release.

One can visualize this process with the aid of Fig. 1.8.1, which shows the sequence of events at such a hypothetical center. For simplicity, we use only a single coordinate to describe the position of the recombination center relative to its neighbors in a crystal with a polar binding contribution. Curve I in Fig. 1.8.1 represents the energy of the ground state, which for the present we assume to represent a neutral center. The electron is excited (e.g., by photon absorption) from A to B while the nuclei surrounding the center are assumed to remain at rest. However, as the center becomes excited (and its charge changes), the neighboring nuclei gradually assume the positions appropriate to the excited state; hence, the electron will move from B to B′ with the energy difference $[E(B) - E(B')]$ being released in the form of phonons. During this rearrangement the center is likely to remain in the excited state for a period much in excess of 10^{-12} to 10^{-13} s needed for the lattice relaxation process. From B′, the electron can fall back with radiative emission $[E(B') - E(A')] <$

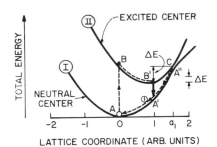

FIG. 1.8.1   Model for the nonradiative recombination process involving a center with rather special properties. The electron transition occurs from A to B. The displacement of the excited atom with respect to its neighbors produces the energy diagram II. The electron recombination process can occur via B′ to A′ with photon emission, or via the nonradiative path C to A″ back to 0, if the electron has energy ΔE allowing it to reach C.

$[E(B) - E(B')]$. Alternatively, there is finite probability, proportional to exp $(-\Delta E/kT)$, that the electron will be thermally excited to C on curve II from which an essentially nonradiative transition occurs to point A″ on curve I. From there, the electron can reach the ground state following curve I when the recombination center returns to the ground state.

From these processes, it is predicted that at *low temperatures,* where the electron is unlikely to acquire the ΔE needed to reach the energy of point C, a radiative transition should be observed, with the energy released lower than the energy needed to excite the recombination center in the first place. However, at *high temperatures,* it is probable that the electronic transition bringing the center back to the ground state will be nonradiative. Evidence for such behavior has been found by Henry and Lang [47, 48], where certain deep levels in GaAs and GaP (such as those introduced by oxygen) exhibit capture cross sections of the form

$$\sigma_t = \sigma_\infty \exp(-E_\infty/kT) \tag{1.8.1}$$

where

$$\sigma_\infty = 10^{-14}\text{--}10^{-15}\ \text{cm}^2 \quad \text{and} \quad E_\infty \cong 0.56\ \text{eV}$$

In this discussion we have been concerned with the nonradiative recombination process at a single atom. It is known that impurity complexes can also produce nonradiative recombination which clearly must involve multiphonon emission as the mechanism for dissipating the energy released in electron–hole recombination. However, the details of the process are likely to be dependent on the nature of the atomic groups. For example, inclusions within crystals provide internal "surfaces" with many states which bridge the bandgap of the host crystal, thus providing an effective means of nonradiative recombination which should be temperature independent.

1.8.2   Nonradiative Processes Involving the Auger Effect

The Auger effect is a mechanism for nonradiative electron–hole recombination that requires relatively large free carrier densities. It is the inverse process to impact ionization. An extensive theoretical literature has evolved on the Auger effect in semiconductors, starting with the work of Beattie and Landsberg [49]. An extensive review of the subject is given by Blakemore [50], Landsberg and Adams [51], and Landsberg [52].

The Auger effect involves the interaction of three carriers. In the band-to-band Auger process, two electrons "collide" while the energy released in the electron–hole recombination is transferred to the remaining electron, which now becomes "hot" and dissipates its energy to the lattice (i.e., nonradiatively). Similarly, two holes and one electron can be involved with the hot hole performing this same function.

The band-to-band Auger process is a complex function of the carrier effective mass, the density of states distribution, and the bandgap energy. Other factors remaining constant, the Auger lifetime $\tau_{Au}^{-1} \propto N^2 P$ or $P^2 N$ in n-type or p-type material, respectively. Therefore, it is a steep function of the majority carrier concentration, a characteristic used to identify whether the Auger effect is responsible for the observed nonradiative lifetime in a given material or device.

In general, the Auger effect becomes of increasing importance, as a limiting factor on the lifetime, with decreasing bandgap energy. At 300 K, it is significant in reducing the carrier lifetime in InAs [53] ($E_g = 0.36$ eV) at the relatively low carrier concentration of 10^{17} cm^{-3}, where $\tau_{Au} \approx 10^{-9}$ s. However, in wider bandgap materials, such as GaAs, the Auger effect is believed to be important only for very high carrier concentrations ($> 10^{19}$ cm^{-3}), for example, in heavily doped p-type material. Several materials have been theoretically analyzed by Takeshima [54]. For example, in GaSb, the Auger lifetime for $P = 10^{18}$ cm^{-3} is calculated to be as low as $\sim 10^{-9}$ s, a value lower than the band-to-band radiative recombination lifetime. Landsberg and Adams [51] have suggested an approximate rule for judging the importance of the Auger effect for a given majority carrier concentration: The ratio of the band-to-band radiative recombination rate to the nonradiative Auger recombination rate is proportional to $E^{7/2}$, where E is the energy released in the electron–hole recombination.

The Auger effect involving impurities provides a means of removing nonradiatively the energy released in free-to-bound carrier recombination or in a donor–acceptor transition [55]. The schematic of the process is shown in Fig. 1.8.2. The probability of the Auger effect occurring follows the rule that the lower the energy released, the more probable the process becomes.

Much caution is needed to identify Auger processes conclusively in the wider bandgap materials because the conditions which give rise to the effect,

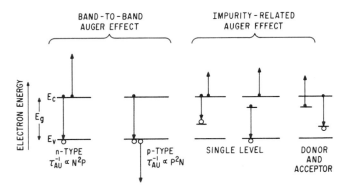

FIG. 1.8.2 Schematic of the simpler Auger processes for nonradiative electron–hole recombination in a semiconductor. The basic process, either band-to-band or impurity related, involves the interaction of two like carriers, one of which carries off the energy released in the electron–hole recombination process. τ_{Au} denotes the nonradiative carrier lifetime due to the Auger process; $\cdot$ = electron, $\bigcirc$ = hole.

i.e., a high free carrier concentration, occur in highly doped materials. The introduction of a high dopant density in many cases leads to the generation of defects and impurity clusters which can account, at least partly, for the nonradiative processes. In general, attempts to identify Auger processes revolve around the fact that the Auger limited lifetime decreases distinctly as the square of the free carrier concentration, a characteristic not shared by the other known nonradiative processes involving defects.

REFERENCES

1. D. J. Stirland and B. W. Straughan, *Thin Solid Films* **31**, 139 (1976).
2. L. Pauling, *The Nature of the Chemical Bond*. Cornell Univ. Press, Ithaca, New York, 1948.
3. D. Long, *Energy Bands in Semiconductors*. Wiley (Interscience), New York, 1968.
4. M. L. Cohen and T. K. Bergstresser, *Phys. Nev.* **141**, 789 (1966).
5. W. Kohn, *Solid State Phys.* **5**, 257 (1957).
6. J. C. Phillips, *Bonds and Bands in Semiconductors*. Academic Press, New York, 1973.
7. A. Baldereschi, *Proc. Int. Conf. Phys. Semicond., 12th*. Teubner, Stuttgart, 1974.
8. D. Redfield, *Phys. Rev.* **130**, 916 (1963;; **140**, A2056 (1965).
9. J. Dow and D. Redfield, *Phys. Rev. B* **5**, 594 (1972).
10. D. Redfield, *Adv. Phys.* **24**, 463 (1975); *J. Electron Mater.* **4**, 945 (1975).
11. D. Redfield, J. P. Wittke, and J. I. Pankove, *Phys. Rev. B* **6**, 1830 (1970).
12. J. I. Pankove, *Phys. Rev.* **140**, A2059 (1965); D. Redfield and M. A. Afromowitz, *Appl. Phys. Lett.* **11**, 138 (1967).
13. B. I. Halperin and M. Lax, *Phys. Nev.* **148**, 722 (1966).
14. J. I. Pankove and E. K. Annavedder, *J. Appl. Phys.* **36**, 3948 (1965).
15. H. C. Casey, Jr. and F. Stern, *J. Appl. Phys.* **47**, 631 (1976).
16. Y. P. Varshni, *Phys. Status Solidi* **19**, 353 (1964).
17. C. J. Hwang and J. C. Dyment, *J. Appl. Phys.* **44**, 3240 (1973).

18. G. A. Acket, W. Nijman, and H. 't Lam, *J. Appl. Phys.* **45**, 3033 (1974).
19. H. Namizaki, H. Kan, M. Ishii, and A. Ito, *Appl. Phys. Lett.* **24**, 486 (1974).
20. R. N. Hall, *Phys. Rev.* **87**, 387 (1952).
21. W. Shockley and W. T. Reed, *Phys. Rev.* **87**, 835 (1952).
22. C. T. Sah, R. N. Noyce, and W. Shockley, *Proc. IRE* **45**, 1228 (1957).
23. P. J. Dean, *in Progress in Solid State Chemistry,* (J. O. McCaldin and G. Somorjai, eds.), Vol. 8. Pergamon, Oxford, 1973.
24. D. M. Eagle, *J. Phys. Chem. Solids* **16**, 76 (1960).
25. H. Kressel, C. J. Nuese, and I. Ladany, *J. Appl. Phys.* **44**, 3266 (1973).
26. T. S. Moss, G. J. Burrell, and B. Ellis, *Semiconductor Optoelectronics.* Wiley, New York, 1973.
27. S. B. Nam, D. C. Reynolds, C. W. Litton, R. J. Almassy, and T. C. Collins, *Phys. Rev. B* **13**, 761 (1976).
28. J. R. Heynes, *Phys. Rev. Lett.* **4**, 361 (1960).
29. R. C. Casella, *J. Appl. Phys.* **34**, 1703 (1963).
30. J. D. Cuthbert and D. G. Thomas, *Phys. Rev.* **154**, 763 (1967).
31. A. Baldereschi, *J. Luminescence* **7**, 79 (1973).
32. P. J. Dean, *J. Luminescence* **7**, 51 (1973).
33. M. I. Wolfe, H. Kressel, T. Halpern, and P. M. Raccah, *Appl. Phys. Lett.* **24**, 279 (1974).
34. R. A. Logan, H. G. White, and W. Wiegmann, *Solid-State Electron.* **14**, 55 (1971).
35. I. Ladany and H. Kressel, *RCA Rev.* **33**, 517 (1972).
36. T. N. Morgan, B. Weber, and R. N. Bhargava, *Phys. Rev.* **166**, 751 (1968).
37. C. H. Henry, P. J. Dean, and J. D. Cuthbert, *Phys. Rev.* **166**, 754 (1966).
38. M. G. Craford, R. W. Shaw, A. H. Herzog, and W. O. Groves, *J. Appl. Phys.* **43**, 4075 (1972).
39. J. C. Campbell, N. Holonyak, Jr., M. G. Craford, and D. L. Keune, *J. Appl. Phys.* **45**, 4543 (1974).
40. J. J. Coleman, N. Holonyak, Jr , A. B. Kunz, W. O. Groves, D. L. Keune, and M. G. Craford, *Solid State Commun.* **16**, 319 (1975).
41. G. G. Kleinman, *J. Appl. Phys.* **47**, 180 (1976).
42. J. J. Coleman *et al., Phys. Rev. Lett.* **33**, 1566 (1974).
43. D. G. Thomas, M. Gershenzon, and F. A. Trumbore, *Phys. Rev.* **133**, A269 (1964).
44. D. G. Thomas, J. J. Hopefield, and K. Colbow, *Proc. Symp. Radiat. Recombination Semicond.* Dunod, Paris, 1964.
45. F. Seitz, *Trans. Faraday Soc.* **35**, 74 (1938).
44. D. G. Thomas, J. J. Hopefield, and K. Colbow, *Proc. Symp. Radiat. Recombination Semicond.* Dunod, Paris, 1964.
45. F. Seitz, *Trans. Faraday Soc.* **35**, 74 (1938).
46. W. B. Fowler and D. L. Dexter, *J. Chem. Phys.* **43**, 768 (1965).
47. C. H. Henry and D. V. Lang, *Proc. Int. Conf. Phys. Semicond., 12th,* p. 411. Teubner, Stuttgart, 1974.
48. C. H. Henry, *J. Electron. Mater.* **4**, 1037 (1975).
49. A. R. Beattie and P. T. Landsberg, *J. Phys. Chem. Solids* **8**, 73 (1959).
50. J. S. Blakemore, *Semiconductor Statistics,* p. 214. Pergamon, New York, 1962.
51. P. T. Landsberg and M. J. Adams, *J. Luminescence* **7**, 3 (1973).
52. P. T. Landsberg, *Phys. Status Solidi* **41**, 457 (1970).
53. V. L. Dalal, W. A. Hicinbothem, Jr., and H. Kressel, *Appl. Phys. Lett.* **24**, 184 (1974).
54. M. Takeshima, *J. Appl. Phys.* **43**, 4114 (1972).
55. K. P. Sinha and M. DiDomenico, *Phys. Rev. B* **1**, 2623 (1970).

BIBLIOGRAPHY

R. A. Smith, *Semiconductors*. Cambridge Univ. Press, London and New York, 1959.

A. J. Dekker, *Solid State Physics*. Macmillan, New York, 1960.

R. A. Smith, *Wave Mechanics of Crystalline Solids*. Chapman and Hall, London, 1961.

H. Jones, *The Theory of Brillouin Zones and Electronic States in Crystals*. North-Holland Pub., Amsterdam, 1962.

R. B. Adler, A. C. Smith, and R. L. Longini, *Introduction to Semiconductor Physics*. Wiley, New York, 1964.

Shyh Wang, *Solid-State Electronics*. McGraw-Hill, New York, 1966.

D. L. Greenaway and G. Harbeke, *Optical Properties and Band Structure of Semiconductors*. Pergamon, Oxford, 1968.

J. I. Pankove, *Optical Processes in Semiconductors*. Prentice-Hall, Englewood Cliffs, New Jersey, 1971 and Dover, New York, 1976.

A. A. Bergh and P. J. Dean, Light-Emitting Diodes, *Proc. IEEE* **60**, 156 (1972).

Chapter 2

p–n Junctions and Heterojunctions

2.1 Current–Voltage Characteristics

2.1.1 Ideal Junctions [1]

A p–n junction is formed by adjoining p- and n-type layers as shown in Fig. 2.1.1. A thin depletion region (i.e., essentially free of mobile carriers) exists at the boundary, the width of which depends on the applied voltage and the carrier concentration in the p- and n-regions. Without external voltage, no current flows because a potential barrier is established at the p–n interface which prevents the net flow of carriers from one region to the next. The magnitude of the barrier is obtained as follows. The Fermi level, in equilibrium, must be equal in both sides of the junction, as indicated in Fig. 2.1.1. Thus, when the materials are joined, the indicated band displacement results in a potential barrier formation which restricts the interdiffusion of the majority carriers. The potential barrier height is determined by the initial positions of the Fermi levels relative to the band edges and the bandgap energy. Assuming nondegenerate materials (i.e., the Fermi level outside the conduction or the valance bands), the barrier height is

$$eV_D = E_g - kT \ln(N_c/N_n) - kT \ln(N_v/P_p) = E_g - kT \ln(N_c N_v / N_n P_p)$$

$$(2.1.1)$$

where N_c and N_v are the effective density of states in the conduction and valence bands, respectively. If the N_D donors/cm^3 are fully ionized, then $N_D = N_n$ and similarly in the p-side of the junction, $N_A = P_p$ for N_A acceptors/cm^3.

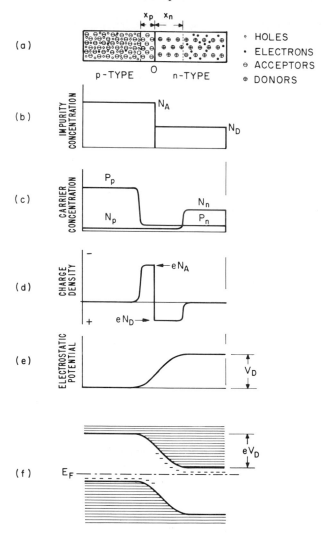

FIG. 2.1.1 Various aspects of the p–n junction without external bias. The Fermi level E_F is constant; the width of the space charge region is divided into widths x_n and x_p as shown.

Since in thermal equilibrium

$$N_i^2 = N_c N_v \exp(-E_g/kT), \qquad E_g = kT \ln(N_c N_v/N_i^2) \qquad (2.1.2)$$

from which it follows that

$$eV_D = kT \ln(N_c N_v/N_i^2) - kT \ln(N_c N_v/N_n N_p) = kT \ln(N_n P_p/N_i^2) \qquad (2.1.3a)$$

Since $N_n P_n = P_p P_p = N_i^2$,

$$V_D = (kT/e) \ln(P_p/P_n) = (kT/e) \ln(N_n/N_p) \qquad (2.1.3b)$$

and we obtain the minority carrier density at the two edges of the space charge region with no applied potential,

$$N_p = N_n \exp(-eV_D/kT), \qquad P_n = P_p \exp(-eV_D/kT) \qquad (2.1.4)$$

The following derivation of the "ideal" diode equation assumes no recombination within the space charge region, a low injection level relative to the background carrier concentration, a field-free region beyond the space charge region, and no carrier generation or recombination processes within the space charge region. As discussed later, modifications are introduced for practical diodes in some portions of the operating range.

When a positive bias V is applied to the p-region (Fig. 2.1.2a), the junction is said to be forward-biased and the potential barrier is reduced. Electrons in the n-type region can now more easily flow into the p-type region, and vice

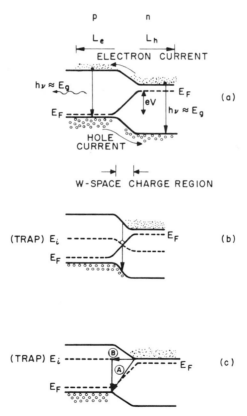

FIG. 2.1.2   Various major current components in a p–n junction with applied voltage V: (a) Diffusion current (thermal emission over the barrier); (b) space charge region recombination via trap with activation energy E_i; (c) tunneling current—either "direct" electron–hole recombination Ⓐ or via a trap in the p-type region with ionization energy E_1 Ⓑ. (Neither side of the junction is doped to degeneracy.)

versa. The additional flow of electrons and holes into the opposite-type regions increases their concentration in the vicinity of the two sides of the p–n interface by $(P_n' - P_n)$ and $(N_p' - N_p)$. These carriers continuously diffuse away from the interface and are replenished by additional carriers. As a result, a current flows. The current flow resulting for a given applied voltage can be calculated from the excess carrier density at the edge of the depletion region. Using an expression similar to (2.1.4), we obtain, for the total hole density in the n-side at the edge of the depletion region,

$$P_n' = P_p \exp[-e(V_D - V)/kT] \tag{2.1.5}$$

Hence, using (2.1.4),

$$P_n' = P_n \exp(eV/kT) \tag{2.1.6}$$

and the *excess hole* density in the n-side of the junction at $x = x_n$, the edge of the space charge region, is the difference between the total hole density P_n' and the value with no applied bias P_n,

$$(\Delta P)_{x_n} = (P_n' - P_n) = P_n[\exp(qV/kT) - 1] \tag{2.1.7}$$

The current density due to holes which diffuse away from the junction is

$$(J_h)_{x_n} = -eD_h(\partial(\Delta P)/\partial x)_{x=x_n} \tag{2.1.8}$$

The excess hole distribution ΔP is assumed to be an exponential function of the distance from the junction,

$$\Delta P = (\Delta P)_{x_n} \exp(-x/L_h) \tag{2.1.9}$$

The current density due to hole flow J_h is given by the product of the carrier charge e, the density of charge $(\Delta P)_{x_h}$, and their velocity = distance/time = L_h/τ. Thus, since $L_n^2 = D_h\tau$, the current density due to holes is

$$J_h = (eD_h/L_h)(\Delta P)_{x_n} = (eD_h P_n/L_h)[\exp(eV/kT) - 1] \tag{2.1.10}$$

Similarly for electrons, their current contribution is

$$J_e = (eD_e N_p/L_e)[\exp(eV/kT) - 1] \tag{2.1.11}$$

Hence the *total* current density due to both electrons and holes is

$$J = e(D_h P_n/L_h) + (D_e N_p/L_e) [\exp(eV/kT) - 1] \tag{2.1.12}$$

The injection efficiency is an important characteristic of p–n junctions since it is generally desirable to enhance either hole or electron injection. The fraction of the total current carried by electrons follows from Eqs. (2.1.10) and (2.1.11);

$$\frac{J_e}{J_e + J_h} = \left(1 + \frac{D_h}{D_e}\frac{P_n}{N_p}\frac{L_e}{L_h}\right)^{-1} \quad \text{or} \quad \frac{J_e}{J_e + J_h} = \left[1 + \left(\frac{D_h}{D_e}\frac{L_h}{L_e}\frac{P_p}{N_n}\right)\right]^{-1} \tag{2.1.13}$$

It is evident that a high electron injection efficiency is achieved by making $N_n \gg P_p$, i.e., a higher donor concentration on the n-side of the junction.

The behavior of the junction under reverse bias can be similarly analyzed and corresponds to a condition of extraction of minority carriers within a diffusion length of the p–n junction. An equation of the following form provides the theoretical basis of the operation of an *ideal* p–n junction:

$$J = J_{s0} \left[\exp(eV/kT) - 1 \right] \qquad (2.1.14)$$

where J_{s0} is the saturation current density given by

$$J_{s0} = e(D_h P_n/L + (D_n N_p/L_n))$$

Under significant reverse bias, the current flow is equal to J_{s0}, but only for applied voltages substantially below the "breakdown voltage." This voltage marks the onset of massive carrier multiplication in the space charge region by impact ionization of valence electrons by energetic electrons or holes. Avalanche multiplication occurs when a carrier traversing the space charge region acquires sufficient energy from the field (in a mean free path of tens of angstroms) to ionize a lattice atom in a subsequent collision, thus creating a new electron–hole pair.

An approximate expression for the dependence of the breakdown voltage V_B of an *abrupt* p^+n junction as a function of bandgap energy and carrier concentration N in the lightly doped side of the junction is [2]

$$V_B \cong 60(E_g/1.1)^{3/2}(N/10^{16})^{-3/4} \qquad (2.1.15)$$

For a graded junction, with impurity gradient a_j, V_B is approximately [2]

$$V_B \cong 60(E_g/1.1)^{6/5} (a_j/3) \times 10^{20})^{-2/5} \qquad (2.1.16)$$

Avalanche multiplication is not the only process leading to a current increase with reverse bias. In very narrow space charge regions (i.e., in diodes made from heavily doped n-and p-type regions) a current increase can occur by an internal field emission process. In this process, the local electric field intensity is so high ($\sim 10^6$ V/cm) that there is a finite probability that some valence electrons can tunnel into the conduction band to form electron–hole pairs which contribute to the current flow.

In diodes containing defects, local carrier multiplication can occur at "microplasma" sites which decrease the observed diode breakdown voltage below the theoretical value. Microplasma sites are formed by dislocations, large inclusions in the space charge region, stacking faults, and so on. In fact, any defect which can give rise to a local enhancement of the field in the space charge region can give rise to microplasma sites. In addition, the presence of a large density of contaminants causes anomallous increases in the diode current with increasing reverse bias. Therefore, the value of the breakdown voltage cannot be indiscriminately taken as are indication of the carrier concentration in the vicinity of the p–n junction.

2.1.2   Nonideal Junctions

The ideal diode [Eq. (2.1.14)] neglects electron–hole recombination *within* the space charge region at defect centers (Fig. 2.1.2b). Most diodes contain such recombination centers which allow space charge region recombination at a rate R_{trap}, an effect reflected in the current–voltage characteristics. In forward bias, the electron loss by recombination in the space charge region W wide gives rise to a current density

$$J_{rec} = e \int_0^W R_{trap} \, dx \tag{2.1.17}$$

R_{trap} is given by (1.5.12) and can be simplified with restrictive assumptions as follows: The trap energy $E_i = E_g/2$; the capture cross sections for electrons and holes are equal to σ_t; and a single lifetime value $\tau = (\sigma_t v_{th} N_t)^{-1}$ can be used for both segments of the space charge region on either side of the metal-lurgical p–n boundary. The electron and hole concentrations in the center of the space charge region, N and P, respectively, are equal and given by $N_i \exp (eV/2kT)$.

With these approximations, and assuming that $\exp(eV/2\,kT) \gg 1$, (1.5.12) reduces to

$$R_{trap} \cong (N_i/2\tau)\exp(eV/2kT) \tag{2.1.18}$$

and from (2.1.17), the resultant forward-bias current density is [4]

$$J_{rec} \approx (eN_i W/2\tau)\exp(eV/2kT) \tag{2.1.19}$$

An important consequence of space charge region recombination is that the forward-bias current–voltage curves of most diodes consist of several regions. At low values of applied bias, the diode current is proportional to $\exp(eV/akT)$ where a is between 1 and 2, whereas at higher bias values, the ideal diode behavior is approached when $a = 1$. Note that the derivation of (2.1.19) is strictly applicable only for a specific set of defects having an ionization energy close to midgap. A more complex behavior may occur with either shallower or deeper traps. Of course, Eq. (1.5.12) can be used for specific defects to calculate R_{trap} and hence the space charge region recombination current density.

In the high current density region, the ideal diode equation again is inadequate because of the voltage drop across the diode series resistance and because of conductivity modulation of the p- and n-type regions. A resistance is contributed by the bulk of the semiconductor and by nonideal "ohmic" contacts. If this diode resistance is fixed at R_s, then the diode equation becomes

$$I = I_{s0} \{\exp[e(V\text{-}IR_s)/akT] - 1\} \tag{2.1.20}$$

where I_{s0} is the saturation current and $1 \le a \le 2$; only the voltage $(V\text{-}IR_s)$ appears across the p–n interface region.

Commonly hidden by the series resistance effects of junctions at high bias is a basic change in the I vs. V dependence of the diode equation when the injected carrier density approaches the background concentration. As discussed in various texts (see the Bibliography) the rate of increase of the minority carrier density with voltage (neglecting the ohmic drop) becomes approximately $\exp(eV/2kT)$, and hence $I \propto \exp(eV/2kT)$. Note that further complication is introduced in the high injection region by the fact that the minority carrier lifetime now depends on the injection level (Section 1.5), which changes the saturation current term.

At sufficiently high values of applied voltage, stimulated emission begins in a laser diode (Chapter 3). Then, the voltage *at the junction* could "lock" if the carrier population in the recombination region no longer increases above lasing threshold, because in the *simplest* model the gain coefficient is fixed above threshold. In practice, however (Appendix B), the carrier population in the recombination region need not be fully built up at the observed lasing threshold, and a sharp "saturation" of the junction voltage therefore is not always observed. However, it is possible to check for junction voltage saturation effects by noting the change in slope of the current versus applied voltage curve, a measurement best performed by determining the derivative of the "terminal" voltage versus current curve. It is evident that with the voltage across the junction fixed, any further increase in applied voltage simply increases the voltage drop across the resistance R_s of the regions external to the junction.

The derivative dV/dI is found from (2.1.20) as follows. Rewriting in terms of voltage at the diode terminals V,

$$V = IR_s + (akT/e)\ln(I/I_{s0} + 1)$$

Hence,

$$dV/dI = R_s + (akT/e)[I/(I + I_{s0})]$$

and since $I \gg I_{s0}$ in the range of interest,

$$I\, dV/dI \cong IR_s + akT/e \qquad\qquad (2.1.21)$$

Measurements of $I\, dV/dI$ have been performed on various double-heterojunction CW laser diodes [3], and evidence has been found in some diodes for the change in slope at lasing threshold indicative of near saturation over a limited current range. Figure 2.1.3a shows the "dip" in the $I\, dV/dI$ curve when lasing starts. Note that this effect does *not* occur in the diode of similar construction, but which is incapable of stimulated emission, where the junction voltage continues to rise with increasing current.

The practical question of the voltage needed to operate a laser diode well above threshold can simply be answered since the I–V curve is generally dominated by the voltage drop across R_s. To illustrate the observed V vs. I behavior of a typical laser diode, we show in Fig. 2.1.3b the V–I curve of a CW

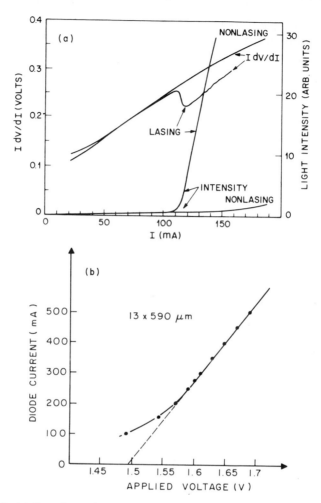

FIG. 2.1.3   (a) Experimental variation of $I\,dI/dV$ versus current I of a CW laser diode and of a diode of similar construction but incapable of lasing. Also shown is the light intensity versus current which shows that the "dip" in $I\,dI/dV$ coincides with the laser threshold, and is absent in the nonlasing diode [3]. (b) Relationship between applied voltage and diode current of a CW laser at 22°C. The linear portion of the curve represents operation in the "ohmic" range when $V > \approx E_g/e$. The slope $dV/dI = 0.44$ ohm $= R_s$.

double-heterojunction laser (with a threshold current of ~ 200 mA) in which the recombination region has bandgap energy ≈ 1.55 eV ($\lambda_L \cong 8200$ Å). Note the slope change when the applied voltage exceeds 1.5 V. The curve becomes linear with $dV/dI = R_s = 0.44$ ohm. Thus, the V–I curves of a laser diode above threshold can be approximated by

$$V \cong IR_s + E_g/e \tag{2.1.22}$$

For example, in a GaAs laser diode operating at a pulsed current of 40 A, with a resistance $R_s - 0.2$ ohm, the voltage which must be applied to the diode $V \cong 1.4 + (0.2)(40) = 9.4$ V.

Tunneling processes can also change the I–V characteristics from the classical diode behavior. In homojunctions made from highly doped p- and n-type regions, electrons can tunnel from the n-region as shown in Fig. 2.1.2c. In practical luminescent diodes this tunneling current is small at reasonable bias values compared to either the current due to space charge region recombination or to the "ideal" injection current. The tunnel current component can be differentiated from these two components by its relative temperature insensitivity, being typically of the form $J \propto \exp(AV)$, where A is a constant which is weakly temperature dependent compared to kT/e, and V is the applied voltage. These tunneling effects are generally significant only in the low bias range of diode operation and are not of practical importance in the electroluminescent devices of interest here.

The direct tunneling process shown in Fig. 2.1.2c (curve Ⓐ), in which an electron in the conduction band of the n-side of the junction recombines with a hole in the valence band of the p-side, can give rise to the emission of a photon with energy approximately equal to the energy separation of the bands as indicated. This *radiative tunneling* [5] process may be seen, usually at low temperatures, in devices having thin (order 100 Å) space charge regions, i.e., in relatively highly doped junctions. Because the separation of the band edges increases with applied voltage V, the peak energy $h\nu_p$ of the emitted radiation shifts with increasing bias, $h\nu_p \cong e(V - V_0)$, where $V_0 \approx 20$ meV [6] in GaAs homojunctions, a value reflecting the presence of the valence bandtail states in the heavily doped p-region.

Note, however, that another mechanism, *band filling* [7], involving bandtail states can also give rise to shifting peaks. Figure 2.1.4 illustrates this process for a heterojunction in which electrons tunnel from the higher bandgap n-type region into conduction bandtail states in the p-side of the heterojunction, a process that is followed by the radiative recombination with a hole in

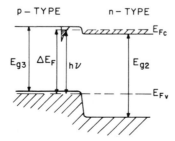

FIG. 2.1.4   Model for "band filling" via a tunneling process of electrons from the conduction band of the n-side of the junction into the conduction bandtail states in the p-side of the junction.

the valence band. As the voltage is increaed, the electrons tunnel into the conduction bandtail states of increasing energy, thus filling them as shown in Fig. 2.1.4. As a result, the separation of the quasi-Fermi levels increases. Note that this band filling mechanism (originally postulated for homojunctions with diffused p-regions) is only appropriate with a significant density of tail states—an effect expected only with highly doped recombination regions. Thus, this band filling process need not be significant in heterojunctions in which, as described in the following sections, the doping level on either side of the junction can be low and still maintain the desired injection efficiency.

Note that band filling can also occur as a result of electron injection. As the electron population increases, the conduction bandtail states gradually become filled, resulting in an upward shift of the emitted peak radiation energy.

2.2   Junction Capacitance

The depletion region consists of a double layer of equal uncompensated positively charged atoms on the n-side of the junction and negatively charged atoms on the p-side of the junction. The effective capacitance due to the change in the depletion layer charge Q with change in applied voltage is

$$C = dQ/dV \qquad (2.2.1)$$

The capacitance can be calculated from an appropriate solution of Poisson's equation which relates the charge density (and distribution) and the potential. The total charge on either side of the junction must be equal to maintain charge neutrality. Hence,

$$N_D x_n = N_A x_p \qquad (2.2.2)$$

where x_n and x_p are the space charge region widths on the n- and p-type sides of the junction. The total width of the space charge region $W = x_n + x_p$ for an abrupt junction is

$$W = [(2\varepsilon/e)[(N_A + N_D)/N_A N_D](V_D - V)]^{1/2} \qquad (2.2.3)$$

The capacitance per unit area is

$$C = \varepsilon/W \qquad (2.2.4)$$

W can be calculated for an arbitrary impurity distribution; the result for various junction types has been given by Lawrence and Warner [8].

A second component of the junction capacitance, due to the injected minority carriers, is important only in forward bias. This "diffusion capacitance" results from the storage of carriers within a diffusion length of the p–n junction interface. As the voltage is changed, the transient flow of carriers provides a flow of charge just as if the junction possessed an additional capacitance value. The diffusion capacitance depends on the lifetime, but in forward-biased junctions it is generally greater than the capacitance due to the space charge region. The effect of the diffusion capacitance can be troublesome when diodes are used as switches since the time required to extract the charge when the junction bias is switched from forward to reverse bias slows down the diode switching speed. A discussion of the limitation this places on the modulation capability of an LED is found in Section 2.5.

With sufficient forward bias, the diffusion capacitance can easily exceed the space charge region capacitance which decreases as the reciprocal of the *square root* of the applied voltage (for an abrupt junction), while the injected carrier density increases *exponentially* with the applied voltage.

2.3 Heterojunctions

2.3.1 General Considerations

A heterojunction, for the present purposes, consists of two adjoining single-crystal semiconductors with dissimilar bandgap energies. Heterojunctions are classified into *isotype* (n–n or p–p) or *anisotype* (p–n). In the ideal heterojunction, most commonly analyzed in the literature, an abrupt interface is assumed between the two semiconductors. In practice, however, some grading is believed present, although graded interface regions less than ~ 100 Å are difficult to measure. As discussed herein, the gradient changes some of the electronic properties of the heterojunction, without, however, eliminating the useful properties.

The most serious problem confronting the fabrication of useful heterojunctions (and the interpretation of heterojunction data) is the presence of interfacial defects resulting from a lattice parameter mismatch between the semiconductors. We defer a discussion of the allowable limit and types of defects observed at heterointerfaces to Chapters 8 and 9. We simply mention that essentially ideal heterojunctions have been produced using semiconductors having a very small lattice parameter mismatch ($< 0.1\%$).

The following basic functions are served by heterojunctions in optoelectronic devices:

1. An isotype heterojunction can be formed between a transparent (higher bandgap) conducting substrate and an epitaxial layer containing the active region of the device. Here, the substrate–epitaxial layer interface serves only a passive role because its electrical properties are not used. Such structures are widely used for LEDs [e.g., Ga(AsP) grown on GaP].

2. Isotype heterojunctions provide a transparent layer in close proximity to an active region in order to lower the surface recombination velocity of an otherwise free surface (Section 8.1.2). Here, the heterojunction interface serves a passivating role.

3. Isotype heterojunctions provide a potential barrier for minority carrier

confinement to effectively reduce their diffusion length (and hence the recombination volume). This heterojunction role plays a key part in the operation of laser diodes and high radiance LEDs.

4.   Anisotype heterojunctions improve the injection efficiency of either electrons or holes, depending on the relative magnitude of the bandgap energy of the two sides of the junction.

5.   Isotype or anisotype heterojunctions provide a dielectric step to form one wall of an optical waveguide. The magnitude of the step is a function of the bandgap energy difference and of the wavelength of the radiation (Chapter 12).

6.   Isotype "caps" are used to facilitate ohmic contacts by providing a small bandgap energy material at the metallized surface.

In the following sections we consider major relevant aspects of the electrical properties of heterojunctions. Comprehensive theoretical and experimental reviews covering many materials can be found in the literature. [9–11].

2.3.2   Heterojunction Band Diagram

A model for the ideal heterojunction with an abrupt interface and which neglects interfacial defect states was proposed by Anderson [12]. Figure 2.3.1 shows the band diagram before and after joining materials with work functions ϕ_1 and ϕ_2, dielectric constants ε_1 and ε_2, and electron affinities χ_1 and χ_2. The *electron affinity* is the energy required to excite an electron from the

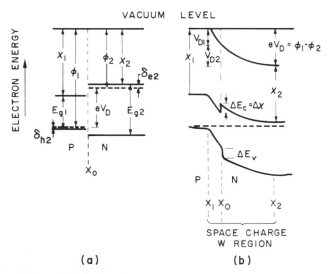

(a)   (b)

FIG. 2.3.1   Model of the ideal anisotype heterojunction, adapted from Anderson [12]. The materials are shown (a) first separated with the vacuum energy level providing the reference energy value, then (b) after they are joined forming a p–n heterojunction with an abrupt interface and no interfacial defects.

bottom of the conduction band into vacuum, while the *work function* is the energy needed to excite the electron from the Fermi level into vacuum. The quantities δ_{h1} and δ_{e2} denote the separation of the Fermi level from the respective band edges in the p- and n-type materials. The key feature of the band diagram after the materials are abruptly joined, Fig. 2.3.1b, is the formation of interfacial energy spikes or steps. The energy reference line is the vacuum level, and the spikes are a natural consequence of the abrupt interface where the Fermi level, in equilibrium with no applied bias, must be constant in the two materials. From the geometrical construction, the amount of band bending after the materials are joined is eV_D, where V_D is the built-in potential of the heterojunction given by

$$eV_D = \phi_1 - \phi_2 = (E_{g1} + \chi_1 - \delta_{h1}) - (\chi_2 + \delta_{e2}) = E_{g1} + \Delta\chi - \delta_{h1} - \delta_{e2}$$

$$(2.3.1)$$

The conduction band energy spike ΔE_c is determined by the electron affinity difference;

$$\Delta E_c = \chi_1 - \chi_2 = \Delta\chi \qquad (2.3.2)$$

The valence band step is

$$\Delta E_v = (\chi_2 + E_{g2}) - (\chi_1 + E_{g1}) = \Delta E_g - \Delta\chi \qquad (2.3.3)$$

Hence,

$$\Delta E_c + \Delta E_v = \Delta E_g \qquad (2.3.4)$$

Table 2.3.1 lists the electron affinity values of some semiconductors of interest here. These values are still uncertain in some cases, since only calculated

TABLE 2.3.1
Electron Affinity[a]

	E_g (eV)	χ (eV)	a_0 (Å)
GaAs	1.424	4.07	5.653
AlAs	2.16	2.62[b]	5.661
GaP	2.2	4.3	5.451
AlSb	1.65	3.65	6.135
GaSb	0.73	4.06	6.095
InAs	0.36	4.9	6.057
InSb	0.17	4.59	6.479
Ge	0.66	4.13	5.658
Si	1.11	4.01	5.431
ZnTe	2.26	3.5	6.103
CdTe	1.44	4.28	6.477
ZnSe	2.67	3.9	5.667
InP	4.38	4.35[b]	5.869
CdS	2.42	4.87[b]	4.137

[a] Data compiled by A. G. Milnes and D. L. Feucht, *Heterojunction and Metal-Semiconductor Junctions*. Academic Press, New York, 1972.
[b] Calculated, J. A. Van Vechten, *Phys. Rev.* **187**, 1007 (1969).

numbers are available (e.g., for AlAs). For alloys, an average variation with composition between the endpoints is assumed. In the hypothetical case where $\chi_1 = \chi_2$, the spike ΔE_c in the conduction band disappears, whereas in the valence band $\Delta E_v = \Delta E_g$. The potential barrier for electron flow from the high bandgap into the low bandgap p-type region then reduces to

$$eV_D = E_{g1} - (kT/e) \ln(N_{c1}/N)(kT/e)\ln(N_{v1}/P) \qquad (2.3.5)$$

This expression is identical to that for a p–n homojunction. However, note from Fig. 2.3.1 that the barrier for hole injection from the low bandgap p-region into the high bandgap n-region is increased by the difference in bandgap energy ΔE_g and is, therefore, higher than in a comparably doped p–n junction. Hence, it is evident that electron injection from the n-region into the is more readily achieved than the inverse process. Therefore, the heterojunction shown constitutes an efficient electron injector, as now discussed in greater detail.

The width of the depletion regions x_1 and x_2 in the two materials as a function of the applied voltage V is

$$x_1 = [2\varepsilon_1\varepsilon_2 N_D/eN_A(\varepsilon_1 N_A + \varepsilon_2 N_D)]^{1/2}(V_D - V)^{1/2} \qquad (2.3.6)$$
$$x_2 = [2\varepsilon_1\varepsilon_2 N_A/eN_D(\varepsilon_1 N_A + \varepsilon_2 N_D)]^{1/2}(V_D - V)^{1/2}$$

The capacitance–voltage relationship is

$$C(V) = [eN_A N_D\varepsilon_1\varepsilon_2/2(\varepsilon_1 N_A + \varepsilon_2 N_D)]^{1/2}(V_D - V)^{1/2} \qquad (2.3.7)$$

where we assume that the N_A acceptors and N_D donors in the uncompensated n-type and p-type regions are ionized: $N_A = P$ and $N_D = N$. Of course, Eq. (2.3.7) reduces to that for a p–n homojunction when $\varepsilon_1 = \varepsilon_2$. Note that the capacitance–voltage curves can be complicated in heterojunctions by interfacial states due to defects [9].

However, in principle, Eq. (2.3.7) allows a determination of V_D from a capacitance–voltage plot (C^{-2} vs V). Hence, using (2.3.1) a value of $\Delta\chi$ can be deduced if the bangap energy E_{g1} and other parameters needed to determine the Fermi level positions with respect to the band edges are known. Then, from (2.3.2) ΔE_c can be calculated, while (2.3.4) yields ΔE_v if ΔE_g is known.

The magnitude of the interfacial spikes is reduced with increasing composition grading at the heterojunction interface because of the reduction in the field magnitude due to the difference in electron affinity. Calculations of this effect for (AlGa)As/GaAs heterojunctions have been made by Cheung [13] and Womac and Rediker [14]. Figure 2.3.2 shows the schematic effect of grading on the interface of isotype and anisotype heterojunctions [13]. Note that isotype heterojunctions with graded interfaces approach ohmic contact behavior.

Figure 2.3.3 shows the effect of grading on the magnitude of the spike in the conduction band of n–n heterojunctions [14]. It is evident that the smaller the

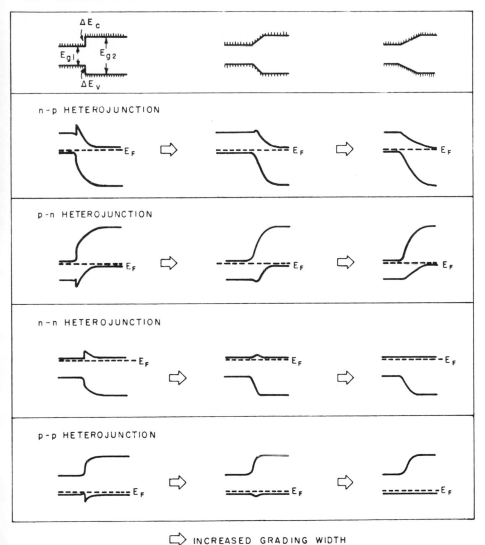

FIG. 2.3.2 Change in the magnitude of the interfacial energy structure of various heterojunctions with increasing bandgap grading in the interface region of the heterojunction [13].

carrier concentration on either side of the heterojunction, the wider the graded region has to be in order to reduce the spike height from 20 to $1kT$. Thus, despite some grading, lightly doped isotype heterojunctions should be expected to be more likely to exhibit nonohmic properties than heavily doped junctions.

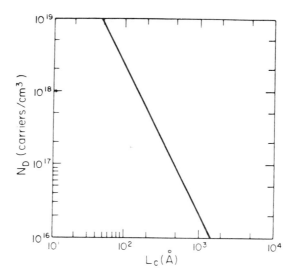

FIG. 2.3.3 Calculated relationship between the donor concentration of an isotype n–n heterojunction (symmetrically doped) and the critical grading width L_c needed to reduce the conduction band spike height ΔE_c from 20 to $1kT$. $N_{D_1} = N_{D_2}$; $\Delta\chi = 20\,kT$ [14].

2.3.3   Current–Voltage Characteristics

Under forward bias, the band diagram of the abrupt heterojunction (n–p or p–n) is changed as shown in Fig. 2.3.4. Because of the complexity introduced by the spikes, as well as the presence of interfacial defects due to lattice mismatch in many of the heterojunctions studied, there is commonly uncertainty concerning the various transport mechanisms. A review of the various models has been presented by Anderson [15] and by Milnes and Feucht [9]. These include thermal emission over the barrier, where $J \propto \exp(eV/kT)$, interfacial recombination, and tunneling through the spikes or via defect states at the interface. Since many heterojunctions are graded, and may not coincide precisely with the p–n interface (because of impurity interdiffusion during heterojunction synthesis), it is not surprising that the agreement between theory and experiment based on the various models has been spotty.

With regard to our present interest in diodes operating at relatively high bias values, it is appropriate to consider some approximations useful in device design. An expression for space charge region recombination current analogous to that for homojunctions (Section 2.2) has been proposed [13] for the forward biased graded interface heterojunction (i.e., neglecting the interfacial energy structure):

$$J_{\rm rec} = (e/2)(x_1 N_{i1}/\tau_1 + x_2 N_{i2}/\tau_2)\exp(eV/akT) \qquad (2.3.8)$$

where x_1 and x_2 are the widths of the space charge region on the two sides,

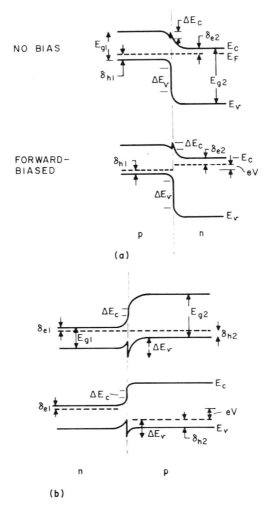

FIG. 2.3.4 Ideal (a) p–n and (b) n–p heterojunction with a no applied bias and with an applied voltage V which forward-biases the junction.

N_{i_1} and N_{i_2} are the intrinsic carrier concentrations, and τ_1 and τ_2 are the lifetimes as limited by the trap densities in the two segments of the space charge region. The value of a will vary between 1 and 2, depending on the trap ionization energies in the two sides of the boundary within the space charge region. If the trap energy is at midgap, then $a = 2$, as in the case of the homojunction.

Also for the graded composition heterojunction, a simple expression can be derived for the ratio of the electron to hole flow across the barrier (i.e., the injection efficiency), based on an extension of the p–n junction analysis of

Section 2.2 but taking into account the different electron and hole effective masses in the two semiconductors and the bandgap energy difference ΔE_g. For a p–n heterojunction, in which the conduction band spike height ΔE_c is neglected, the ratio of electron to hole current is

$$J_e/J_h = D_e N_{p1} L_h/D_h P_{n2} L_e \qquad (2.3.9)$$

Since $N_{p1} P_{p1} = N_{i1}^2$ and $N_{n2} P_{n2} = N_{i2}^2$, then

$$N_{i1}^2/N_{i2}^2 = (m_{c1}^* m_{v1}^*/m_{c2}^* m_{v2}^*)^{3/2} \exp(\Delta E_g/kT)$$

$$J_e/J_h = (D_e L_h N_{D2}/D_h L_e N_{A1})(m_{c1}^* m_{v1}^*/m_{c2}^* m_{v2}^*)^{3/2} \exp(\Delta E_g/kT) \qquad (2.3.10)$$

where we have assumed no difference in basic band structure of the two semiconductors.

The exponential term is the most important in (2.3.10) and for $\Delta E_g = 0.2$ eV, for example, the ratio of electron to hole flow is already in excess of 10^3 at room temperature. Therefore, doping level differences play a minor role in affecting the heterojunction injection efficiency as long as the barrier height is sufficiently large.

Many of the anisotype heterojunction studies with significant lattice mismatch show that tunneling processes (via defects, most probably) are important in the low to moderate current density range (<100 A/cm^2). The current–voltage characteristics are then of the familiar form

$$J = J_0 \exp(AV) \qquad (2.3.11)$$

where A is weakly temperature dependent, and J_0 depends in an ill defined way on the temperature, the defect density, the width of the space charge region, and the bandgap energies of the materials involved.

Turning our attention to the experimental impact of these theoretical considerations, we will consider the (AlGa)As/GaAs heterojunction, since it is the most important one for the devices discussed in this text. Consider an abrupt heterojunction based on the estimate of the electron affinity of GaAs and AlAs, (Table 2.3.1), and assuming a linear dependence of χ on Al fraction x, then $\Delta\chi = 1.45x$ eV for an Al$_x$Ga$_{1-x}$As/GaAs heterojunction. Thus, from (2.3.2) with $x = 0.5$, $\Delta E_c = 0.73$ eV. Since the bandgap energy difference (see Chapter 11) $\Delta E_g = 2 - 1.42 = 0.58$ eV, from (2.3.4) we estimate $\Delta E_v = 0.58 - 0.73 = -0.15$ eV.

As noted, the electron affinity value for AlAs is uncertain, but in any case a substantial conduction band step ΔE_c is expected which should be reflected in the transport properties of isotype heterojunctions by providing an impedance to the flow of electrons across the boundary (i.e. nonohmic behavior). Similarly, in anisotype heterojunctions, this spike represents a barrier to electron flow which can either be thermally overcome or, if the barrier is thin, allow tunneling to occur through it.

Detailed experiments to determine experimentally the magnitude of the spike by transport and photoelectric excitation experiments yielded negative results [13]. Isotype heterojunctions were found to be ohmic for the most part (even with light doping) and it was therefore suggested that grading effects at the heterojunction boundary reduced the magnitude of ΔE_c as discussed earlier [13,14].

With regard to isotype heterojunctions, no clear conclusions can be reached concerning the presence of the interfacial "structure." Capacitance–voltage measurements yield inconclusive estimates of $\Delta \chi$ (on the basis of V_D), whereas the current–voltage curves suggest thermal injection and space charge region recombination as dominant mechanisms. This is illustrated in Fig. 2.3.5 which shows the I–V curves of an $Al_{0.5}Ga_{0.5}As/GaAs$:Ge, n–p double-heterojunction diode between 20 and 100°C. The active region of the diode, 0.1 μm thick, was p-type (10^{18} cm^{-3}). The current density range is limited to a maximum of 150 A/cm^2, and the bending at the high end of the curves is believed due mainly to the resistance of the diode. The table inserted in Fig. 2.3.5

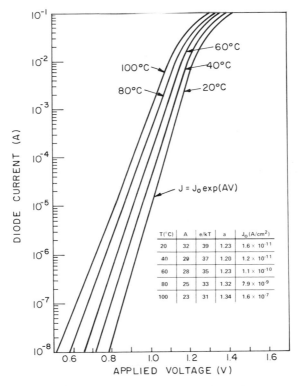

T(°C)	A	e/kT	a	J_0 (A/cm^2)
20	32	39	1.23	1.6×10^{-11}
40	29	37	1.20	1.2×10^{-11}
60	28	35	1.23	1.1×10^{-10}
80	25	33	1.32	7.9×10^{-9}
100	23	31	1.34	1.6×10^{-7}

FIG. 2.3.5 Current–voltage characteristics in forward bias of an $Al_{0.5}Ga_{0.5}As/GaAs$: Ge double-heterojunction diode having a recombination region width $d_3 = 0.1$ μm (6.45 × 10^{-4} cm^2). The curves are taken at various temperatures, and the bending at high bias involves diode series resistance effects. The inserted table shows the variation of A and J_0 with temperature (Kressel and Ettenberg, unpublished).

shows that A in Eq. (2.3.11) changes with temperature, and that the ratio $kT/Ae = a$ is between 1.23 and $\sim$1.34. This suggests that no single transport mechanism accounts for the observed behavior, but thermal injection appears dominant with probable contributions from recombination in the space charge region.

With regard to the practical applications of heterojunctions, we can conclude the following on the basis of the available studies of (AlGa) As devices:

1. Isotype heterojunctions can be used to provide improved contacting procedures, by reducing the bandgap energy at the surface, without any real concern for rectification at the heterojunction boundaries.

2. The current–voltage curves in forward bias look very similar to those of homojunction devices, except that high injection efficiency is obtained for either electrons or holes, as desired. Thus, the benefits of the use of heterojunctions are obtained with no detrimental factors due to interfacial energy structure which would impair the current–voltage characteristics.

3. The understanding of heterojunctions is inadequate. Perhaps experiments conducted with molecular beam epitaxy (Chapter 9), which produces truly abrupt junctions, will help elucidate the properties of the interface in (AlGa)As heterojunctions. It is particularly important in such experiments to ensure that no dopant diffusion occurs beyond the metallurgical interface of the materials with dissimilar bandgap energies. It is very likely that such effects, in addition to grading of the compositions, make the analysis of the heterojunction properties difficult.

2.4   Light–Current Relationships in Spontaneous Emission

The quality of a nonlasing p–n junction is commonly judged by the linearity of the light output as a function of junction current. In the case of injection into a region with a radiative lifetime independent of the injected carrier concentration, for instance in the homojunction shown in Fig. 2.1.2a, the light output is a linear function of the current since each injected carrier is assumed to lead, via recombination with a hole, to the emission of a photon. However, in such a device, if nonradiative recombination occurs in the *space charge region* due to defects ($E_i \cong E_g/2$), the light output power P_θ will remain proportional to the carrier injection flow over the barrier, and thus vary with applied voltage:

$$P_\theta \propto \exp(eV/kT) \tag{2.4.1}$$

whereas the current will increase with voltage as $I \propto \exp(eV/2\,kT)$. Hence,

$$P_\theta^2 \propto I \tag{2.4.2}$$

The presence of tunneling currents, frequently nonradiative if defects are involved, also leads to a nonlinear P_θ vs. I behavior, and the power law will depend on the position of the defects in the space charge region.

Of course, even for injection, an internal quantum efficiency which increases with the density of injected carriers will also give rise to a nonlinear light output versus current curve. Since heterojunctions which contain misfit dislocations (see Section 9.4) are also likely to contain defects within the *bulk* regions of the device, as well as at the interfaces, complex nonlinear effects are expected which are not easily assigned to any one of these mechanisms.

For illustration of the observed light output versus current in a good quality (AlGa)As double-heterojunction laser we show in Fig. 2.4.1 the various regimes of P_θ vs. I. At very low currents, we find that $P_\theta^2 \propto I$, suggestive of nonradiative space charge region recombination. At higher currents we find $P_\theta \propto I$ (suggesting injection and recombination in a constant quantum efficiency region) until the lasing threshold is reached, at which point the light output increases steeply with current because of the improved external efficiency resulting from stimulated emission (Chapter 3). The inserted spectral

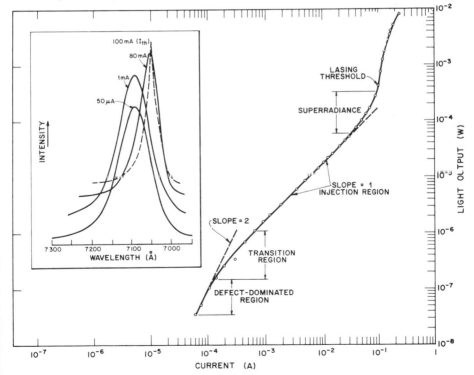

FIG. 2.4.1 Dependence of the power emission P_θ as a function of the diode current of an (AlGa)As double-heterojunction laser diode operating CW at 77 K. The inserted curves show the spectra at various current levels. The laser threshold current is 0.1 A.

emission curves in Fig. 2.4.1 show the line narrowing at the onset of lasing. Note that below the superradiant region starting at 80 mA, the spectral emission curves, including the very low current region, are invariant with respect to peak energy, indicative of no change in the radiative recombination process, i.e., probably carrier recombination *within* the active region rather than via centers in the space charge region.

To illustrate the role of defects on the light output versus diode current characteristics, we show two curves in Fig. 2.4.2 for double-heterojunction (InGa)P/GaAs diodes, one of which has a significantly smaller lattice parameter mismatch (hence lower defect density) than the other. Not only is the efficiency of the diode with the larger mismatch lower, but its slope of $\ln(P_\theta)$

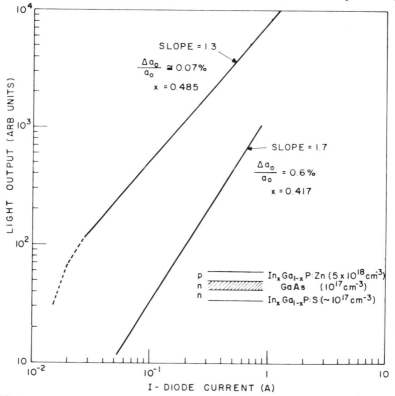

FIG. 2.4.2 Light output as a function of current of two double-heterojunction In_x $Ga_{1-x}P$/GaAs diodes at 300 K. In one diode, the lattice parameter mismatch is $\Delta a_0/a_0 = 0.07\%$, and in the other it is 0.6%. The resultant interfacial and bulk defect densities vary greatly and affect the curves. The efficiency scale is arbitrary, but the relationship between the two curves is scaled. The diode with the large lattice parameter mismatch not only has a lower overall efficiency, but its light output versus diode current curve is substantially more superlinear (slope = 1.7) than for the device with the smaller lattice mismatch (slope = 1.3) (C. J. Nuese, unpublished).

vs. $\ln(I)$ is steeper than for the diode containing fewer defects. It is probable that nonradiative space charge region recombination and tunneling contribute to the transport properties of such diodes, both of which contain a substantially higher dislocation density (and associated defects) than the (AlGa)As heterojunctions of Figs. 2.3.5 and 2.4.1.

Finally, we call attention to experimental studies of heavily doped (AlGa)As heterojunctions for which tunneling processes of a radiative nature were indicated. Alferov *et al.* [16] found that the polarization effects of the spontaneous radiation may be used to identify the nature of the shifting peaks. An analysis of shifting peaks in heterojunction structures has also been made by Constantinescu and Goldenblum [17] in which various models are compared.

2.5 Diode Frequency Response as Limited by Carrier Lifetime

The diffusion capacitance limits the frequency response of an LED, in the simple one dimensional model, because of storage of injected carriers in the active region of the device. In the following derivation linking the frequency response of the optical output from an LED to the minority carrier lifetime, we shall assume injection of electrons into a p-type region of width d_3. The electron density as a function of position x in the recombination region $(\Delta N)_x$ is determined by the equation of continuity together with boundary conditions at the p–n junction (or heterojunction) placed at $x = 0$, and at the other boundary placed at $x = d_3$. (We ignore the thin space charge region.) The frequency response of the diode $R(\omega)$ is the ratio of the photon flux $F_1(\omega)$ to the ac electron flux $(1/e)J_1(\omega)$ as a function of the modulating frequency ω. In effect, $R(\omega)$ represents the ratio of the optical power emitted at frequency ω for a given current pulse amplitude to the power which would be emitted under a very slow current change of the same magnitude.

Consider a one-dimensional case with electron injection into p-type material [18]. When injection ceases, the rate of change of the excess carrier density is

$$\frac{\partial(\Delta N)_x}{\partial t} = -R_{sp} + \frac{D_e}{e}\frac{\partial^2 J}{\partial x^2} \qquad (2.5.1)$$

where R_{sp} is the recombination rate. For simplicity we assume that the recombination is given by a single lifetime τ, and the following derivation is therefore only strictly true if bimolecular recombination is *not* dominant. (As discussed in Section 1.5, in the case of bimolecular recombination a single lifetime cannot be defined, although an average carrier lifetime is reasonable.) Then

$$R_{sp} = \frac{(\Delta N)_x}{\tau} \quad \text{and} \quad \frac{\partial(\Delta N)_x}{\partial t} = -\frac{(\Delta N)_x}{\tau} + \frac{D_e}{e}\frac{\partial^2 J}{\partial x^2} \qquad (2.5.2)$$

We assume in (2.5.1) that the current flow is due only to diffusion, neglecting drift fields in the recombination region. We also assume that the diode is not fully debiased, superimposing a time-dependent current component on a dc value.

We therefore divide the carriers into a *steady state* and *frequency-dependent* part which depend on position x within the recombination region,

$$(\Delta N)_x = (\Delta N)_{0x} + (\Delta N)_{1x}\, e^{j\omega t} \qquad (2.5.3)$$

Substituting into (2.5.1) and collecting terms, we obtain

$$D_e \frac{\partial^2 (\Delta N)_{0x}}{\partial x^2} - \frac{(\Delta N)_{0x}}{\tau} = 0 \qquad \text{(static)} \qquad (2.5.4a)$$

$$D_e \frac{\partial^2 (\Delta N)_{1x}}{\partial x^2} - \frac{(\Delta N)_{1x}(1 + j\omega \tau)}{\tau} = 0 \qquad \text{(frequency dependent)} \quad (2.5.4b)$$

Our concern is with the frequency dependent part. We can define a *complex* electron diffusion length analogous to the static value $L_e = (D_e \tau)^{1/2}$ as $L_e^* = [D_e \tau/(1 + j\omega \tau)]^{1/2}$, which makes (2.5.4a) and (2.5.4b) analogous in form:

$$\frac{\partial^2 (\Delta N)_{0x}}{\partial x^2} - \frac{(\Delta N)_{0x}}{L_e^2} = 0 \qquad (2.5.5a)$$

$$\frac{\partial^2 (\Delta N)_{1x}}{\partial x^2} - \frac{(\Delta N)_{1x}}{L_e^{*2}} = 0 \qquad (2.5.5b)$$

We now consider the boundary conditions. At the p–n junction or heterojunction, we require that only electrons cross the boundary, and the static and time-dependent carrier concentrations are $(\Delta N)_{00}$ and $(\Delta N)_{10}$. At the other boundary of the active region $x = d_3$, the surface recombination velocity S is given by

$$S = - \frac{D_e}{(\Delta N)_x} \frac{\partial (\Delta N)_x}{\partial x}\bigg|_{x=d_3}$$

For a completely reflecting boundary, $S = 0$, $S = \infty$ is an ohmic contact and $S = D_e/L_e$ is an interface which cannot be distinguished from a continuation of the bulk. The quantity SL_e/D_e, commonly used to characterize a heterojunction, is the ratio of the interfacial recombination velocity S and the bulk diffusion velocity $D_e/L_e = L_e/\tau$ (surface recombination velocity in heterojunction structures is discussed in Section 8.1). Subject to these boundary conditions, the solution to (2.5.3) is, with the notation $S^* = SL_e^*/D_e$,

$$(\Delta N)_{0x} = (\Delta N)_{00} \left[\frac{\cosh[(d_3 - x)/L_e] + (SL_e/D_e)\sinh[(d_3 - x)/L_e]}{\cosh(d_3/L_e) + (SL_e/D_e)\sinh(d_3/L_e)}\right] \quad (2.5.6a)$$

$$(\Delta N)_{1x} = (\Delta N)_{10} \left[\frac{\cosh[(d_3 - x)/L_e^*] + S^* \sinh[(d_3 - x)/L_e^*]}{\cosh(d_3/L_e^*) + S^* \sinh(d_3/L_e^*)}\right] \qquad (2.5.6b)$$

Equations (2.5.6) are of course equivalent for $\omega = 0$ when $L_e^* = L_e$.

To calculate the frequency-dependent photon flux $F_1(\omega)$ we integrate the recombination rate term of (2.5.2) over the width of the recombination region to obtain the photon density emitted/cm^2-s:

$$F_1(\omega) = \frac{1}{\tau} \int_0^{d_3} (\Delta N)_{1x} \, dx$$

$$F_1(\omega) = \frac{(\Delta N)_{10}}{\tau} \left[\frac{L_e^* \sinh(d_3/L_e^*) + S^* L_e^* \cosh(d_3/L_e^*) - S^* L_e^*}{\cosh(d_3/L_e^*) + S^* \sinh(d_3/L_e^*)} \right]$$

(2.5.7)

The frequency-dependent current flow across the p–n junction is determined by the concentration gradient of carriers at the junction:

$$J_1(\omega) = eD_e \left. \frac{\partial(\Delta N)_{1x}}{\partial x} \right|_{x=0}$$

$$J_1(\omega) = -eD_e(\Delta N)_{10} \left[\frac{1/L_e^* \sinh(d_3/L_e^*) + S^*/L_e^* \cosh(d_3/L_e^*)}{\cosh(d_3/L_e^*) + S^* \sinh(d_3/L_e^*)} \right] \quad (2.5.8)$$

The frequency response is then

$$R(\omega) = \frac{eF_1(\omega)}{J_1(\omega)} = \frac{1}{D_e \tau} \left| \frac{L_e^* \sinh(d_3/L_e^*) + S^* L_e^* \cosh(d_3/L_e^*) - S^* L_e^*}{1/L_e^* \sinh(d_3/L_e^*) + S/D_e \cosh(d_3/L_e^*)} \right|$$

(2.5.9)

Two important limiting cases simplify (2.5.9): For both the case of the ideal reflecting heterojunction barrier at $x = d_3$ where $S = 0$ as well as for a wide heterojunction spacing where $d_3 \gg L_e$, we obtain the simple result

$$R(\omega) = |L_e^*|^2/D_e\tau = |L_e^*|^2/L_e^2 = (1 + \omega^2\tau^2)^{-1/2} \qquad (2.5.10)$$

which is independent of the width of the recombination region. Good agreement with experiment is obtained as discussed in Chapter 14.

REFERENCES

1. R. A. Smith, *Semiconductors*. Cambridge Univ. Press, London and New York, 1959.
2. S. M. Sze and G. Gibbons, *Appl. Phys. Lett.* **8**, 111 (1966); a review of microplasma effects is given by H. Kressel, *RCA Rev.* **28**, 175 (1967).
3. T. L. Paoli and P. A. Barnes, *Appl. Phys. Lett.* **28**, 714 (1976).
4. C. T. Sah, R. N. Noyce, and W. Shockley, *Proc. IRE* **45**, 1228 (1957).
5. J. I. Pankove, *Phys. Rev. Lett.* **9**, 283 (1962).
6. H. C. Casey, Jr., and D. J. Silversmith, *J. Appl. Phys.* **40**, 241 (1969).
7. R. J. Archer, R. C. Leite, A. Yariv, S. P. S. Porto, and J. M. Whelan, *Phys. Rev. Lett.* **10**, 483 (1963).
8. H. Lawrence and R. M. Warner, *Bell Syst. Tech. J.* **39**, 389 (1960).
9. A. G. Milnes and D. L. Feucht, *Heterojunctions and Metal–Semiconductor Junctions*. Academic Press, New York, 1972.
10. B. L. Sharma and R. K. Purohit, *Semiconductor Heterojunctions*. Pergamon, Oxford, 1974.

11. L. J. van Ruyven, in *Annual Review of Materials Science*. Annual Reviews, Palo Alto, California, 1972.
12. R. L. Anderson, *Solid-State Electron.* **5**, 341 (1962).
13. D. T. Cheung, Thesis, Stanford Univ. Stanford, California (Tech. Rep. 5124–1; April 1975).
14. J. F. Womac and R. H. Rediker, *J. Appl. Phys.* **43**, 4129 (1972).
15. R. L. Anderson, *Proc. Int. Conf. Phys. Chem. Semicond. Heterojunctions Layer Struct.* Vol. II. Akademiai Kiado, Budapest, 1971.
16. Zh. I. Alferov, D. Z. Garbuzov, E. P. Morozov, and E. L. Portnoi, *Sov. Phys.-Semicond.* **3**, 885 (1970).
17. C. Constantinescu and A. Goldenblum, *Phys. Status Solidi (a)* **1**, 551 (1970).
18. The derivations in this section follow those of J. P. Wittke and M. D. Miller, RCA Laboratories, 1974, unpublished. A similar result was obtained by Y. S. Liu and D. A. Smith, *Proc. IEEE* **63**, 542 (1975).

BIBLIOGRAPHY

W. Shockley, *Electrons and Holes in Semiconductors*. Van Nostrand-Reinhold, Princeton, New Jersey, 1950.
A. G. Grove, *Physics and Technology of Semiconductor Devices*. Wiley, New York, 1967.
S. M. Sze, *Physics of Semiconductor Devices*. Wiley, New York, 1969.

Chapter 3

Stimulated Emission and Gain

3.1 Introduction

This chapter is devoted to a description of the optical gain process and of the conditions needed to obtain a useful lasing structure using a semiconductor. We begin with a description of the simplest configuration, which consists of a box containing isolated atoms having two energy levels, the ground state electron energy E_1 and the excited state energy E_2. (The choice of zero energy is arbitrary because we will be concerned only with the difference in energy $E_2 - E_1$). A detailed description of the stimulated emission process in this system is given in Section 3.2, and the extension to a semiconductor is treated in Section 3.3.

The atomic system consisting of the atoms of Fig. 3.1.1 is, in thermal equilibrium, mostly in the ground state, with very few atoms having the upper level populated. The distribution of atoms in the excited and in the ground state follows a Boltzmann distribution. Consider now a photon with energy $h\nu_{12} = E_2 - E_1$ incident on our box. It will typically be *absorbed* within a path length α^{-1}, giving rise to an additional electron in the upper level. This electron will fall back into the ground level after a mean time τ_{sp}, the spontaneous carrier lifetime.

The photon incident on the system can also produce a process inverse to the absorption process; i.e., it may induce the *downward* transition of an electron in the upper level into the lower level. In this case, which is called *stimulated emission*, the induced photon is emitted into the same mode as the incident photon. Since in thermal equilibrium the density of excited atoms is very small

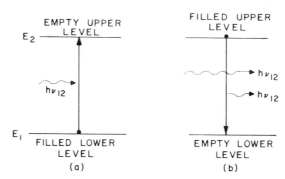

FIG. 3.1.1   Two-level atom showing (a) the photon absorption process and (b) the stimulated emission process.

the stimulated emission rate is likewise vanishingly small. Therefore a photon incident on the system will most likely be absorbed. It is only if we produce a condition of *population inversion*, in which the excited atom population exceeds the density of atoms in the ground state, that optical gain becomes possible.

These concepts are general but semiconductor lasers differ from gas or other types of solid state lasers in which the radiative transitions occur between discrete levels of spatially isolated excited atoms. The spontaneous radiation produced by transitions between the isolated atoms extends over a very narrow spectral range, whereas in semiconductors the active atoms are very closely packed, causing their energy levels to overlap into bands. For example, the high packing density of atoms in a semiconductor laser compared to only about 10^{10} cm^{-3} in a gas laser it advantageous because the semiconductor optical gain coefficient is therefore relatively high (50 cm^{-1} in typical laser diodes), thus allowing for much shorter optical cavities.

Population inversion in a semiconductor is illustrated in Fig. 3.1.2 which shows the electron energy as a function of the density of states in a pure semiconductor at $T = 0$ K. The electrons injected into the material fill the lower energy states of the conduction band to E_{Fc}, the quasi-Fermi level for electrons. Since an equal density of holes is generated to conserve charge neutrality in the material, the states in the valence band to E_{Fv} are empty of electrons. Photons with energy greater than E_g but less than $\Delta E_F = E_{Fc} - E_{Fc}$ cannot be absorbed because the conduction band states are occupied, but these photons can induce downward electron transitions from the filled conduction band states into the empty valence band states. With increasing temperature, a redistribution of the electrons and holes occurs, which smears out the sharply defined carrier distribution of Fig. 3.1.2. However, the basic condition for stimulated emission remains, in terms of the separation of the quasi-Fermi levels,

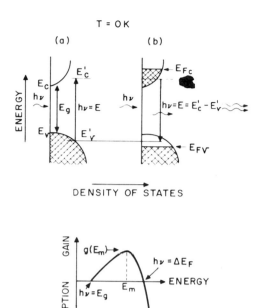

FIG. 3.1.2 Absorption and stimulated emission in a pure direct bandgap semiconductor at very low temperatures. (a) Absorption of incident photon with energy greater than the bandgap energy E_g. (b) Stimulated emission when the conduction band is filled to the quasi-Fermi level E_{Fc} and the valence band is empty to the quasi-Fermi level E_{Fc}. (c) Absorption or gain coefficient, depending on the wavelength of the incident photon, when the bands are populated as shown in (b). The gain coefficient is a maximum for a photon energy E_m. An incident photon with energy greater than the quasi-Fermi level separation ΔE_F is absorbed. (Bandgap contraction effects are neglected.)

$$E_{Fc} - E_{Fv} > h\nu \qquad (3.1.1)$$

The requirement for lasing in a given optical cavity is that the gain matches the optical losses at some photon energy within the spontaneous radiation spectrum. Typically this occurs near the peak of the spontaneous emission. However, as indicated in Section 3.5, matters are generally complicated by changes in the conduction and valence band states induced by a high injected carrier density which perturbs the density of states at the band edges.

In the case of highly doped semiconductors, the lasing transitions can involve impurities as initial or terminal states, and bandtail effects lead to substantial reductions in the observed photon energy because of the effective bandgap shrinkage discussed in Section 1.4. For instance, in GaAs doped with shallow ($\sim$30 meV) acceptors to $N_A > 10^{18}$ cm^{-3}, the radiative transitions at

300 K involve mostly the impurity states, and the lasing peak energy is therefore *below* the bandgap energy. In n-type GaAs, on the other hand, because
n-type dopants with ionization energies of 5–6 meV merge with the conduction band in the usual concentration range, the Fermi level shifts with doping
into the conduction band and the photon energy *exceeds* the bandgap energy.
If the material is compensated but p-type, the lasing photon energy is always
below the bandgap energy. With dopant variations, the lasing wavelength at
room temperature can be varied over an approximate range of 0.85–0.95 μm
in GaAs, going from heavy n-type to heavy compensated p-type but the device performance is usually best in the 0.88–0.91 μm range. A detailed discussion of dopant effects is given in Section 3.5.

   A unique feature of the laser diode, not present in other laser types, is the
ability to obtain stimulated emission by minority carrier injection using a
p–n junction or heterojunction. However, efficient operation of the laser diode
does require effective carrier and radiation confinement to the vicinity of the
junction. These subjects are covered subsequently.

   In the following discussion, we will frequently refer to modes, radiation
density, and photon density. To clarify the nomenclature, we briefly review
the relevant concepts.

   The number of electromagnetic modes with resonant frequencies between
ν and $\nu + d\nu$ can be calculated as follows in the case in which the enclosing
walls of the cavity are widely separated compared to the confined radiation
wavelength. The size of the enclosure is then arbitrary and the desired density
relationships are readily derived. Consider, then, a cubic enclosure with refractive index n and sides L. The propagation characteristic of a mode (i.e.,
wave with characteristics determined by boundary conditions) is described
by $\exp(i\mathbf{k} \cdot \mathbf{r})$, with $\mathbf{r} = x\hat{\mathbf{x}} + y\hat{\mathbf{y}} + z\hat{\mathbf{z}}$, and the wave vector $\mathbf{k}$ has the three
components

$$\mathbf{k}_x = (2\pi/L)q\hat{\mathbf{x}}, \qquad \mathbf{k}_y = (2\pi/L)s\hat{\mathbf{y}}, \qquad \mathbf{k}_z = (2\pi/L)m\hat{\mathbf{z}} \qquad (3.1.2a)$$

and

$$k^2 = k_x^2 + k_y^2 + k_z^2 = (2\pi/\lambda)^2 = (2\pi\nu n/c)^2 \qquad (3.1.2b)$$

A combination of integers q, s, and m describes a mode.

   From (3.1.2a) we can associate a volume $(2\pi/L)^3$ in $\mathbf{k}$ space with each mode.
The number of modes N_ν per unit volume which have wave vectors between
0 and a selected k (or frequency ν) value is obtained by dividing the volume of
the sphere with radius k in $\mathbf{k}$ space ($\tfrac{4}{3}\pi k^3$) by the volume per mode $(2\pi/L)^3$:

$$N_\nu = k^3 L^3/3\pi^2 = 8\pi^3\nu^3 n^3 L^3/3c^3\pi^2. \qquad (3.1.3)$$

Equation (3.1.3) includes a factor of 2 to account for the two possible polarizations per mode.

Since the volume of the enclosure is L^3, the number of modes per unit enclosure volume in the frequency range from 0 to ν is

$$N_\nu/V = 8\pi\nu^3 n^3/3c^3 = 8\pi n^3 E^3/3h^3 c^3 \quad (\text{cm}^{-3}) \tag{3.1.4}$$

For a very large mode density closely spaced in frequency (a result of our assumption of a large enclosure relative to the wavelength of the enclosed radiation), we can take the derivative of (3.1.4) and obtain the *mode density per unit frequency interval per unit volume* between ν and $\nu + d\nu$:

$$\tilde{n}_\nu = \frac{1}{V}\frac{dN_\nu}{d\nu} = \frac{8\pi\nu^2 n^3}{c^3} \quad (\text{s/cm}^3) \tag{3.1.5}$$

Equation (3.1.5) is the number of waves per unit volume which have different combinations of integers q, s, and m, and yet have a frequency in the interval between ν and $\nu + d\nu$.

The equivalent expression for the *mode density per unit wave energy* interval is

$$\tilde{n}_E = 8\pi n^3 E^2/c^3 h^3 \quad (\text{erg}^{-1}\,\text{cm}^{-3}) \tag{3.1.6}$$

The *energy density* (in the optical field) in an energy interval between E and $E + dE$ is

Energy density = (energy/photon) (mode density) (photons/mode)$_{\text{av. no.}}$
$$u_\nu = \quad (h\nu) \quad\quad (\tilde{n}_\nu) \quad\quad (\tilde{N})$$

$$= (h\nu)(\tilde{n}_\nu)(\tilde{N}) \quad (\text{ergs/cm}^3) \tag{3.1.7}$$

The field intensity for light velocity in the medium c/n is

$$I_\nu = (c/n)u_\nu \quad (\text{Watts/cm}^2) \tag{3.1.8}$$

Under conditions of *thermal equilibrium*, the average energy per mode is

$$\bar{E} = h\nu[1/2 + (\exp(h\nu/kT) - 1)^{-1}] \tag{3.1.9}$$

where

$$\tilde{N}_0 = [\exp(h\nu/kT) - 1]^{-1}$$

is the average photon density per mode.

The energy density of a "blackbody" between ν and $\nu + d\nu$ is then conventionally written

$$u_\nu = \bar{E}\tilde{n}_\nu = (8\pi hn^3\nu^3/c^3)[1/2 + (\exp(h\nu/kT) - 1)^{-1}] \tag{3.1.10}$$

The term 1/2 in the bracket results from an arbitrary choice of zero energy and has no physical significance. The blackbody radiation density at temperature T is then

$$u_\nu\,d\nu = (8\pi hn^3\nu^3/c^3)\,(\exp(h\nu/kT) - 1)^{-1}\,d\nu$$
$$u_E\,dE = (8\pi n^3 E^3/h^3 c^3)(\exp(E/kT) - 1)^{-1}\,dE \tag{3.1.11}$$

3.2   Optical Gain in the Two-Level Atomic System

In this section we review the semiclassical treatment of optical amplification in a two-level atomic system. The basic treatment conceived by Einstein, [1] provides the most useful introduction to the concepts needed to understand the operation of more complex lasing systems. In Section 3.3 we extend the treatment to a semiconductor in which additional complications are introduced by the density of states distribution.

We begin by analyzing the system in thermal equilibrium, since this provides the means for deriving the relationships among the key parameters. Since the coupling constants between the atoms and the field are independent of the nature of the field with which they interact, their values can be deduced from thermal equilibrium conditions and applied to monochromatic fields (with adjustment for line shape).

Consider, then, a system consisting of isolated atoms in an enclosure. The distribution of the atoms between the excited state in which there is an electron in level 2 with energy E_2, and atoms in which the electron is in the ground state 1 with energy E_1, is described by the Boltzmann statistics

$$N_2/N_1 = (g_2/g_1) \exp[-(E_2 - E_1)/kT] \qquad (3.2.1)$$

where N_2 and N_1 represent the density of atoms in states 2 and 1, respectively, and g_1 and g_2 are the degeneracies of the levels.

An atom in the excited state can undergo an electron transition from level 2 to level 1 either *spontaneously* or in a process *stimulated* by the radiation field. In either case, energy $E_2 - E_1$ is released in the form of a photon $h\nu_{12}$. For the spontaneous transition, the spontaneous lifetime τ_{sp} is the average time that the atom stays in the excited state before the electron transition from 2 to 1 occurs *independent* of the radiation field. Therefore, the spontaneous transition rate (i.e., number of transitions per unit time per unit volume) is the product of the density of atoms in the excited state N_2 and $1/\tau_{sp}$.

The *stimulated downward* transition of an electron from level 2 to level 1 is proportional to a constant B_{21}, the radiation density at $E = h\nu_{12}$ given in thermal equilibrium by u_ν [Eq. (3.1.11)], and N_2. Therefore, the *total* transition rate from 2 to 1, which includes the spontaneous and stimulated process, is

$$R_{21} = N_2/\tau_{sp} + N_2 B_{21} u_\nu \qquad (3.2.2)$$

The radiation field can also stimulate an *upward* transition of an electron from the ground state 1 into the higher state (absorption). We define another constant B_{12} for this process and then obtain the upward transition rate

$$R_{12} = B_{12} N_1 u_\nu \qquad (3.2.3)$$

In thermal equilibrium, the upward and downward transition rates must be equal, maintaining the population ratio of atoms among ground and excited states according to the Boltzmann distribution. Therefore,

$$R_{21} = R_{12} \tag{3.2.4}$$

and using (3.1.11) for u_ν, we obtain

$$(8\pi h\nu_{12}^3/c^3)\,[\exp(h\nu_{12}/kT) - 1]^{-1} = (N_2/N_1 B_{12}\tau_{sp})\,[1 - B_{21}(N_2/N_1)]^{-1} \tag{3.2.5}$$

From (3.2.5), using (3.2.1) for N_2/N_1, we obtain the relationships

$$B_{12} = B_{21}(g_2/g_1), \qquad B_{21} = (c^3/(8\pi\tau_{sp}h\nu_{12}^3)) \quad (\text{cm}^3/\text{ergs-s}) \tag{3.2.6}$$

Equation (3.2.6) and the resultant relationships represent the only consistent solution to the problem of the atomic interaction with the radiation field valid under all conditions including thermal equilibrium. Therefore, while these relationships for the averaged coefficients were derived under conditions of thermal equilibrium and for isotropic radiation averaged over all polarizations, we are free to apply them when a deviation from thermal equilibrium is brought about by the incidence of a monochromatic radiation field (photon energy $h\nu_{12}$) on the atomic system because these coefficients are properties of the atom and not of the radiation field (as averaged). However, we must modify our analysis to take into account the fact that in the case of the *thermal* radiation field analysis, the field intensity changes only slowly with frequency. We therefore implicitly assumed that the field is constant over the narrow spectral response range of the atoms. In the case of the monochromatic field, on the other hand, the field intensity is by definition described by a delta function. As a result, we need to introduce a normalized atomic response function* $A(\nu_{12})$ of an assembly of atoms with resonance frequency ν_{12}. In the following, we will assume that the stimulated transition rates associated with each frequency component are additive, and the expressions (3.2.2) and (3.2.3) for R_{21} and R_{12} in the presence of the monochromatic field can be modified by multiplication by the response function.

Our next task is to compute the change in intensity of the monochromatic field as it traverses the system in a given direction. The intensity of the field (W/cm^2) is given by

$$I_\nu = \tilde{n}_\nu \tilde{N}(h\nu_{12})c \tag{3.2.7}$$

---

* Response functions for the general case are discussed in detail in standard texts on quantum electronics (see the Bibliography). Spectral broadening is conventionally divided into two types. The term *homogeneous broadening* is applied to the assembly of indistinguishable atoms all having the same center frequency and assumed to share a common environment. The term *inhomogeneous broadening* is used for an assembly of atoms having differing resonant frequencies (e.g., due to local variations in their environment). The overall inhomogeneous line width results from the summation of the statistical distribution of resonant frequencies and individual line widths.

where $\tilde{n}_\nu \tilde{N}$ is the photon density.

The interaction of this field with atoms produces a *net* stimulated transition rate (upward minus downward) which is proportional to the *energy density* $\tilde{n}_\nu \tilde{N} h\nu_{12}$ in the field. Therefore, the *net* rate of stimulated transitions is given by $(\tilde{N}\tilde{n}_\nu)(h\nu_{12})A(\nu_{12})[B_{21}N_2 - B_{12}N_1]$. Since each stimulated transition involves a photon of energy $h\nu_{12}$ either emitted or absorbed, the power change per unit volume (or the rate of change of the field intensity per centimeter) is

$$dI_\nu/dz = (\tilde{N}\tilde{n}_\nu)(h\nu_{12})A(\nu_{12})[B_{21}N_2 - B_{12}N_1](h\nu_{12})$$
$$= (I_\nu/c)A(\nu_{12})[B_{21}N_2 - B_{12}N_1](h\nu_{12}) \qquad (3.2.8)$$

Using our previously derived values for B_{21} and B_{12} [Eq. (3.2.6)], we obtain the desired gain coefficient $g(\nu_{12})$, or absorption coefficient $\alpha(\nu_{12})$ which are the central quantities we need to understand optical gain:

$$\left.\begin{matrix} g(\nu_{12}) \\ \alpha(\nu_{12}) \end{matrix}\right\} = \frac{1}{I_\nu}\frac{dI_\nu}{dz} = \frac{c^2 A(\nu_{12})}{8\pi\tau_{sp}\nu_{12}^2}\left[N_2 - \frac{g_2}{g_1}N_1\right] \qquad (3.2.9)$$

This key equation defines the condition for optical amplification in terms of the density of excited atoms relative to the density in the ground state. If $N_2 > (g_2/g_1)N_1$, then the gain coefficient at the frequency ν_{12} is $g(\nu_{12})$, and the radiation intensity *grows* exponentially with distance traversed

$$I_\nu \propto \exp[g(\nu_{12})z] \qquad (3.2.10)$$

if no optical losses are present, and no reduction of the gain occurs. On the other hand, if the density of excited atoms is relatively low, $N_2 < (g_2/g_1)N_1$, then the radiation is absorbed and it *decreases* exponentially with distance,

$$I_\nu \propto \exp[-\alpha(\nu_{12})z] \qquad (3.2.11)$$

Because in thermal equilibrium N_2 is always negligible compared to N_1 absorption is the normal state of affairs. The production of the high density of excited atoms may be accomplished in gases by an ionization process. In insulating solids, it may be produced by the use of intense external light sources with strongly absorbed radiation, as a result of which a high density of atoms can have electrons occupying the higher energy levels. In semiconductors, excess carriers may be injected at suitable junctions.

3.3 Optical Gain in a Direct Bandgap Semiconductor

The preceding review of the simple two-level atomic system was intended to provide an introductory treatment of the gain processes and the basic requirements which have to be satisfied. In this section we turn our attention to the more complex situation of a semiconductor in which the two-energy-level concept remains, but in which these energy levels (the conduction and valence band states) are distributed over an energy range described by density of states functions. In addition, conservation of momentum requirements must be considered, and the occupancy of the states is now described by the Fermi–Dirac statistics rather than the Boltzmann equation used in the simple two-level model.

We begin by discussing, with the aid of Fig. 3.1.2, a semiconductor with the simplest density of states distribution, the parabolic one. The quasi-Fermi level for electrons is at E_{Fc}, and the hole quasi-Fermi level is at E_{Fv}. We define interaction parameters for upward and downward transitions: B_{cv}, B_{vc}, and C_{cv}, which involve, respectively, the *stimulated* conduction to valence transition, *stimulated* valence to conduction band transition, and the *spontaneous* conduction to valence band transition.* Our first tasks will be to obtain the interrelationship of these parameters in a manner analogous to the procedure used for the two-level atom case. We will use the single-electron approximation in which each electron–hole recombination process is unaffected by other transitions. It is assumed that equilibrium *within* each band is maintained by appropriate carrier redistribution in a time short compared to their lifetime.

To calculate the transition rates, we must take into account the occupancy of the conduction and valence band states. For this purpose we introduce the following nomenclature:

1. The term p_c denotes the probability that an electron is available in the conduction band at energy E_c'.

2. q_v denotes the probability that the state at E_v' is capable of capturing an electron (i.e., contains a hole).

Therefore, the *spontaneous* transition rate between two states at E_c' and E_v', with $E_c' - E_v' = E$, is

$$r_{sp}'(E) = C_{cv}p_cq_v \qquad (3.3.1)$$

$r_{st}^d(E)$, the *stimulated* downward transition rate (per photon and per unit energy interval) into a given mode with energy E, is proportional to the photon density in that mode $\tilde{N}$,

$$\tilde{N} r_{st}^d(E) = B_{cv}p_cq_v\tilde{N} \qquad (3.3.2)$$

The *upward stimulated transition rate* $r_{st}^u(E)$ (photon absorption) per incident photon is similarly

$$\tilde{N}r_{st}^u(E) = B_{vc}p_vq_c\tilde{N} \qquad (3.3.3)$$

where p_v denotes the probability that an appropriate state in the valence band contains an electron, and q_c denotes the probability that the required state in conduction band is empty.

From the Fermi–Dirac statistics, the occupancy factors are related as

* These parameters will depend on the states involved.

follows:

$$q_c = 1 - p_c, \qquad q_v = 1 - p_v \tag{3.3.4}$$

$$p_c = \{\exp[(E_c' - E_{Fc})/kT] + 1\}^{-1},$$
$$p_v = \{\exp[(E_v' - E_{Fv})/kT] + 1\}^{-1} \tag{3.3.5}$$

$$q_c/p_c = \exp[(E_c' - E_{Fc})/kT], \qquad q_v/p_v = \exp[(E_v' - E_{Fv})/kT]$$

$$(q_c/p_c)(p_v/q_v) = \exp\{[(E_c' - E_v')/kT] - [(E_{Fc} - E_{Fv})/kT]\} \tag{3.3.6}$$

To determine the relationship between the B coefficients, we use the detailed balance concept, as we did for the two-level atomic system, which consists of analyzing the semiconductor in thermal equilibrium. This will allow us to form the appropriate balance between upward and downward transitions using the average photon density per mode in thermal equilibrium. Hence,

$$r_{sp}'(E) + \tilde{N}_0 r_{st}^b(E) = \tilde{N}_0 r_{st}^u(E) \tag{3.3.7}$$

where $\tilde{N}_0 = [\exp(E/kT) - 1]^{-1}$ from (3.1.9). Therefore,

$$\tilde{N}_0 B_{cv} p_c q_v + C_{cv} p_c q_v = \tilde{N}_0 B_{vc} p_v q_c$$

$$\tilde{N}_0 = \frac{C_{cv}/B_{cv}}{(B_{vc}/B_{cv})(p_v q_c/p_c q_v) - 1} = \frac{1}{\exp(E/kT) - 1} \tag{3.3.8}$$

Since in thermal equilibrium $E_{Fc} - E_{Fv} = 0$,

$$\frac{q_c}{p_c}\frac{q_v}{p_v} = \exp\left(\frac{E_c' - E_v'}{kT}\right) = \exp\left(\frac{E}{kT}\right) \tag{3.3.9}$$

Hence,

$$\frac{C_{cv}/B_{cv}}{(B_{vc}/B_{cv})\exp(E/kT) - 1} = \frac{1}{\exp(E/kT) - 1} \tag{3.3.10}$$

from which it follows that $C_{cv} = B_{cv}$, $B_{vc} = B_{cv}$. Therefore, a single averaged coefficient $B(E)$, dependent on the energy separation of the states involved, can be used.

Having deduced these relationships, we are in a position to calculate the rate $r'(E)$ at which photons are emitted per unit volume and per unit solid angle and within an energy interval between E and $E + dE$, assuming an optically isotropic medium,

$$r'(E)\,dE = [r_{st}'(E) + \tilde{N} r_{st}'(E)]\,dE \tag{3.3.11}$$

$r_{st}'(E)$ is the net stimulated rate per incident photon per unit energy found by taking the difference between the downward stimulated rate $r_{st}^d(E)$ and the upward stimulated rate $r_{st}^u(E)$. Therefore, from (3.3.2) and (3.3.3),

$$\tilde{N} r_{st}'(E) = \tilde{N}[r_{st}^d(E) - r_{st}^u(E)] = B(E)\tilde{N}[p_c q_v - p_v q_c] \tag{3.3.12}$$

Since from (3.3.1), $r_{sp}'(E) = B(E)p_c q_v$,

$$r_{st}'(E) = r_{sp}'(E)[1 - (p_v q_c/p_c q_v)]$$

Using (3.3.6),

$$r'_{st}(E) = r'_{sp}(E)\{1 - \exp[(E - \Delta E_F)/kT]\} \qquad (3.3.13)$$

where $\Delta E_F = E_{Fc} - E_{Fv}$. It is evident from (3.3.13) that the condition for stimulated emission is that the photon energy $E < \Delta E_F$ [2]. We must therefore introduce a sufficient density of excess carriers into the semiconductor to produce this desired quasi-Fermi level separation. This requirement is analogous to the one deduced in Section 3.2 for the two-level atomic system that the population of excited atoms $N_2 > g_2 N_1/g_1$.

To account for all the possible transitions between the conduction and valence band states separated by energy E, we must sum over all the relevant states so separated,

$$r_{sp}(E) = \sum r'_{sp}(E) \qquad \text{and} \qquad r_{st}(E) = \sum r'_{st}(E) \qquad (3.3.14)$$

Hence, from (3.3.1) and (3.3.4),

$$r_{sp}(E) = \sum B(E)p_c q_v = \sum B(E)p_c(1 - p_v) \qquad (3.3.15)$$

$$r_{st}(E) = \sum B(E)[p_c q_v - p_v q_c] = \sum B(E)(p_c - p_v)$$

The value of $B(E)$ depends on band structure parameters. The expression obtained by Kane [3] when $B(E)$ is evaluated at $E = E_g$ is

$$B(E_g) = (8\pi^2 n e^2 E_g/m_0^2 h^2 c^3)|M|^2_{av} \qquad (3.3.16)$$

where the averaged matrix element $|M|^2_{av}$ for parabolic density of states is

$$|M|^2_{av} = (m_0 E_g/12)[(E_g + \Delta)/(E_g + 2/3\Delta)](m_0/m_c^* - 1) \qquad (3.3.17)$$

where m_0 is the free electron mass, and Δ is the spin–orbit coupling energy (0.33 eV in GaAs), with $m_c^* = 0.068\, m_0$,

$$|M|^2_{av} = 1.3\, m_0 E_g$$

At this point we have established the basic expressions needed to calculate the optical gain coefficient, although we must later return to the evaluation of the various terms. The gain (or absorption) coefficient is defined as follows: We denote $g(E)$ the optical gain coefficient at a photon energy E, and $\alpha(E)$ the band-to-band absorption coefficient

$$\left.\begin{matrix} g(E) \\ \alpha(E) \end{matrix}\right| = \frac{\text{power emitted (absorbed) per unit volume}}{\text{power crossing per unit area}}$$

Since the net stimulated transition rate summed over all states in unit energy interval separated by E is $r_{st}(E)\tilde{N}$ and the energy emitted (or absorbed) per transition is E, the power emitted per unit volume is $\tilde{N}Er_{st}(E)$. Consider power flow in a given direction. The power crossing a unit area is given by the product of the mode density $\tilde{n}_E$ between E and $E + dE$, the photon density per mode $\tilde{N}$, the energy per photon E, and the speed of light c/n. Hence,

$$\frac{g(E)}{\alpha(E)} \bigg| = \frac{E\tilde{N}r_{st}(E)}{(c/n)E\tilde{N}\tilde{n}_E} = \frac{r_{st}(E)}{(c/n)\tilde{n}_E} \tag{3.3.18}$$

Using (3.3.13) and (3.1.6),

$$\frac{g(E)}{\alpha(E)} \bigg| = \frac{c^2 h^3}{8\pi n^2 E^2} r_{sp}(E) \left[1 - \exp\left(\frac{E - \Delta E_F}{kT}\right) \right] \tag{3.3.19}$$

Equation (3.3.19) is similar to (3.2.9) derived for the two-level atom system and it shows that $g(E)$ is positive for incident photon energies $E < \Delta E_F$, but we must keep in mind that the bandgap energy E_g is the minimum photon energy under discussion, since a single photon with lower energy cannot stimulate band-to-band absorption.* Basically, (3.3.19) allows us to calculate the degree of population inversion (another way of viewing an increasing separation between the quasi-Fermi level which results from injected carriers) needed to obtain gain in a given cavity structure. As discussed in Section 3.4 the gain coefficient at threshold must equal the absorption coefficient due to various optical losses.

We now consider the various ways of calculating $r_{sp}(E)$, $r_{st}(E)$ [Eq. (3.3.13)] and hence the gain coefficient. The summation of the relevant states can be performed under two sets of assumptions: Either we consider that only "direct" transitions where **k** is conserved are allowed, or we sum over all states without concern for **k** conservation. The **k** conservation condition appears appropriate in relatively pure materials† where dopants are insignificant as initial or terminal states for the radiative transitions of interest. On the other hand the neglect of **k** conservation is justified in highly doped materials where momentum is conserved in electron–hole recombination because of elastic scattering by the impurities.

Consider first the **k** conservation assumption. The density of states distributions in the conduction and valence bands uniquely determine the density of initial and terminal states separated by the energy E. Lasher and Stern [4] used a "reduced" density of states distribution $\tilde{\rho}(E)$ (for one spin direction) of the form

$$\tilde{\rho}(E) = \frac{1}{(2\pi^2)} \frac{1}{k_{cv}^2} \left[\frac{\partial(E_c' - E_v')}{\partial k_{cv}} \right]_{E=E_c'-E_v'} \tag{3.3.20}$$

where k_{cv} is the k value corresponding to the vertical transition separating two states by energy E at which point the derivative in the brackets is evaluated. The reason for using the "reduced" density of states distrubution is that the conduction and valence band densities of states must be considered simultaneously in order to accommodate the **k** conservation requirement. The

---

* We ignore for the moment bandgap shrinkage.
† This assumption has been questioned under conditions of high injected carrier density (Section 3.5).

summation over the states separated by E [Eqs. (3.3.14) and (3.3.15)] can now be replaced by an expression including the density of states distribution:

$$r_{sp}(E) = B(E)\tilde{p}(E)\,p_c(1 - p_v), \qquad r_{st}(E) = B(E)\tilde{p}(E)\,(p_c - p_v) \quad (3.3.21)$$

We obtain the *total* spontaneous emission rate by integration over *all* energy values to include the states in the conduction and valence bands relevant to the luminescent processes:

$$R_{sp} = \int r_{sp}(E)\,dE \qquad (3.3.22)$$

Turning now to the case in which **k** is *not* conserved the choice of available states separated by energy E is increased relative to the **k** conservation assumption because all electrons and holes can now freely recombine independent of momentum. This amounts to a summation over the conduction and valence band states independently with appropriate occupation factors. The spontaneous recombination rate due to all electrons and holes separated by E is from (3.3.15)

$$r_{sp}(E) = \int B(E)\rho_c(E')\rho_v(E' - E)p_c[1 - p_v]\,dE' \qquad (3.3.23)$$

The total recombination rate is found from (3.3.22). With the electron and hole concentrations $N = N_0 + \Delta N$ and $P = P_0 + \Delta N$ we obtain the simple result

$$R_{sp} = B_r NP \qquad (3.3.24)$$

where B_r (cm^3/s) represents $B(E)$ evaluated at $E = E_g$.

Before proceeding with the evaluation of the gain coefficient we pause to relate (3.3.22), (3.3.24), and (3.3.19) in order to show how the recombination coefficient B_r can be calculated semiempirically on the basis of the experimental absorption coefficient [5]. Turning back to (3.3.19) we note that in thermal equilibrium (i.e., no carrier injection) the quasi-Fermi level separation $\Delta E_F = 0$. Hence, rewriting (3.3.19)

$$r^0_{sp}(E) = (8\pi n^2 E^2 \alpha(E)/c^2 h^3)[1 - \exp(E/kT)]^{-1} \qquad (3.3.25)$$

The total *thermal equilibrium* spontaneous recombination rate R^0_{sp} from (3.3.22) is

$$R^0_{sp} = \int_0^\infty r^0_{sp}(E)\,dE = \frac{8\pi n^2}{c^2 h^3} \int_0^\infty \frac{E^2 \alpha(E)\,dE}{[1 - \exp(E/kT)]} \qquad (3.3.26)$$

If we assume that independent summation of all the conduction and valence band states is appropriate (i.e., no selection rule) then

$$R^0_{sp} = B_r N_0 P_0 = B_r N_i^2 \qquad (3.3.27)$$

where N_0 and P_0 are majority and minority carriers in thermal equilibrium and N_i is the intrinsic carrier concentration. Hence,

$$B_r = R^0_{sp}/N_i^2 \qquad (3.3.28)$$

We see from (3.3.28) that B_r can be calculated by integrating the experimental $\alpha(E)$ curve using (3.3.26) with the intrinsic carrier concentration calculated from (1.3.5). Once B_r is calculated, the dependence of the spontaneous radiative lifetime on carrier concentration can be estimated as discussed in Section 1.5.* The B_r values in Table 1.5.1 were calculated by this procedure. It must be noted, however that uncertainty in the experimental absorption data can lead to large differences in the calculated B_r values as we had occasion to mention in Section 1.5.

Turning back to our laser formulation, the calculation of R_{sp} is now shown to be a key step in relating the diode current density to the gain coefficient which is the useful information needed to predict the laser threshold current density. The density of states chosen in the integration of (3.3.22) may be varied and the bandtail states included.

The relationship between the total spontaneous emission rate and the diode current density J is determined as follows. Assuming that the recombination occurs within a region d_3 wide, and unidirectional injection,

$$J = eR_{st}d_3 \qquad (3.3.29)$$

where we assume that all the injected carriers result in radiative recombination. It is conventional to compute the current density for $d_3 = 1 \ \mu m$, and the resultant quantity is denoted J_{nom}. Hence,

$$J_{nom} = eR_{sp} \qquad (3.3.30)$$

To calculate the gain coefficient, it is assumed that R_{sp} at threshold accounts for all the luminescent processes [4]. The neglect of stimulated recombination introduces a small error in the calculated J_{th} which, in view of other approximations, is not serious.

To relate J_{nom} to the gain coefficient $g(E)$, we determine R_{sp} for varying injected carrier densities from (3.3.22) using appropriate values of $r_{sp}(E)$ dependent on the choice of band structure and k selection requirement. Then, from (3.3.19), we determine the variation of the gain coefficient with photon energy for a given injected carrier level, i.e., quasi-Fermi level separation. The gain will peak at some energy E_m between E_g and ΔE_F. Thus, from (3.3.30) we have J_{nom} for a given injection level and from (3.3.19) we have determined the $g(E)$ curve. This procedure is repeated, producing a curve of the maximum gain coefficient $g(E_m)$ vs. J_{nom}. Henceforth, g will refer to $g(E_m)$, since this is the value of practical interest in determining the laser diode threshold.

It is intuitively evident that the curve of g vs. J_{nom} will show a zero value for low injection where $\Delta E_F = E_g$ in the case of a parabolic density of states function because of its sharply defined edge. However, if bandtail states are

* $N_0 P_0 = N_i^2$ is true only for nondegenerately doped material.

present (or a significant density of impurities), there will no longer be a sharp cutoff at E_g, since states exist which extend into the gap, and a more gradual g vs. J_{nom} curve will be obtained. Furthermore, bandgap contraction effects resulting from carrier injection will displace the curves downward in energy.

Figure 3.3.1 shows the result of several calculations [6] of the gain coefficient (or absorption coefficient) as a function of J_{nom} at 297 and 77 K. The GaAs is p-type, being doped with typical 0.03 eV shallow acceptors which are assumed to have merged with the valence band. With increasing injected carrier density (J_{nom}), the peak gain coefficient increases as does the energy E_m where the gain is maximum. This upward shift reflects the increasing separation of the quasi-Fermi levels, which, however, is partly compensated by the assumed contraction of the bandgap energy due to the injected carrier density (Section 3.5.1),

$$\Delta E_g = -1.42 \times 10^{-8}(P^{1/3} + N^{1/3}) \quad (eV) \tag{3.3.31}$$

where P and N represent the total hole and electron concentrations, respectively. Thus, for an initial hole concentration of $4 \times 10^{17} \, cm^{-3}$ and an injected pair density of $2 \times 10^{18} \, cm^{-3}$, the bandgap contraction is 37 meV. It is evident in Fig. 3.3.1 that because of the valence bandtail states and the assumed bandgap contraction, the gain coefficient can peak well below the nominal bandgap energy of 1.424 eV at 297 K and 1.51 eV at 77 K. Thus, the lasing photon energy will be below these bandgaps, as indeed experimentally observed (Section 3.5).

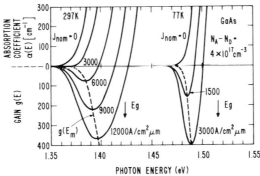

FIG. 3.3.1 Calculated gain or absorption coefficient at 297 and 77 K as a function of photon energy for several values of the nominal current density J_{nom}. The dashed line is the photon energy at which the gain coefficient is maximum. The sample is p-type, with a net hole concentration of $4 \times 10^{17} \, cm^{-3}$, and it is assumed that the acceptor states have merged with the valence band [6].

Stern [7] has calculated g vs. J_{nom} as a function of temperature for undoped GaAs which corresponds most closely to the situation in a pure material, or in a heterojunction laser diode with a lightly doped recombination region.

He took into account nonparabolicity and warping of the bands and includes the **k** selection rule. Figure 3.3.2a shows the g vs. J_{nom} plots at temperatures between 80 and 400 K.

In general, the calculated maximum gain coefficient versus J_{nom} is super-linear (above a minimum J_{nom}),

$$g \propto J_{nom}^b \tag{3.3.32}$$

where b increases with temperature from a value of ~1 at a very low temperature to ~3 at room temperature. In specific gain ranges, however, a linear relationship can sometimes be established between g and J_{nom}. For undoped GaAs material, the gain between 30 and 100 cm^{-1} at 300 K is approximated by the form shown in Fig. 3.3.2b,

$$g = \beta_s(J_{nom} - J_1) \tag{3.3.33}$$

where the constants β_s and J_1 vary with temperature as shown in Table 3.3.1. Also shown in this table is the injected carrier density needed for $g = 50$

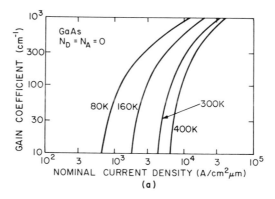

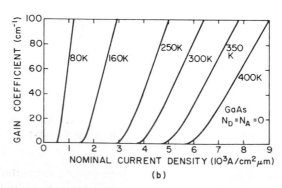

FIG. 3.3.2 (a) Plot of the gain coefficient g versus the nominal current density J_{nom} for undoped GaAs. (b) Linear plot for approximate fit in the gain range 30–100 cm^{-1} [7].

TABLE 3.3.1[a]

Temperature Dependence of Parameters Characterizing Undoped GaAs[b]

T (K)	B_s (cm/A)	J_1 (A/cm^2)	$J_{nom, 50}$ (A/cm^2)	$N = P$ (cm^{-3})	$B_{eff, 50}$ (cm^3/s)
80	0.16	900	600	2.7×10^{17}	7.8×10^{-10}
160	0.080	2300	1600	7.2×10^{17}	2.7×10^{-10}
250	0.057	4100	3200	1.4×10^{18}	1.3×10^{-10}
300	0.044	5300	4100	1.8×10^{18}	9.5×10^{-11}
350	0.039	6500	5200	2.3×20^{18}	7.5×10^{-11}
400	0.036	7600	6200	2.9×10^{18}	5.8×10^{-11}

[a] F. Stern, *IEEE J. Quantum Electron.* **9**, 290 (1973).

[b] β_s is a nominal gain coefficient for the gain range $30 < g < 100$ cm . The last three columns give the nominal current density, the concentration of electrons (and holes), and the effective recombination constant $B_{eff} = R_{sp}/NP$, all for $g = 50$ cm^{-1}.

cm^{-1} as well as the effective value of B_r. [Note that the B_r value used at 300 K is consistent with other data (Section 1.5).]

The choice of models for the states involved changes the numerical values of the g vs. J_{nom} curves. Calculations based on the Halperin and Lax [8] band-tail states approximation (for heavily doped materials) have been made by Stern [6, 7, 9] and Hwang [10] on the assumption that the material is so heavily doped that the impurity states have merged with the unperturbed band states. Then the **k** conservation condition is relaxed because of the elastic interaction between the carriers and the impurities. Figure 3.3.3 shows curves of g vs. J_{nom} for n-type GaAs compensated with acceptors [7] and p-type GaAs compensated with donors [9]. Figure 3.3.4 shows the temperature dependence of J_{nom}, for $g = 50$ cm^{-1}, for both n-type and p-type compensated GaAs. Finally, Fig. 3.3.5 shows the exponent b in (3.3.32) for $g = 30$–100 cm^{-1} as a function of temperature. The superlinearity increases with temperature as more of the states close to the unperturbed states in the valence and conduction bands participate in the radiative transitions.

The temperature dependence of the current density needed to maintain a given gain coefficient will evidently vary depending on the assumed material parameters. A relatively simple temperature dependence is calculated for undoped GaAs as shown in Fig. 3.3.6, where $J_{nom} \propto T^{1.4}$ (with $g = 50$ cm^{-1}). Contributing to the temperature dependence of J_{nom} is the change in the carrier distribution in the bands which is spread over a large energy range with increasing temperature. Thus, the quasi-Fermi level separation for a given injected carrier density is reduced. The temperature dependence of the threshold current density of laser diodes is discussed in detail in Chapter 8. Other factors besides the J_{nom} change contribute, including changes in the internal losses and carrier and optical confinement loss. However, other factors remaining constant, the J_{nom} vs. T dependence represents the lowest possible threshold current density change with temperature.

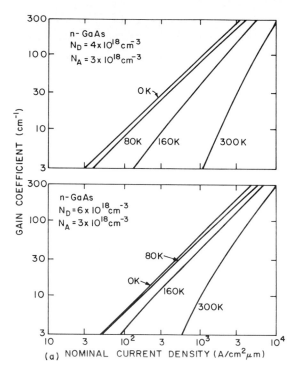

FIG. 3.3.3 Gain coefficient gversus nominal current density at 0,80,160, and 300 K for (a) compensated n-type GaAs with the dopant concentrations indicated [7].

In fact, Fig. 3.3.6 shows the variation of the threshold current density of a double-heterojunction (AlGa)As/GaAs laser with an active region which is relatively lightly doped (2×10^{16} electrons/cm^3). Its temperature dependence to 300 K is seen to follow the theoretically expected behavior quite closely.

We have so far not mentioned possible reductions in the gain coefficient as the intensity of the electromagnetic field is increased. This is not likely to be a problem near threshold, but only in the strong excitation lasing region. The models used for the gain coefficient calculations assume that the carrier population equilibrium is very rapidly reestablished following a stimulated recombination process. However, we can visualize a situation in which the field intensity (i.e., photon density) is so high that the carrier lifetime for stimulated recombination into a mode (which is inversely proportional to the photon number in a mode) becomes comparable to the time needed to replenish the relevant population in the conduction band. Gain saturation has been observed, in optically excited GaAs [6a] homogeneous samples, to occur initially with increasing pump rate on the *high energy side* of the curve of gain

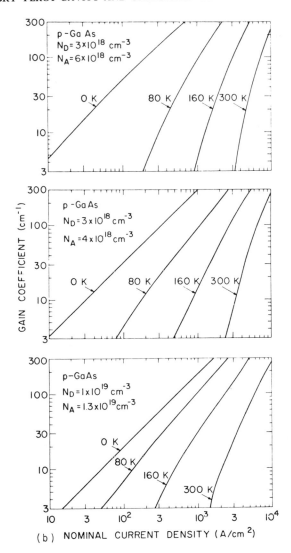

FIG. 3.3.3   Gain coefficient gversus nominal current density at 0, 80, 160, and 300 K for (b) ptype GaAs with the concentrations indicated [9].

versus photon energy (which is basically of the type shown in Fig. 3.1.2c or 3.3.1).

3.4   The Fabry–Perot Cavity and Threshold Condition

The commonly used resonator for semiconductor lasers is of the Fabry–Perot type in which a pair of flat, partially reflecting mirrors directed toward

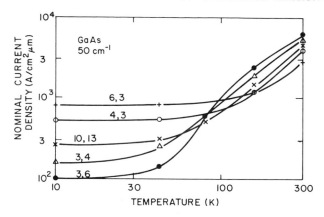

FIG. 3.3.4 Nominal current density required to reach a gain coefficient of 50 cm^{-1} for the two n-type samples and for three p-type samples versus temperature. The integers labeling each curve give the donor and acceptor concentrations, respectively, in units of 10^{18} cm^{-3} [7].

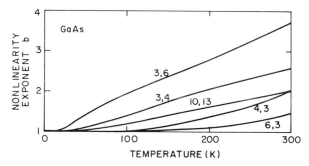

FIG. 3.3.5 Nonlinearity exponent b in the relation $g \propto J^b$ between gain and current. The values are for the range $30 < g < 100$ cm^{-1}. Labeling as for Fig. 3.3.4 [7].

each other enclose the cavity. The lateral dimensions are usually smaller than the mirror spacing. The actual formation of these mirrors occurs by cleaving the facets on parallel {110} planes, which are the natural cleavage planes of the zinc-blende materials. Therefore, the mirrors are only partially reflecting (unless deliberately coated). In the case of GaAs, the reflectivity of the GaAs–air interface is 0.32 (see Section 4.8) for the radiation emitted by that material. The topic of modes which the cavity can sustain is rather involved, and is discussed in Chapter 5. For the moment, we are concerned with the specific concepts needed to relate the gain calculation of the preceding section to the threshold current density.

The longitudinal dimension of the cavity L (i.e., the distance between the cleaved facets) is much larger than the lasing wavelength of about 1 μm, and the many modes which can therefore exist are denoted *longitudinal modes*

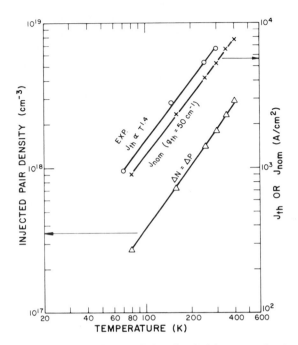

FIG. 3.3.6 Temperature dependence of the threshold current density of a double-heterojunction laser diode with a lightly doped GaAs ($N_0 = 2 \times 10^{16}$ cm^{-3}) recombination region of width 1.3 μm (0). Also shown are the theoretical dependence of the nominal current density J_{nom} needed to maintain a gain coefficient of 50 cm^{-1} in undoped GaAs (x), and the corresponding injected carrier pair density.

(see Chapter 5). Each of these modes has a slightly different wavelength resulting from the fact that the round trip over the cavity length L must produce a phase shift of 2π. Therefore, the number of *nodes q* between the mirrors of the cavity is

$$q\lambda_q/2n_q = L \qquad (3.4.1)$$

where n_q is the refractive index at the wavelength λ_q.

As evident from Section 3.3, the stimulated emission rate into a mode is proportional to the intensity of the radiation in that mode. The optical cavity provides the essential feedback mechanism for optical amplification of selected modes because in the repeated reflections between the two parallel and partially reflecting mirrors, part of the radiation associated with modes having the highest optical gain coefficient is retained and further amplified at each pass. Lasing occurs when the gain is sufficient to overcome the optical losses.

The condition for lasing in a cavity of length L with mirror reflectivities R_1

and R_2 is derived as follows. The gain coefficient at a photon energy E is $g(E)$. The material in the optical path is assumed to have an absorption coefficient $\bar{\alpha}(E)$ specified to be of a *nonresonant* nature (e.g., *intraband* electron transitions) in which the carriers generated by photon absorption do not contribute to the inverted population in the active region. (The subject is discussed in detail in Chapter 8.) Of course, *interband* transitions within the active region, which are the *inverse* of the stimulated downward transitions, are not included in $\bar{\alpha}(E)$.

Assuming that the gain coefficient does not saturate, the radiation intensity grows exponentially with distance z between the mirrors,

$$I_{\mathrm{E}}(z) = I_{\mathrm{E}}(0)\,\exp[(g(E) - \bar{\alpha}(E))z] \tag{3.4.2}$$

The lasing threshold condition is for the wave to make a round trip traversal ($z = 2L$) of the cavity without attenuation; i.e., the optical gain and loss are matched. Since a fraction of the incident radiation R_1 and R_2 is reflected at each incidence on the mirrors, the wave intensity at the end of the complete pass is

$$I_{\mathrm{E}}(2L) = I_{\mathrm{E}}(0)R_1 R_2\,\exp[2L(g(E) - \bar{\alpha}(E))] \tag{3.4.3}$$

At the lasing threshold, $I_E(2L) = I_E(0)$,

$$1 = R_1 R_2\,\exp[2L(g(E) - \bar{\alpha}(E))] \tag{3.4.4}$$

Therefore,

$$g(E) - \bar{\alpha}(E) = (2L)^{-1}\,\ln[(R_1 R_2)^{-1}]$$

At threshold, then

$$g(E) = g_{\mathrm{th}} = (2L)^{-1}\,\ln[(R_1 R_2)^{-1}] + \bar{\alpha}(E) \tag{3.4.5}$$

The mode that satisfies (3.4.5) reaches threshold first, and in principle all the subsequent energy fed into the device should promote the growth of that mode. Therefore, the spontaneous radiation intensity should cease to grow above threshold. In practice, one rarely finds a single longitudinal mode diode laser because of various phenomena which may limit the growth in intensity of any one mode and mechanisms which exist for power sharing among modes. A discussion is found in Appendix B. For the moment, we continue our discussion with a relationship between the gain coefficient and the threshold current density. For simplicity, we assume that the stimulated radiation is *fully* confined to the recombination region by a waveguide mechanism—deferring partial radiation confinement to Chapter 8—and furthermore, that the injected carriers are fully confined to that region. Then, from (3.4.5) we can relate J_{nom} to g, in the range where the linear equation (3.3. 33) is valid,

$$\beta_{\mathrm{s}}(J_{\mathrm{nom}} - J_1) = L^{-1}\,\ln R^{-1} + \bar{\alpha} \tag{3.4.6}$$

where $R = R_1 = R_2$. Then.

$$J_{\text{nom}} = \beta_s^{-1}(L^{-1} \ln R^{-1} + \bar{\alpha}) + J_1 \qquad (3.4.7)$$

At threshold, assuming that a fraction η_i of the electron–hole pair recombination is radiative, from the definition of J_{nom},

$$J_{\text{nom}} = \eta_i J_{\text{th}}/d_3 \qquad (3.4.8)$$

Therefore,

$$J_{\text{th}} = (d_3/\eta_i) [\beta_s^{-1}(L^{-1} \ln R^{-1} + \bar{\alpha}) + J_1] \qquad (3.4.9)$$

Using the reasonable values of $L = 500 \ \mu$m and $\bar{\alpha} = 10 \ \text{cm}^{-1}$, J_{th} is approximately 5000 A/cm^2 at 300 K for a 1-μm-wide recombination region using the β_s and J_1 values of Table 3.3.1. This is in good agreement with experiment as shown in Section 9.2 for double-heterojunction laser diodes at room temperature.

It is instructive to illustrate the laser diode behavior in the vicinity of threshold. As shown in Fig. 3.4.1a, the onset of threshold at $I \cong 250$ mA corresponds to a sharp increase in the power output with diode current. At 100 mA (much below threshold), only spontaneous radiation is emitted and the spectrum is broad, as shown in Fig. 3.4.1b. At 200 mA, as threshold is approached, the spectrum begins to narrow as portions of the spontaneous emission are amplified. At the same time, the emitted beam width narrows (particularly

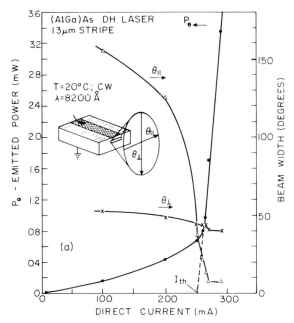

FIG. 3.4.1a

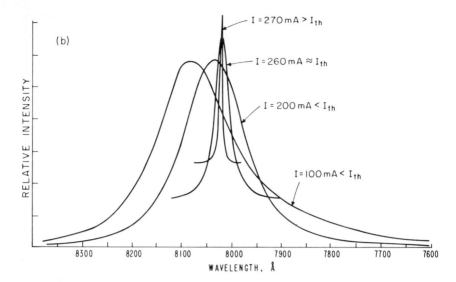

FIG. 3.4.1 Variation of key laser diode parameters at threshold. (a) Curve of the power emitted P_θ versus diode current, as well as the beam width at half-intensity in the direction perpendicular to the junction plane $\theta_\perp$ and parallel to the junction $\theta_\parallel$ as the device begins to lase. Note the strong narrowing of $\theta_\parallel$. The dashed line indicates the conventional method of estimating the threshold current from measurements of the power emission versus diode current. (b) Emission spectra of the diode below the threshold current, just at threshold, and slightly above it, indicating the narrowing of the emission when lasing is initiated.

in the plane of the junction) as an increasing fraction of the radiation emitted is stimulated. The "knee" portion of the power output versus current curve is the region of mixed operation (spontaneous plus stimulated radiation). Finally, for $I \leq 260$ mA, the spontaneous emission approaches a saturation value* and stimulated emission dominates. The beam is then fully narrowed as determined by the near-field distribution, mode content, and so on (Chapter 6). The threshold current density is conventionally defined on the basis of the extrapolation of the curve to $I_{th} = 250$ mA as shown in Fig. 3.4.1a. This agrees within 10% with the spectral and far-field narrowing criteria of full stimulated emission.

Although below threshold most of the spontaneously generated radiation is internally absorbed in the absorbing passive regions of the device, above threshold the directional nature of the stimulated radiation ensures that it is incident at normal or nearly normal incidence to the facets. As a result, the fraction of the radiation emitted is determined by the reflectivity of the facets for a given mode, and the absorption coefficient for that mode.

The number of photons emitted per radiative electron–hole pair recombina-

* The common observation is that the rate of increase of the spontaneous emission with current decreases (Appendix B).

tion above threshold is the *differential quantum efficiency* η_{ext}. Assuming that the gain coefficient at threshold and above remains fixed at the threshold value g_{th}, and that the absorption coefficient is $\bar{\alpha}$ [as in (3.4.5)], the fraction of the radiation emitted is [11]

$$\eta_{\text{ext}}/\eta_{\text{i}} = (g_{\text{th}} - \bar{\alpha})/g_{\text{th}} \tag{3.4.10}$$

Using (3.4.5), it follows from (3.4.10),

$$\eta_{\text{ext}}/\eta_{\text{i}} = (L^{-1} \ln R^{-1})/(\bar{\alpha} + L^{-1} \ln R^{-1}) \tag{3.4.11}$$

The value of η_{ext} is experimentally determined from the linear slope of power emitted P_θ versus the current I,

$$\eta_{\text{ext}} = P_\theta/[(I - I_{\text{th}})(E_g/e)] \tag{3.4.12}$$

where $h\nu \cong E_g$, P_θ is the power in watts, E_g is in electronvolts and I_{th} is the threshold current. With increasing current above I_{th}, a slope decrease due to junction heating is eventually observed. Therefore, η_{ext} is best determined in pulsed operation where the power dissipated is low.

Having completed the "proper" treatment of the gain problem in semiconductors, we now return to Section 3.2 and use Eq. (3.2.9) to derive a simple expression for the relationship between the gain coefficient and the threshold current density of a lser diode [12]. This approximate expression simply treats the semiconductor in terms of a two-level atomic system. The spontaneous emission line width is approximated by $A(h\nu_{12}) \cong (\Delta\nu)^{-1}$. We assume that the injected carrier density $N_2 \gg (g_1/g_2)N_1$. Then, the current density at threshold is

$$J_{\text{th}} \cong e(N_2/\tau_{\text{sp}})d_3 \tag{3.4.13}$$

Hence (under vacuum), with unity internal quantum efficiency and with full radiation confinement,

$$g_{\text{th}} = (J_{\text{th}}c^2(\Delta\nu)^{-1})/(8\pi ed_3\nu_{12}^2) \tag{3.4.14}$$

where ν_{12} is the center frequency of the emission. Using $g_{\text{th}} = \bar{\alpha} + L^{-1} \ln R^{-1}$, and the light speed in the medium c/n,

$$J_{\text{th}} = d_3[(8\pi e\nu_{12}^2(\Delta\nu)n^2)/c^2][\bar{\alpha} + L^{-1} \ln R^{-1}] \tag{3.4.15}$$

This expression is strictly correct only at very low temperatures since carrier distribution among the states of the bands is ignored. It is nevertheless instructive because it shows how J_{th} varies with the basic parameters. For example, a reduction in the bandgap energy (and hence ν_{12}) and a reduction in the spontaneous line width $\Delta\nu$ are beneficial in reducing the threshold current density, other factors being equal. Note also that (3.4.15) shows a linear relationship between the threshold current density and the gain coefficient, a result that is obtained at very low temperatures with the sophisticated calculations taking into account band parameters (Fig. 3.3.5).

In closing this section it is appropriate to review the three "lifetime" parameters relevant to the operation of the laser: the spontaneous (radiative) and stimulated carrier lifetimes and the photon lifetime.

We have extensively discussed the spontaneous lifetime and its relationship to band structure and carrier concentration in Chapter 1. The limiting value of the radiative lifetime is about 1 ns in GaAs at room temperature, a value reached with dopant concentrations on the order of 10^{19} cm^{-3}.

The *stimulated* carrier lifetime decreases with the optical density in the cavity, and values on the order of 10^{-11} s are suggested by delay data. In the experiments of Basov *et al.* [13] the delay between the application of a current pulse and the onset of stimulated light emission was measured, with the diode already "biased" to threshold. Figure 3.4.2 shows the dependence of the delay as a function of the ratio of the current through the diode to the threshold current. The reduction in the delay (which it related to the stimulated carrier lifetime) with increasing I/I_{th} is evident. At $17 = I/I_{th}$ the delay time is reduced to 6×10^{-11} s, although the delay time is already substantially below 1 ns just above threshold. These results are of prime importance in the ability to modulate a laser diode, as discussed further in Section 14.3.

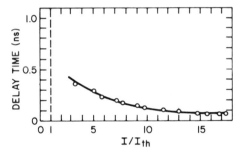

FIG. 3.4.2   Delay time between the current pulse and the onset of stimulated emission as a function of the ratio of the current I to the threshold current I_{th}. The decrease in the delay time is related to the reduction in the carrier lifetime with increasing photon density above threshold [1.3]

The third quantity is the *photon lifetime* τ_{ph} with which we will have occasion to be concerned when fluctuation phenomena are discussed in Chapter 17. The photon lifetime is the average time that the photon remains in the cavity prior to its loss by either absorption or emission through the facets. In a Fabry–Perot cavity it is given by

$$\tau_{ph}^{-1} = (c/n)[\bar{\alpha} + L^{-1} \ln R^{-1}] \tag{3.4.16}$$

where c is the light velocity and n the index of refraction in the medium, and the other quantities are those used earlier. With the quantity in brackets typically 50 cm^{-1}, $\tau_{ph} \approx 2 \times 10^{-12}$ s, which is the upper limit to the modulation capability of the device.

3.5 Laser Transitions

3.5.1 Pure Materials

Important lasing transitions in III–V compounds involve free carrier to impurity transitions, band-to-band transitions, and transitions involving bandtail states in heavily doped materials. At very low temperatures and low excitation levels, excitonic effects have also been observed in pure materials. The most important transitions in laser diodes at room temperature involve bandtail states (in very heavily doped, i.e., $\gg 10^{18}$ cm^{-3}, recombination regions) and band-to-band transitions (with modifications due to injection) in moderately and lightly doped material. The nature of the transition can frequently be estimated from the lasing photon energy relative to the bandgap energy and the spontaneous emission peak, and the temperature dependence of the lasing peak. In general, the energy of the first one or two modes observed at threshold is used as reference. However, in the study of diodes care is needed, as now discussed, to avoid erroneous interpretations arising from selective absorption.

Before discussing effects in laser diodes, we briefly review observations made on optically pumped platelet lasers at very low temperatures (~ 2 K) [14]. Figure 3.5.1 shows the *spontaneous* emission spectrum of a GaAs sample of exceptional purity with $N_A - N_D = 3 \times 10^{13}$ cm^{-3}. The highest energy lines (1.5122 and 1.5124 eV) are due to free exciton emission, whereas the other lines involve either excitons bound to impurities or donor-to-acceptor transitions.

The excitonic lines disappear with substantial injection because of free

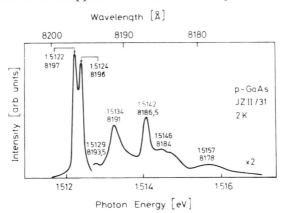

FIG. 3.5.1 Photoluminescence of a high purity ($N_A - N_D = 3 \times 10^{13}$ cm^{-3}) GaAs sample at 2 K showing the complex structure seen with low excitation levels. This structure is associated with various excitonic recombination processes and residual impurity-related recombination processes [14].

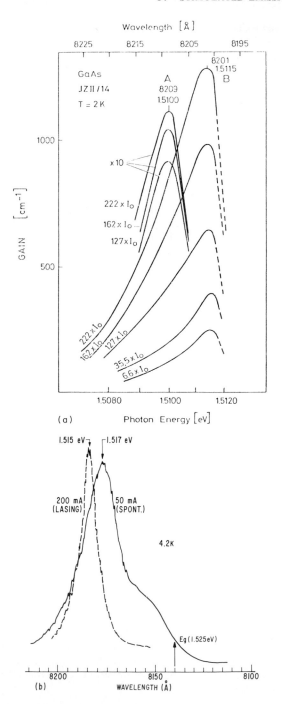

(a)

(b)

carrier screening (Section 1.7.2). Nevertheless, it is found that of the two processes producing gain at 2 K in optically pumped platelet lasers, one is believed to involve an excitonic effect, although its nature is still uncertain. The second, and dominant process, involves a band-to-band lasing transition with band modifications introduced by the high injected carrier density (see below). Figure 3.5.2a shows the gain versus photon energy of the two processes in stimulated emission. Line B is the dominant band-to-band process (which is the only one which remains at higher temperatures). Line A is the line believed associated with the excitonic process. Note that it saturates at a gain value of the order of only $\sim$100 cm^{-1}, whereas the maximum gain of line B is 1500 cm^{-1}. The fact that *both* lines are simultaneously seen it believed due to their origin from different regions below the surface of the sample. The highly excited region *near the surface* produces line B, whereas line A originates substantially *below* the surface, where the carrier density is lower.

In Section 3.3 we mentioned that the **k** conservation requirement appears a reasonable requirement in relatively pure materials. However, analysis of the gain versus E line shape obtained at 2 K from the high purity samples suggests that better agreement is obtained by assuming that **k** is *not* conserved in the stimulated emission transitions, possibly as a consequence of the presence of the "hot" free carrier plasma in the material [14]. It is possible that the same arguments would also limit the **k** conservation requirements in pure materials at high temperatures, and this clearly represents an area of uncertainty. Concerning the relationship between g and J_{nom}, we shall see in Chapter 8 that reasonable quantitative agreement between theory and experiment is obtained assuming **k** conservation for the threshold current density of double-heterojunction diodes having lightly doped recombination regions. However, this agreement may not be a sufficiently sensitive test of the model.

Turning our attention to the lasing properties of laser diodes at very low temperatures, we show in Fig. 3.5.2b the emission seen from a (AlGa)As/GaAs double-heterojunction laser diode in which the lightly doped (2×10^{16} cm^{-3}, n-type) recombination region actually contains a small Al concentration which increases the bandgap energy by 4 meV above that of GaAs [16]. At 50 mA, spontaneous emission is observed which peaks at 1.517 eV. At 200

FIG. 3.5.2   (a) Optical gain versus wavelength for a p-type sample ($P = 1 \times 10^{14}$ cm^{-3}, $\mu_h = 9000$ cm^2/V-s at 77 K) for different excitation levels. The sample was excited by a nitrogen laser; I_0 corresponds to a power density of 4.5 kW/cm^2. Band B is the band-to-band process, whereas A is believes excitonic in origin [14]. (b) Lasing and spontaneous emission from a double-heterojunction (AlGa)As laser diode with (essentially) GaAs in the recombination region ($N_0 = 2 \times 10^{16}$ cm^{-3} at 300 K). The nominal bandgap energy is at 1.525 eV because of the presence of a very small amount of Al in the recombination region. The lasing peak is seen to be 10 meV below E_g [15].

mA (just at the laser threshold), the emission is at 1.515 eV and no obvious structure which could be attributed to other than the dominant band-to-band lasing process is seen.

We now turn to the interesting observation that the lasing peak B in Fig. 3.5.2a and that in the diode of Fig. 3.5.2b are substantially below the nominal bandgap energy* despite the low doping level which precludes significant dopant-related bandtail states. In the case of line B, the energy of 1.512 is 9 meV below the GaAs bandgap energy of 1.521 eV. In the case of the diode, the lasing line at 1.515 is 10 meV below the bandgap energy. In fact, the displacement of the lasing photon energy below the nominal bandgap energy of the material is a general effect due to perturbations of the conduction and valence band edges by the high injected carrier density. Although the precise magnitude of the relevant effects is still uncertain, two factors have been postulated to explain the observation: a "rigid" contraction of the bandgap, proportional to the cube root of the free carrier density (i.e., the average carrier spacing) [17–19], and the formation of bandtail states due to the random fluctuations in the distribution of free carriers [20]. The estimated bandtail depth is about kT for typical carrier densities in lasing GaAs structures while Eq. (3.3.31) is one expression for estimating the effective rigid contraction. At very low temperatures, only the rigid band contraction is therefore present since kT is very small, which explains the 9–10 meV shift seen at 2 and 4.2 K [21]. Because of the increasing carrier density needed for lasing with increasing temperature, the separation between the bandgap energy and the lasing peak energy will increase. This is in fact observed. Figure 3.5.3 shows data obtained with GaAs (2×10^{16} cm^{-3}) laser diodes [16] and optically excited high purity GaAs platelet lasers [24]. At 300 K, the lasing peak is 24–30 meV below the nominal bandgap energy E_g.

It is important to note that this displacement below E_g is the sum of two factors which affect the lasing energy $h\nu_L$: (1) the bandgap shrinkage and induced bandtail formation which *depresses* $h\nu_L$; (2) filling of the conduction band with electrons and the valence band with holes, an effect which tends to *increase* $h\nu_L$. Therefore, the prediction of the lasing energy must take into account these two factors which depend on injected carrier density via the gain needed to reach threshold, i.e., J_{nom}. As shown in the calculated results of Fig. 3.5.1 (which considers both effects in a doped material), the energy at which the maximum gain is observed does shift upward with increasing J_{nom}. Therefore, if a laser diode is very "lossy" and requires a gain coefficient of, say, 300 cm^{-1} to reach threshold, then the separation between E_g and $h\nu_L$

---

* By "nominal bandgap energy" we mean the value determined in pure materials by conventional methods, such as absorption and electroreflectance, where the excess carrier density is negligible. The term "one electron" bandgap is also used.

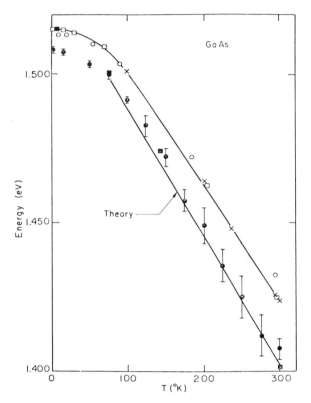

FIG. 3.5.3 Temperature dependence of the "one electron" or nominal (i.e., low injection level) bandgap energy of GaAs as determined by Camassel *et al.* [19] (x); Sell [22] (□); Sturge [23] (○). The experimentally determined variations of the lasing photon energy in "pure" GaAs are from the data of Kressel and Lockwood [15] (■); and Chinn *et al.* [24] (●). The theoretical lasing energy curve is calculated by Camassel *et al.* [19] on the basis of a rigid band contraction model proportional to the cube root of the free carrier concentration at threshold.

may be much less than the 24–30 meV value observed in Fig. 3.5.3 at room temperature for conditions where $g \lesssim 50$ cm^{-1}.

We now turn to some important problems in diode optical measurements due to selective absorption of the below-threshold radiation, which can complicate data analysis, and particularly the identification of the origin of laser transitions from a study of the spontaneous emission spectra.

Because of the high internal absorption coefficient of the spontaneous radiation, the emission viewed from the diode *edge* is distorted because the lower energy portion of the band is preferentially emitted from the diode. Thus, a comparison of the stimulated and spontaneous emission peaks is more often than not difficult to interpret because of "ghost" effects in which the spontaneous emission peaks reflect the selective internal absorption rather than fundamental processes. To minimize these effects, it is possible to construct heterojunction structures in which the surface layer is transparent to the internally emitted radiation as shown in Fig. 3.5.4 [16]. A small ohmic contact is provided, leaving much of the surface exposed. A structure of this type can lase if the facets are cleaved. Thus, it is possible to image the surface of the diode and obtain the spontaneous emission spectra, while the edge emission provides the position of the stimulated emission peak. Figure 3.5.5a shows the spontaneous emission spectra as viewed through the surface of the diode below threshold ($I = 5$ mA) and above threshold ($I = 6$ and 10 A, measured pulsed). The lasing peak is seen to be located on the *low* energy side of the spontaneous emission spectrum, as expected. The broadening of the spontaneous spectra at high currents is the combined result of the shift of the quasi-Fermi levels and of the formation of states within the bandgap as discussed earlier in regard to lightly doped GaAs.

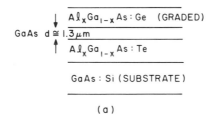

(a)

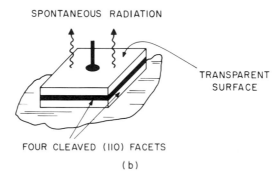

(b)

FIG. 3.5.4 (a) Schematic cross section of double-heterojunction laser diode showing active region with width of 1.3 μm. (b) Diode structure used for simultaneous study of spontaneous surface emission and lasing in internal reflection mode [16].

Figure 3.5.5b shows the spontaneous spectra under the same conditions as viewed below and above threshold from the *edge* of the diode. Note the structure seen which one could erroneously interpret as due to impurity levels.

Finally, Fig. 3.5.6 shows the spontaneous emission *intensity* as a function of the diode current. At threshold, the intensity begins to saturate because of the increased stimulated emission process, but full saturation is not observed. Nonuniform population inversion is one factor that can change the observed spontaneous emission above threshold.

3.5.2 Effect of Dopants on the Emission Wavelength

For a given semiconductor, the lasing wavelength shifts with the dopant type and concentration. For instance, the GaAs lasing wavelength at 300 K can be as short as 0.85 μm (1.46 eV) for highly Te-doped GaAs (3–4 $\times$ 10^{18} cm^{-3}), or as long as 0.95 μm (1.31 eV) with heavy Si doping (order 10^{19} cm^{-3}) [25]. It is clear from the preceding discussion that the emission wavelength, even for a single dopant concentration in the recombination region, can vary depending on the gain needed at threshold. However, order of magnitude differences in dopant concentration, particularly the use of heavily compensated material, produce significant differences in lasing wavelength. In this section we review first some results obtained which illustrate the role of dopants. These studies have been conducted using optically pumped platelet lasers which can be conveniently characterized without the complexity introduced by having to incorporate the recombination region in a diode structure.

Figure 3.5.7 shows the lasing peaks observed at 77 K in p-type GaAs doped with Ge or Cd [26]. The injected carrier pair concentration is estimated to be about 5 $\times$ 10^{17} cm^{-3} (see Fig. 3.3.5), a number to keep in mind as we observe the lasing transitions with increasing dopant concentrations. Note in Fig. 3.5.7 that for a background hole concentration below $\sim$4 $\times$ 10^{17} cm^{-3}, two lasing peaks are seen—the higher energy line at 1.495 eV (the band-to-band process reduced in energy by the bandgap contraction effect), and the lower energy line at 1.48 eV, which involves the shallow acceptors as terminal states. As the hole concentration of the sample is increased with doping, the band-to-band lasing energy is gradually decreased (reflecting the effect of the higher free carrier concentration) and the remaining lasing line becomes the one involving the acceptor states which merged with the valence band edge. The gradual reduction in the lasing energy above the mid—10^{18} cm^{-3} dopant range is the result of deepening bandtail states.

Note that at room temperature these effects involving *distinct* acceptor and

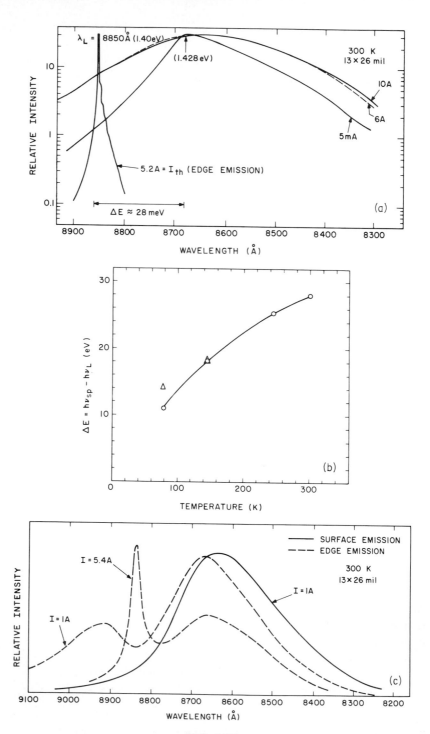

FIG. 3.5.5

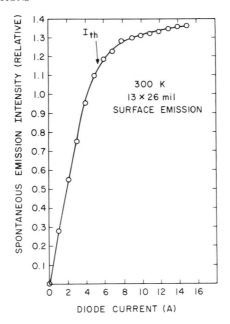

FIG. 3.5.6 Intensity of spontaneous emission as a function of current below and above lasing threshold as viewed through surface of diode lasing in internal reflection mode (diode of Fig. 3.5.4) [16].

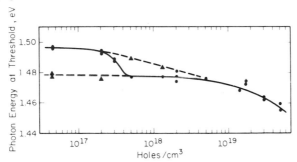

FIG. 3.5.7 Photon energy at threshold (77 K) of optically pumped p-type GaAs platelets as a function of the hole concentration: ● (solid curve), laser photon energy at threshold; ▲ (dashed curve), the photon energy of secondary transitions, which may or may not lase depending on pumping intensity and geometry [26].

FIG. 3.5.5 (a) Spontaneous spectra at 300 K below and above lasing threshold as viewed through surface of diode. Lasing spectrum was observed by viewing the edge of the diode. (b) Energy separation (o) between diode spontaneous emission band peak $h\nu_{sp}$ and lasing peak at threshold $h\nu_L$ between 77 and 300 K. Also shown for comparison are two data points (Δ) for electron-beam-pumped laser (EBP) made from GaAs similar to that in active region of heterojunction laser diode. (c) Same diode, but the emission is now viewed through the edge, with the surface covered with black wax. Note the additional structure seen, an effect due to selective absorption of the spontaneous radiation within the diode, particularly in the GaAs substrate. However, the lasing peak energy is undistorted [16].

band edge transitions are unlikely. The two major reasons for this difference are first, the much higher injected carrier density at threshold which would tend to produce a band contraction or bandtailing of a magnitude (20–30 meV) sufficient to effectively merge the band-to-band and the band-to-acceptor transitions; second, because of the higher injected carrier density, a small acceptor concentration (i.e., substantially below 2×10^{18} cm^{-3}) would have a negligible impact on the stimulated emission "traffic" since most of the holes would be in the valence band.

To return to the 77 K study of platelet lasers, Fig. 3.5.8 shows the lasing energy compared for n-type, p-type, and compensated (denoted p–n) GaAs [27]. The inserts in the figure illustrate the nature of the transitions. In the n-type material, the Fermi level is within the conduction band for initial electron concentrations in excess of about 10^{18} cm^{-3}, and therefore the lasing transitions are above the nominal bandgap energy E_g. As the electron concentration increases, the Fermi level shifts further into the conduction band, resulting in an increase in the lasing energy.

For p-type material, as already mentioned, the deepening of the valence band states associated with the acceptors results in lasing transitions which are below E_g and which decrease with increasing acceptor concentration.

In the case of the compensated samples, bandtail states are formed on both the conduction and valence bands which deepen with increasing doping. As a result, the lasing transitions are well below the bandgap energy, and the lasing energy is reduced with increasing dopant concentration.

The lasing wavelength of a diode at 77 K should follow the results obtained from optically excited samples. However, the radiation emitted from a diode in the *spontaneous* region, particularly in edge emission, is, as mentioned earlier, dependent on the degree of internal absorption as well as on the dopant concentration and temperature. In general, the emitted peak energy will decrease as the dopant concentration increases, whereas the spectral emission will broaden. Some examples for diodes with GaAs: Ge in the recombination region are presented in Section 14.6.2.

Striking effects with regard to shifting spontaneous peaks are observed in diodes having very highly doped and compensated recombination regions. The use of Si provides such compensated regions (Chapter 10) when liquid phase epitaxy is used to grow the recombination region. Even higher doping can be achieved with the simultaneous introduction of Si and Zn into the recombination region, a process which provides deep bandtail states when the total dopant concentration is greater than 10^{19} cm^{-3}. The effect of such high doping levels and simultaneous introduction of donors and acceptors is to reduce the lasing photon energy noticeably, as indeed expected from Fig. 3.5.8.

We consider for illustration [28] an (AlGa)As/GaAs heterojunction laser

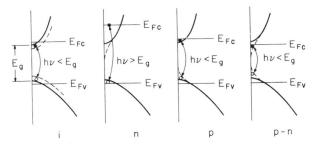

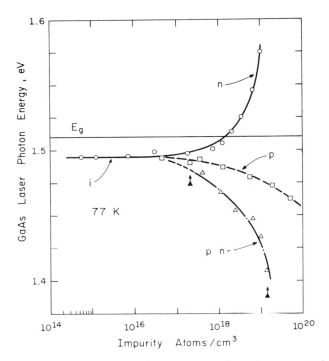

FIG. 3.5.8 Dependence of the laser photon energy on impurity concentration in an optically pumped GaAs laser at 77 K. The n-type samples are Se, Sn, or Te doped; the p-type samples are Cd or Zn doped. The compensated material is Zn–Sn, Sn–Te, or Sn–Se doped. The top diagrams illustrate the recombination processes appropriate to the various curves. Sketch i is appropriate to undoped or lightly doped material where the injected carrier pair density substantially exceeds the background concentration [27].

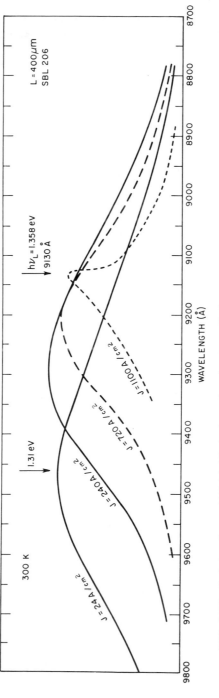

FIG. 3.5.9 Emission from (AlGa)As/GaAs heterojunction laser diodes (as viewed through the diode edge) with p-type recombination region closely compensated and highly doped ($>10^{19}$ cm^{-3}) with Si and Zn (grown by liquid phase epitaxy). Note the relatively large shifts of the spontaneous peak energy with current, an effect caused by the presence of deep bandtail states in the material of the recombination region [28].

diode in which the recombination was doped with Si and Zn to a level of at least 10^{19} cm^{-3}. The consequence of the band filling process, in which the injected carriers gradually fill the bandtail states in the recombination region, thus increasing the peak photon energy (Section 2.1), is evident from Fig. 3.5.9. Note the increase in the peak energy from 1.31 eV at 24 A/cm^2 to 1.35 eV at 720 A/cm^2. The lasing peak is at 1.358 eV at 300 K, a value 66 meV below the nominal GaAs bandgap energy of 1.424 eV. At 77 K the same diode lases at 1.43 eV ($E_g - 0.08$ eV), a value consistent with compensated GaAs (from Fig. 3.5.8) with a doping level of about 10^{19} cm^{-3}. At both temperatures, the bandtail states are clearly involved in reducing the lasing photon energy below E_g.

The *shape* of the diode *edge emission* spectrum of Fig. 3.5.9 is affected by three elements which contribute to its narrowing: (1) As the injected carrier density increases, more states with equivalent energy separation between the two bands become filled and hence contribute to the emission, leading to a sharpening of the spectrum. (2) As the spectrum shifts to higher energy more of the upper portion of the emission can be internally absorbed in the GaAs regions of the device. (3) As threshold is approached, the spectrum is selectively amplified following the gain dependence on photon energy outlined in Section 3.3.

It is evident from this that analysis of such data is complex since the specific contributions of the three factors outlined above are not easily distinguished. However, it is evident that recombination regions with high doping levels do exhibit behavior different from those with moderately (uncompensated) doped p-type regions. For example, in a DH laser with only 10^{18} Ge acceptors/cm^3 there is a small peak shift of the spontaneous emission spectrum with current at room temperature–a shift in the peak that does not exceed the range from 1.38 (at 21 A/cm^2) to 1.395 eV, which is the lasing photon energy.

REFERENCES

1. A. Einstein, *Phys. Z.* **18**, 121 (1917).
2. M. G. A. Bernard and G. Duraffourg, *Phys. Status Solidi* **1**, 659 (1961).
3. E. O. Kane, *J. Phys. Chem. Solids* **1**, 249 (1957).
4. G. Lasher and F. Stern, *Phys. Rev.* **133**, A553 (1964).
5. W. Van Roosbroeck and W. Shockley, *Phys. Rev.* **94**, 1558 (1954).
6. F. Stern, *J. Appl. Phys.* **42**, 5382 (1976).
6a. O. Hildebrand and E. Göbel, *Proc. Int. Conf. Phys. Semicond.*, 12th, p. 147. Stuttgart, 1974.
7. F. Stern, *IEEE J. Quantum Electron.* **9**, 290 (1973).
8. B. I. Halperin and M. Lax, *Phys. Rev.* **148**, 722 (1966).
9. F. Stern, *in Laser Handbook* (F. T. Arecchi and E. O. Schulz-DuBois, eds.). North-Holland Publ., Amsterdam, 1972.
10. C. J. Hwang, *Phys. Rev. B* **2**, 4117, 4126 (1971).

11. J. R. Biard, W. N. Carr, and B. S. Reed, *Trans. Met. Soc.* **230**, 286 (1964).
12. G. J. Lasher, *IBM J. Res. Rev.* **7**, 58 (1963).
13. N. G. Basov *et al.*, *Sov. Phys.-Solid State* **8**, 2254 (1967)
14. E. Göbel and M. H. Pilkuhn, *J. Phys. Suppl.* C-3, **35**, 194 (1974) [Earlier data are presented by E. Göbel, H. Herzog, and M. H. Pilkuhn, *Solid State Commun.* **13**, 719 (1973).]
15. H. Kressel and H. F. Lockwood, *Appl. Phys. Lett.* **20**, 175 (1972).
16. H. Kressel, H. F. Lockwood, F. H. Nicoll, and M. Ettenberg, *IEEE J. Quantum Electron.* **9**, 383 (1973).
17. P. A. Wolff, *Phys. Rev.* **126**, 405 (1962).
18. J. A. Rossi, D. L. Keune, N. Holonyak, Jr., P. D. Dapkus, and R. D. Burnham, *J. Appl. Phys.* **41**, 312 (1970).
19. J. Camassel, D. Auvergne, and H. Mathieu, *J. Appl. Phys.* **46**, 2684 (1975).
20. W. F. Brinkman and P. A. Lee, *Phys. Rev. Lett.* **31**, 237 (1973).
21. O. Hildebrand, B. O. Faltermeier, and M. H. Pilkuhn, *Solid State Commun.* **19**, 841 (1976).
22. D. D. Sell, *Proc. Int. Conf. Phys. Semicond.* 11th, *Warsaw* 1972.
23. M. D. Sturge, *Phys. Rev.* **127**, 768 (1962).
24. S. R. Chinn, J. A. Rossi, and C. M. Wolfe, *Appl. Phys. Lett.* **23** 599, (1973).
25. J. A. Rossi and J. J. Hsieh, *Appl. Phys. Lett.* **21**, 287 (1972).
26. J. A. Rossi, N. Holonyak, Jr., P. D. Dapkus, J. B. McNeely, and F. V. Williams, *Appl. Phys. Lett.* **15**, 109 (1969).
27. P. D. Dapkus, N. Holonyak, Jr., J. A. Rossi, F. V. Williams, and D. A. High, *J. Appl. Phys.* **40**, 3300 (1969).
28. H. Kressel, H. F. Lockwood, and F. Z. Hawrylo, *J. Appl. Phys.* **43**, 561 (1972).

BIBLIOGRAPHY

F. Stern, Stimulated emission in semiconductors, *in Semiconductors and Semimetals* (R. K. Willardson and A. C. Beer, eds.), Vol. 2. Academic Press, New York, 1966.

M. H. Pilkuhn, *Phys. Status Solidi* **25**, 9 (1967).

A. Yariv, *Quantum Electronics.* Wiley, New York, 1975.

M. Adams and P. Landsberg, *in GaAs Lasers* (C. H. Gooch, ed.), Wiley, New York, 1969.

H. Kressel, Semiconductor lasers, *in Lasers* (A. K. Levine and A. J. DeMaria, eds.), Vol. 3. Dekker, New York, 1971.

J. I. Pankove, *Optical Processes in Semiconductors.* Prentice-Hall, Englewood Cliffs, New Jersey, 1971 and Dover, New York, 1976.

H. Kressel, Semiconductor lasers: Devices; F. Stern, Semiconductor lasers: Theory, *in Laser Handbook* (F. T. Arecchi and E. O. Schulz-DuBois, eds.). North-Holland Publ., Amsterdam, 1972.

C. H. Gooch, *Injection Electroluminescent Devices.* Wiley, New York, 1973.

T. S. Moss, G. J. Burrell, and B. Ellis, *Semiconductor Optoelectronics.* Wiley, New York, 1973.

Chapter 4

Relevant Concepts in Electromagnetic Field Theory

4.1 Introduction

This chapter deals with some of the more fundamental aspects of classical electromagnetic theory, with the emphasis placed on those results applicable to wave phenomena in the optical frequency spectrum. Since wave phenomena can be derived from Maxwell's equations it is appropriate to consider some of the more fundamental aspects of these equations.

For the most general case, the electric and magnetic fields are generally written as a function of both spatial variables, x, y, z and time t as follows

$$\mathbf{e} = \mathbf{e}(x, y, z; t) \tag{4.1.1}$$

$$\mathbf{h} = \mathbf{h}(x, y, z; t) \tag{4.1.2}$$

Because mathematical tools such as Fourier analysis can be applied to an arbitrary time varying signal, we can assume without loss of generality the harmonic time varying signals

$$\mathbf{e} = \text{Re}[\mathbf{E}(x, y, z)e^{i\omega t}] \tag{4.1.3}$$

$$\mathbf{h} = \text{Re}[\mathbf{H}(x, y, z)e^{i\omega t}] \tag{4.1.4}$$

where Re means the real part of the term in brackets. In these expressions, the quantities $\mathbf{E}$ and $\mathbf{H}$ are complex functions. To simplify the field expressions, the Re designation is dropped, and the resulting field expressions become

$$\mathbf{e} = \mathbf{E}(x, y, z)e^{i\omega t} \tag{4.1.5}$$

$$\mathbf{h} = \mathbf{H}(x, y, z)e^{i\omega t} \tag{4.1.6}$$

117

The complex notation illustrated here is very useful in analysis; however, certain basic precautions should be taken with some algebraic manipulations such as multiplication of two complex quantities. This situation arises when energy and power are derived from products of the electric and magnetic fields. To discuss the complex number manipulations, consider the electric

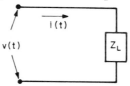

FIG. 4.1.1   Power considerations in an electric circuit. The instantaneous voltage and current are shown in the circuit.

circuit shown in Fig. 4.1.1. The time average power flowing to the load Z_L is given by [1]

$$\langle p(t) \rangle = \frac{1}{T} \int_0^T i(t)v(t) \, dt \tag{4.1.7}$$

where the brackets enclosing $p(t)$ indicate the time average. If the voltage and current are sinusoidal varying quantities, then

$$v(t) = V_0 \cos \omega t \tag{4.1.8a}$$

$$i(t) = I_0 \cos(\omega t + \phi) \tag{4.1.8b}$$

where ϕ is the phase angle between the current and voltage, and the power becomes

$$\langle p(t) \rangle = \tfrac{1}{2} (V_0 I_0) \cos \phi \tag{4.1.9}$$

On the other hand, if the voltage and current are written in the complex notation, then

$$v(t) = V_0 e^{i\omega t} \tag{4.1.10a}$$

$$i(t) = I_0 e^{i(\omega t + \phi)} \tag{4.1.10b}$$

In the complex notation, the time average power simply becomes

$$\langle p(t) \rangle = \tfrac{1}{2} \, \text{Re}[v(t) \, i^*(t)] \tag{4.1.11}$$

where $i^*(t)$ is the complex conjugate of $i(t)$:

$$i^*(t) = I_0 \exp[-i(\omega t + \phi)]$$

Note that operators such as time derivatives are simplified; for example, dv/dt from (4.1.8a) is

$$dv/dt = -\omega v_0 \sin \omega t \tag{4.1.12}$$

whereas the time derivative of (4.1.10a) is

$$dv/dt = i\omega v_0 e^{i\omega t} \tag{4.1.13}$$

It is seen that d/dt is replaced by $i\omega$. It is easy to show that the right-hand side of (4.1.12) is identical to the real part of right-hand side of (4.1.13)

4.2   Maxwell's Equations

Maxwell's equations, which can be deduced from fundamental concepts such as Faraday's law and the Ampere circuital theorem by including both conduction and displacement currents, form the basis for a majority of the material covered in this book. In the MKS system of units, the field equations become

$$\nabla \times \mathbf{e} = -\partial \mathbf{b}/\partial t \tag{4.2.1}$$

$$\nabla \times \mathbf{h} - \mathbf{j} + \partial \mathbf{d}/\partial t \tag{4.2.2}$$

$$\nabla \cdot \mathbf{d} = \rho \tag{4.2.3}$$

$$\nabla \cdot \mathbf{b} = 0 \tag{4.2.4}$$

The first and second equations are derived from Faraday's law and Ampere's circuital theorem, respectively. The quantities $\mathbf{e}$ and $\mathbf{h}$ are the electric and magnetic field intensities, respectively, and $\mathbf{b}$ and $\mathbf{d}$ are the corresponding magnetic and electric flux densities. The electromagnetic field sources are the current density $\mathbf{j}$ and the charge density ρ which are not independent since they are related through the continuity equation

$$\nabla \cdot \mathbf{j} + \partial \rho/\partial t = 0 \tag{4.2.5}$$

It is interesting to note that the continuity equation is not independent of Maxwell's equations and can be derived by taking the divergence of (4.2.2) and using (4.2.3).

Maxwell's equations in their present form are incomplete until the relations between the various field quantities such as $\mathbf{e}$, $\mathbf{d}$, $\mathbf{b}$, and $\mathbf{h}$ are related to the medium. The physics of the medium or material must be investigated to find the relation between the various quantities. (These relationships are generally referred to as the constitutive relations.) Before we discuss some of the more general constitutive relationships, it is advantageous to consider the field quantities under the assumption of harmonic time variation. For arbitrary time varying signals, the constitutive relationships are relatively complicated and involve the convolution of different functions.

When all field quantities vary as $e^{i\omega t}$, the field equations take on the forms

$$\nabla \times \mathbf{E} = -i\omega \mathbf{B} \tag{4.2.6}$$

$$\nabla \times \mathbf{H} = \mathbf{J} + i\omega\mathbf{D} \qquad (4.2.7)$$

$$\nabla \cdot \mathbf{D} = \rho \qquad (4.2.8)$$

$$\nabla \cdot \mathbf{B} = 0 \qquad (4.2.9)$$

$$\nabla \cdot \mathbf{J} + j\omega\rho = 0 \qquad (4.2.10)$$

Now for the situation in which the field quantities are small in amplitude so that there is a linear relation between various field quantities, the most general constitutive relations are given by [2]

$$\mathbf{D} = (\varepsilon)\mathbf{E} \qquad (4.2.11)$$

$$\mathbf{B} = (\mu)\mathbf{H} \qquad (4.2.12)$$

$$\mathbf{J} = (\sigma)\mathbf{E} \qquad (4.2.13)$$

The terms (ε), (μ), and (σ) are the permittivity, permeability, and conductivity tensors. When the tensor quantities can be written as a unit tensor times a scalar multiplier, the medium is said to be isotropic, otherwise it is anisotropic.

The relation (4.2.11) can be written in the form

$$\mathbf{D} = \varepsilon_0\mathbf{E} + \mathbf{P} \qquad (4.2.14)$$

where $\mathbf{P}$ is the polarization vector resulting from the applied electric field $\mathbf{E}$. This polarization is due to a modification of the charge distribution within the material; the individual atoms become small electric dipoles where the positive charge is being effectively separated from the negative portion.

4.3 Complex Dielectric Constant

The Maxwell equation (4.2.7) can be written in a form for a lossy or conducting medium which is similar to the case for a reactive medium. Instead of being real, the dielectric constant is complex [3]. This equivalent form is useful for obtaining solutions to various boundary value problems with lossy regions from those solutions obtained for reactive material. For harmonically time varying fields, the current density term $\mathbf{J}$ in (4.2.7) is replaced by $\sigma\mathbf{E}$ as

$$\nabla \times \mathbf{H} = (\sigma + i\omega\varepsilon)\mathbf{E} \qquad (4.3.1)$$

where σ is the wavelength-dependent conductivity. Equation (4.3.1) is rewritten as

$$\nabla \times \mathbf{H} = i\omega\varepsilon_0(\kappa - i\sigma/\omega\varepsilon_0)\mathbf{E} \qquad (4.3.2)$$

The relative dielectric constant $\kappa = \varepsilon/\varepsilon_0$. The relative *complex* dielectric constant $\bar{\kappa}$ is

$$\bar{\kappa} = \kappa - i(\sigma/\omega\varepsilon_0) \equiv \kappa' - i\kappa'' \qquad (4.3.3)$$

Note that when $\sigma > 0$, as is the case for a nonactive medium, the imaginary part of $\bar{\kappa}$ is negative. This arises because the time dependence $e^{+i\omega t}$ has a positive exponential argument. The complex dielectric constant $\bar{\varepsilon} = \varepsilon_0 \bar{\kappa}$, where $\varepsilon_0 \cong 10^{-9}/36\pi$ farads/m.

The optical properties of a semiconductor can be described by the complex dielectric constant. The nature of the electromagnetic wave propagation in a semiconductor is dependent on the optical constants of the material. The two optical constants totally responsible for the propagation characteristics in the material discussed here are (1) the index of refraction $n = \sqrt{\kappa'}$, and (2) the absorption constant α.* The two optical quantities n and α are more commonplace than the real and imaginary parts of the complex dielectric constant.

Consider a plane wave propagating in a semiconductor in the positive z direction as $\exp(i\omega t - \gamma z)$, where

$$\gamma = i(\omega/\bar{v}) \tag{4.3.4}$$

$$\bar{v} = (\mu\varepsilon)^{-1/2} \tag{4.3.5}$$

where $\bar{v}$ is the complex phase velocity. Substituting the expression for the complex dielectric constant into (4.3.5), the propagation constant becomes

$$\gamma = ik_0(\kappa' - i\kappa'')^{1/2} \tag{4.3.6}$$

where $k_0 = \omega(\mu_0\varepsilon_0)^{1/2}$, and it is assumed that $\mu = \mu_0$. Equation (4.3.6) can be written as

$$\gamma = ik_0\sqrt{\kappa'}[1 - i(\kappa''/\kappa')]^{1/2} \tag{4.3.7}$$

Assuming $\kappa' \gg \kappa''$, one obtains

$$\gamma \simeq ik_0[\sqrt{\kappa'} - i\kappa''/2\sqrt{\kappa'}] \tag{4.3.8}$$

If γ is written as

$$\gamma = \tfrac{1}{2}\alpha + i\beta = k_0(\tfrac{1}{2}A + iB) \tag{4.3.9}$$

then

$$B = \sqrt{\kappa'} \tag{4.3.10}$$

and

$$A = \kappa''/\sqrt{\kappa'} \tag{4.3.11}$$

Equation (4.3.5) can be written as

$$\bar{v} = \frac{1}{(\mu_0\varepsilon_0)^{-1/2}}\frac{1}{\bar{\kappa}^{-1/2}} = c/\sqrt{\bar{\kappa}} \tag{4.3.12}$$

where c is the velocity of light in free space. Using (4.3.12)

$$c/\bar{v} = \sqrt{\bar{\kappa}} \equiv \tilde{N} \equiv n - ik \tag{4.3.13}$$

* Generally, the magnetic permeability μ may be complex; however, when $\mu = \mu_0 = 4\pi \times 10^{-7}$ henrys/m, the material is said to be nonmagnetic.

where $\tilde{N}$ is the complex refractive index, n the index of refraction, and k the extinction coefficient. The real and imaginary parts of (4.3.13) give the relations

$$\kappa' = n^2 - k^2 \tag{4.3.14}$$

$$\kappa'' = 2nk \tag{4.3.15}$$

Let us write k and κ'' in terms of the power attenuation coefficient α and the free space wavelength λ_0. Using (4.3.11) and (4.3.15)

$$k = \sqrt{\kappa'}\,\alpha\lambda_0/4\pi n \tag{4.3.16}$$

$$\kappa'' = \sqrt{\kappa'}\,\alpha\lambda_0/2\pi \tag{4.3.17}$$

where $\lambda_0 = 2\pi/k_0$. Let us now examine the magnitude of k and κ'' for GaAs. Assuming $\kappa' \simeq 13$, $n \simeq 3.6$, $\lambda_0 \simeq 0.9$ μm, and $\alpha = 20$ cm^{-1}, the magnitudes of k and κ'' are of the order of 10^{-4} and 10^{-3}, respectively; hence $\kappa'' \ll \kappa'$ and $k \ll n$. Equations (4.3.14) and (4.3.15), considering k^2 as being negligible compared to n^2, are reduced to

$$\kappa' = n^2 \tag{4.3.18}$$

$$\kappa'' = n\alpha/k_0 \tag{4.3.19}$$

Then, from Eqs. (4.3.10), (4.3.11), and (4.3.15),

$$B = \sqrt{\kappa'} = n \tag{4.3.20}$$

and

$$A = 2k \tag{4.3.21}$$

The important result here is the relationship between the components of the complex dielectric constant and the familiar optical constants n and α. Consequently, if we know α and n, the complex dielectric constant can be determined. It should be noted that α represents the intensity or power attenuation whereas $\alpha/2$ is the field attenuation coefficient.

4.4 Boundary Conditions

The solution of Maxwell's equations in a given region of space is matched to the solution is another region of space by appropriately fitting the fields at the boundary. The material characteristics of the two regions are illustrated in Fig. 4.4.1 where each region has its corresponding material constants. For simplicity we will assume that the material constants are scalar quantities. The vector $\hat{\mathbf{n}}$, the unit vector which points from region 1 to region 2, is used here to write the boundary in a simplified form

$$\hat{\mathbf{n}} \cdot (\mathbf{B}_1 - \mathbf{B}_2) = 0 \tag{4.4.1}$$

$$\hat{\mathbf{n}} \cdot (\mathbf{D}_1 - \mathbf{D}_2) = \rho_s \tag{4.4.2}$$

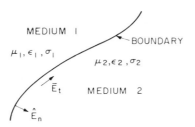

FIG. 4.4.1 The boundary between two different materials. The tangential component lies parallel to the interface whereas the normal vector component is perpendicular.

$$\hat{n} \times (\mathbf{E}_1 - \mathbf{E}_2) = 0 \qquad (4.4.3)$$

$$\hat{n} \times (\mathbf{H}_1 - \mathbf{H}_2) = \mathbf{J}_s \qquad (4.4.4)$$

where ρ_s is the surface charge density and $\mathbf{J}_s$ is the surface current density. We note here that (4.4.1) indicates that the normal component of the magnetic field is continuous across the boundary, and (4.4.2) indicates that the normal component of electric flux density $\mathbf{D}$ is discontinuous by an amount equivalent to the surface electric charge density. The tangential field components are governed by (4.4.3), which indicates that the tangential electric field is continuous across the boundary, and (4.4.4), indicating the tangential magnetic field intensity is discontinuous by an amount equivalent to the surface current density.

The condition (4.4.1) results from the fact that there are no magnetic changes, and condition (4.4.2) is derived from Gauss's law. On the other hand, condition (4.4.3) is due to the fact that the electric field is conservative, i.e., the integral of the electric field around a closed path is zero. Condition (4.4.4) is derived from Ampere's circuital theorem.

For the case in which the surface charge densities and surface current densities are nonexistent, the boundary conditions reduce to

$$B_{1_n} = B_{2_n} \qquad (4.4.5)$$

$$D_{1_n} = D_{2_n} \qquad (4.4.6)$$

$$E_{1_t} = E_{2_t} \qquad (4.4.7)$$

$$H_{1_t} = H_{2_t} \qquad (4.4.8)$$

where the subscripts n and t refer to the normal and transverse components, respectively.

4.5 Poynting's Theorem

The propagation or flow of electromagnetic energy can be determined from Maxwell's equations. Generally, the discussion of the Poynting theorem is associated with the conservation of energy: The total energy flowing into a given volume in space is equal to the energy dissipated within the volume. Assuming harmonic time variation Maxwell's equations can be written as

$$\mathbf{H}^* \cdot \nabla \times \mathbf{E} = -i\omega \mathbf{H}^* \cdot \mathbf{B} \tag{4.5.1}$$

$$\mathbf{E} \cdot \nabla \times \mathbf{H}^* = \mathbf{E} \cdot \mathbf{J}^* + i\omega \mathbf{E} \cdot \mathbf{D}^* \tag{4.5.2}$$

where $\mathbf{H}^*$ is the complex conjugate of $\mathbf{H}$. Subtracting (4.5.2) from (4.5.1) and using the vector identity

$$\nabla \cdot (\mathbf{E} \times \mathbf{H}^*) = \mathbf{H}^* \cdot \nabla \times \mathbf{E} - \mathbf{E} \cdot \nabla \times \mathbf{H}^*$$

we obtain

$$\nabla \cdot (\mathbf{E} \times \mathbf{H}^*) = -\mathbf{E} \cdot \mathbf{J}^* - i\omega(\mathbf{E} \cdot \mathbf{D}^* - \mathbf{H}^* \cdot \mathbf{B}) \tag{4.5.3}$$

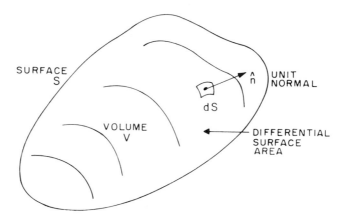

FIG. 4.5.1   Arbitrary volume V enclosed by the surface S.

Integrating this expression over an arbitrary volume, shown in Fig. 4.5.1, and applying the divergence theorem, we obtain

$$\iint_s \mathbf{E} \times \mathbf{H}^* \cdot \hat{\mathbf{n}} \, ds = -\iiint_v \mathbf{E} \cdot \mathbf{J}^* \, dv - i2\omega \iiint_v \left(\frac{\mathbf{E} \cdot \mathbf{D}^*}{2} - \frac{\mathbf{H}^* \cdot \mathbf{B}}{2} \right) dv \tag{4.5.4}$$

We now consider a physical intrepretation of the right-hand side of (4.5.4). If we assume $\mathbf{J} = \sigma\mathbf{E}$, $\mathbf{D} = \varepsilon\mathbf{E}$, $\mathbf{B} = \mu\mathbf{H}$ with σ, μ, ε being real, the quantity $\mathbf{E} \cdot \mathbf{J}^*$ represents the total ohmic losses within the volume and $(\mathbf{E} \cdot \mathbf{D}^*)/2$ and $(\mathbf{H}^* \cdot \mathbf{B})/2$ are the total electric and magnetic energies stored in the fields. Defining the Poynting vector

$$\mathbf{S} = \mathbf{E} \times \mathbf{H}^* \tag{4.5.5}$$

we obtain

$$\tfrac{1}{2} \operatorname{Re} \iint_s \mathbf{S} \cdot \mathbf{n} \, ds = \tfrac{1}{2} \iiint_v \mathbf{E} \cdot \mathbf{J}^* \, dv = -\text{total power dissipated in } V$$

and

$$\tfrac{1}{2} \, \text{Im} \iint_s \mathbf{S} \cdot \hat{\mathbf{n}} \, ds = \text{(difference of mean values of total magnetic and electric energy inside } V) \, \omega$$

Note that the unit normal is defined in the outward direction so that the real part of the normal component of the Poynting vector integrated over the surface gives negative power dissipated. This means that if $\mathbf{E} \times \mathbf{H}^*$ is directed inward, power is dissipated, i.e., there is a "sink" inside. On the other hand, if $\mathbf{E} \times \mathbf{H}^*$ is directed outward, power is generated inside, giving a "source."

Since $\mathbf{E}$ and $\mathbf{H}$ have dimensions of volts per meter and amperes per meter, $\mathbf{S}$ has dimensions of watts per square meter. From these results $\mathbf{S}$ is interpreted as a power density vector; the magnitude of $\mathbf{S}$ represents the total power crossing a unit surface whose normal is defined by the direction of $\mathbf{S}$. For example, if $\mathbf{E} = \hat{\mathbf{x}} \, E_x$ and $\mathbf{H} = \hat{\mathbf{y}} \, H_y$, the power in the wave is flowing in the positive z direction.

4.6   Vector Wave Equation

The equations defining the wave phenomena of the electromagnetic fields can be derived from the basic time-dependent Maxwell's equations. First we will derive the general wave equation for arbitrary time-dependent fields and then consider the special case of harmonically time varying fields.

Using the time-dependent Maxwell's equations we take the curl of (4.2.1)

$$\nabla \times (\nabla \times \mathbf{e}) = -\frac{\partial}{\partial t} (\nabla \times \mathbf{b}) \tag{4.6.1}$$

where the space and time derivatives have been interchanged. Since we are restricting our discussion to nonmagnetic materials $\mathbf{b} = \mu_0 \mathbf{h}$. Substituting (4.2.2) into (4.6.1) gives

$$\nabla \times (\nabla \times \mathbf{e}) = -\mu_0 \frac{\partial}{\partial t} \left(\mathbf{j} + \frac{\partial \mathbf{d}}{\partial t} \right) \tag{4.6.2}$$

Putting $\mathbf{j} = \sigma \mathbf{e}$ and $\mathbf{d} = \varepsilon \mathbf{e}$, this becomes

$$\nabla \times (\nabla \times \mathbf{e}) = -\mu_0 \sigma \frac{\partial \mathbf{e}}{\partial t} - \mu_0 \varepsilon \frac{\partial^2 \mathbf{e}}{\partial t^2} \tag{4.6.3}$$

The left-hand side of (4.6.3) can be simplified to

$$\nabla \times (\nabla \times \mathbf{e}) = \nabla(\nabla \cdot \mathbf{e}) - \nabla \cdot \nabla \mathbf{e}$$

in rectangular coordinated $\nabla \cdot \nabla \equiv \nabla^2$, the Laplacian. If the medium is free of charge, i.e., $\rho = 0$, then

$$\nabla \cdot \mathbf{d} = \nabla(\varepsilon \mathbf{e}) = 0 \tag{4.6.4}$$

For a homogeneous medium where the dielectric constant is independent of position one has $\nabla \cdot \mathbf{e} = 0$, whereas for an inhomogeneous medium

$$\nabla \cdot \mathbf{e} = -\mathbf{e} \cdot \frac{\nabla \varepsilon}{\varepsilon} \tag{4.6.5}$$

Equation (4.6.3) now reduces to

$$\nabla^2 \mathbf{e} + \nabla\left(\mathbf{e} \cdot \frac{\nabla \varepsilon}{\varepsilon}\right) = \mu_0 \varepsilon \frac{\partial^2 \mathbf{e}}{\partial t^2} + \mu_0 \sigma \frac{\partial \mathbf{e}}{\partial t} \tag{4.6.6}$$

the general wave equation. For the case of a homogeneous medium

$$\nabla^2 \mathbf{e} = \mu_0 \varepsilon \frac{\partial^2 \mathbf{e}}{\partial t^2} + \mu_0 \sigma \frac{\partial \mathbf{e}}{\partial t} \tag{4.6.7}$$

and when $\sigma = 0$ one gets the familiar result

$$\nabla^2 \mathbf{e} = \mu_0 \varepsilon \frac{\partial^2 \mathbf{e}}{\partial t^2} \tag{4.6.8}$$

For harmonic time variation $e^{i\omega t}$ the time derivative $\partial/\partial t \to i\omega$, so that (4.6.7) and (4.6.8) can be simplified to

$$\nabla^2 \mathbf{E} + (\omega^2 \mu_0 \varepsilon - i\omega\mu_0\sigma)\mathbf{E} = 0 \tag{4.6.9}$$

and

$$\nabla^2 \mathbf{E} + \omega^2 \mu_0 \varepsilon \mathbf{E} = 0 \tag{4.6.10}$$

where we have assumed $\mathbf{e} = \mathbf{E}e^{i\omega t}$.

Note that (4.6.9) has a form similar to (4.6.10) if we use the complex dielectric constant determined by (4.3.3), so that

$$\nabla^2 \mathbf{E} + \omega^2 \mu_0 \,\tilde{\varepsilon}\, \mathbf{E} = 0 \tag{4.6.11}$$

This equation is a vector differential equation which is valid for each component of the electric field. Indeed, we can have

$$\nabla^2 \psi + \omega^2 \mu_0 \,\tilde{\varepsilon}\, \psi = 0 \tag{4.6.12}$$

where ψ can represent any component of the electromagnetic field such as E_x, E_y, E_z, H_x, H_y, H_z. Consequently, each field component obeys (4.6.12); however, it should be noted that specific solutions for each field component for a given problem are determined from the boundary conditions. To obtain insight into the solution of the wave equation, we consider the simple case where $\sigma = 0$ so that (4.6.7) may be written as

$$\nabla^2 \phi = \mu_0 \varepsilon \frac{\partial^2 \phi}{\partial t^2} \tag{4.6.13}$$

where ϕ represents any time varying component of the electromagnetic field. For a harmonically time varying field

$$\phi(x, y, z, t) = \psi(x, y, z)e^{i\omega t}$$

In rectangular coordinates the Laplacian operator

$$\mathbf{V}^2 = \frac{\partial^2}{\partial x^2} + \frac{\partial^2}{\partial y^2} + \frac{\partial^2}{\partial z^2}$$

Equation (4.6.13) may be solved by separation of variables with a typical solution of the form

$$\phi = \exp[i(\omega t - k_x x - k_y y - k_z z)] \tag{4.6.14}$$

where ω, k_x, k_y, and k_z are the separation constants which satisfy

$$k_x^2 + k_y^2 + k_z^2 = \omega^2 \mu_0 \varepsilon \tag{4.6.15}$$

Note that the spatial argument of the exponential function may be written as $\mathbf{k} \cdot \mathbf{r}$. A more general solution to the wave equation will be composed of a superposition of the plane waves where the vector $\mathbf{k}$ is variable:

$$\phi(x, y, z, t) = \int\!\!\!\int\!\!\!\int_{-\infty}^{\infty} \Phi(\mathbf{k}) \exp[i(\omega t - \mathbf{k} \cdot \mathbf{r})] \, d^3 k \tag{4.6.16}$$

where we define $\Phi(\mathbf{k}) = \Phi(k_x, k_y, k_z)$, and $d^3 k = dk_x \, dk_y \, dk_z$ is the volume integral in k space. The variable ω is constrained by (4.6.15). The function $\Phi(\mathbf{k})$ can be determined from $\phi(x, y, z, t)$ at time $t = 0$ by using the inverse Fourier transform

$$\Phi(\mathbf{k}) = \frac{1}{(2\pi)^3} \int\!\!\!\int\!\!\!\int_{-\infty}^{\infty} \phi(\mathbf{r}, \, 0) \, \exp(i\mathbf{k} \cdot \mathbf{r}) \, d^3 r \tag{4.6.17}$$

Several points should be made regarding the solution given in (4.6.16). The solution is obtained by integrating over the three components of the $\mathbf{k}$ vector as shown in Fig. 4.6.1. Note that we have restricted our integration to real values of k_x, k_y, and k_z, however, the variables may in fact be complex. When $\mathbf{k}$ is strictly real, then $\mathbf{k}/|\mathbf{k}|$ represents the direction of the plane wave component while $\lambda = 2\pi/|\mathbf{k}|$ is the wavelength of the plane wave. On the other hand, when $\mathbf{k}$ has complex values, the plane wave will also be attenuated. Finally, instead of integrating over k_x, k_y, and k_z, we can treat k_x, k_y, and ω as the integration variables with k_z constrained according to (4.6.15). In this case, the "transfrom" or plane wave weighting factor $\Phi = \Phi(k_x, k_y, \omega)$ is determined by the boundary function $\phi(x, y, 0, t)$ which represents the value of the field in the $x\,y$ plane as a function of time.

4.7   Plane Waves

Since any solution of the wave equation can be written as a linear super-position of plane waves, it is important to understand some of the elementary properties of plane waves. Basically, we define a plane wave as one which is

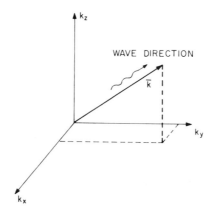

FIG. 4.6.1   A plane wave propagating in the direction defined by the **k** vector. A general solution to the wave equation is obtained from a linear superposition of plane waves.

dependent only on one space variable if we make a suitable transformation of coordinates.

Without loss of generality we assume that all field quantities vary only with respect to z and t, i.e., $\mathbf{E} = \mathbf{E}(z, t)$, $\mathbf{H} = \mathbf{H}(z, t)$. The two Maxwell curl equations become

$$\partial E_y/\partial z = \mu \ \partial H_x/\partial t \qquad (4.7.1a)$$

$$\partial E_x/\partial z = -\mu \ \partial H_y/\partial t \qquad (4.7.1b)$$

$$0 = \mu \ \partial H_z/\partial t \qquad (4.7.1c)$$

and

$$\partial H_y/\partial z = -\varepsilon \ \partial E_x/\partial t \qquad (4.7.2a)$$

$$\partial H_x/\partial z = \varepsilon \ \partial E_y/\partial t \qquad (4.7.2b)$$

$$0 = \varepsilon \ \partial E_z/\partial t \qquad (4.7.2c)$$

From Eqs. (4.7.1c) and (4.7.2c) we see that the z components of the electromagnetic field are independent of time. Here we will only be interested in dynamic quantities; consequently, place E_z, $H_z = 0$. With the remaining four equations we obtain simple wave equations for each field component. For example, if H_x is eliminated in Eqs. (4.7.1a) and (4.7.2b), we obtain

$$\partial^2 E_y/\partial z^2 = \mu\varepsilon \ \partial^2 E_y/\partial t^2 \qquad (4.7.3)$$

If E_x, E_y, H_x, $H_y = \phi(z, t)$, then ϕ satisfies

$$\partial^2 \phi/\partial z^2 = v^{-2} \partial^2 \phi/\partial t^2 \qquad (4.7.4)$$

where $v = (\mu\varepsilon)^{-1/2}$.

The general solution of (4.7.4) is

$$\phi^+ = f_1(t - z/v) \tag{4.7.5a}$$
$$\phi^- = f_2(t + z/v) \tag{4.7.5b}$$

The first solution represents a wave traveling in the positive z direction and the latter represents wave travel in the negative z direction. The quantities f_1 and f_2 are general functions.

If we put

$$E_x^+ = f_1(t - z/v) \tag{4.7.6}$$

and substitute into Eq. (4.7.1b), then we find

$$H_y^+ = (\mu v)^{-1} f_1(t - z/v) \tag{4.7.7}$$

which says that the ratio

$$E_x^+/H_y^+ = (\mu/\varepsilon)^{1/2} \equiv \eta \tag{4.7.8}$$

The quantity η is called the *free-space wave impedance*. For a vacuum $\eta = \eta_0 \simeq 120\pi$ ohms. On the other hand, if

$$E_x^- = f_2(t + z/v) \tag{4.7.9}$$

then the magnetic field is given by

$$H_y^- = -(\mu v)^{-1} f_2(t + z/v) \tag{4.7.10}$$

and the ratio of E_x^- and H_y^- is

$$E_x^-/H_y^- = -\eta \tag{4.7.11}$$

These relations can be understood also by considering the Poynting vector. For example, $\mathbf{E} \times \mathbf{H}$ of positive traveling waves is

$$P_z^+ = E_x^+ H_y^+ = \frac{|f_1(t - z/v)|^2}{\eta} \tag{4.7.12}$$

which means that power is flowing in the positive z direction, while

$$P_z^- = -\frac{|f_2(t + z/v)|^2}{\eta} \tag{4.7.13}$$

gives power flowing in the negative z direction.

Another property of plane waves is the fact that the electric field $\mathbf{E}$ is perpendicular to the magnetic field $\mathbf{H}$. We take the electric field for a positive traveling wave as $\mathbf{E} = \hat{\mathbf{x}} E_x^+ + \hat{\mathbf{y}} E_y^+$ and the magnetic field $\mathbf{H} = \hat{\mathbf{x}} H_x^+ + \hat{\mathbf{y}} H_y^+$. The inner product is

$$\mathbf{E} \cdot \mathbf{H} = E_x^+ H_x^+ + E_y^- H_y^- \tag{4.7.14}$$

Using the expressions (4.7.8) and (4.7.11), we get $\mathbf{E} \cdot \mathbf{H} = 0$, which implies that the electric and magnetic fields are orthogonal.

In certain conditions it is important to understand the nature of the polarization of the electric field as it propagates along a given direction. For optical systems, it is often easy to measure the polarization of the field using simple device configurations known as polarizers. For a wave propagating in the positive z direction, the nature of the polarization is described by the path traced by the electric field vector in the xy plane as time elapses. For example, in Fig. 4.7.1a the electric field traces a path along a line indicating linear polarization, in Fig. 4.7.1b the field describes a circular path which gives circular polarization, and in Fig. 4.7.1c the field is said to be elliptically polarized.

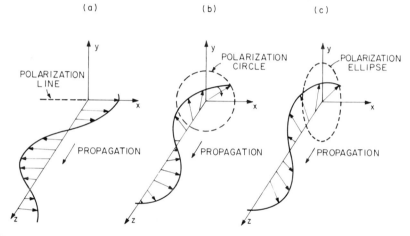

FIG. 4.7.1   The polarization of different types of plane waves. (a) Linear polarization: the electric field lies in the xz plane with the tip of the electric field vector tracing a line along the x axis in the xy plane. (b) Circular polarization: the electric field vector tends to rotate about the z axis as it propagates with the tip of the field vector tracing a circle in the xy plane. (c) Elliptical polarization the tip of the field vector traces an ellipse in the xy plane.

A linear polarized wave will have the electric field vector always lying in one plane whereas for circular and elliptical polarization, the field vector will always lie in a sort of "twisted" plane (similar to an auger bit) which is rotated about the z axis. Generally, circular and linear polarization are considered as special cases of elliptical polarization. An analytical description is determined from the instantaneous fields

$$e_x = E_1 \cos (\omega t - \beta z) \qquad (4.7.15a)$$

$$e_y = E_2 \cos (\omega t - \beta z + \theta) \qquad (4.7.15b)$$

where θ in the general case is a function of time, and E_1 and E_2 are the amplitudes of x and y components. For linear polarization, $\theta = 0$; for circular polarization, $\theta = \pi/2$, $E_1 = E_2$. Elliptical polarization occurs when E_1 is different from E_2 and when the phase term is nonzero.

4.8   Plane Wave Reflection and Transmission at Plane Boundaries

The reflection and radiation characteristics of heterostructure injection lasers can be understood from the wave reflection and transmission properties of plane waves incident upon a plane boundary separating two dielectric media. Figure 4.8.1 shows an incident wave on an interface with the reflected and transmitted waves. The incident wave is directed at the interface at an angle θ_1 with respect to the normal of the interface (here the x axis is normal to the interface). The reflected wave propagates away from the interface in the direction $\mathbf{k_1}'$ (the wave vector) with $\mathbf{k_1}' \cdot \hat{\mathbf{n}}/|\mathbf{k_1}'| = \cos \theta_1$ and the transmitted wave propagating in medium 2 travels at an angle θ_2 with respect to the interface normal.

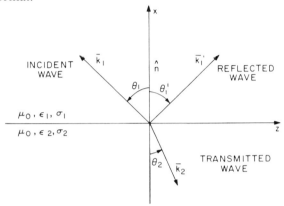

FIG. 4.8.1   A plane wave at oblique incidence on the interface between the two media. For $\perp$ polarization, the electric field is perpendicular to the xz plane, and for $||$ polarization the field is parallel to the xz plane.

There are basically two types of electric field polarization which we consider in this discussion:

1.   the electric field of the incident wave is perpendicular to the xz plane (this is called $\perp$ polarization) or the plane of incidence and
2.   the electric field is parallel to the xz plane ($||$ polarization).

Note that for the first case the electric field lies totally along the y axis, whereas for the second case there are two components E_x and E_z.

First we consider case 1 where the incident electric and magnetic fields are

$$\mathbf{E_i} = \hat{\mathbf{y}} E_0 \exp(-i\mathbf{k_1} \cdot \mathbf{r}) \tag{4.8.1a}$$

and

$$\mathbf{H_i} = -(E_0/\eta_1) [\hat{\mathbf{x}} \sin \theta_1 + \hat{\mathbf{z}} \cos \theta_1] \exp(-i\mathbf{k_1} \cdot \mathbf{r}) \tag{4.8.1b}$$

where the position vector $\mathbf{r} = \hat{\mathbf{x}}x + \hat{\mathbf{y}}y + \hat{\mathbf{z}}z$. Since $\mathbf{k}_1 = k_1(-\hat{\mathbf{x}} \cos \theta_1 + \hat{\mathbf{z}} \sin \theta_1)$, the inner product $\mathbf{k}_1 \cdot \mathbf{r}$ is independent of y. The ratio $|\mathbf{E}_i|/|\mathbf{H}_i| = \eta_1$, the intrinsic wave impedance of medium 1. The reflected fields are given by

$$\mathbf{E}_r = \hat{\mathbf{y}}E_0' \exp(-i\mathbf{k}_1' \cdot \mathbf{r}) \tag{4.8.2a}$$

and

$$\mathbf{H}_r = (E_0'/\eta_1)[-\hat{\mathbf{x}} \sin \theta_1' + \hat{\mathbf{z}} \cos \theta_1'] \exp(-i\mathbf{k}_1' \cdot \mathbf{r}) \tag{4.8.2b}$$

where $\mathbf{k}_1' = k_1[\hat{\mathbf{x}} \cos \theta_1' + \hat{\mathbf{z}} \sin \theta_1']$. The transmitted fields are

$$\mathbf{E}_t = \hat{\mathbf{y}}E_0'' \exp(-i\mathbf{k}_2 \cdot \mathbf{r}) \tag{4.8.3a}$$

$$\mathbf{H}_t = -(E_0''/\eta_2) [\hat{\mathbf{x}} \sin \theta_2 + \hat{\mathbf{z}} \cos \theta_2] \exp(-i\mathbf{k}_2 \cdot \mathbf{r}) \tag{4.8.3b}$$

The boundary conditions for the three fields are

$$(\mathbf{E}_i + \mathbf{E}_r)_y = (\mathbf{E}_t)_y \tag{4.8.4a}$$

$$(\mathbf{H}_i + \mathbf{H}_r)_z = (\mathbf{H}_t)_z \tag{4.8.4b}$$

which gives continuity of the tangential field components at $x = 0$. Condition (4.8.4a) gives

$$E_0 \exp(-ik_1 \sin \theta_1 z) + E_0' \exp(-ik_1 \sin \theta_1' z) = E_0'' \exp(-ik_2 \sin \theta_2 z) \tag{4.8.5}$$

whereas Eq. (4.8.4b) gives

$$(E_0/\eta_2) \cos \theta_1 \exp(-ik_1 \sin \theta_1 z) - (E_0'/\eta_1) \cos \theta_1' \exp(-ik_1 \sin \theta_1' z)$$
$$= (E_0''/\eta_2) \cos \theta_2 \exp(-ik_2 \sin \theta_2) \tag{4.8.6}$$

Equations (4.8.5) and (4.8.6) can be satisfied for all values of z if

(a) $\theta_1 = \theta_1'$, the angle of incidence is equal to the angle of reflection,
(b) $k_1 \sin \theta_1 = k_2 \sin \theta_2$,
(c) $E_0 + E_0' = E_0''$, $\tag{4.8.7a}$

(d) $(E_0/\eta_1) \cos \theta_1 - (E_0'/\eta_1) \cos \theta_1' = (E_0''/\eta_2) \cos \theta_2$. $\tag{4.8.7b}$

Condition (b) is the familiar Snell's law

$$(\sin \theta_1)/(\sin \theta_2) = \sqrt{\varepsilon_2}/\sqrt{\varepsilon_1} = n_2/n_1 \tag{4.8.8}$$

We note that if $n_1 > n_2$, $\theta_2 > \theta_1$, which implies that the waves or light rays are bent away from the normal. When θ_1 satisfies the condition $\theta_1 > \theta_c \equiv \sin^{-1}(n_2/n_1)$, all the power is reflected at the interface and there will be no power transmitted into medium 2. However, there will exist an electric field in region 2 but the field will decay exponentially along the negative x direction.

The power in the incident, reflected, and transmitted waves is given by the Poynting vector

$$\mathbf{S} = \tfrac{1}{2} \mathrm{Re}\,(\mathbf{E} \times \mathbf{H}^*) \tag{4.8.9}$$

The direction of $\mathbf{E}_i \times \mathbf{H}_i^*$ of the incident wave is of course directed along the

$\mathbf{k}_1$ direction, whereas $\mathbf{E}_r \times \mathbf{H}_r^*$ is directed along $\mathbf{k}_1'$. The respective magnitudes of the various vectors are

$$S_i = \tfrac{1}{2} \operatorname{Re}(E_0^2/\eta_1^*) \tag{4.8.10a}$$

$$S_r = \tfrac{1}{2} \operatorname{Re}(E_0'^2/\eta_1^*) \tag{4.8.10b}$$

$$S_t = \tfrac{1}{2} \operatorname{Re}(E_0''^2/\eta_2^*) \tag{4.8.10c}$$

The wave impedances will be complex if the dielectric constants are complex. The power directed along the x direction of the various components is

$$S_{ix} = \tfrac{1}{2} \operatorname{Re}(E_0^2/\eta_1^*) \cos \theta_1 \tag{4.8.11a}$$

$$S_{rx} = \tfrac{1}{2} \operatorname{Re}(E_0'^2/\eta_1^*) \cos \theta_1 \tag{4.8.11b}$$

$$S_{tx} = \tfrac{1}{2} \operatorname{Re}(E_0''^2/\eta_2^*) \cos \theta_2 \tag{4.8.11c}$$

Energy conservation gives

$$S_{ix} = S_{rx} + S_{tx} \tag{4.8.12}$$

The power reflection R and transmission T coefficients are given by

$$R \equiv S_{rx}/S_{ix} \tag{4.8.13}$$

$$T \equiv S_t/S_i \tag{4.8.14}$$

Note that $R = E_0'^2/E_0^2$.

The magnitude of the various field components relative to E_0 can be determined from Eq. (4.8.7). Dividing both equations by E_0, we have

$$1 + \rho = \tau \tag{4.8.15a}$$

$$[(\cos \theta_1)/\eta_1](1 - \rho) = [(\cos \theta_2)/\eta_2]\,\tau \tag{4.8.15b}$$

where $\rho = E_0'/E_0$ and $\tau = E_0''/E_0$ are the field reflection and transmission coefficients, respectively. From Eq. (4.8.15) we determine ρ and τ in terms of the intrinsic impedances and the angles θ_1 and θ_2 (for $\perp$ polarization)

$$\rho_\perp = \frac{\eta_2/(\cos \theta_2) - \eta_1/(\cos \theta_1)}{\eta_2/(\cos \theta_2) + \eta_1/(\cos \theta_1)} \tag{4.8.16a}$$

$$\tau_\perp = 2\frac{\eta_2/(\cos \theta_2)}{\eta_2/(\cos \theta_2) + \eta_1/(\cos \theta_1)} \tag{4.8.16b}$$

Note that if we define $Z_{1x} = \eta_1/(\cos \theta_1)$ and $Z_{2x} = \eta_2/(\cos \theta_2)$, then

$$\rho = (Z_2 - Z_1)/(Z_2 + Z_1) \tag{4.8.17a}$$

$$\tau = 2Z_2/(Z_2 + Z_1) \tag{4.8.17b}$$

which are the standard voltage reflection and transmission coefficients of a transmission line of impedance Z_1 terminated with a load impedance Z_2. The power reflection coefficient $R = \rho^2$ is

$$R_\perp = \frac{|n_1 \cos \theta_1 - n_2 \cos \theta_2|^2}{|n_1 \cos \theta_1 + n_2 \cos \theta_2|^2} \tag{4.8.18}$$

where we have used the indices of refraction instead of the wave impedances. From Eq. (4.8.8) the refraction angle θ_2 can be written in terms of θ_1, giving

$$R_\perp = \frac{|n_1 \cos \theta_1 - (n_2{}^2 - n_1{}^2 \sin^2 \theta_1)^{1/2}|^2}{|n_1 \cos \theta_1 + (n_2{}^2 - n_1{}^2 \sin^2 \theta_1)^{1/2}|^2} \tag{4.8.19}$$

At the critical angle $\cos \theta_2 = 0$ so that $R = 1$. At angles θ_1 greater than the critical angle, $\cos \theta_2$ becomes imaginary so that $R = 1$ since the absolute values of the two complex numbers $|u - iv| = |u + iv|$.

The reflection and transmission coefficients of the fields for parallel polarization are calculated similar to the case just given. In the preceding example there was only one component of the electric field and two components of the magnetic field, whereas for parallel polarization there is only one component of $\mathbf{H}$ and two components of $\mathbf{E}$. We will still reference our results to the total electric field strength E_0 with

$$\mathbf{E}_i = E_0(\hat{\mathbf{x}} \sin \theta_1 + \hat{\mathbf{z}} \cos \theta_1) \exp(-i\mathbf{k}_1 \cdot \mathbf{r}) \tag{4.8.20a}$$

$$\mathbf{H}_i = (E_0/\eta_1)\hat{\mathbf{y}} \exp(-i\mathbf{k}_1 \cdot \mathbf{r}) \tag{4.8.20b}$$

The reflected fields are

$$\mathbf{E}_r = E_0{}'(\hat{\mathbf{x}} \sin \theta_1{}' - \hat{\mathbf{z}} \cos \theta_1{}') \exp(-i\mathbf{k}_1{}' \cdot \mathbf{r}) \tag{4.8.21a}$$

$$\mathbf{H}_r = (E_0{}'/\eta_1)\hat{\mathbf{y}} \exp(-i\mathbf{k}_1{}' \cdot \mathbf{r}) \tag{4.8.21b}$$

and the transmitted fields are

$$\mathbf{E}_t = E_0{}''(\hat{\mathbf{x}} \sin \theta_2 + \hat{\mathbf{z}} \cos \theta_2) \exp(-i\mathbf{k}_2 \cdot \mathbf{r}) \tag{4.8.22a}$$

$$\mathbf{H}_t = (E_0{}''/\eta_2)\hat{\mathbf{y}} \exp(-i\mathbf{k}_2 \cdot \mathbf{r}) \tag{4.8.22b}$$

Matching the tangential fields at the boundary $x = 0$ gives $\theta_1 = \theta_1{}'$ and Snell's law. To calculate the field reflection coefficient we will use the "x component" wave impedance

$$Z_1 = E_{zi}/H_{yi} = \eta_1 \cos \theta_1 \tag{4.8.23}$$

Note that the components E_{zi} and H_{yi} are the two values associated with the component of the Poynting vector of the incident wave directed toward the interface. The x component of the wave impedance in region 2 is

$$Z_2 = \eta_2 \cos \theta_2 \tag{4.8.24}$$

The reflection coefficient ρ can be calculated simply by using Eq. (4.8.17a) (for $||$ polarization)

$$\rho_{||} = \frac{\eta_2 \cos \theta_2 - \eta_1 \cos \theta_1}{\eta_2 \cos \theta_2 + \eta_1 \cos \theta_1} \tag{4.8.25}$$

Again $\eta_1 = \eta_0/n_1$ and the angle θ_2 can be written in terms of θ_1, n_1, n_2 using Snell's law, giving

$$\rho_{||} = \frac{n_1(n_2{}^2 - n_1{}^2 \sin^2 \theta_1)^{1/2} - n_2{}^2 \cos \theta_1}{n_1(n_2{}^2 - n_1{}^2 \sin^2 \theta_1)^{1/2} + n_2{}^2 \cos \theta_1} \tag{4.8.26}$$

The power reflection $R_{||} = \rho_{||}\rho_{||}^{*}$.

At angles $\theta \geq \theta_c$, $R_{||} \rightleftharpoons 1$ since $\cos \theta_2$ is either zero or imaginary. An important distinction between $R_{\perp}$ and $R_{||}$ is that there is an angle θ_1 which gives $R_{||} = 0$ provided the media are lossless, i.e., n_1 and n_2 are real. When this condition is satisfied, all the power incident on the interface is transmitted into medium 2. The angle $\theta = \theta_B$, the Brewster angle, when total transmission occurs is given by

$$\theta_B = \sin^{-1}[n_2/(n_1{}^2 + n_2{}^2)^{1/2}] \tag{4.8.27}$$

When the angle of incidence $\theta_1 = 0$, $R_{\perp} = R_{||} \equiv R$, and R is given by

$$R = (n_2 - n_1)^2/(n_2 + n_1)^2 \tag{4.8.28}$$

As an example illustrating these results consider the transmission and reflection of light out of a semiconductor such as GaAs into free space [4]. We take $n_1 = 3.6$ and $n_2 = 1$. The value of $\theta_c = 16.13°$ and the Brewster angle $\theta_B = 15.52°$. When the incident angle $\theta_1 = 0$, the reflection coefficient $R = 0.319$. In Fig. 4.8.2 the reflection coefficients $R_{||}$ and $R_{\perp}$ are shown as a function of the incident angle. It should be noted that the reflection coefficient of perpendicular-polarized waves is larger than that of parallel-polarized waves.

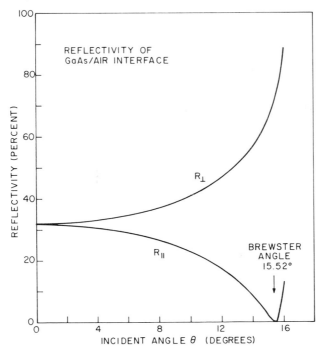

FIG. 4.8.2 The reflectivity for a plane wave incident upon a GaAs–air interface. At normal incidence, the parallel and perpendicular reflectivities are equal. At angles larger than the critical angle (~16.1), both reflectivities are 100%.

REFERENCES

1. H. H. Skilling, *Electrical Engineering Circuits*, p. 145. Wiley, New York, 1965.
2. S. Ramo, J. R. Whinnery, and T. Van Duzer, *Fields and Waves in Communication Electronics*, p. 486. Wiley, New York, 1965.
3. F. Stern, *Solid State Phys.* **15**, 327–342 (1963).
4. M. J. Adams and M. Cross, *Electron. Lett.* **7**, 569 (1971).

BIBLIOGRAPHY

M. Born and E. Wolf, *Principles of Optics*, 3rd ed. Pergamon, Oxford, 1964.

R. E. Collin, *Field Theory of Guided Waves*. McGraw-Hill, New York, 1960.

D. Marcuse, *Light Transmission Optics*. Van Nostrand-Reinhold, Princeton, New Jersey, 1972.

S. A. Schelkunoff, *Electromagnetic Waves*. Van Nostrand-Reinhold, Princeton, New Jersey, 1943.

J. A. Stratton, *Electromagnetic Theory*. McGraw-Hill, New York, 1941.

S. Ramo, J. R. Whinnery, and T. Van Duzer, *Fields and Waves in Communication Electronics*. Wiley, New York, 1965.

Chapter 5

Modes in Laser Structures: Mainly Theory

This chapter is devoted to a comprehensive theoretical discussion of the modal properties of laser diodes. We begin by a brief introduction of the horizontal and vertical laser diode geometry to place the analysis in proper structural context. Detailed discussions of structures and technology can be found in later chapters.

5.1 Laser Topology and Modes

Contemporary laser topologies are shown in Fig. 5.1.1. In general a Fabry–Perot resonator is formed by cleaving two parallel facets which produces a resonant condition for optical lasing along the cavity axis (direction perpendicular to the facets). A reflecting metal film is commonly placed on one facet to improve the useful output at the opposite one.

5.1.1 Vertical Geometry

Considering the internal device, the laser diode requires an active region in which an electron–hole pair recombination generates the optical flux and a mode confinement region which overlaps the active region; more generally, the mode confinement region extends beyond the active volume. The optical confinement is controlled by the changes in refractive index. The extent of the recombination region is limited by either the minority carrier diffusion length or by a potential barrier to the minority carriers. In heterojunction lasers, the potential barrier at the interface is several kT high, whereas in homojunctions

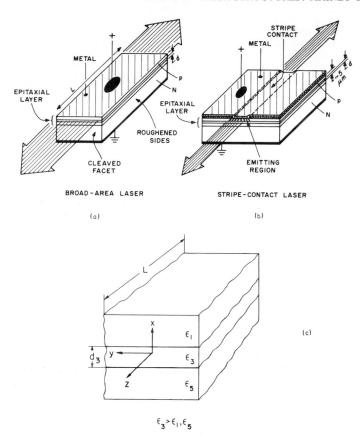

FIG. 5.1.1 Laser diode geometries: (a) Broad-area diode with sawed sides and cleaved facets; (b) planar stripe-contact diode; (c) model for dielectric waveguide. A description of various stripe structures is given in Chapter 12.

there is a small change in potential associated with p^+p or n^+n impurity distributions which provide limited carrier confinement.

The realization that an internally formed dielectric waveguide was essential for laser operation came early in the history of the semiconductor laser [1–4]. However, it was only with the development of lattice-matching AlAs–GaAs alloys that heterojunction structures could be constructed in which the magnitude of the dielectric discontinuity was greatly increased (without lattice defect formation), thus greatly increasing the optical confinement to the vicinity of the recombination region. With the flexibility now made possible with the multilayer epitaxial technology (Chapter 9–12), it is possible to construct lasers in which the waveguide region either overlaps the recombination region or controllably extends beyond it.

Figure 5.1.2 shows a section through the five-layer structure which can be considered the generalized laser diode. The laser consists of a radiative recombination (active) region 3 (width d_3)* in which the inverted carrier population produces the required optical gain, and a waveguide region for optical confinement of thickness $d^\circ = d_2 + d_3 + d_4$. The higher bandgap regions 1 and 5 provide optical barriers because of their reduced index of refraction at the lasing photon energy of the recombination region.

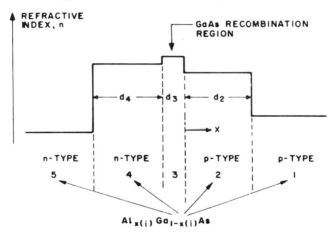

FIG. 5.1.2 Cross section of generalized laser structure showing the refractive index at the lasing wavelength. The radiative recombination occurs in region 3, and regions 2, 3, and 4 constitute the nominal waveguide.

Figure 5.1.3 shows the idealized cross section of important classes of laser diodes using from one to four heterojunctions. For each structure, we show the energy diagram, the refractive index profile, the distribution of the optical energy, and the position of the recombination region. These structures (listed in historical stage of evolution) are of increasing complexity.

1. In the homojunction laser [5–7] there are no abrupt refractive index steps for optical confinement or high potential barriers for carrier confinement. The recombination region width is essentially set by the minority carrier diffusion length. The radiation confinement is the result of refractive index gradients and carrier concentration differences. Typically a p^+–p–n configuration is used, where the p^+–p interface provides a small potential barrier.

2. In the single-heterojunction (close-confinement) [8, 9] diode, a p^+–p heterojunction forms one boundary of the waveguide as well as a potential barrier for carrier confinement within the p-type recombination region. The refractive index step at the p^+–p heterojunction is much larger (typically a

*The nomenclature of d_3 is used throughout for the recombination region width.

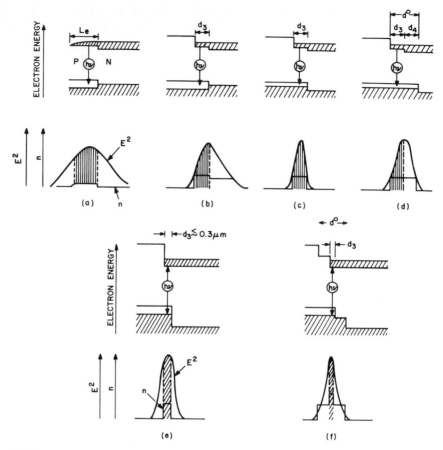

FIG. 5.1.3   Schematic cross section of various laser structures showing the electric field distribution E in the active region, and variation of the bandgap energy E_g and of the refractive index n at the lasing photon energy: (a) Homojunction laser, (b) single-heterojunction close-confinement laser, (c) double-heterojunction laser, (d) large optical cavity (LOC) laser, (e) narrow optical cavity laser, and (f) five-layer heterojunction laser with centered recombination region (four heterojunctions).

factor of 5) than that at the p–n homojunction. Thus, this is an asymmetrical waveguide. The threshold current densities are typically one-fourth to one-fifth the homojunction values at room temperature (~ 10 kA/cm^2 vs. ~ 50 kA/cm^2).

3.   In the double-heterojunction (DH) laser the recombination region is bounded by two higher bandgap regions to confine the carriers and the radiation. The device can be made either symmetrical or asymmetrical. In the symmetrical heterojunction barrier case, referring to Fig. 5.1.2, $d_4 = d_2 = 0$,

$n_1 = n_5$, and $d_3 = d°$. The first reported DH laser had $J_{th} \approx 4000$ A/cm^2 [10]. The reduction to a threshold current density at room temperature of about 2000 A/cm^2 was thereafter achieved with these devices with GaAs [11] and with (AlGa)As in the recombination region [12].

4. In the large optical cavity (LOC) laser, $d_2 = 0, n_3 \simeq n_4$, and $d° = d_3 + d_4$. The waveguide region is wider than the recombination region, which occupies one side of the space between the two major heterojunctions [13]. The device was basically intended for efficient pulsed power operation.

5. The very narrowly spaced double-heterojunction laser is a subclass of the basic DH device, but it is designed with an extremely thin recombination region $d_3 < 0.3$ μm, with n_1 and n_5 adjusted to permit the wave to spread somewhat outside d_3 but still provide full carrier confinement [14]. This is to minimize the beam divergence while keeping $J_{th} < 2000$ A/cm^2, a value desirable for room temperature CW operation.

6. Four-heterojunction (FH) laser: Five regions are included, usually with $n_3 > n_2 = n_4 > n_1 = n_5$. A submicron thick recombination region is bracketed by two heterojunctions which are further enclosed within two outer heterojunctions [15]. The basic concept of an extended waveguide region is similar to the thin DH concept. The recombination region is generally centered within the waveguide region. By adjusting the refractive index step between the recombination region and the adjoining regions 2 and 4, the fraction of radiation within d_3 and the interaction with the two outer heterojunctions can be adjusted. This structure allows the maximum design flexibility.

The properties of the various heterojunction structures are discussed in detail in the subsequent sections of this chapter and elsewhere in the book.

5.1.2 Horizontal Geometry

Waves propagating parallel to the cleaved facets must be suppressed by the introduction of high losses peculiar to them. For broad-area contacts, sawing the sidewalls achieves this. In the stripe-contact diode (also called stripe geometry), the lateral active junction area is restricted by the carrier flow from a stripe. This restriction produces a shallow maximum in the dielectric constant which forms a dielectric waveguide confining the optical field to a region below the stripe. Various methods of forming stripe-contact structures which differ in the degree of lateral confinement are discussed in Section 12.3.

5.1.3 Waveguide Modes

The cavity modes of the injection laser are conveniently separated into two independent sets of TE (transverse electric, $E_z = 0$) and TM (transverse magnetic, $H_z = 0$) modes. The modes of each set are characterized by three mode numbers, q, s, m, which define the number of "half-sinusoidal" variations of the field along the major axes of the cavity. By *longitudinal* (or *axial*) *modes* we mean those associated with change in q at fixed m and s. In particular, q determines the principal structure in the frequency spectrum. Similarly, *lateral* modes are associated with changes in s which give the character of the lateral profile of the laser beam. A major concern in this chapter is with the *transverse* modes associated with the index m, which involve the electromagnetic field and beam profile in the direction perpendicular to the junction plane.

Throughout the discussion of the modal behavior of laser diodes, we will not concern ourselves with the internal dynamics of the lasing process.

Axial modes are related to the length L of the cavity and the index of refraction and its dispersion as seen by the propagating wave. Since the optical cavity is composed of regions with different indices of refraction, the propagating mode sees an averaged index. The allowed longitudinal modes are determined from elementary considerations for a cavity of length L.

The *lateral modes in the plane of the junction* are dependent on the preparation of the sidewalls and the diode width. These modes generally have differing s numbers for sawed sidewalls and for the stripe-contact laser diodes. The wavelength separation due to the lateral modes is only a fraction of an angstrom unit, compared to a few angstrom units for the wavelength spacing of the longitudinal modes.

Transverse modes (direction perpendicular to the junction plane) depend on the dielectric variations perpendicular to the junction plane. The theoretical analysis of this problem is very important since the interaction between the propagating wave along the waveguide and the optical gain region (recombination region) within the waveguide is a controlling factor in the laser characteristics, including the radiation pattern and threshold current density.

The refractive index variation across the optical cavity is of major importance. Several factors contribute to the profile at the lasing wavelength. Carrier density controls the plasma resonance frequency, whose contribution to the index can be predicted by considering the simple classical oscillator. Most of the major factors affecting the index can be understood from the Kramers–Kronig relation between the absorption coefficient and the refractive index [16–18]. If the absorption coefficient varies from region to region across a laser structure, then there is a corresponding variation of the index. Some of the specific factors affecting the index profile are as follows:

1. The free carrier concentration differs in the recombination region. For example, the dielectric discontinuity between a depleted region and one containing a density P of free holes is $\Delta\varepsilon/\varepsilon \sim \omega_p^2/\omega^2$ where ω_p is the plasma frequency $(Pe^2/m_v^*)^{1/2}$ and m_v^* is the effective hole mass. A similar expression holds for electrons.

2. Above threshold the active region has a negative absorption coefficient whereas it is positive for the neighboring regions. Although a relatively exact

calculation for the gain of the active region can be made at the lasing wavelength, the frequency dependence of the absorption coefficient is uncertain. Consequently, it is difficult to estimate the contribution to the index of refraction from the population inversion in the active region.

3.   The shape of the absorption edge depends on the doping level, and there is a related dependence of the refractive index in the vicinity of the bandgap energy. The dependence of the GaAs refractive index on energy and doping level has been directly measured and also calculated from available absorption data (see Section 12.2.1).

4.   The variation of the nominal bandgap introduces the largest differences in the refractive index. It is easy to change the refractive index by many percent by changing the Al content of (AlGa)As (see Section 12.2.1). The very large changes in refractive index with bandgap are the basis of heterojunction laser design.

5.2 Waveguide Equations

The prominent feature that distinguishes a laser source from ordinary light is the narrow line width of the radiation and the coherent nature of the beam [19]. The optical field characterized by (5.2.1) is both spatially and time coherent. Time coherence implies that the field will be in phase with itself after some time interval whereas spatial coherence implies that the field will be in phase in space at different times. If we add a random phase to the terms in Eqs. (5.2.1), the fields become incoherent although they oscillate at a single frequency. Our characterization of the cavity modal fields will apply only to coherent sources.

Maxwell's equations can be written in a simplified form when they are applied to systems of cylindrical structures. In particular, we will consider the cylindrical structures with wave propagation along the axis of the cylinder. Consequently, the electromagnetic fields will have a functional dependence of the form

$$\mathbf{e} = \mathbf{E}(x, y) \exp(i\omega t - \gamma z) \tag{5.2.1a}$$

$$\mathbf{h} = \mathbf{H}(x, y) \exp(i\omega t - \gamma z) \tag{5.2.1b}$$

where $\gamma = \alpha/2 + i\beta$ is the complex propagation constant. For purely propagating waves $\alpha = 0$, and for attenuating waves $\beta = 0$. When we write the fields as in Eqs. (5.2.1), it should be noted that this is a special solution to Maxwell's equations and is true only for specific values of γ at a given frequency ω. The value of the propagation constant γ can be determined only after the geometry of the waveguide structure is specified. The mathematical technique for determining γ is obtained through application of the boundary conditions of the field quantities.

When the fields [Eqs. (5.2.1)] are substituted into Maxwell's curl equations, we obtain

$$\partial E_z/\partial y + \gamma E_y = -i\omega\mu H_x \qquad (5.2.2a)$$

$$-\gamma E_x - \partial E_z/\partial x = -i\omega\mu H_y \qquad (5.2.2b)$$

$$\partial E_y/\partial x - \partial E_x/\partial y = -i\omega\mu H_z \qquad (5.2.2c)$$

and

$$\partial H_z/\partial y + \gamma H_y = i\omega\varepsilon E_x \qquad (5.2.3a)$$

$$-\gamma H_x - \partial H_z/\partial x = i\omega\varepsilon E_y \qquad (5.2.3b)$$

$$\partial H_y/\partial x - \partial H_x/\partial y = i\omega\varepsilon E_z \qquad (5.2.3c)$$

These equations can be written in a form such that when E_z and H_z are determined the remaining transverse (x and y) components can be found. For example E_y or H_x can be eliminated from (5.2.2a) and (5.2.3b) and the remaining component H_x or E_y can be found in terms of E_z and H_z. Consequently, E_z and H_z play the roles of a type of potential function. Although (5.2.2) and (5.2.3) are Maxwell's equations in rectangular coordinates, these arguments can be applied to other cylindrical coordinate systems such as in polar coordinates (r, θ) where the transformed components E_r, E_θ, H_r, and H_θ can be written in terms of E_z and H_z. In rectangular coordinates (5.2.2) and (5.2.3) reduce to

$$E_x = -(\gamma^2 + k^2)^{-1} [\gamma \, \partial E_z/\partial x + i\omega\mu \, \partial H_z/\partial y] \qquad (5.2.4a)$$

$$E_y = (\gamma^2 + k^2)^{-1} [-\gamma \, \partial E_z/\partial y + i\omega\mu \, \partial H_z/\partial x] \qquad (5.2.4b)$$

$$H_x = (\gamma^2 + k^2)^{-1} [i\omega\varepsilon \, \partial E_z/\partial y - \gamma \, \partial H_z/\partial x] \qquad (5.2.4c)$$

$$H_y = -(\gamma^2 + k^2)^{-1} [i\omega\varepsilon \, \partial E_z/\partial x + \gamma \, \partial H_z/\partial y] \qquad (5.2.4d)$$

When the material has a finite conductivity, the form of Maxwell's equations will not change. The dielectric constant ε can be replaced by the complex dielectric constant $\bar{\varepsilon}$.

The longitudinal field components E_z and H_z are determined from the solution of the wave equation with appropriate boundary conditions. For example, all field components obey Eq. (4.6.12) so that we find

$$\mathbf{\nabla}^2_{xy}E_z + (k^2 + \gamma^2)E_z = 0 \qquad (5.2.5a)$$

and

$$\mathbf{\nabla}^2_{xy}H_z + (k^2 + \gamma^2)H_z = 0 \qquad (5.2.5b)$$

where we have replaced the operator $\mathbf{\nabla}^2$ by $\mathbf{\nabla}^2_{xy} + \gamma^2$. Since the field z dependence is of the form $e^{-\gamma z}$, $\partial/\partial z \to -\gamma$.

Again we point out that these manipulations of Maxwell's equations are fairly standard. Although we can write field solutions in terms of other functions such as Hertzian potentials, the intrinsic character of Maxwell's equations when applied to guided waves are borne out in Eqs. (5.2.4) and (5.2.5).

5.3 Wave Definitions

For certain geometrical structures, the solution to Eq. (5.2.5a) is independent of the solution to Eq. (5.2.5b). This means that E_z is independent of H_z. For example, in a metallic waveguide (rectangular, circular, etc.) the longitudinal E_z can be found by solving (5.2.5a) and applying the boundary conditions ($E_z = 0$ at the conducting surface). This procedure allows us to determine the propagation constant and other characteristics of the longitudinal E_z. Consequently, we can have a guided wave with $H_z = 0$ while $E_z \neq 0$. There are basically four possible field arrangements defined as follows:

1. Transverse electromagnetic waves (TEM) which have E_z, $H_z = 0$. The total field quantities lie in the transverse plane. These waves are usually associated with twin conductors such as coaxial cables.

2. Transverse magnetic waves which have $H_z = 0$ and $E_z \neq 0$.

3. Transverse electric waves which have $E_z = 0$ and $H_z \neq 0$.

4. Hybrid waves occur when both $E_z \neq 0$ and $H_z \neq 0$, since both field components are required to satisfy the field boundary conditions. We need to distinguish the hybrid waves from those conditions when both E_z and H_z can exist independently.

As mentioned previously, TEM waves exist mainly for two-conductor cable systems. These waves can exist only if $\gamma^2 + k^2 = 0$, so that there is a nontrivial solution to the transverse field components. Consequently, the propagation constant $\gamma - ik = i\omega(\mu\varepsilon)^{1/2}$. TEM waves are discussed very briefly here since they are very seldom found in optical waveguides.

The transverse electric and magnetic waves are frequently found in metallic waveguides such as in microwave systems. These waves can also exist in two-conductor coaxial cables; however their cutoff frequencies are very high in such cables. The most frequent appearance of TE and TM waves in optical systems occurs in dielectric slab waveguides. In these structures the electromagnetic field quantities are constant in the direction parallel to the slab.

Finally, hybrid waves are found in the more complicated waveguide systems. For example, in a rectangular waveguide which is partially loaded with some dielectric material both E_z and H_z are present in a modal field. Hybrid waves exist in optical waveguides such as optical fibers, optical stripelines, and in any high dielectric stripe embedded in a lower dielectric medium. Since optical fibers will play an important role in most future optical communication systems, it is imperative that hybrid modes be well understood [20–21].

5.4   Slab Waveguides

Three-layer slab waveguides [22] are mathematically simple and easy to understand compared to the multiple-layer waveguides and optical fibers. However, the physical waveguide phenomena of three-layer structures are applicable to the more complicated structures. The three-layer slab waveguide is formed by three layers of dielectric material with the center layer having the largest index of refraction.

Before discussing the mathematical and physical concepts, we need to mention the various types of modes associated with slab waveguides. A *trapped* or *bounded mode* is one whose field energy is located in the neighborhood of the waveguide or center slab. The mode being a propagating wave implies that the electromagnetic energy travels along the waveguide. The electromagnetic energy stays predominantly in the high dielectric region. The other type of field satisfying Maxwell's equations is called a *radiation mode*. Radiation modes have field intensities that do not vanish at large distances from the slab.

The fundamental slab structure is shown in Fig. 5.4.1. Ultimately, we will discuss the field solutions of a five-layer slab waveguide structure; however, some of the wave concepts pertaining to slab waveguides can be more easily explained using the three-layer slab guides. For the sake of uniformity, we will discuss the three-layer geometry by assuming that the layer regions 2 and 4 of Fig. 5.1.2 have thicknesses $d_2, d_4 = 0$. The three slabs have indices of refraction n_1, n_3, n_5 where $n_3 > n_1, n_5$. The regions 1 and 5 extend to infinity in the positive and negative x directions, respectively. The slab width is d_3. In Fig. 5.4.1b we show the profile of the index of refraction.

The electromagnetic modes of the slab waveguide can be composed of plane waves propagating along the positive z direction and cocked at an angle with

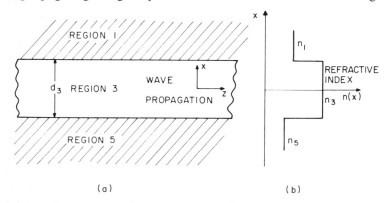

(a)   (b)

FIG. 5.4.1   Schematic cross section of the three-layer optical waveguide. (a) The wave propagates along the z direction, and (b) the refractive index as a function of the x coordinate.

respect to the z axis. For example, in Fig. 5.4.2, the plane wave is propagating at an angle θ with respect to z. When the value of $\theta' = \pi/2 - \theta$ is larger than the critical angle, the plane wave will be totally reflected at the boundary between regions 3 and 5. This reflection in turn sets up a standing wave along the x direction; however, there will be a traveling wave in the z direction. For a given plane wave inclination θ and a waveguide width d_3, the plane wave will be reflected from the boundary at the region 1–3 interface, thus confining the majority of the wave energy to region 3. There will be a field extension into regions 1 and 5, but it decays exponentially since the refracted angle θ'' (Section 4.8) is imaginary with a corresponding imaginary propagation constant.

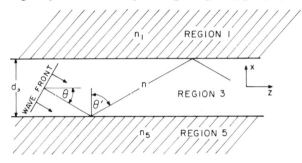

FIG. 5.4.2 The trapped waveguide mode representation using ray optics and the superposition of plane waves.

To determine the waveguide modes of the three-layer slab, Maxwell's equations as developed in Section 5.2 will be used. Since the fields are independent of y, the derivatives of all field components with respect to y are zero. The expressions in Eq. (5.2.4) become

$$E_x = -\frac{\gamma}{\gamma^2 + k^2}\frac{\partial E_z}{\partial x} \tag{5.4.1a}$$

$$E_y = -\frac{i\omega\mu}{\gamma^2 + k^2}\frac{\partial H_z}{\partial x} \tag{5.4.1b}$$

$$H_x = -\frac{\gamma}{\gamma^2 + k^2}\frac{\partial H_z}{\partial x} \tag{5.4.1c}$$

$$H_y = \frac{-i\omega\varepsilon}{\gamma^2 + k^2}\frac{\partial E_z}{\partial x} \tag{5.4.1d}$$

where E_z and H_z satisfy Eq. (5.2.5). It is easy to see that TE waves have E_x, $H_y = 0$, whereas TM waves have H_x, $E_y = 0$. In the preceding discussion the longitudinal field component is first calculated while transverse components are determined from Eq. (5.4.1). Frequently, it is advantageous to write the field components in terms of a transverse component. For example, E_y is the only electric field component in TE waves, while H_y is the only magnetic component for TM waves. All field components satisfying the wave equations E_y and H_y can be treated as "potential functions" and the remaining fields determined from them.

5.4.1 Transverse Electric Modes

The component E_y satisfies

$$\frac{d^2E_y}{dx^2} + (k^2 + \gamma^2)E_y = 0 \tag{5.4.2}$$

The remaining field components are

$$H_x = \frac{i\gamma}{\omega\mu} E_y \tag{5.4.3a}$$

$$H_z = \frac{i}{\omega\mu} \frac{\partial E_y}{\partial x} \tag{5.4.3b}$$

For wave propagation $\gamma = i\beta$. The quantity $\omega\mu = k_0\eta_0$, where $\eta_0 = 120\pi$ ohms, is the free-space wave impedance.

The solution to Eqs. (5.4.2) and (5.4.3) can be separated into four categories of modes. If the propagation constant $\gamma = i\beta$ is purely imaginary, then the modes represent traveling waves in the positive z direction. The value of the propagation constant β lies between k_0n_2 and 0 whereas the attenuation α lies between 0 and ∞. For propagating modes there are three types of field distributions, as presented in Fig. 5.4.3b:

Case I The mode is completely trapped. There is exponential field decay in both regions 1 and 5. There are a finite number of trapped modes with discrete β values, $n_1 < \beta/k_0 < n_3$.

Case II The mode is not trapped with field extension in the positive x direction and exponential decay in the negative x direction. The propagation constant β is continuous with $n_5 < \beta/k_0 < n_1$.

Case III The mode is not trapped with field extension in both the positive and negative x directions. The propagation constant β is continuous with $0 < \beta/k_0 < n_5$.

Case I Trapped modes (TE) The electric field E_y in (5.4.2) is determined in each of the three regions with ($\gamma = i\beta$)

$$E_y = e^{-i\beta z} \begin{cases} A_1 \exp[h_1(d_3/2 - x)], & x > d_3/2 \\ A_2 \cos h_3x + B_2 \sin h_3x, & |x| < d_3/2 \\ A_3 \exp[h_5(d_3/2 + x)], & x < -d_3/2 \end{cases} \tag{5.4.4}$$

where

$$\beta^2 - k_1^2 = h_1^2 \tag{5.4.5a}$$

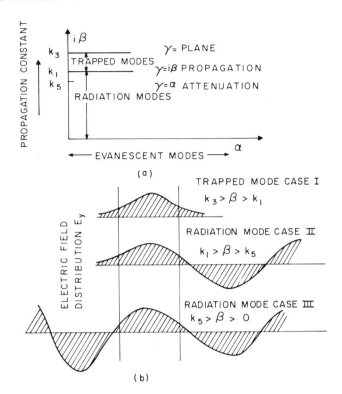

FIG. 5.4.3 Representation of the various modes supported by a lossless three-layer waveguide. (a) The value of the complex propagation constant γ for the various modes, and (b) the electric field distribution in the transverse direction.

$$k_3^2 - \beta^2 = h_3^2 \tag{5.4.5b}$$

$$\beta^2 - k_5^2 = h_5^2 \tag{5.4.5c}$$

Note that $h_1, h_5 > 0$ so that the field decays exponentially, i.e., the mode is trapped. The boundary conditions require that E_y and H_z be continuous at the two interfaces $x = \pm d_3/2$. This leads to the secular equation

$$\tan h_3 d_3 = \frac{h_3(h_1 + h_5)}{h_3^2 - h_1 h_5} \tag{5.4.6}$$

Thus, (5.4.5) and (5.4.6) form four equations with the four unknowns h_1, h_3, h_5, and β. Equation (5.4.4) can be written in a more simple form

$$E_y = A e^{-i\beta z} \begin{cases} \cos(h_3(d_3/2) - \phi) \exp[h_1(d_3/2 - x)], & x > d_3/2 \\ \cos(h_3 x - \phi), & |x| < d_3/2 \\ \cos(h_3(d_3/2) + \phi) \exp[h_5(d_3/2 + x)], & x < -d_3/2 \end{cases} \tag{5.4.7}$$

where ϕ satisfies the relation

$$\tan 2\phi = \frac{(h_5 - h_1)h_3}{h_1 h_5 + h_3{}^2} \tag{5.4.8}$$

The solution of Eqs. (5.4.5) and (5.4.6) determines the eigenfunctions or normal trapped modes when $\mathrm{Re}(h_1, h_5) > 0$, i.e., exponential decay of the fields. We associate the integer m with the trapped eigenmodes and write Eq. (5.4.7) as

$$E_y = \psi_m(x) \exp(-i\beta_m z) \tag{5.4.9}$$

The wave functions can be normalized according to the power flow in the mode; however, here we normalize the wave functions to unity such that

$$\int_{-\infty}^{\infty} \psi_m{}^*(x)\psi_n(x)\, dx = \delta_{mn} \tag{5.4.10}$$

where δ_{mn} is the Kronecker delta function. The quantity A in Eq. (5.4.7) becomes

$$A^{-2} = 2\left[d_3 + \frac{\cos^2[h_3(d_3/2) - \phi]}{h_1} + \frac{\cos^2[h_3(d_3/2) + \phi]}{h_5} + \frac{\sin h_3 d_3 \cos 2\phi}{h_3}\right] \tag{5.4.11}$$

Case II   Radiation modes, positive x (TE)   The radiation modes here have field quantities which extend to infinity in the positive x direction and decay exponentially in the negative x direction. The trapped modes of the preceding section have exponential field decay in both the positive and negative x directions. For the trapped modes $n_1 < \beta/k_0 < n_3$, giving positive values of $h_1{}^2, h_3{}^2, h_5{}^2$ of Eqs. (5.4.5). However, the radiation modes here have $n_5 < \beta/k_0 < n_1$, so that if $h_1{}^2$ is defined as in Eq. (5.4.5a), h_1 would be completely imaginary. Consequently, we define a new set of relations

$$k_1{}^2 - \beta^2 = h_1{}^2 \tag{5.4.12a}$$
$$k_3{}^2 - \beta^2 = h_3{}^2 \tag{5.4.12b}$$
$$\beta^2 - k_5{}^2 = h_5{}^2 \tag{5.4.12c}$$

Now the electric field solution of Eq. (5.4.2) for propagating modes is

$$E_y = Ae^{-i\beta z}\begin{cases} a(h_1)\cos h_1 x + b(h_1)\sin h_1 x, & d_3/2 < x \\ \cos(h_3 x - \phi), & d_3/2 < x < d_3/2 \\ \cos(h_3(d/2) + \phi)\exp[h_5(d_3/2 + x)], & x < -\tfrac{1}{2}d_3 \end{cases} \tag{5.4.13}$$

Now the field in region 1 is oscillating because $\beta^2 < k_1{}^2$; i.e., in region 1, E_y satisfies

$$\frac{d^2 E_y}{dx^2} + h_1{}^2 E_y = 0 \tag{5.4.14}$$

The field expressions in region 1 could be written as $E_y = A[(a - ib)/2 \exp(ih_1 x) + (a + ib)/2 \exp(-ih_1 x)]e^{-i\beta z}$, which is composed of two plane waves: one traveling in the direction defined by the vector $-\hat{x}h_1 + \hat{z}\beta$ and the other in the direction $\hat{x}h_1 + \hat{z}\beta$. Since both waves have the same amplitude, this implies that the power propagating away from the waveguide is equal to the power propagating toward the center slab region. This is a consequence of the fact that the wave or mode traveling in the positive z direction is neither attenuated nor amplified.

In (5.4.13) the fields have been matched at the boundary $x = -d_3/2$. The fields must also be matched at $x = d_3/2$. In addition, H_z of (5.4.3b) must be matched at both the upper and lower interfaces. Matching E_y and its x derivative at $x = d_3/2$ gives

$$a(h_1) = \cos\frac{h_1 d_3}{2}\cos\left(\frac{h_3 d_3}{2} - \phi\right) + \frac{h_3}{h_1}\sin\frac{h_3 d_3}{2}\sin\left(\frac{h_3 d_3}{2} - \phi\right) \qquad (5.4.15a)$$

$$b(h_1) = \sin\frac{h_1 d_3}{2}\cos\left(\frac{h_3 d_3}{2} - \phi\right) + \frac{h_3}{h_1}\cos\frac{h_3 d_3}{2}\sin\left(\frac{h_3 d_3}{2} - \phi\right) \qquad (5.4.15b)$$

The boundary condition on H_z at $x = -d_3/2$ gives

$$\tan[h_3 d_3/2 + \phi] = h_5/h_3 \qquad (5.4.16)$$

Equations (5.4.12) and (5.4.16) are used to determine h_1, h_3, h_5, and ϕ in terms of β. Here we see that β takes on all values between k_3 and k_2 whereas for the trapped modes β takes on discrete values between k_1 and k_2. The normalization constant A is given by

$$A^{-2} = (\pi/2)[a^2(h_1) + b^2(h_1)](h_1/\beta) \qquad (5.4.17)$$

and the transverse wave functions satisfy

$$\int_{-\infty}^{\infty} \psi^*(\beta', x)\psi(\beta, x)\, dx = \delta(\beta - \beta') \qquad (5.4.18)$$

where $\delta(\beta - \beta')$ is the Dirac delta function, defined as

$$\delta(\beta - \beta') = \begin{cases} 0, & \beta \neq \beta' \\ \infty, & \beta = \beta' \end{cases}$$

Case III Radiation modes (TE) In the preceding case the radiation modes extended to infinity only in the positive x direction. The modes here extend to infinity in both the positive and negative x directions. The propagation constant β/k_0 lies between 0 and n_3. The solution of Eq. (5.4.2) is

$$E_y = Ae^{-i\beta z}\begin{cases} a(h_1)\cos h_1 x + b(h_1)\sin h_1 x, & x > d_3/2 \\ \cos(h_3 x - \phi), & |x| < d_3/2 \\ c(h_5)\cos h_5 x - d(h_5)\sin h_5 x, & x < -d_3/2 \end{cases} \qquad (5.4.19)$$

where the transverse field parameters satisfy

$$k_1^2 - \beta^2 = h_1^2 \qquad (5.4.20a)$$

$$k_3{}^2 - \beta^2 = h_3{}^2 \tag{5.4.20b}$$

$$k_5{}^2 - \beta^2 = h_5{}^2 \tag{5.4.20c}$$

It is important to note that h_1, h_3, h_5 satisfy different equations for each of the three cases.

The boundary conditions at $x = \pm d_3/2$ give

$$a(h_1) = \cos h_1 \frac{d_3}{2} \cos\left(h_3 \frac{d_3}{2} - \phi\right) + \frac{h_3}{h_1} \sin h_1 \frac{d_3}{2} \sin\left(h_3 \frac{d_3}{2} - \phi\right) \tag{5.4.21a}$$

$$b(h_1) = \sin h_1 \frac{d_3}{2} \cos\left(h_3 \frac{d_3}{2} - \phi\right) - \frac{h_3}{h_1} \cos h_1 \frac{d_3}{2} \sin\left(h_3 \frac{d_3}{2} - \phi\right) \tag{5.4.21b}$$

and

$$c(h_5) = \cos h_5 \frac{d_3}{2} \cos\left(h_3 \frac{d_3}{2} + \phi\right) + \frac{h_3}{h_5} \sin h_5 \frac{d_3}{2} \sin\left(h_3 \frac{d_3}{2} + \phi\right) \tag{5.4.22a}$$

$$d(h_5) = \sin h_5 \frac{d_3}{2} \cos\left(h_3 \frac{d_3}{2} + \phi\right) - \frac{h_3}{h_5} \cos h_5 \frac{d_3}{2} \sin\left(h_3 \frac{d_3}{2} + \phi\right) \tag{5.4.22b}$$

If we assume that the propagation constant β is continuous, h_1, h_3, h_5 can be found from Eq. (5.4.20). However, the field is not completely specified since ϕ cannot be found because there are two independent sets of modes which can be made orthogonal by appropriately specifying ϕ for both sets of modes [23]. To determine ϕ consider first the case when $k_1 = k_5$ so that $h_1 = h_5$. The value of $\phi = 0$ gives the "even" modes while $\phi = \pi/2$ gives the odd modes. (The fields are either even or odd with respect to $x = 0$.) Now for the asymmetrical waveguide put $\phi = \phi_0$ for set S_a and $\phi = \phi_0 + \pi/2$ for the other set, say S_b. The equation giving ϕ_0 is found by making the two sets orthogonal:

$$\int_{-\infty}^{\infty} \psi_a(x, \beta)\psi_b(x, \beta')\, dx = \delta(\beta - \beta')\delta_{ab} \tag{5.4.23}$$

The value of the normalization constant A is

$$A^{-2} = \tfrac{1}{2}\pi[a^2(h_1) + b^2(h_1)](h_1/\beta) + \tfrac{1}{2}\pi[c^2(h_5) + d^2(h_5)](h_5/\beta) \tag{5.4.24}$$

and ϕ_0 satisfies

$$\tan 2\phi_0 = [(h_5 - \eta h_1)/(h_5 + \eta h_1)] \tan h_3 d_3 \tag{5.4.25}$$

The asymmetry factor η satisfies

$$\eta = (k_3{}^2 - k_5{}^2)/(k_3{}^2 - k_1{}^2) > 1 \tag{5.4.26}$$

In Fig. 5.4.3 the fields of the various modes are plotted as a function along x. It is interesting to relate the various trapped and radiation modes in terms of a plane wave propagating at angles with respect to the z axis. In Fig. 5.4.2 the trapped modes are composed of two plane waves propagating predominantly in region 3. The fields of the radiation modes of region 1 (Case II) are represented by the plane waves of Fig. 5.4.4a. The power of the reflected wave is equivalent to that of the incident wave, and the angle θ is related to the value of β. The fields of the radiation modes of regions 1 and 5 are represented by the plane waves of Fig. 5.4.4b. The powers of both the incident waves in regions 1 and 5 are equal to the respective powers of the transmitted–reflected waves.

The angle θ of Figs. 5.4.2 and 5.4.4 relates to the value of β. The θ of Fig. 5.4.2 is less than that of Fig. 5.4.4a, and θ of Fig. 5.4.4a is less than that of Fig. 5.4.4b. For the trapped modes θ' (the complement of θ) is larger than the critical angle so that all energy is confined to the slab region. Obviously, it appears that trapped modes can only be excited from the end of the waveguides. However, the glass prism can be used to excite the trapped modes for waveguide structures where region 1 is air. The requirement is that the index of the glass prism n_g must be greater than n_3 so that the light enters the waveguide at an angle $\theta > \theta_c$. Figure 5.4.5a shows the case for $n_g < n_3$ whereas Fig. 5.4.5b shows $n_g > n_3$. In Fig. 5.4.5a it is obvious that the waveguide

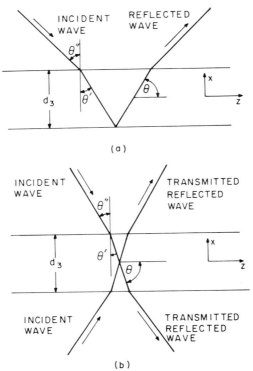

FIG. 5.4.4 The radiation mode representation using ray optics and the superposition of plane waves. (a) Case II radiation modes where the fields extend to ∞ along the positive x direction, and (b) case III radiation modes with fields extending to $\pm\infty$ along the x direction.

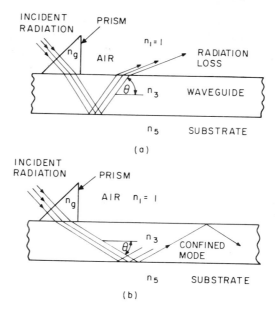

FIG. 5.4.5 The glass prism used to excite the trapped waveguide modes. (a) The waveguide index $n_3 > n_g$ producing inefficient coupling, and (b) $n_3 < n_g$ producing efficient coupling to the trapped modes.

cannot be excited with the prism index $n_g < n_3$ since the structure is similar to the basic guide structures with n_3 being the largest index of refraction. However, in Fig. 5.4.5b the light entering region 3 is bent away from the interface normal so that it is possible to obtain angles θ' which are larger than the critical angle θ_c.

5.4.2   Transverse Magnetic Modes

The field solution for the TM modes is similar to that obtained for TE modes. The magnetic field H_y satisfies the wave equation, and E_x and E_z are obtained by substituting E_x, E_z, H_y for H_x, H_z, E_y and $-\varepsilon$ for μ in Eq. (5.4.3).

Case I   Trapped modes (TM)   The field solution is

$$H_y = Ae^{-i\beta z} \begin{cases} \cos(h_3(d_3/2) - \phi) \exp[h_1(d_3/2 - x)] \\ \cos(h_3 x - \phi) \\ \cos(h_3(d_3/2) + \phi) \exp[h_5(d_3/2 + x)] \end{cases} \tag{5.4.27}$$

where

$$\tan h_3 d = \frac{(h_3/\kappa_3)(h_1/\kappa_1 + h_5/\kappa_5)}{(h_3/\kappa_3)^2 - h_1 h_5/\kappa_1 \kappa_5} \tag{5.4.28a}$$

$$\tan 2\phi = \frac{(h_3/\kappa_3)(h_1/\kappa_1 - h_5/\kappa_5)}{(h_3/\kappa_3)^2 + h_1 h_5/\kappa_1 \kappa_5} \tag{5.4.28b}$$

The field H_y is written as

$$H_y = \psi_m(x) \exp(-i\beta_m z) \qquad (5.4.29)$$

where the ψ_m satisfy the orthogonality condition (5.4.10) and the normalization coefficient in Eq. (5.4.27) is given in Eq. (5.4.11).

Case II   Radiation modes, positive x (TM)   The transverse field is

$$H_y = A e^{-i\beta z} \begin{cases} a(h_1) \cos h_1 x + b(h_1) \sin h_1 x, & x > d_3/2 \\ \cos(h_3 x - \phi), & |x| < d_3/2 \\ \cos((h_3/2)d_3 + \phi) \exp[h_5(d_3/2 + x)], & x < d_3/2 \quad (5.4.30) \end{cases}$$

where

$$a(h_1) = \cos h_1 \frac{d_3}{2} \cos\left(h_3 \frac{d_3}{2} - \phi\right) + \frac{\kappa_1 h_3}{\kappa_3 h_1} \sin h_3 \frac{d_3}{2} \sin\left(h_3 \frac{d_3}{2} - \phi\right) \qquad (5.4.31a)$$

$$b(h_1) = \sin h_1 \frac{d_3}{2} \cos\left(h_3 \frac{d_3}{2} - \phi\right) - \frac{\kappa_5 h_3}{\kappa_3 h_1} \cos h_3 \frac{d_3}{2} \sin\left(h_3 \frac{d_3}{2} - \phi\right) \qquad (5.4.31b)$$

$$\tan\left(h_3 \frac{d_3}{2} + \phi\right) = \frac{\kappa_3 h_5}{\kappa_5 h_3} \qquad (5.4.31c)$$

The fields are normalized as

$$\int_{-\infty}^{\infty} \psi^*(\beta', x)\psi(\beta, x)\, dx = \delta(\beta - \beta')$$

where A is given by Eq. (5.4.17).

Case III   Radiation modes (TM)   Again the transverse field H_y satisfies a condition similar to that for TE fields:

$$H_y = A e^{-i\beta z} \begin{cases} a(h_1) \cos h_1 x + b(h_1) \sin h_1 x \\ \cos(h_3 x - \phi) \\ c(h_5) \cos h_5 x - d(h_5) \sin h_5 x \end{cases} \qquad (5.4.32)$$

Matching the appropriate fields at $x = d_3/2$ gives $a(h_1)$ and $b(h_1)$ as in Eq. (5.4.31), whereas matching at $x = -d_3/2$ gives

$$c(h_5) = \cos h_5 \frac{d_3}{2} \cos\left(h_3 \frac{d_3}{2} + \phi\right) + \frac{\kappa_5 h_3}{\kappa_3 h_5} \sin h_5 \frac{d_3}{2} \sin\left(h_3 \frac{d_3}{2} + \phi\right) \qquad (5.4.33a)$$

$$d(h_5) = \sin h_5 \frac{d_3}{2} \cos\left(h_3 \frac{d_3}{2} + \phi\right) - \frac{\kappa_5 h_3}{\kappa_3 h_5} \cos h_5 \frac{d_3}{2} \sin\left(h_3 \frac{d_3}{2} + \phi\right) \qquad (5.4.33b)$$

Normalizing the fields over the transverse direction gives A identical to Eq. (5.4.24).

5.5   Slab Waveguide Mode Characteristics

In this section we determine the field parameters used for a discussion of the trapped waveguide modes defined by Eq. (5.4.4). In addition, the modal cut-off conditions can be determined in terms of the waveguide geometry such as the guide width and two dielectric discontinuities. The modal confinement factor which is a measure of the optical field propagating in the waveguide region d_3 is also given. Finally, we discuss the modal dispersion properties of laser modes in two-dimensional waveguides.

5.5.1   Field Parameters

The field characteristics of the trapped TE modes can be determined for any set of dielectric discontinuities if the waveguide geometry is normalized [24]. In particular, the quantities h_1, h_3, h_5, and d_3 are normalized as

$$H_i = \frac{h_i}{k_0^*(\kappa_3 - \kappa_1)^{1/2}}, \qquad i = 1,3,5 \tag{5.5.1a}$$

$$D_3 = d_3 k_0 (\kappa_3 - \kappa_1)^{1/2} \tag{5.5.1b}$$

The asymmetry factor η is

$$\eta = (\kappa_3 - \kappa_5)/(\kappa_3 - \kappa_1) > 1 \tag{5.5.2}$$

The secular equation (5.4.6) becomes

$$\tan H_3 D = H_3(H_1 + H_5)/(H_3^2 - H_1 H_5) \tag{5.5.3}$$

The relations between the normalized parameters are obtained from Eq. (5.4.5) as

$$B = H_1 \tag{5.5.4a}$$

$$H_3^2 + B^2 = 1 \tag{5.5.4b}$$

$$H_5^2 - B^2 = \eta - 1 \tag{5.5.4c}$$

where the propagation constant is normalized as

$$B^2 = \frac{\beta^2 - k_1^2}{k_0^2(\kappa_3 - \kappa_1)} \tag{5.5.4d}$$

In Fig. 5.5.1 we show the various parameters as a function of the waveguide width D_3 where η has been treated as a parameter.

5.5.2   Modal Cutoff Conditions

When the value of H_1 is zero, the field extension along the positive x axis is infinite. This condition defines cutoff for the various trapped modes. To determine the value of D_3 defining cutoff the values of H_3 and H_5 in Eq. (5.5.4) are substituted into Eq. (5.5.3), giving

$$\tan D_3 = (\eta - 1)^{1/2} \tag{5.5.5}$$

For symmetrical structures, $\eta = 1$ so that $\tan D_3 = 0$. The fundamental mode

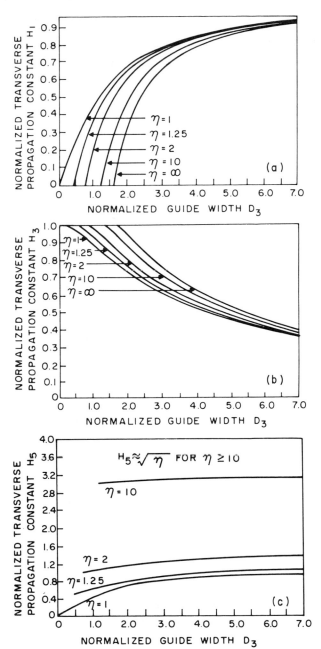

FIG. 5.5.1 Normalized transverse propagation constants of the fundamental mode versus normalized cavity width [from Eq. (5.5.1b)]. The asymmetry factor η is a parameter [24].

has no cutoff D_3 value, whereas for mode 2, $D_3 = \pi$. In general, the cutoff D_3 value for the m_{th} transverse mode is

$$D_3^{(m)} = (m - 1)\pi \tag{5.5.6}$$

For a given value of D_3, the number M of transverse modes is

$$M = \text{In}\{1 + D_3/\pi\} \tag{5.5.7}$$

where In is the integer truncation of the term in braces.

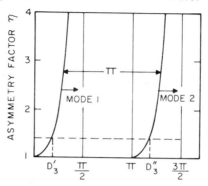

NORMALIZED GUIDE WIDTH D_3

FIG. 5.5.2 Cutoff conditions for the first and second waveguide modes. A waveguide geometry defined by a point to the right of each curve implies that the mode can propagate in the guide.

For asymmetrical waveguides, the relation (5.5.5) is shown in Fig. 5.5.2. For a given η value we find from Fig. 5.5.2 the value D_3' giving the smallest waveguide width at which the fundamental waveguide mode can propagate. The cutoff width for the second mode is $D_3'' = D_3' + \pi$, or in general for the m_{th} mode $D_3^{(m)} + D_3' + (m - 1)\pi$. The maximum number of propagating modes in a waveguide of width D_3 is

$$M = \text{In}\{1 + (D_3 - D_3')/\pi\} \tag{5.5.8}$$

As an example, take $d = 5~\mu\text{m}$, $\lambda_0 = 0.9~\mu\text{m}$, $n_1 = 3.5$, $n_3 = 3.6$, $n_5 = 3.4$. The asymmetry factor $\eta = 1.96$, and the normalized width $D_3 = 29.4$ and $D_3' = 0.7782$. The number of possible modes M is 10. On the other hand, suppose we wish to design a structure that supports only the fundamental waveguide mode. This means that D_3 should be a value just less than D_3'', or $D_3 < D_3' + \pi$. Using the definition of D_3, we find

$$d_3 < \frac{\tan^{-1}(\eta - 1)^{1/2} + \pi}{2\pi(\kappa_3 - \kappa_1)^{1/2}}\lambda_0 \tag{5.5.9}$$

If we use the index steps of the preceding example, then $d_3 < 0.67~\mu\text{m}$.

5.5.3 Field Confinement Factor

Another important parameter associated with the simple slab structures is the confinement factor Γ, which is defined as the fraction of the transverse modal intensity distribution lying in the slab region. Since the wave functions are normalized according to Eq. (5.5.10), the confinement factor is given by

$$\Gamma_m = \int_{-d_3/2}^{d_3/2} \psi_m{}^2(x)\, dx \qquad (5.5.10)$$

In Fig. 5.5.3 we show the confinement factor as a function of the normalized cavity width D_3 for various values of the asymmetry factor η.

5.5.4 Axial (q) and Transverse (m) Modes

The axial and transverse modes in a Fabry–Perot cavity are interdependent. The basic resonent modes can be determined without considering the details of the cavity losses since the modal structure is almost totally related to the reactive nature of the waveguide material. In Fig. 5.5.4 we show the cavity enclosed by two reflection planes located at $z = 0$ and $z = L$.

Before we discuss the spectral emission characteristics of a guided structure

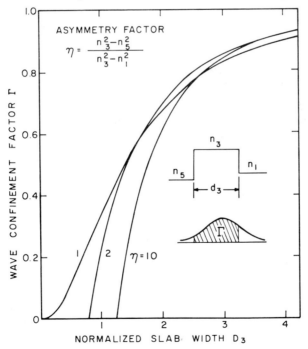

FIG. 5.5.3 The wave confinement factor Γ for the fundamental mode. D_3 is obtained from Eq. (5.5.1b).

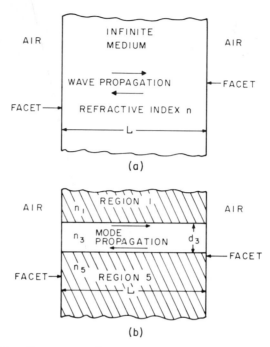

FIG. 5.5.4 Fabry–Perot geometries which produce a resonant condition along the propagation direction. (a) Plane waves propagating in an infinite medium, and (b) mode propagation in a three-layer slab waveguide.

we consider the simple case of an index medium n bounded by the two reflecting planes as in Fig. 5.5.4a. The fundamental resonant condition for plane waves propagating along the z direction is

$$k_0 nL = q\pi \tag{5.5.11}$$

where q is the axial mode number and n is the material index. The number q is very large for typical Fabry–Perot cavities; for example, with $L = 200 \ \mu\text{m}$, $\lambda = 0.9 \ \mu\text{m}$, $n = 3.6$, one obtains $q = 1600$. The mode wavelength separation is found by differentiating (5.5.11)

$$\frac{2}{\lambda} L\delta n - \frac{2}{\lambda^2} Ln\delta\lambda = \delta q \tag{5.5.12}$$

For large values of q, (5.5.12) can be written as

$$\frac{2L}{\lambda^2} \frac{\delta\lambda}{\delta q} = -\frac{1}{n(1 - (\lambda/n)(dn/d\lambda))} \tag{5.5.13}$$

The denominator on the right-hand side of (5.5.13) contains the expression

$dn/d\lambda$, which arises from the dispersion of the index near the bandgap The quantity

$$n_e = n\left(1 - \frac{\lambda}{n}\frac{dn}{d\lambda}\right) \tag{5.5.14}$$

is the equivalent index of the material.

When $\delta q = -1$, we obtain the modal spacing between adjacent axial modes

$$\delta\lambda = \lambda_q - \lambda_{q+1} = \lambda^2/2Ln_e \tag{5.5.15}$$

Conversely, we can determine the equivalent index n_e from the output spectral characteristics.

In a slab waveguide the form of (5.5.13) is slightly different because the waveguide itself introduces *geometrical dispersion*. Geometrical dispersion is inherent in most waveguide systems and occurs because the wave velocity is frequency dependent. The plane waves of Fig. 5.4.2 are inclined at angles θ with respect to the axis of propagation and, since θ is frequency dependent, it follows that modes at different frequencies travel at different velocities. It is important to note that the waveguide structures with a continuously (parabolic) varying index do not exhibit geometrical dispersion.

The resonant condition for the axial and transverse modes satisfies (5.4.5b)

$$((2\pi/\lambda_{mq})n_3)^2 = (q\pi/L)^2 + h_{3m}^2 \tag{5.5.16}$$

where h_{3m} corresponds to the mth transverse mode and $\beta L = q\pi$ is the longitudinal resonant condition. The transverse mode number m is small compared to q. In fact, the more useful laser structures are designed to operate in the fundamental $m = 1$ transverse mode (Chapter 6). Consequently, to determine the mode spacing as in (5.5.15) we consider only the specific sets of transverse (vertical) modes, and differentiate (5.5.16). The resulting expression is rather complicated, but it can be simplified by assuming

$$n_3 \gg H_{3m}(n_3^2 - n_1^2)^{1/2}, \qquad n_3^2 - n_1^2 \sim 2n_3(n_3 - n_1)$$

$$\frac{d}{d\lambda}(n_3^2 - n_1^2) \sim 2(n_3 - n_1)\frac{dn_3}{d\lambda}$$

where H_{3m} is given in Fig. 5.5.1. The approximate expression becomes

$$\left(\frac{2L}{\lambda^2}\right)\frac{\delta\lambda_{mq}}{\delta q} = -\left\{n_3\left[\left(1 + \frac{2(n_3 - n_1)}{n_3}G_d\right) - \frac{\lambda}{n_3}\left(1 + \frac{(n_3 - n_1)}{n_3}G_d\right)\frac{dn_3}{d\lambda}\right]\right\}^{-1}$$

$$\tag{5.5.17}$$

where G_d is given by

$$G_d = -H_{3m}D_3\frac{dH_{3m}}{dD_3} \tag{5.5.18}$$

Figure 5.5.5 shows the dependence of G_d on the normalized width D_3. For the fundamental transverse mode, the maximum separation between the axial modes occurs when $D_3 \sim 2$ and for the second-order transverse mode, the maximum separation between axial modes occurs when $D_3 \sim 4.75$. It is important to note that axial mode separation is dependent on the transverse mode order m. In most cases, however, geometrical dispersion is only a second-order effect compared to the index dispersion. For example, in a GaAs/(AlGa)As DH laser with $n_3 - n_5 = 0.2$, $d_3 = 0.25\ \mu m$, $\lambda = 0.9\ \mu m$, we find $(\lambda/n_3)(dn_3/d\lambda) \sim 0.38$. From (5.5.14) the value of $n_e \approx 4.97$, and the effective index determined from (5.5.17) is approximately 5.07. If the cavity width is increased to $d_3 = 0.55\ \mu m$, the laser with $m = 2$ has an effective index [from (5.5.17)] of 5.25.

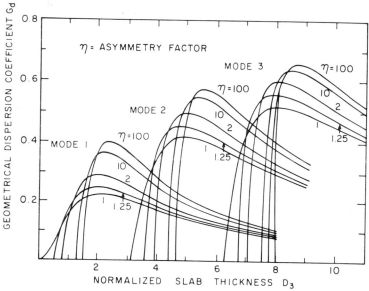

FIG. 5.5.5 The geometrical dispersion coefficient G_d for the first three modes as a function of normalized cavity width.

5.6   Propagation in a Dissipative/Gain Medium

Except for some special geometries it is possible to use approximate techniques to determine the attenuation of modes in a lossy medium. The theory used for finding the basic field distribution across the optical cavity of the various laser structures will be incorporated in the calculations of the modal threshold gain relations. The field calculations are cogent to the gain calculations because a standard perturbation theory will be used to determine the wave attenuation using the field distributions found in a completely reactive waveguide. In particular, assume that the field distribution in a reactive structure is

$$E(x,y,z) = E_0\psi(x,y) \exp(-i\beta z) \tag{5.6.1}$$

When losses are introduced in the structure and if the transverse field distribution is only slightly changed, then the propagating wave takes the form

$$E(x,y,z) = E_0\psi(x,y) \exp(-\tfrac{1}{2}\alpha z - i\beta z) \tag{5.6.2}$$

where $\alpha/2$ is the wave attenuation. If $\sigma(x,y)$ is the inhomogeneous optical conductivity of the material, then the wave attenuation can be written as

$$\alpha = \frac{\iint \sigma(x,y)\psi^2(x,y)\,dx\,dy}{\beta\varepsilon_0 c/2k_0} \tag{5.6.3}$$

where the wave functions have been normalized to unity. For the special case when there is a small percentage change in the index of refraction over all waveguide regions, then (5.6.3) can be approximated using (4.3.3), (4.3.19), and the relation $\beta \simeq k_0 n$:

$$\alpha = \iint \alpha_i(x,y)\psi^2(x,y)\,dx\,dy \tag{5.6.4}$$

where $\alpha_i(x,y)$ is the *local* plane wave absorption as opposed to the *wave modal absorption*.

For TE modes the Poynting vector along z is

$$S_z = (E_0^2/2\eta_0)\,\psi^2(x)n(x)\exp(-\alpha z) \tag{5.6.5}$$

The total power flowing in the positive z direction per unit length along the y direction is obtained by integrating S_z

$$P_z = \int_{-\infty}^{\infty} S_z(x)\,dx \tag{5.6.6}$$

In Fig. 5.6.1 we show P_z as a function of z, the direction of propagation. The longitudinal power flow has been separated into that flowing in the positive and negative directions. This particular example illustrates the results peculiar to a laser with cleaved ends at $z = 0$ and $z = L$. The power incident upon the facets is $P_z^+ (z = L)$ and $P_z^-(z = 0)$. The reflected power $P_r = RP_z^+(z = L)$, where $R \simeq 0.3$ for a GaAs–air interface.

The value of α illustrated in Fig. 5.6.1 is related to the active region gain, the attenuation in all regions, and the cavity geometry. The electric field satisfies

$$E_y^+(z = 0) = \rho E_y^-(z = 0) = \rho E_y^-(z = L)\exp(-\gamma L)$$
$$= \rho^2 E_y^+(z = L)\exp(-\gamma L) = \rho^2 E_y^+(z = 0)\exp(-2\gamma L) \tag{5.6.7}$$

where ρ is the field reflection coefficient of the facet and $\gamma = \tfrac{1}{2}\alpha/2 + i\beta$.

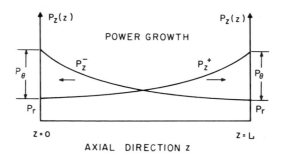

FIG. 5.6.1 The power growth of a laser mode as it propagates. The value P_θ is the radiated power at each facet while P_r is the reflected power.

Putting $R = \rho^2$ and eliminating E_y^+, the real and imaginary parts of the complex equation reduce to

$$R \exp(-\alpha L) = 1 \qquad (5.6.8a)$$

$$\exp(-i2\beta L) = 1 \qquad (5.6.8b)$$

The attenuation constant α satisfies

$$\alpha = -L^{-1} \ln(R^{-1}) \qquad (5.6.9)$$

and the propagation constant β satisfies

$$\beta L = q\pi, \qquad q = \ldots, -1, 0, 1, \ldots \qquad (5.6.10)$$

Since the complex propagation constant γ is modal dependent, these equations will be modal dependent. The reflection coefficient R_{ms} has a value less than unity so that α_{ms} determined from (5.6.9) will be negative.

In a laser of length $L = \infty$ we see from (5.6.9) that the modal attenuation constant $\alpha = 0$. (For the sake of simplicity we assume a three-layer slab waveguide.) However, if regions 1, 3, and 5 have $\alpha_i \neq 0$, then from (5.6.4)

$$\alpha = \alpha_1 a_1 + \alpha_3 a_3 + \alpha_5 a_5 \qquad (5.6.11)$$

where

$$a_i = \int_i \psi^2(x) \, dx \qquad (5.6.12)$$

is the fraction of the field in the ith layer. (Note that $a_3 \equiv \Gamma$ in Section 5.5.3.) Obviously, if $\alpha_i > 0$, then it is impossible to have the condition $\alpha = 0$ in an infinitely long laser. Consequently, the "absorption" α_3 of the active region must be negative.

Before discussing the numerical conditions on α_3 we pause to consider the actual nature of the active region 3. First, it is important to realize that the active region will have a high density of electron–hole pairs due to injection of carriers as discussed in Chapter 3. Since an electromagnetic field looses energy to the free carriers, a plane wave propagating in such a medium has a corresponding *free carrier absorption coefficient* α_{fc}. Second, since the active region is a generator due to stimulated emission, a plane wave propagating in such a medium has a *gain coefficient g*. If we neglect the absorption due to free carriers, the wave propagates with an increasing amplitude, proportional to exp(gz). Including losses due to free carriers, a plane wave propagates in an inverted region as exp $[-(\alpha_{fc} - g)z]$.

Because of its convenience for later calculations (Chapter 8), we now determine the active region gain at threshold G_{th}, for a laser of *infinite length without free carrier losses*. Since the modal $\alpha = 0$ we have from (5.6.11)

$$a_1 a_1 + (-G_{th})a_3 + a_5 a_5 = 0 \qquad (5.6.13)$$

or

$$\Gamma G_{th} = a_1 a_1 + a_5 a_5 \qquad (5.6.14)$$

Consider now the special case when the waveguide is symmetrical with $\alpha_1 = \alpha_5$ and $n_1 = n_5$. Owing to normalization of the transverse wave functions, $a_1 + a_5 = 1 - \Gamma$. The gain at threshold becomes

$$G_{th} = [(1 - \Gamma)/\Gamma]\alpha_1 \qquad (5.6.15)$$

For total confinement $\Gamma = 1$. Specific confinement factors can be found from Fig. 5.5.3. For example, assume $\alpha_1 = 10 \text{ cm}^{-1}$, $n_3 = 3.6$, $n_3 - n_1 = 0.1$, $\lambda = 0.9 \text{ } \mu m$, and $d_3 = 0.2 \text{ } \mu m$. The normalized guide width $D_3 = 1.18$. From Fig. 5.5.3 we find $\Gamma = 0.42$ so that $G_{th} = 13.8 \text{ cm}^{-1}$.

For a laser of finite length and with free carrier absorption, α must satisfy (5.6.9), which leads to the definition of gain at threshold g_{th}:

$$\Gamma g_{th} = \Gamma(G_{th} + \alpha_{fc}) + L^{-1} \ln R^{-1} \qquad (5.6.16)$$

where we have written $\alpha_3 = g_{th} - \alpha_{fc}$, which is the net gain of the active region. Using this example and for the time being assuming $\alpha_{fc} = 10 \text{ cm}^{-1}$ and $L^{-1} \ln R^{-1} = 30 \text{ cm}^{-1}$, we find $g_{th} = 95 \text{ cm}^{-1}$.

Further discussion of G_{th} in various structures is given in Chapter 8 where we apply these concepts to practical devices.

5.7   Three-Dimensional Modes in Practical Structures

The modes used to describe accurately the three-dimensional fields in laser cavities are the "box" and Hermite–Gaussian modes. The box modes which are used to define the laser fields in a Fabry–Perot resonator are similar to the resonant modes of a rectangular microwave cavity. The fields are confined to the active region by the two cleaved facets along the direction of propagation, the two heterojunctions along the vertical x direction, and the two sawed sidewalls along the lateral y direction. The modes of the stripe-geometry laser are similar to the box modes except that the fields along the lateral y direction are confined by dielectric differences because carrier injection into the active region is restricted by the contact (for planar stripe lasers). Furthermore, the functional dependence of the index of refraction in the vicinity of the active region is different for each of the mode sets. In particular, the box modes are derived from an index of refraction which has *abrupt discontinuities* while the stripe-geometry modes of diffused lasers are derived from a *continuously changing index* which can be assumed to vary parabolically along both the x and y directions. For planar heterojunction stripe-geometry lasers, only the y direction is so characterized.

Since the dielectric constant for the two-dimensional modes may vary continuously with position, the wave equation (4.6.6) must be used. However, the gradient of the dielectric constant can be neglected when the index variations with position are slow compared to the field variation. Quantitatively, this means that the index must vary only slightly over the distance of an optical wavelength in the material. Under this assumption the vector wave equation is simplified, allowing us to use the scalar wave equation. The optical fields are divided into two sets of modes, E_{ms}^x and E_{ms}^y as discussed by Marcatili [25]. The main field components of the E_{ms}^x modes are E_x and H_y and the major components of the E_{ms}^y modes are E_y and H_x. Both sets are hybrid modes and are basically of the TEM type since the main field components are perpendicular to the direction of propagation. In the slab waveguides discussed previously the E_{ms}^y fields are similar to the TE waves, whereas the E_{ms}^x fields are related to TM waves. If we assume waveguide modes of the form $\exp(i\omega t - \gamma z)$ where γ is the complex propagation constant, then the E_{ms}^y modes are determined from the set of equations (the superscript y is dropped)

$$E_x = 0 \tag{5.7.1a}$$

$$E_z = \frac{1}{\gamma}\frac{\partial E_y}{\partial y} \tag{5.7.1b}$$

$$H_x = \frac{-i}{k_0\eta_0\gamma}\left[k_0^2\kappa + \frac{\partial^2}{\partial y^2}\right]E_y \tag{5.7.1c}$$

$$H_y = \frac{-i}{k_0\eta_0\gamma}\frac{\partial^2 E_y}{\partial x\partial y} \tag{5.7.1d}$$

$$H_z = \frac{i}{k_0\eta_0}\frac{\partial E_y}{\partial x} \tag{5.7.1e}$$

where E_y is found from the wave equation. The E^x modes are found from a set of equations similar to those just given. Those equations are obtained by simply making the transformations $\mathbf{E} \to \mathbf{H}$, $\mu \to -\varepsilon$, and vice versa. The scalar wave equation defining the transverse dependence of the fields assumes the form

$$\mathbf{V}_t{}^2\psi + [k_0{}^2\kappa(x,y) + \gamma^2]\psi = 0 \tag{5.7.2}$$

The operator $\mathbf{V}_t{}^2$ is the transverse Laplacian. The transverse field component E_y becomes

$$E_{y_{ms}} = \psi(x,y)\,\exp(-\gamma_{ms}\,z) \tag{5.7.3}$$

5.7.1 Box Modes of Dielectric Rectangular Waveguides

The box modes derived here use the results of the two-dimensional modes of the preceding section. Since the field solutions in the rectangular waveguide have two-dimensional variations, the transverse field components h_i will be subscripted as h_{xi} and h_{yi} to denote the transverse field propagation constants along the x and y directions, respectively.

For the waveguide structure shown in Fig. 5.7.1, the dielectric constant κ (x, y) will be constant in the various regions. The solution of the wave equation (5.7.2) becomes [25]

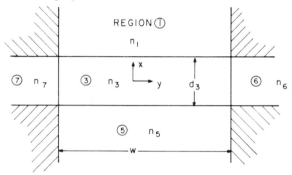

FIG. 5.7.1 The two-dimensional waveguide geometry used for the analysis of box modes.

$$\psi(x, y) = A_e \begin{cases} \cos(h_{x3}(d_3/2) + \phi)\,\exp[h_{x1}(d_3/2 - x)]\cos(h_{y3}y), & \text{region 1} \\ \cos(h_{x3}x + \phi)\cos(h_{y3}y), & \text{region 3} \\ \cos(h_{x3}(d_3/2) - \phi)\,\exp[h_{y5}(d_3/2 + x)]\cos(h_{y3}y), & \text{region 5} \\ \dfrac{\kappa_3}{\kappa_6}\cos(h_{x3}x + \phi)\cos(h_{y3}W/2)\,\exp[h_{y6}(W/2 - y)], & \text{region 6} \end{cases}$$

$$\tag{5.7.4}$$

The constant A_e is determined from the normlization condition. In the ith medium, the propagation constants h_{xi} and h_{yi} are related by

$$-h_{x1}^2 + h_{y1}^2 = k_1{}^2 + \gamma^2 \tag{5.7.5a}$$

$$h_{x3}^2 + h_{y3}^2 = k_3{}^2 + \gamma^2 \tag{5.7.5b}$$

$$-h_{x5}^2 + h_{y5}^2 = k_5{}^2 + \gamma^2 \tag{5.7.5c}$$

$$h_{x6}^2 - h_{y6}^2 = k_6{}^2 + \gamma^2 \tag{5.7.5d}$$

To match the fields at the boundaries between regions 1, 3, and 5, we place $h_{y1} = h_{y3} = h_{y5}$, whereas the fields in regions 3 and 6 are matched by assuming $h_{x3} = h_{x6}$. The form of the solution in (5.7.4) implies that region 6 is identical to region 7. The boundary condition making E_y continuous across regions 1, 3, and 5 and D_y continuous across regions 3 and 6 is satisfied by (5.7.4). Matching H_z across regions 1, 3, and 5 gives

$$\tan (h_{x3} d_3) = \frac{h_{x3}(h_{x1} + h_{x5})}{h_{x3}^2 - h_{x1}h_{x5}} \tag{5.7.6a}$$

where ϕ satisfies

$$\tan (2\phi) = \frac{h_{x3}(h_{x1} - h_{x5})}{h_{x3}^2 + h_{x1}h_{x5}} \tag{5.7.6b}$$

Matching E_z at the 3–6 interface gives

$$\tan (h_{y3} \, W/2) = \frac{\kappa_3 h_{y6}}{\kappa_6 h_{y3}} \tag{5.7.7}$$

The transverse propagation constants h_{xi} and h_{yi} can now be found from the simultaneous solution of (5.7.5), (5.7.6), and (5.7.7). It is important to note that the h_{xi} can be determined from (5.7.6a) along with (5.7.5a)–(5.7.5c), while the h_{yi} can be found from (5.7.7), (5.7.5b), and (5.7.5d). With h_{x3} and h_{y3} calculated, one can calculate the propagation constant from (5.7.5b).

The field solutions (5.7.4) are even functions with respect to y. There are of course another set of modes that have field solutions which are odd functions about the x axis. The field solutions for the odd modes are given as

$$\psi(x, y) = A_o \begin{cases} \cos(h_{x3}(d_3/2) + \phi) \exp[h_{x1}(d_3/2 - x)] \sin(h_{y3}y), & \text{region 1} \\ \cos(h_{x3}x + \phi) \sin(h_{y3}y), & \text{region 3} \\ \cos(h_{x3}(d_3/2) - \phi) \exp[h_{y5}(d_3/2 + x)] \sin(h_{y3}y), & \text{region 5} \\ \dfrac{\kappa_3}{\kappa_6} \cos(h_{x3}x + \phi) \sin(h_{y3}W/2) \exp[h_{y6}(W/2 - y)], & \text{region 6} \end{cases}$$

$$\tag{5.7.8}$$

The secular equations (5.7.5) and (5.7.6) also give the modal eigenvalues for the odd modes; however, the application of the boundary conditions at $y = W/2$ gives

$$\cot(h_{y3}W/2) = -(\kappa_3 h_{y6})/(\kappa_6 h_{y3}) \tag{5.7.9}$$

It is important to note that the secular equations governing the modal eigenvalues for the rectangular waveguide are identical to those equations obtained for simple slab waveguides.

5.7.2   Hermite–Gaussian Modes

The resonant modes of the stripe-geometry lasers with weak perpendicular and lateral confinement can be given in terms of the Hermite–Gaussian functions. This formulation is applicable only to stripe-geometry laser devices (Section 12.3) which do not have abrupt dielectric changes between the active waveguiding region and the passive regions.

Hermite–Gaussian functions are well known since they are solutions of the Schrödinger wave equation for the harmonic oscillator. Hermite–Gaussian functions occur as solutions of Maxwell's equations in a dielectric medium under the assumption that the dielectric constant has a spatial dependence which is parabolic. In the oxide-isolated stripe-geometry configuration, it is assumed that the maximum value of the dielectric constant occurs at a point located below the stripe contact in the active region; however, it does not vary along the direction of propagation [26]. Assuming that the dielectric constant is spatially symmetric both horizontally (y) and vertically (x) about the peak, it can be expanded in a power series with only even terms. Retaining only the zero and second-order terms, one gets

$$\kappa(x, y) = \bar{\kappa}[1 - (x/x_0)^2 - (y/y_0)^2] \qquad (5.7.10)$$

where $\bar{\kappa}$ is the peak value and x_0 and y_0 determine the decay rate in the respective directions. In laser devices the variation of the index along x is due to the fact that the material characteristics are changing. (This is discussed in Chapter 12.) The small index variation in the horizontal direction occurs because the injection current is restricted due to the nature of the stripe-contact design of the type shown in Fig. 5.1.1b.

Obviously there is a limit to the validity of (5.7.10) in view of the fact that for $x > x_0$ or $y > y_0$ the dielectric constant given by (5.7.10) becomes negative. Hence the usefulness of (5.7.10) is restricted to small x and y values since it is indeed a power series expression. Consequently, the Maxwell equation solutions will be restricted to modes with fields confined to the region of validity of (5.7.10). The resulting modes are generally the very low order ones.

Equation (5.7.2) can be solved by separation of variables by assuming

$$\psi(x, y) = X(x)Y(y) \qquad (5.7.11)$$

The lateral field becomes

$$E_{yms} = X_m(x)Y_s(y)\exp(-\gamma_{ms}z) \qquad (5.7.12)$$

Substituting the product solution (5.7.11) into (5.7.2) and separating the x and y dependence, one gets

$$\left\{\frac{1}{X}\frac{d^2X}{dx^2} + k_0^2\bar{\kappa}\left[1 - \left(\frac{x}{x_0}\right)^2\right] - \beta^2\right\} + \left\{\frac{1}{Y}\frac{d^2Y}{dy^2} - k_0^2\bar{\kappa}\left(\frac{y}{y_0}\right)^2\right\} = 0$$

$$(5.7.13)$$

where γ has been replaced by $i\beta$ ($\alpha = 0$) since we are interested in propagating modes. The first term is a function of x and the second depends only on y. Therefore, we have

$$\frac{d^2 X}{dx^2} + \left\{ k_0{}^2 \bar{\kappa} \left[1 - \left(\frac{x}{x_0} \right)^2 \right] - \beta^2 - K^2 \right\} X = 0 \qquad (5.7.14a)$$

$$\frac{d^2 Y}{dy^2} + \left\{ K^2 - k_0{}^2 \bar{\kappa} \left(\frac{y}{y_0} \right)^2 \right\} Y = 0 \qquad (5.7.14b)$$

The value K^2 is the separation constant. To transform (5.7.14) to a more useful form we make the transformations

$$\xi = [k_0{}^2 \bar{\kappa}/x_0{}^2]^{1/4} x \qquad (5.7.15a)$$

$$\eta = [k_0{}^2 \bar{\kappa}/y_0{}^2]^{1/4} y \qquad (5.7.15b)$$

$$\rho = x_0 (k_0{}^2 \bar{\kappa} - \beta^2 - K^2)/k_0(\kappa)^{1/2} \qquad (5.7.15c)$$

$$\chi = y_0 K^2 / k_0(\bar{\kappa})^{1/2} \qquad (5.7.15d)$$

which gives

$$d^2 X/d\xi^2 + (\rho - \xi^2) X = 0 \qquad (5.7.16a)$$

$$d^2 Y/d\eta^2 + (\chi - \eta^2) Y = 0 \qquad (5.7.16b)$$

For large values of ξ and η the values ρ and χ can be neglected so that X and Y have a Gaussian functional dependence. However, the details of the complete solution of these equations involving Hermite polynomials can be found in quantum mechanical treatments of the harmonic oscillator. The complete solution of (5.7.16a) is

$$X(\xi) = H_{m-1}(\xi) \exp(-\xi^2/2) \qquad (5.7.17)$$

where

$$\rho = 2m - 1, \qquad m = 1,2,3, \ldots \qquad (5.7.18)$$

The Hermite polynomial

$$H_m(\xi) = (-1)^m \exp(\xi^2) \frac{d^m}{d\xi^m} \exp(-\xi^2) \qquad (5.7.19)$$

of order m has $H_0(\xi) = 1$, $H_1(\xi) = 2\xi$, $H_2(\xi) = 4\xi^2 - 2$, and $H_3(\xi) = 8\xi^3 - 12\xi$. Substituting the appropriate values of ξ and η from (5.7.15), the field solution becomes

$$\psi_{ms}(x,y) = N_{ms} H_{m-1}(\sqrt{2}\, x/\bar{x})\, H_{s-1}(\sqrt{2}\, y/\bar{y}) \exp[-(x/\bar{x})^2 - (y/\bar{y})^2] \quad (5.7.20)$$

where

$$\bar{x} = [\lambda x_0/\pi \bar{n}]^{1/2}, \qquad \bar{y} = [\lambda y_0/\pi \bar{n}]^{1/2} \qquad (5.7.21)$$

and we have placed $\kappa = \bar{n}^2$. The normalization constant N_{ms} determined from

$$\int_{-\infty}^{\infty} \int_{-\infty}^{\infty} \psi_{ms}(x,y) \psi_{m's'}(x,y)\, dx\, dy = \delta_{mm'} \delta_{ss'} \qquad (5.7.22)$$

is given by

$$N_{ms} = 2[\pi 2^{m+s}(m-1)!\,(s-1)!]^{-1/2} \tag{5.7.23}$$

Eliminating the separation constant K in (5.7.15c) and (5.7.15d) and substituting $\rho = 2m-1$ and $\chi = 2s-1$, we find the propagation constant

$$\beta_{ms} = k_0\bar{n}\left[1 - \frac{2m-1}{k_0\bar{n}x_0} - \frac{2s-1}{k_0\bar{n}y_0}\right]^{1/2} \tag{5.7.24}$$

The resonant condition for longitudinal modes is $\beta L = q\pi$. By solving for the free-space wave number $k_0 = 2\pi\nu/c$ in (5.7.24) we determine the resonant frequencies

$$\nu_{msq} = \frac{c}{4\pi\bar{n}}\left[\frac{2m-1}{x_0} + \frac{2s-1}{y_0}\right] + \frac{cq}{2L\bar{n}}\left\{1 + \left[\frac{L}{2\pi q}\left(\frac{2m-1}{x_0} + \frac{2s-1}{y_0}\right)\right]^2\right\}^{1/2} \tag{5.7.25}$$

For low order transverse modes and large x_0, y_0 values, the quantity

$$\frac{L}{2\pi q}\left(\frac{2m-1}{x_0} + \frac{2s-1}{y_0}\right) \ll 1$$

and condition (5.7.25) can be approximated as

$$\nu_{msq} = \frac{c}{4\pi\bar{n}}\left(\frac{2m-1}{x_0} + \frac{2s-1}{y_0} + \frac{2\pi q}{L}\right) \tag{5.7.26}$$

To determine the separation in wavelength between the various modes, we differentiate (5.7.26), which gives

$$L\frac{\delta\lambda}{\lambda^2} = -\frac{1}{2\bar{n}_e}\left(\frac{L}{\pi x_0}\delta m + \frac{L}{\pi y_0}\delta s + \delta q\right) \tag{5.7.27}$$

where $\bar{n}_e$ is given by (5.5.14). The longitudinal mode spacing for a given transverse mode ($\delta m, \delta s = 0$) can now be determined from Eq. (5.7.27). It is important to note that there is no geometrical dispersion since the axial mode separation is identical to that obtained for plane wave propagation in an infinite dielectric medium with two reflecting mirrors spaced a distance L apart.

Zachos and Ripper [26] were able to fit the modal properties of homojunction (diffused) GaAs lasers operating CW at 77 K to the Hermite–Gaussian result (5.7.27). The reason is that for both directions of the stripe-geometry devices they studied, a rather gradual variation of the refractive index with distance following (5.7.10) could be postulated. They found that values of $y_0 = 1100$–2000 μm and $x_0 = 17$ μm were appropriate to fit the observed radiation patterns and spectra as shown in Fig. 5.7.2. Note the groups corresponding to longitudinal modes q (separated by 1.8 Å), each with a cluster of associated modes s separated by ~ 0.18 Å. Only a single transverse mode was excited, the fundamental mode.

It is common to find in laser diodes with planar stripe-contact widths

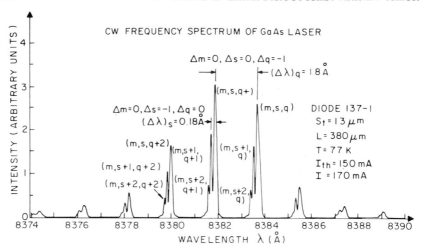

FIG. 5.7.2   Spectrum from homojunction CW stripe-geometry laser diode, formed with oxide isolation, operating at 77 K. The structure due to the longitudinal mode groups (q) is clearly seen with associated structure due to the lateral modes (s). The stripe width of the laser is 13 μm, and it is operating in the fundamental ($m = 1$) transverse mode [26].

of ≤ 13 μm that near threshold only a single (fundamental) lateral mode is excited (Chapter 7). In this case, as discussed in Section 7.7 only individual lines due to the longitudinal modes q are observed.

5.8   Five-Layer Slab Waveguide Modes

The five-layer waveguide structure is useful for modeling the more complicated lasers such as the LOC, four-heterojunction, and narrow DH devices [27,28]. The field quantities in the lateral and axial directions are of course tied to the vertical modes described by the five-layer structure, but frequently the main characteristics of the vertical modes can be obtained without delving into the complete modal picture.

For the five-layer model used here to describe the vertical modes, the optical cavity, which constitutes regions 2–4 of Fig. 5.1.2, is bounded by two thick passive regions, 1 and 5. The variation of the field in the y direction is neglected. The solution to the wave equation for the electric field **E** is sought in each of the five regions and the wave equation for the transverse modes can be written as

$$d^2\psi/dx^2 + (k_0{}^2\kappa_i - \beta^2)\psi = 0 \tag{5.8.1}$$

where κ_i is the dielectric constant of the ith layer. The assumed solutions of the wave equation in the five regions are

$$\psi_1 = A_1 \exp[h_1(d_2 - x)] \tag{5.8.2a}$$

$$\psi_i = A_i \sin(h_i x) + B_i \cos(h_i x), \qquad i = 2,3,4 \tag{5.8.2b}$$

$$\psi_5 = A_5 \exp[h_5(d_3 + d_4 + x)] \tag{5.8.2c}$$

where

$$k_0^2 \kappa_1 - \beta^2 = -h_1^2 \tag{5.8.3a}$$

$$k_0^2 \kappa_i - \beta^2 = h_i^2, \qquad i = 2,3,4 \tag{5.8.3b}$$

$$k_0^2 \kappa_5 - \beta^2 = -h_5^2 \tag{5.8.3c}$$

Equations (5.8.3) are obtained by substituting the assumed solutions (5.8.2) into the wave equation (5.8.1). The corresponding equations governing the TM fields are similar to those governing the TE fields. The forms of the appropriate field components of both TE and TM modes are given in Table 5.8.1.

TABLE 5.8.1
The Field Components in the Five Regions of Fig. 5.1.2[a]

Mode	1	$i = 2, 3, 4$	5
		Region	
TE	$E_y\ A_1 \exp[h_1(d_2-x)]$	$A_i \sin(h_i x) + B_i \cos(h_i x)$	$A_5 \exp[h_5(d_3 + d_4 + x)]$
	$H_x -\dfrac{\gamma}{i\omega\mu} A_1 \exp[h_1(d_2-x)]$	$-\dfrac{\gamma}{i\omega\mu}[A_i \sin(h_i x)+B_i\cos(h_i x)]$	$-\dfrac{\gamma}{i\omega\mu} A_5 \exp[h_5(d_3+d_4+x)]$
	$H_z\ \dfrac{h_1}{i\omega\mu} A_1 \exp[h_1(d_2-x)]$	$-\dfrac{h_i}{i\omega\mu}[A_i \cos(h_i x)-B_i \sin(h_i x)]$	$-\dfrac{h_5}{i\omega\mu} A_5 \exp[h_5(d_3+d_4+x)]$
TM	$E_x\ A_1 \exp[h_1(d_2-x)]$	$A_i \sin(h_i x)+B_i \cos(h_i x)$	$A_5 \exp[ih_5(d_3+d_4+x)]$
	$H_y\ \dfrac{i\omega\varepsilon_1}{\gamma} A_1 \exp[h_1(d_2-x)]$	$\dfrac{i\omega\varepsilon_i}{\gamma}[A_i \sin(h_i x)+B_i\cos(h_i x)]$	$\dfrac{i\omega\varepsilon_5}{\gamma} A_5 \exp[h_5(d_3+d_4+x)]$
	$E_z -\dfrac{h_1}{\gamma} A_1 \exp[h_1(d_2-x)]$	$\dfrac{h_i}{\gamma}[A_i \cos(h_1 x)-B_i \sin(h_i x)]$	$\dfrac{h_5}{\gamma} A_5 \exp[h_5(d_3 +d_4 +x)]$

[a] The term $\exp(i\omega t - \gamma z)$ has been dropped.

The continuity of the transverse field components, E_y and H_z, at the various boundaries at $x = d_2,\ 0,\ -d_3$, and $-(d_3 + d_4)$ gives the following secular equation for TE modes:

$$(\bar{c}_3 A - \bar{s}_3 B)(s_4 h_5 + c_4 h_4) + (\bar{s}_3 A + \bar{c}_3 B)(c_4 h_5 - s_4 h_4) = 0 \tag{5.8.4}$$

where

$$s_i = \sin(h_i d_i), \qquad i = 2,3,4 \tag{5.8.5a}$$

$$c_i = \cos(h_i d_i), \qquad i = 2,3,4 \tag{5.8.5b}$$

$$\bar{s}_3 = \sin(h_4 d_3) \tag{5.8.5c}$$

$$\bar{c}_3 = \cos(h_4 d_3) \tag{5.8.5d}$$

$$\tilde{s}_3 = \sin[h_4(d_3 + d_4)] = \bar{s}_3 c_4 + \bar{c}_3 s_4 \tag{5.8.5e}$$

$$\tilde{c}_3 = \cos[h_4(d_3 + d_4)] = \bar{c}_3 c_4 + \bar{s}_3 s_4 \tag{5.8.5f}$$

$$A = U(\bar{s}_3 s_3 h_4 + \bar{c}_3 c_3 h_3) - V(\bar{s}_3 c_3 h_4 - \bar{c}_3 s_3 h_3) \qquad (5.8.5\text{g})$$

$$B = U(\bar{c}_3 s_3 h_4 - \bar{s}_3 c_3 h_3) - V(\bar{c}_3 c_3 h_4 - \bar{s}_3 s_3 h_3) \qquad (5.8.5\text{h})$$

$$U = h_2(s_2 h_2 - c_2 h_1) \qquad (5.8.5\text{i})$$

$$V = h_3(s_2 h_1 + c_2 h_2) \qquad (5.8.5\text{j})$$

The constants A_1, A_i, and B_i of the field expressions can be determined from the appropriate boundary equations. The amplitude constants are written in terms of the amplitude constant A_5, which may be evaluated by an appropriate normalization procecure:

$$A_4 = h_4^{-1}(h_5 \bar{c}_3 - h_4 \bar{s}_3)A_5 \qquad (5.8.6\text{a})$$

$$B_4 = h_4^{-1}(h_5 \bar{s}_3 + h_4 \bar{c}_3)A_5 \qquad (5.8.6\text{b})$$

$$A_3 = h_3^{-1}(h_4 c_3 \bar{c}_3 + h_3 s_3 \bar{s}_3)A_4 + (h_4 c_3 \bar{s}_3 - h_3 s_3 \bar{c}_3)B_3 \qquad (5.8.6\text{c})$$

$$B_3 = h_3^{-1}(h_4 s_3 \bar{c}_3 - h_3 c_3 \bar{s}_3)A_4 + (h_4 s_3 \bar{s}_3 + h_3 c_3 \bar{c}_3)B_4 \qquad (5.8.6\text{d})$$

$$A_2 = (h_3/h_2)A_3 \qquad (5.8.6\text{e})$$

$$B_2 = B_3 \qquad (5.8.6\text{f})$$

$$A_1 = s_2 A_2 + c_2 B_2 \qquad (5.8.6\text{g})$$

The field structure for TM modes is determined similarly to that for TE modes.

5.9 Modal Facet Reflectivity

A simple understanding of the mode reflectivity can be obtained by considering the Fresnel reflection coefficient of a plane wave as discussed in Section 4.8. A plane wave with oblique incidence on an interface has a reflection coefficient depending on (1) the angle of incidence and (2) the polarization of the electric field. The electric field polarized parallel to the interface ($\perp$ polarization) is similar to the case of TE modes, whereas the electric field having a component perpendicular to the interface ($||$ polarization) is like TM modes ($\perp$ and $||$ mean that the electric field is either perpendicular or parallel to the plane of incidence). For $\perp$ polarization, the facet reflectivities increase monotonically with incident angle [29]. It is approximately 30% at a zero incident angle with the facet normal and 100% at an angle of $\sim 16.1°$, the critical angle. For $||$ polarization, the reflectivity decreases monotonically to zero at the Brewster angle ($\sim 15.5°$) and then increases to 100% at the critical angle. Consequently, the reflectivity for $||$-polarized waves is always less than that for $\perp$-polarized waves.

A mode in a slab waveguide can be decomposed into a set of plane waves propagating at different angles with respect to the direction of propagation or facet normal. The reflectivity of the mode can be estimated by appropriately weighing or averaging the Fresnel reflectivity according to the angular spectra of the mode [30,31]. Accordingly, it is easy to see that the reflectivity of TE modes is greater than that of TM modes. Consequently, the *equivalent* absorption coefficient associated with cavity end losses satisfies $\alpha_{\text{endTE}} < \alpha_{\text{endTM}}$.

The facet reflectivity for a given mode can be derived by a more rigorous technique which includes the effects of coupling to other waveguide modes, including the radiation modes. Basically, when a given mode strikes the waveguide–air interface, the reflected energy is distributed among all modes. The "air modes," which form a continuous spectrum, will of course be different from waveguide modes. The distribution of the incident energy across all the reflected and transmitted modes is determined from the solution of a rather complicated boundary value problem obtained by matching the tangential fields on each side of the facet [32,33]. The reflectivity R_m of the mth trapped mode is then defined as the ratio of the reflected energy in the mode and of the energy of the incident mode.

Mathematically, we find using the conservation of energy condition that $R_m + T + S_s = 1$, where T is the transmitted power and S_s the scattered power distributed over all waveguide modes except the mth one. When the dielectric step between the active region 3 and the passive regions 1 and 5 is small to moderate, as in typical GaAs/(AlGa)As lasers, the value of $S_s \ll 1$. On the other hand, for large dielectric steps the value of S_s can be relatively large, as we will see. Since the power scattered into the nonresonating modes is lost internally, the device external quantum efficiency is limited by $T/(T + S_s)$.

For TE modes consider the mth mode incident on the waveguide–air interface in Fig. 5.9.1. Because the mode sees a waveguide discontinuity, power will be scattered into all waveguide modes traveling in the negative z direction

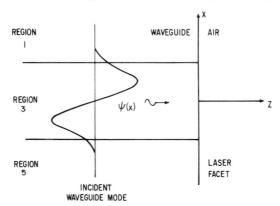

FIG. 5.9.1   Waveguide mode incident on the laser facet. Region 3 defines the optical cavity.

as well as transmitted to the region $z > 0$. Consequently, the transverse field in the region $z < 0$ is given by

$$E_y = \psi_m(x) \exp(-i\beta_m z) + \sum_{m'=1}^{M} \rho_{mm'}\psi_{m'}(x) \exp(i\beta_{m'}z)$$

$$+ \int \rho_m(\beta)\psi(\beta,x) \exp(i\beta z) \, d\beta \tag{5.9.1}$$

where we have assumed that there are only M trapped modes. The integral includes the radiation as well as the evanescent modes. In this formulation ρ_{mm} is the mth modal reflection coefficient and $\rho_{mm'}(m \neq m')$ represents the coupling or conversion coefficient which is a measure of power scatter from the incident mode m into the m' mode. The power reflection coefficient $R_m = |\rho_{mm}|^2$. For the sake of briefness we use the summation $\sum_{m'=1}^{\infty}$ to include both trapped and continuous modes.

Since we are discussing a waveguide with an array of modes (varying propagation constants), Eq. (5.4.3) cannot be used to determine the magnetic field components. However, we find

$$i\omega\mu H_x = \partial E_y/\partial z \tag{5.9.2}$$

so that

$$\omega\mu H_x = -\beta_m\psi_m(x) \exp(-i\beta_m z) + \sum_{m'=1}^{\infty} \rho_{mm'}\beta_{m'}\psi_{m'}(x) \exp(i\beta_{m'}z) \tag{5.9.3}$$

Outside the waveguide, $z > 0$, the tangential field components are

$$E_y = \int_{\infty}^{\infty} \tau(p) \exp[-i(px + qz)] \, dp \tag{5.9.4a}$$

$$\omega\mu H_y = -\int_{-\infty}^{\infty} q\tau(p) \exp[-i(px + qz)] \, dp \tag{5.9.4b}$$

where $p^2 + q^2 = k_0^2$ [see Eq. (4.6.16)]. The condition on the variable p is Im $\{q\} < 0$ so that the fields remain finite at $z = \infty$. Note that at $z = 0$, (5.9.4a) indicates that $\tau(p)$ is the Fourier transform of the facet field E_y.

In the discussion that follows we make frequent use of the Fourier transform pair, $\psi_m(x)$ and $\bar{\psi}_m(p)$, given by

$$\psi_m(x) = \int_{-\infty}^{\infty} \bar{\psi}_m(p) \exp(-ipx) \, dp \tag{5.9.5a}$$

$$\bar{\psi}_m(p) = \frac{1}{2\pi} \int_{-\infty}^{\infty} \psi_m(x) \exp(ipx) \, dx \tag{5.9.5b}$$

For the trapped TE modes (5.4.7), we have

$$\bar{\psi}_m(p) = \frac{A_m}{2\pi} \left\{ \frac{k_0^2(\kappa_3 - \kappa_1) \cos(h_3 d_3/2 - \phi) \exp(ip \, d_3/2)}{(h_1 - ip)(h_3^2 - p^2)} \right.$$

$$\left. + \frac{k_0^2(\kappa_3 - \kappa_5) \cos(h_3 d_3/2 + \phi) \exp(-ip \, d_3/2)}{(h_5 + ip)(h_3^2 - p^2)} \right\} \tag{5.9.6}$$

For a symmetric waveguide, $\eta = 1$, this simplifies. The $\bar{\psi}_m(p)$ functions are normalized according to

$$\int_{-\infty}^{\infty} \bar{\psi}_l^*(p)\bar{\psi}_m(p)\, dp = \frac{1}{2\pi}\delta_{lm} \tag{5.9.7}$$

Matching the tangential fields at the $z = 0$ interface, we obtain

$$\tau(p) = \bar{\psi}_m(p) + \sum_{m'=1}^{\infty} \rho_{mm'}\bar{\psi}_{m'}(p) \tag{5.9.8a}$$

$$q\tau(p) = \beta_m\bar{\psi}_m(p) - \sum_{m'=1}^{\infty} \rho_{mm'}\beta_{m'}\bar{\psi}_{m'}(p) \tag{5.9.8b}$$

In principle these two equations can be used to calculate the reflection and transmission coefficients. The difficulty arises because there are an infinite number (discrete and continuum) of coefficients to calculate. Consequently, we use approximate methods for calculating $\rho_{mm'}$ by truncating the series and using only the trapped modes, since for small dielectric steps there is very little power scattered into the continuous modes. Multiplying (5.9.8b) by $\bar{\psi}_l^*(p)$ and using the orthogonality relations (5.9.7), we obtain

$$\int_{-\infty}^{\infty} q\tau(p)\bar{\psi}_l^*(p)\, dp = \frac{1}{2\pi}\beta_m\,\delta_{lm} - \frac{1}{2\pi}\rho_{ml}\beta_l \tag{5.9.9}$$

We now substitute $\tau(p)$ from (5.9.8a) into (5.9.9), obtaining

$$\sum_{m'=1}^{M} \rho_{mm'}(q_{lm'} + \frac{1}{2\pi}\beta_l\delta_{lm'}) = \frac{1}{2\pi}\beta_m\delta_{lm} - q_{lm} \tag{5.9.10}$$

where the matrix element $q_{lm'}$ is

$$q_{lm'} = \int_{-\infty}^{\infty} \bar{\psi}_l^*(p)q\,\bar{\psi}_{m'}(p)\, dp \tag{5.9.11}$$

The results (5.9.10) form a linear set of equations, allowing us to determine the elements $\rho_{mm'}$. Using the following matrix definition

$$B = \frac{1}{2\pi}\begin{pmatrix} \beta_1 & 0 & \cdots & 0 \\ 0 & \beta_2 & \cdots & 0 \\ 0 & 0 & \cdots & \beta_M \end{pmatrix} \tag{5.9.12}$$

we get the reflection matrix

$$P = (B - Q^t)(B + Q^t)^{-1} \tag{5.9.13}$$

where we use $P = (\rho_{ij})$, $Q = (q_{ij})$, $Q^t = (q_{ji})$. For the case $M = 1$, we find

$$\rho_{11} = (-\beta_1 - 2\pi q_{11})/(\beta_1 + 2\pi q_{11}) \tag{5.9.14}$$

In Fig. 5.9.2 we show the facet reflectivity of a waveguide–air interface for the fundamental mode as a function of the waveguide parameters. The field solutions are determined for a simple symmetrical double-heterojunction structure as a function of the cavity width d_3 and Δn. The lasing wavelength

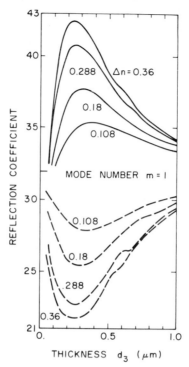

FIG. 5.9.2   Facet reflection coefficient for the fundamental transverse waveguide mode of a double-heterojunction laser as a function of the thickness of the active layer d_3. Parameter Δn is the index discontinuity between the waveguide and the surrounding material. Solid lines represent TE waves, broken lines indicate TM waves [32].

$\lambda_L = 0.86\ \mu$m. Note that the reflectivity for the TE modes increases with the dielectric discontinuity whereas the reflectivity decreases for the TM modes.

To determine the role played by the facet reflectivity in modal discrimination, we show in Fig. 5.9.3 the normalized end loss $\alpha_L = \ln\,(1/R_m)$ for the trapped waveguide modes as a function of cavity width d_3. An index discontinuity of 5% gives $\Delta n = 0.18$. It is clear that the high order TE modes have the smallest end losses and that $\alpha_{\mathrm{endTE}} < \alpha_{\mathrm{endTM}}$.

The power scattered into the radiation modes can of course be calculated by not truncating the continuous mode terms of (5.9.8). This power can be determined theoretically by a rather lengthy mathematical formulation. Consequently, we show only the results obtained from the computer calculations [34]. Figure 5.9.4 shows the contours of constant S_s for various waveguide thicknesses and dielectric steps. The value κ_3 pertains to PbSnTe lasers. In the calculations, it is assumed that the fundamental mode is incident on the laser facet. For normalized thicknesses $D_3 > \pi$, the second-order mode can

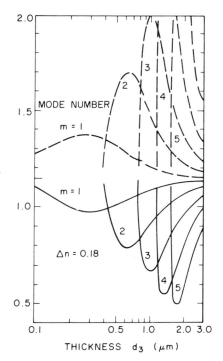

FIG. 5.9.3   Plots of ln $(1/R_m)$ for the mth transverse mode as a function of the active layer thickness of a double-heterojunction laser. The index step $\Delta n = 0.18$ [32].

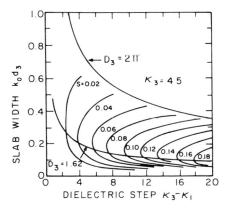

FIG. 5.9.4   Contours of constant S_s, the fraction of power incident on the mirror in the TE mode which is coupled into the radiation modes of the laser waveguide, for various normalized thicknesses of the guiding region $k_0 d_3$ and dielectric steps $\kappa_3 - \kappa_1$. The dielectric constant $\kappa_3 = 45$. Above the curve labeled $D_3 = 2\pi$, the TE$_3$ mode propagates and the theory does not apply. The curve labeled $D_3 = 1.62$ is the locus of minimum effective width for the fundamental mode [34].

propagate; however, there will be no scatter into the TE_2 mode since there is no power conversion between even and odd modes. Consequently, only one trapped mode is used in the calculations. The curve $k_0 d_3 (\kappa_3 - \kappa_1)^{1/2} = 1.62$ is the locus of the effective guide width for the TE_1 mode, defined by

$$D_{\text{eff}} = (D_3 + 2/H_1)$$

The waveguide is symmetrical. Note that for small index steps, the scattering coefficient $S_s \ll 1$.

5.10   Mode Selection in Laser Structures

The gain distribution and the end facet refleetivity play major roles in selecting the cavity mode operation. The gain distribution produces mode discrimination because of the way the modes interact with the active region. For example, the mode which has the largest fraction of its field intensity in the gain region will have the largest optical gain, assuming that the remaining passive regions have the same absorption coefficient. The facet reflectivity affects the order of mode operation; however, its major effect is on the mode group operation, i.e., TE or TM.

For the purpose of illustration, we analyze the threshold gain characteristic of two large cavity devices: the LOC, where the active region is located adjacent to the $p-p^+$ heterojunction, and a modified LOC device, where the active region is moved further into the optical cavity. The modified LOC consists of three regions within the two outer heterojunctions (spaced d^0). Within the large optical cavity the recombination region is surrounded by two lossy regions: region 2 is p-GaAs, and region 4 is n-GaAs. Threshold gain characteristics of the LOC are obtained by varying the total width d^0 while keeping the width d_3 constant. In the modified LOC, we keep the total width d^0 constant and vary d_2 and d_4, the displacement of the active region (within the optical cavity) from the $p-p^+$ heterojunction. In particular, it is found that when the active region is placed in the center of the optical cavity, the active region has a tendency to interact strongly with those electromagnetic modes that have peaks in the center of the cavity, whereas those modes that have null points at the center of the cavity interact weakly with the active region.

For the five-layer model, the threshold gain G_{th} of the active region for a device with $\alpha_{\text{end}} = 0$, $\alpha_{\text{fc}} = 0$ is

$$a_3 G_{\text{th}} = \sum_{i \neq 3} \alpha_i a_i \qquad (5.10.1)$$

Let us now consider a simplified case where in the five-layer model we assume $d_2 = 0$, $n_3 = n_4$, and $n_1 = n_5$. The variation of the index of refraction, for this simplified model, as a function of position across the LOC is shown in Fig. 5.10.1. In the calculation of G_{th}, the active region width is kept constant,

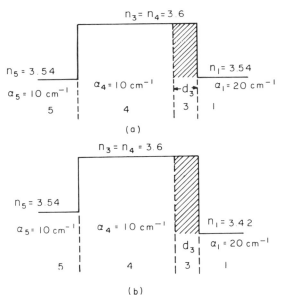

FIG. 5.10.1   The simplified model of the index of refraction as a function of position across the optical cavity: (a) Symmetrical waveguide $(n_1 = n_5)$, and (b) asymmetrical waveguide $(n_1 < n_5)$.

$d_3 = 0.5\ \mu$m, and the width of the optical cavity is varied. The threshold gain curves for the various modes as a function of cavity width are shown in Fig. 5.10.2a. Note that for a heterojunction index discontinuity of 0.06, the gain curves show that the second mode reaches threshold first in a 2-μm cavity, the third mode reaches threshold first in a 3-μm cavity, and so on. Also for large cavity widths at or near the crossover points of the G_{th} curves, the modal selection between the high order modes becomes less pronounced, and other factors such as cavity end losses should be considered as a competing factor in modal selection. For example, we have shown earlier that the mirror reflectivity for TE modes increases with increasing order whereas for TM modes it decreases with increasing mode order. In addition, the mirror reflectivity of TE modes is larger than that for TM modes. Therefore, considering reflectivity, higher order TE modes are preferred. It is clear that the threshold gain for the fundamental mode becomes extremely large in wide optical cavities, making their dominance unlikely. The fact that G_{th} for a particular mode is infinite below certain cavity widths simply indicates that the mode cannot propagate in the cavity.

   In the preceding paragraph, we discussed the threshold gain curves for a symmetrical LOC structure. Let us now consider the gain curves for an *asymmetrical* LOC structure, shown in Fig. 5.10.1b with the waveguide parameters

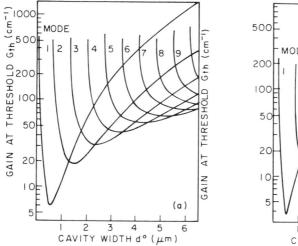
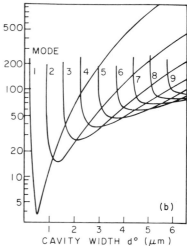

FIG. 5.10.2 Threshold gain curves for the different transverse cavity modes of the LOC structure of Fig. 5.10.1: (a) symmetrical structure and (b) asymmetrical structure.

used in the calculations. Note that the asymmetry is 3 : 1 with more of the mode energy leaking toward region 5. The threshold gain curves for the asymmetrical cavity are shown in Fig. 5.10.2b. The major difference between the two sets of curves of Fig. 5.10.2 occurs near the cutoff region for the different modes; the asymmetrical cavity produces sharper cutoff curves.

Consider next the effect of displacing the active region toward the center of the cavity (i.e., away from the outer heterojunctions), and observe the change in the modal selection. When $d_2 = 0$, the active region is at the edge of the cavity, and when $d_2 = (d^0 - d_3)/2$. the active region is centered within the cavity. Note that we neglect any index differences *between* the outer heterojunctions. We assume $n_2 = n_3$ and $\alpha_2 = \alpha_1$; the total guide width $d^0 = 4\,\mu m$. The threshold gains for different modes as a function of displacement of the active region toward the center of the cavity are plotted in Fig. 5.10.3. In Fig. 5.10. 3a, we see that as d_2 increases, the required gain of the fundamental mode decreases whereas the gain of all higher order modes goes through oscillations. Note that for the symmetrical cavity, fundamental mode operation is possible if d_2 ranges from 0.95 to 1.75 μm, the best possibility for obtaining fundamental mode operation is when $d_2 = 1.4\,\mu m$, where the difference in gain between the fundamental mode and the high order modes is approximately 35 cm^{-1}. In Fig. 5.10.3b, d_2 ranges from 0.9 to 1.5 μm for the fundamental mode operation; the optimum value of $d_2 = 1.1\,\mu m$ with a difference in gain between the fundamental mode and the lowest high order mode of 90 cm^{-1}. Thus while the active region is at the edge of the cavity, the propagation of the fundamental mode is not possible because of the high threshold gain. However, by displacing the active region we can encourage fundamental mode operation in thick

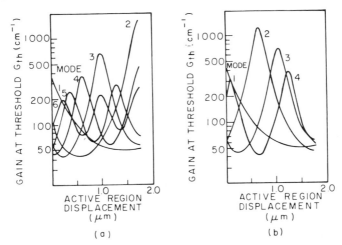

FIG. 5.10.3 The effect of active region displacement on the gain at threshold for (a) symmetrical structure and (b) asymmetrical structure. Parameters are shown in Fig. 5.10.1, with $d_3 = 0.5\ \mu m$, $d^\circ = 4\ \mu m$, and active region displacement obtained by varying d_2.

structures. As we will see in Chapter 7, the four-heterojunction structure incorporates these concepts (Fig. 5.1.3f).

Threshold gain is also a function of the absorption coefficient of the different regions and the thickness of the active region. The larger the absorption coefficients of the passive regions or the narrower the active region, the larger is the threshold gain, which means that higher threshold current will be needed for lasing. Even though the variation of the absorption coefficients or the change in thickness of the active region changes the threshold gain and, as a result, alters the mode selection, the overall shape of the gain curves remains similar to those of Fig. 5.10.3. In the following chapter, we discuss practical devices which behave similarly to those discussed herein. In fact, the four-heterojunction device minimizes the absorption coefficient within the waveguide by making regions 2 and 4 of a slightly higher bandgap material than the active region 3.

REFERENCES

1. F. Stern, Stimulated emission in semiconductors, *in Semiconductors and Semimetals* (R. K. Willardson and A. C. Beer, eds.), Vol. 2. Academic Press, New York, 1966.
2. A. L. McWhorter, *Solid State Electron.* **6**, 417 (1963).
3. A. L. McWhorter, H. J. Zeiger, and B. Lax, *J. Appl. Phys.* **34**, 235 (1963).
4. A. Yariv and R. C. C. Leite, *Appl. Phys. Lett.* **2**, 55 (1963).
5. R. N. Hall, G. E. Fenner, J. D. Kingsley, T. J. Soltys, and R. O. Carlson, *Phys. Rev. Lett.* **9**, 366 (1962).
6. M. I. Mathan, W. P. Dumke, G. Burns, F. H. Dill, Jr., and G. Lasher, *Appl. Phys. Lett.* **1**, 63 (1962).
7. T. M. Quist *et al.*, *Appl. Phys. Lett.* **1**, 91 (1962).

8.   H. Kressel and H. Nelson, *RCA Rev.* **30**, 106 (1969).
9.   I. Hayashi, M. B. Panish, and P. W. Foy, *IEEE J. Quantum Electron.* **5**, 211 (1969).
10. Zh. I. Alferov, V. M. Andreev, E. L. Portni, and M. K. Trukhan, *Sov. Phys.—Semi-cond.* **3**, 1328 (1969). *English Trans*: **3**, 1107 (1970)].
11. M. B. Panish, I. Hayashi, and S. Sumski, *Appl. Phys. Lett.* **16**, 326 (1970).
12. H. Kressel and F. Z. Hawrylo, *Appl. Phys. Lett.* **17**, 169 (1970).
13. H. F. Lockwood, H. Kressel, H. S. Sommers, Jr., and F. Z. Hawrylo, *Appl. Phys. Lett.* **17**, 499 (1970).
14. H. Kressel, J. K. Butler, F. Z. Hawrylo, H. F. Lockwood, and M. Ettenberg, *RCA Rev.* **32**, 393 (1971).
15. G. H. B. Thompson and P. A. Kirkby, *IEEE J. Quantum Electron.* **9**, 311 (1973).
16. F. Stern, *Solid State Phys.* **15**, 299 (1963).
17. F. Stern, *Phys. Rev.* **133A**, 1653 (1964).
18. J. Zoroofchi and J. K. Butler, *J. Appl. Phys.* **44**, 3697 (1973).
19. L. Mandel and E. Wolf, *Rev. Mod. Phys.* **37**, 231 (1965).
20. R. B. Adler, *Proc. IRE* **40**, 339 (1952).
21. E. Snitzer, *J. Opt. Soc. Am.* **51**, 491 (1961).
22. V. V. Shevchenko, *Continuous Transitions in Open Waveguides*. Golem Press, Boulder, Colorado, 1971.
23. K. Ogawa, W. S. C. Chang, B. L. Sopri, and F. Rosenbaum, *IEEE Quantum. Electron.* **9**, 29 (1973).
24. W. W. Anderson, *IEEE J. Quantum Electron.* **1**, 228 (1965).
25. E. A. J. Marcatili, *Bell Syst. Tech. J.* **48**, 2071 (1969).
26. T. H. Zachos and J. E. Ripper, *IEEE J. Quantum Electron.* **5**, 29 (1969).
27. J. K. Butler, *J. Appl. Phys.* **42**, 4447 (1971).
28. M. Cross, *IEEE J. Quantum Electron.* **9**, 517 (1973).
29. M. J. Adams and M. Cross, *Electron. Lett.* **7**, 569 (1971).
30. F. K. Reinhart, I. Hayashi, and M. B. Panish, *J. Appl. Phys.* **42**, 4466 (1971).
31. E. I. Gordon, *IEEE J. Quantum Electron.* **9**, 772 (1973).
32. T. Ikegami, *IEEE J. Quantum Electron.* **8**, 470 (1972).
33. L. Lewin, *IEEE Trans. Microwave Th. Tech.* **23**, 576 (1975).
34. R. W. Davies and J. N. Walpole, *IEEE J. Quantum Electron.* **12**, 291 (1976).

BIBLIOGRAPHY

R. E. Collin, *Field Theory of Guided Waves*. McGraw-Hill, New York, 1960.
N. S. Kapany and J. J. Burke, *Optical Waveguides*. Academic Press, New York, 1972.
D. Marcuse, *Light Transmission Optics*. Van Nostrand-Rienhold, Princeton New Jersey, 1972.
D. Marcuse, *Theory of Dielectric Optical Waveguides*. Academic Press, New York, 1974.
S. Ramo, J. R. Whinnery and T. Van Duzer, *Fields and Waves in Communcation Electronics*. Wiley, New York, 1960.

Chapter 6

Laser Radiation Fields

6.1 Introduction

The radiation pattern characteristics of different semiconductor lasers are discussed in this chapter. The radiation fields are obtained from the development of the two-and three-dimensional waveguide structures discussed in Chapter 5. When a dielectric waveguide is terminated by cleaving, the modal field incident on the cleaved facet produces the radiation field. Consequently, the radiation field is modal dependent and the modal fields depend on the waveguide geometry.

For slab waveguides, the radiation pattern characteristics depend mainly on the dielectric discontinuities and the width of the guiding slab. The radiation pattern of the fundamental mode has a major lobe and several small subsidiary side lobes. On the other hand, if the laser is operating in a high order transverse mode, one expects to find the "rabbit ear" radiation pattern.

The pattern characteristics derived can be used for either of two purposes: (1) to design a laser device which will produce a prescribed radiation pattern and (2) to analyze laser devices which have been fabricated in the laboratory. For example, it is occasionally difficult to determine the exact waveguide discontinuities from fabrication information. However, the radiation pattern characteristics can be used to obtain index of refraction steps. In Fig. 6.1.1 we show the relevant parameters associated with the pattern characteristics. The y axis is directed along the junction plane whereas the x axis is perpendicular to the junction plane. The figure illustrates the radiation field of the fundamental mode. The half-power beam width in the junction plane is $\theta_{\parallel}$ and the pattern beam width perpendicular to the junction plane is $\theta_{\perp}$.

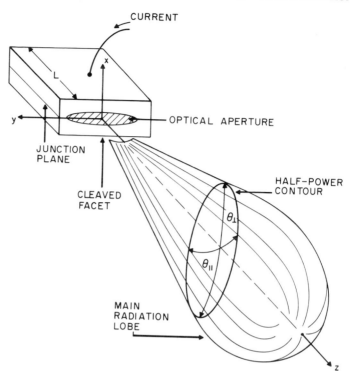

FIG. 6.1.1 Radiation from the end facet of an injection laser. The half-power beam widths $\theta_\perp$ and $\theta_\parallel$ are measured perpendicular and parallel to the junction plane, respectively.

6.2 Radiation from Slab Waveguides

In this section we develop the pattern characteristics produced by simple slab waveguides. This is presented as an aid to understanding some of the pattern characteristics due to the refraction properties of plane waves. In the next section we develop the radiation fields on a more rigorous basis.

A first-order approximation of the radiation pattern in the plane perpendicular to the p–n junction is obtained mathematically by taking the Fourier transform of the electric field at the emitting laser facet. [1–5]. If the laser is operating in a single waveguide mode, then the field at the facet is assumed to have a distribution identical to that of the mode. This simple approach, which treats the laser facet as an antenna aperture, can be used to determine some of the important characteristics of the radiation fields, but a more refined method is needed in order to deduce some of the fine structure of the pattern and to obtain more accurate predictions of $\theta_\perp$.

The method discussed here is sufficient for engineering approximations and it can be used for the calculation of radiation patterns of multiple-layer devices as well as other complicated index of refraction graded slab waveguides. The effects of mode conversion at the waveguide–air interface are neglected in the theory presented here [6].

For the sake of simplicity, we consider only the radiation of TE waves (electric field parallel to the junction plane). The modal field transmitted across the waveguide–air interface is found by decomposing the modal field into a spectrum of plane waves and then determining the transmission characteristics of each plane wave member of the spectrum. It is found that the radiation pattern in the plane perpendicular to the junction plane is the product of the Fourier transform of the waveguide modal field and an angular function which is called the Huygens obliquity factor. The Huygens obliquity factor has an effect of reducing the radiation intensity at large angles from the facet normal and consequently reducing the radiation pattern beam width from that obtained using only the Fourier transform of the near-field distribution.

As a model for studying the radiation characteristics of simple laser structures we consider a slab waveguide radiating into free space. The coordinate system and its orientation relative to the slab guide are shown in Fig. 5.9.1.

A discussion of the radiation fields is related to the modal fields on the laser–air interface. When the fields on the laser facet are completely specifièd, the radiation pattern can be found using the simple Kirchhoff–Huygens approximation. This method does not adequately describe the pattern at angles approaching 90° with respect to the normal to the laser facet (along the x axis), because it does not yield the sharp nulls in the experimental profiles at $\pm 90°$ (Fig. 6.2.1) [7]. (The discrepancy is due to insufficient field specification on the laser facet.) To understand these nulls consider the waveguide modal fields radiated by a pair of plane waves propagating in the dielectric slab. Figure 6.2.1 shows the slab and one of the single plane waves with the corresponding reflected and transmitted waves. When the angle of incidence θ' is

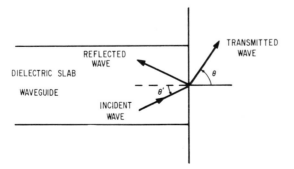

FIG. 6.2.1 A plane wave component incident on the waveguide–air interface. In GaAs waveguides where the index of refraction is 3.6, an incident angle $\theta' \sim 16.1°$ gives $\theta = 90°$.

greater than the critical angle (16.1° for GaAs–air interface) there is no transmitted power. Consequently for $\theta \sim 90°$ ($\theta' \sim 16.1°$), the radiation field
should have a null. The theoretical derivation given here predicts the nulls
and consequently allows an accurate method of analyzing far-field readiation
patterns [8].

For TE waves the component E_y can be written

$$E_y = E_0\psi(x) \exp(i\omega t - \gamma z) \tag{6.2.1}$$

The cross section function $\psi(x)$ can be expressed as

$$\psi(x) = \int_{-\infty}^{\infty} \bar{\psi}(p) e^{-ipx} dp \tag{6.2.2a}$$

where

$$\bar{\psi}(p) = \frac{1}{2\pi} \int_{-\infty}^{\infty} \psi(x) e^{ipx} dx \tag{6.2.2b}$$

A plane wave integral representation of the waveguide mode is given by

$$E_y = E_0 e^{i\omega t} \int_{-\infty}^{\infty} \bar{\psi}(p) \exp(-ipx - \gamma z) dp \tag{6.2.3a}$$

The magnetic field components become

$$H_z = E_0 \frac{e^{i\omega t}}{k_0\eta_0} \int_{-\infty}^{\infty} p\bar{\psi}(p) \exp(-ipx - \gamma z) dp \tag{6.2.3b}$$

$$H_x = \frac{iE_0\gamma}{k_0\eta_0} e^{i\omega t} \int_{-\infty}^{\infty} \bar{\psi}(p) \exp(-ipx - \gamma z) dp \tag{6.2.3c}$$

The magnetic field is determined from E_y using (5.4.3a). A plane wave component of the representation in (6.2.3) is

$$E_y(p) = E_0 e^{i\omega t} \bar{\psi}(p) \exp[-i(px + \beta z)] e^{-\alpha z} \tag{6.2.4}$$

Equation (6.2.4) represents a plane wave propagating in a homogeneous
medium with a propagation constant $k' = (p^2 + \beta^2)^{1/2}$. The wave front is
directed at an angle θ' with respect to the z axis as illustrated in Fig. 6.2.2.
(We also show the magnetic field impinging on an interface with the corresponding reflected and transmitted fields.) The angle $\theta' = \cos^{-1}(\beta/k')$ is
determined from (6.2.4). Snell's law is used to find θ, $\sin \theta / \sin \theta' = \bar{n}$, where
$\bar{n} = k'/k_0$ so that $\sin \theta = p/k_0$. In region 1, $\eta_1 = E_y^i/H_x^i = -i\eta_0 k_0/\gamma$, in
region 2, $\eta_2 = E_y^t/H_x^t = -\eta_0 k_0/(k_0^2 - p^2)^{1/2}$ and η_1, η_2 are the wave impedances in regions 1 and 2, respectively, of Fig. 6.2.2. The field reflection and
transmission coefficients are

$$\rho = (\eta_2 - \eta_1)/(\eta_2 + \eta_1), \qquad \tau = 2\eta_2/(\eta_2 + \eta_1)$$

so that $E_y^r = \rho E_y^i$ and $E_y^t = \tau E_y^i$. The resulting fields are

$$E_y^r = \frac{-(k_0^2 - p^2)^{1/2} - i\gamma}{(k_0^2 - p^2)^{1/2} - i\gamma} E_0 \bar{\psi}(p) \exp[-i(px - \beta z) e^{\alpha z}] \tag{6.2.5a}$$

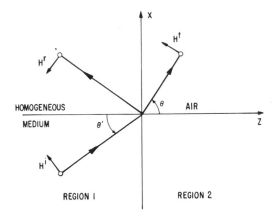

FIG. 6.2.2 Incident plane wave in a homogeneous medium with the transmitted and reflected waves. The electric field is perpendicular to the xz plane, along the y axis.

$$E_y^t = \frac{-2i\gamma}{(k_0^2 - p^2)^{1/2} - i\gamma} E_0 \,\bar{\psi}(p)\, \exp[-i(px + qz)] \qquad (6.2.5b)$$

where $p^2 + q^2 = k_0^2$. The time variation $e^{i\omega t}$ has been omitted. The integral forms of the reflected and transmitted fields become

$$E_y^r = E_0 \, e^{+\gamma z} \int_{-\infty}^{\infty} \frac{q + i\gamma}{q - i\gamma} \bar{\psi}(p)\, e^{-ipx}\, dp \qquad (6.2.6a)$$

$$E_y^t = -2i\gamma E_0 \int_{-\infty}^{\infty} \frac{1}{q - i\gamma} \bar{\psi}(p)\, \exp[-i(px + qz)]\, dp \qquad (6.2.6b)$$

where $[k_0^2 - p^2]^{1/2}$ has been replaced by q. The conditions on p and q require $\mathrm{Im}[q] < 0$, where Im is the imaginary part of the term in braces. Equation (6.2.6) gives the reflected and transmitted fields when there is no modal conversion at the waveguide discontinuity (waveguide–air interface). In general, there will be small amounts of power going into other waveguide modes (both continuous and discrete) in the reflected field (6.2.6a); however, this modal conversion has been estimated to be less than 0.5%.

If the integration variable p in (6.2.6b) is changed to w by the transformation

$$p = k_0 \sin w \qquad (6.2.7)$$

where $w = u + iv$, and we put $z = r \cos \theta$, $x = r \sin \theta$, the transmitted fields become

$$E_y^t = -i2E_0 k_0 \gamma \int_c \frac{\cos w \, \bar{\psi}(k_0 \sin w)\, \exp[-ik_0 r \cos(\theta - w)]}{k_0 \cos w - i\gamma}\, dw \qquad (6.2.8)$$

Integration is carried out over the contour c in Fig. 6.2.3. Note that on c $\mathrm{Im}\{q\} = -k_0 \sin u \sinh v < 0$. The point $p = -\infty$ corresponds to a point in

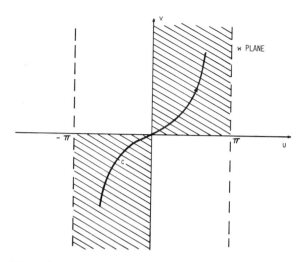

FIG. 6.2.3 Integration contour in the w plane used for the calculation of the radiation fields. The contour is along the path of steepest descent.

the shaded region where $v = -\infty$, whereas the point $p = +\infty$ corresponds to a point in the shaded region and $v = +\infty$.

In the radiation zone, $k_0 r \gg 1$, the integral (6.2.8) can be approximated by saddle point integration or by the stationary phase method:

$$E_y^t(r,\theta) = -ik_0\gamma E_0 \frac{4\pi \exp(ik_0 r)}{(k_0 r)^{1/2}} \frac{\cos\theta\,\bar{\psi}(k_0\sin\theta)}{k_0\cos\theta - i\gamma} \qquad (6.2.9)$$

Note that in (6.2.9) the field decays as $r^{-1/2}$, which is the usual condition for the radiation zone in cylindrical systems. Theoretically, a finite source can be treated as infinite provided the radial distance from the line source is small compared to the length of the source. Also, the transverse dimension of the aperture must be small compared to its width. (For example, the facet width W is of the order of 100 μm parallel to the junction, and has a thickness which is ≤ 10 μm.) When the observation point is a large distance from the source ($r \gg W$), the approximation (6.2.9) becomes poor. In this case the field strengths should not only decay as r^{-1} but in addition have a field variation in the plane of the junction. On the other hand, the behavior of the pattern in the plane perpendicular to the junction will have a functional dependence on θ as given by (6.2.9).

The intensity pattern is

$$I(\theta) = I_0 \frac{\cos^2\theta\,|\bar{\psi}(k_0\sin\theta)|^2}{|k_0\cos\theta - i\gamma|^2} \qquad (6.2.10)$$

Since $\gamma = i\beta$, and n_1, $n_5 < \beta/k_0 < n_3$, the intensity pattern can be approximated as

$$I(\theta) \simeq I_0 \frac{\cos^2 \theta}{(\cos \theta + n_3)^2} \, |\bar{\psi}(k_0 \sin \theta)|^2 \tag{6.2.11}$$

The term $\cos \theta + n_3 \simeq n_3$ so that the intensity pattern is the square of the product of $\cos \theta$ with the Fourier transform of the modal field distribution. For the trapped modes in a three-layer structure, $\bar{\psi}$ is given by (5.9.6).

6.3   Boundary Solution of the Radiation Fields

The radiation field produced by an injection laser can be derived by treating the facet as a standard antenna aperture [9,10]. Both the trapped and radiation modes have field distributions that extend to infinity along both the x and y directions of the aperture, as shown in Fig. 6.3.1. For the one-dimensional modes of slab waveguides treated in Chapter 5, the field quantities will not vary along the y direction. The angular variables θ and ϕ and also indicated in the figure.

In the region $z > 0$, the field quantities satisfy the wave equation; in particular, for $\exp(i\omega t)$ time variation

$$\nabla^2 \mathbf{E} + k_0^2 \mathbf{E} = 0 \tag{6.3.1}$$

where $\mathbf{E}$ may be directed in an arbitrary direction, and k_0 is the free-space

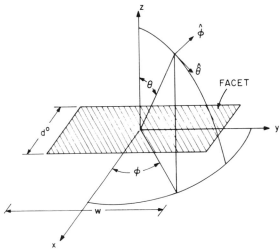

FIG. 6.3.1   The orientation of the coordinate system with respect to the laser facet. The z axis is directed normal to the facet whereas the x and y coordinates lie in the plane of the facet.

wave number. As in Chapter 4, we write the solution of (6.3.1) as a linear superposition of plane waves of the form*

$$E(x,y,z) = \int_{-\infty}^{\infty} \int_{-\infty}^{\infty} e(k_x,k_y) \exp[-i(k_x x + k_y y + k_z z)] \, dk_x \, dk_y \quad (6.3.2)$$

where

$$k_z^2 = k_0^2 - k_x^2 - k_y^2 \quad (6.3.3)$$

Note that (6.3.2) contains only two integration variables, k_x and k_y, since the other, k_z in our case, is constrained by (6.3.3). When $k_x^2 + k_y^2 > k_0^2$, $\text{Im}\{k_z\}$ < 0, so that the fields remain finite at $z = \infty$. The components k_x, k_y, k_z form the wave vector $\mathbf{k} = \hat{\mathbf{x}}k_x + \hat{\mathbf{y}}k_y + \hat{\mathbf{z}}k_z$, so that (6.3.2) can be written as

$$E(x,y,z) = \int_{-\infty}^{\infty} \int_{-\infty}^{\infty} e(k_x, k_y) \exp(-i\mathbf{k} \cdot \mathbf{r}) \, dk_x \, dk_y \quad (6.3.4)$$

Since the region $z > 0$ is source free, $\mathbf{V} \cdot \mathbf{E} = 0$. This implies that the three vector components of $\mathbf{e}$ satisfy

$$\mathbf{e} \cdot \mathbf{k} = 0 \quad (6.3.5)$$

so that strictly speaking, the radiation field has only two independent components. For example,

$$e_z = (\mathbf{e}_t \cdot \mathbf{k}_t)/k_z \quad (6.3.6)$$

where the subscript t implies the transverse x and y components.

At $z = 0$, it is seen that $\mathbf{E}(x,y,0)$ is the Fourier transform of $e(k_x, k_y)$. For the inverse transform, we obtain

$$e(k_x, k_y) = \frac{1}{4\pi^2} \int_{-\infty}^{\infty} \int_{-\infty}^{\infty} \mathbf{E}(x,y,0) \exp(i\mathbf{k}_t \cdot \mathbf{r}_t) \, dx \, dy \quad (6.3.7)$$

Because of the dependence of e_z on $\mathbf{e}_t$ [Eq. (6.3.6)], it is clear that the radiation field can be determined from only the *transverse facet* electric field $\mathbf{E}_f(x,y) = \mathbf{E}_t(x,y,0)$

$$e_t(k_x, k_y) = \frac{1}{4\pi^2} \int_{-\infty}^{\infty} \int_{-\infty}^{\infty} \mathbf{E}_f(x,y) \exp(i\mathbf{k}_t \cdot \mathbf{r}_t) \, dx \, dy \quad (6.3.8)$$

Thus, $\mathbf{e}(k_x, k_y)$ is the Fourier transform of the tangential electric field on the laser facet.

From Maxwell's equation $H = (i/k_0\eta_0) \nabla \times E$, the magnetic field is determined from (6.3.4):

$$H(x,y,z) = \frac{1}{k_0\eta_0} \int_{-\infty}^{\infty} \int_{-\infty}^{\infty} \mathbf{k} \times e(k_x, k_y) \exp(-i\mathbf{k} \cdot \mathbf{r}) \, dk_x \, dk_y \quad (6.3.9)$$

*Here we use k_x, k_y, and k_z as the plane wave propagation constants along the directions x, y, and z, respectively.

If the magnetic field is given on the laser facet, then

$$\mathbf{k} \times \mathbf{e}(k_x, k_y) = \frac{k_0 \eta_0}{4\pi^2} \int_{-\infty}^{\infty} \int_{-\infty}^{\infty} \mathbf{H}(x,y,0) \exp(i\mathbf{k}_t \cdot \mathbf{r}_t) \, dx \, dy \quad (6.3.10)$$

The far-zone fields can be determined from (6.3.4). Transforming to spherical coordinates, $x = r \sin \theta \cos \phi$, $y = r \sin \theta \sin \phi$ and $z = r \cos \theta$, the argument of the exponential becomes

$$\mathbf{k} \cdot \mathbf{r} = r(k_x \sin \theta \cos \phi + k_y \sin \theta \sin \phi + k_z \cos \theta)$$

In the radiation zone, r is very large, so that (6.3.4) can be evaluated by the stationary phase method:

$$\mathbf{E}(r, \theta, \phi) = \frac{2\pi i k_0 \exp(-ik_0 r)}{r} [\hat{\phi}(e_y \cos \phi - e_x \sin \phi) \cos \theta$$

$$+ \hat{\theta}(e_x \cos \phi + e_y \sin \phi)] \quad (6.3.11)$$

where $\mathbf{e}(k_x, k_y) = \mathbf{e}(k_0 \cos \phi \sin \theta, k_0 \sin \phi \sin \theta)$. Since the radiation pattern is the angular distribution of the electric field at a constant distance r from the radiating facet it is written as

$$\mathbf{E}(\theta, \phi) = C[\hat{\phi}(e_y \cos \phi - e_x \sin \phi) \cos \theta + \hat{\theta}(e_x \cos \phi + e_y \sin \phi)] \quad (6.3.12)$$

In the xz plane, $\phi = 0$, and the radiation pattern becomes

$$\mathbf{E}(\theta, \phi = 0) = C(\hat{\phi} \cos \theta e_y + \hat{\theta} e_x) \quad (6.3.13)$$

The unit vector $\hat{\phi}$ points along the positive y axis for all values of θ whereas the unit vector $\hat{\theta}$ points along the x axis when $\theta = 0$ and points along the negative z axis when $\theta = \pi/2$. For example, if the facet field has only an e_y component, then the pattern in the xz plane is

$$E_\phi = C \cos \theta e_y(k_0 \sin \theta, 0) \quad (6.3.14)$$

while for a field polarized along x, e, the pattern in the zx plane becomes

$$E_\theta = C e_x(k_0 \sin \theta, 0) \quad (6.3.15)$$

The field behavior in the yz plane is found by placing $\phi = \pi/2$. Now the unit vector $\hat{\phi}$ points along the negative x axis for all θ values whereas $\hat{\theta}$ is directed along positive y when $\theta = 0$ and along negative z when $\theta = \pi/2$.

For the special case of a one-dimensional aperture when, for example, the field quantities are independent of y, a similar derivation of the radiation fields can be obtained. Expression (6.3.2) becomes

$$\mathbf{E}(x, z) = \int_{-\infty}^{\infty} \mathbf{e}(k_x) \exp[-i(k_x x + k_z z)] \, dk_x \quad (6.3.16)$$

and at $z = 0$, $\mathbf{e}(k_x)$ given in terms of the aperture electric and magnetic fields satisfies

$$e(k_x) = \frac{1}{2\pi} \int_{-\infty}^{\infty} E(x, 0) \exp(ik_x x) \, dx \qquad (6.3.17a)$$

$$k \times e(k_x) = \frac{k_0 \eta_0}{2\pi} \int_{-\infty}^{\infty} H(x, 0) \exp(ik_x x) \, dx \qquad (6.3.17b)$$

The transform e satisfies $e \cdot k = 0$ since $\nabla \cdot E = 0$. Note that (6.3.16) is similar to (6.2.6b). The radiation field is obtained by placing $x = r \cos \theta$ and $y = r \sin \theta$. For large r values, (6.3.16) evaluated by the stationary phase method becomes

$$E(r, \theta) = (2\pi i k_0 / r)^{1/2} \cos \theta e(k_0 \sin \theta) \exp(-ik_0 r) \qquad (6.3.18)$$

The radiation pattern has the form

$$E(\theta) = C \cos \theta e(k_0 \sin \theta) \qquad (6.3.19)$$

When the facet field is polarized along y, $e_t = \hat{y} e_y$, then the radiation field

$$E_y(\theta) = C \cos \theta e_y(k_0 \sin \theta) \qquad (6.3.20)$$

On the other hand, for $e_t = \hat{x} e_x$, the θ component of the radiation pattern becomes

$$E_\theta(\theta) = C e_x(k_0 \sin \theta) \qquad (6.3.21)$$

In the derivation of (6.3.21) we use the relation $e_z = -\sin \theta / \cos \theta e_x$. Note that expressions (6.3.20) and (6.3.21) are similar to (6.3.14) and (6.3.15), respectively. The radiation pattern (6.3.20) corresponds to the radiation of TE modes whereas (6.3.21) is for TM modes.

The radiation field in the xz plane for fields polarized along y is given by (6.3.14) and (6.3.20). The quantity e_y is the Fourier transform of the facet field. The radiation pattern is thus the product of $\cos \theta$ and the Fourier transform e_y. On the other hand, for fields polarized along the x direction, the xz plane radiation pattern is given by (6.3.15) and (6.3.21). In this case, the radiation pattern is just the Fourier transform e_x of the facet field distribution.

The facet field distribution is determined from a solution of the boundary value problem resulting from a continuity of the tangential field components at the waveguide–air interface. The tangential electric field Fourier transform for TE slab waveguide modes is given by (5.9.6), which is of course related to the modal facet reflectivities. Consequently, the radiation fields are determined completely only when the exact boundary value problem is solved. However, it is often practical to approximate the radiation pattern for certain cases. For example, if we assume that the TE_m slab waveguide mode $\psi_m(x) \exp(-i\beta_m z)$ is incident on the laser facet, then the tangential electric field is assumed to be $E_y(x, 0) = \psi_m(x)$ and the Fourier transform $e_y(k_x) = \bar{\psi}_m(k_x)$.

6.4   Modal Radiation Patterns from Slab Waveguides

In the preceding section we developed the expression for the radiation fields from the facet field distribution. In this section the approximate expressions for the radiation pattern due to the different trapped waveguide modes are developed [11–13]. In particular, the approximate pattern expressions are determined from the Fourier transform of the laser modal field distribution.

6.4.1   TE Slab Mode Radiation

Assuming that the mth waveguide mode is incident upon the laser facet, then the transverse electric and magnetic fields given by (5.9.1) and (5.9.3) are

$$E_y(x,z) = \psi_m(x) \exp(-i\beta_m z) + \sum_{m'=1}^{\infty} \rho_{mm'}\psi_{m'}(x) \exp(i\beta_{m'} z) \qquad (6.4.1a)$$

$$k_0\eta_0 H_x(x,z) = -\beta_m\psi_m(x) \exp(-i\beta_m z) + \sum_{m'=1}^{\infty} \rho_{mm'}\beta_{m'}\psi_{m'}(x) \exp(i\beta_{m'} z)$$

$$(6.4.1b)$$

As mentioned previously, the summation $\sum_{m'=1}^{\infty}$ implies summation over both the trapped and radiation modes. When $z = 0$ in (6.4.1), we obtain the transverse electric and magnetic fields on the laser facet. Consequently, using (6.3. 17) the aperture transform $\mathbf{e}\,(k_x)$ can be determined from either the tangential electric or magnetic field. For TE modes e_y is the only nonzero component of the facet field. Consequently, we find

$$e_y(k_x) = \bar{\psi}_m(k_x) + \sum_{m'=1}^{\infty} \rho_{mm'}\bar{\psi}_{m'}(k_x) \qquad (6.4.2a)$$

$$k_z e_y(k_x) = \beta_m\bar{\psi}_m(k_x) - \sum_{m'=1}^{\infty} \rho_{mm'}\beta_{m'}\bar{\psi}_{m'}(k_x) \qquad (6.4.2b)$$

where $\bar{\psi}_m(k_x)$ is the Fourier transform of the mth waveguide mode, and $k_z = (k_0^2 - k_x^2)^{1/2}$. In an exact analysis of the boundary value problem, the aperture transform $e_y(k_x)$ can be determined from either of Eqs. (6.4.2). However, it is frequently useful to approximate the facet field from the transform $\bar{\psi}_m(k_x)$ of the incident waveguide mode. In an approximate method which uses either (6.4.2a) or (6.4.2b), one formula may yield a much better approximation than the other. Lewin [13] has discussed an approximate method which is concerned with extracting from the rigorous equations the best results possible for a given order of approximation. If we multiply (6.4.2a) by N, a function of k_x, and add the results to (6.4.2b), we obtain the weighted average

$$e_y(k_x) = \frac{(N + \beta_m)\,\bar{\psi}_m(k_x) + \varDelta}{k_z + N} \qquad (6.4.3)$$

where

$$\Delta = N \sum_{m'=1}^{\infty} \rho_{mm'} \bar{\psi}_{m'}(k_x) - \sum_{m'=1}^{\infty} \rho_{mm'} \beta_{m'} \bar{\psi}_{m'}(k_x) \qquad (6.4.4)$$

The value $\Delta = 0$ when N is given by

$$N = \left[\sum_{m'=1}^{\infty} \rho_{mm'} \beta_{m'} \bar{\psi}_{m'}(k_x) \right] / \left[\sum_{m'=1}^{\infty} \rho_{mm'} \bar{\psi}_{m'}(k_x) \right] \qquad (6.4.5)$$

At this point, (6.4.3) is an exact expression for the aperture field; no approximations have been made. Further, if we retain an expression for N which includes only the radiation modes, then

$$e_y(k_x) = \left[(N + \beta_m) \bar{\psi}_m(k_x) + \sum_{m'=1}^{M} \rho_{mm'} (N - \beta_{m'}) \bar{\psi}_{m'}(k_x) \right] / (k_z + N) \quad (6.4.6)$$

where N is given by

$$N = \left[\sum_{m'=M+1}^{\infty} \rho_{mm'} \beta_{m'} \bar{\psi}_{m'}(k_x) \right] / \left[\sum_{m'=M+1}^{\infty} \rho_{mm'} \bar{\psi}_{m'}(k_x) \right] \qquad (6.4.7)$$

where the summations in (6.4.7) are integrals over the waveguide radiation modes. Determination of the value of N can be made by using the approximate value of the Fourier transform for the radiation mode fields. For example, the radiation modes defined by Case II have an approximate transform

$$\bar{\psi}(k_x) = (A/4\pi)[(a - ib) \delta(k_x + h_1) + (a + ib) \delta(k_x - h_1)]$$

where $\delta(k_x + h_1)$ is the Dirac delta peaking at $k_x = -h_1$. The transform of the Case III mode is also approximated by a series of delta functions. The resulting integrals in (6.4.7) can be evaluated with an approximate value

$$N \simeq (k_1^2 - k_x^2)^{1/2} \qquad (6.4.8)$$

The wave number k_1 is determined from the waveguide dielectic value. Actually, the value of N should be obtained by an average of the form $N = s (k_1^2 - k_x^2)^{1/2} + (1 - s) (k_s^2 - k_x^2)^{1/2}$ where s is a constant. Since most of the laser structures discussed here have index discontinuities less than 20%, we conclude that the N value given by (6.4.8) is relatively accurate.

When a waveguide structure supports only the fundamental cavity mode, $m = M = 1$, (6.4.6) becomes

$$e_y(k_x) = \frac{(1 + \rho_{11})}{k_z + N} \left[N + \frac{1 - \rho_{11}}{1 + \rho_{11}} \beta_1 \right] \psi_1(k_x) \qquad (6.4.9)$$

The radiation pattern is now obtained by substituting (6.4.9) into (6.3.20) where $k_x = k_0 \sin \theta$ in Eq. (6.4.9). The value $N = k_0 [\kappa_1 - \sin^2 \theta]^{1/2}$ will of course vary between $k_0 n_1$ and $k_0 (n_1^2 - 1)^{1/2}$. And since $k_z \ll N$, we conclude that the coefficient of $\bar{\psi}_1 (k_0 \sin \theta)$ in (6.4.9) has only a small variation between $0 < \theta < 90°$. Hence, the radiation pattern is essentially given as the product of $\cos \theta$ and the Fourier transform of the aperture field.

6.4.2   TM Slab Mode Radiation

The radiation characteristics of TM modes can be obtained in a manner similar to that used previously. The field components at the facet are H_y, E_x, and E_z. Assuming that the mth mode is incident upon the waveguide–air interface, the magnetic field in the cavity is

$$H_y(x, z) = \psi_m(x) \exp(-i\beta_m z) + \sum_{m'} \rho_{mm'}\psi_{m'}(x) \exp(i\beta_{m'}z) \qquad (6.4.10a)$$

and the electric field satisfies

$$\frac{k_0}{\eta_0} \kappa(x)E_x(x, z) = \beta_m\psi_m(x) \exp(-i\beta_m z) - \sum_{m'} \rho_{mm'}\beta_{m'}\psi_{m'}(x) \exp(i\beta_{m'}z') $$

$$(6.4.10b)$$

Substituting (6.4.10a) into (6.3.17b), we obtain

$$\frac{k_0}{\eta_0} e_x(k_x) = k_z[\bar{\psi}_m(k_x) + \sum_{m'=1}^{\infty} \rho_{mm'}\bar{\psi}_{m'}(k_x)] \qquad (6.4.11a)$$

while substituting (6.4.10b) into (6.3.17a),

$$\frac{k_0}{\eta_0} e_x(k_x) = \beta_m\bar{\phi}_m(k_x) - \sum_{m'=1}^{\infty} \rho_{mm'}\beta_{m'}\bar{\phi}_{m'}(k_x) \qquad (6.4.11b)$$

Again, $\bar{\psi}_m(k_x)$ is the Fourier transform of $\psi_m(x)$, and $\bar{\phi}_m(k_x)$ is the transform of $\psi_m(x)/\kappa(x)$. The aperture transform $e_x(k_x)$ can be determined from either of these equations provided the reflection coefficients $\rho_{mm'}$ are known. For an approximate solution $e_x(k_x)$ is found from a weighted average of Eq. (6.4.11). Multiplying (6.4.11a) by $N(k_x)$ and adding (6.4.11b), the facet field becomes

$$\frac{k_0}{\eta_0} e_x(k_x) = \frac{k_z[N\bar{\psi}_m(k_x) + \beta_m\bar{\phi}_m(k_x) + \Delta]}{k_z + N} \qquad (6.4.12)$$

where

$$\Delta = N \sum_{m'=1}^{\infty} \rho_{mm'}\bar{\psi}_{m'}(k_x) - \sum_{m=1'}^{\infty} \rho_{mm'}\beta_{m'}\bar{\phi}_{m'}(k_x) \qquad (6.4.13)$$

and $\Delta = 0$ when

$$N = \frac{\sum \rho_{mm'}\beta_{m'}\bar{\phi}_{m'}(k_x)}{\sum \rho_{mm'}\bar{\psi}_{m'}(k_x)} \qquad (6.4.14)$$

When the waveguide supports only the fundamental mode, (6.4.12) can be approximated as discussed in the preceding section:

$$\frac{k_0}{\eta_0} e_x(k_x) = \frac{1 + \rho_{11}}{k_z + N}\left[N\bar{\psi}_1(k_x) + \beta_1 \frac{1 + \rho_{11}}{1 + \rho_{11}} \bar{\phi}_1(k_x)\right] \qquad (6.4.15)$$

where

$$N(k_x) \simeq (k_1^2 - k_x^2)^{1/2}/k_1 \qquad (6.4.16)$$

The radiation pattern is obtained by substituting (6.4.15) into (6.3.21).

6.5   Radiation of Three-Layer Slab Modes

To illustrate the radiation characteristics of the laser modes in the preceding section, patterns obtained from machine calculations are discussed here. In particular, we compare the radiation patterns of TE and TM modes for a narrow symmetric waveguide which supports only the fundamental modes. The appropriate transform for TE modes is

$$\bar{\psi}_1{}^{\mathrm{TE}}(k_x) = \frac{A_1}{\pi} k_0{}^2 (\kappa_3 - \kappa_1) \cos\left[h_3 \frac{d_3}{2}\right] \frac{h_1 \cos[k_x d_3/2] - k_x \sin[k_x d_3/2}{(h_1{}^2 + k_x{}^2)(h_3{}^2 - k_x{}^2)}$$

(6.5.1)

and for TM modes,

$$\bar{\psi}_1{}^{\mathrm{TM}}(k_x) = \frac{A_1}{\pi} \cos\left[h_3 \frac{d_3}{2}\right]\left\{\frac{h_1\cos[k_x d_3/2] - k_x \sin[k_x d_3/2]}{h_1{}^2 + p^2}\right.$$
$$\left. + \frac{(\kappa_3/\kappa_1)\, h_1 \cos[k_x d_3/2] - k_x \sin[k_x d_3/2]}{h_3{}^2 - k_x{}^2}\right\}$$

(6.5.2)

and

$$\bar{\phi}_1{}^{\mathrm{TM}}(k_x) = \frac{A_1}{\kappa_1 \pi} \cos\left[h_3 \frac{d_3}{2}\right]\left\{\frac{h_1 \cos[k_x d_3/2] - k_x \sin[k_x d_3/2]}{h_1{}^2 + k_x{}^2}\right.$$
$$\left. + \frac{h_1 \cos[k_x d_3/2] - (\kappa_1/\kappa_3)\, k_x \sin[k_x d_3/2]}{h_3{}^2 - k_x{}^2}\right\}$$

(6.5.3)

For specific waveguide geometries, h_1 and h_3 can be found from Fig. 5.5.1. Also, the values $h_i{}^{\mathrm{TE}} \simeq h_i{}^{\mathrm{TM}}$ for the usual laser structures fabricated with GaAs–(AlGa)As.

In Fig. 6.5.1 we show the pattern characteristics. Note that the major differences between the TE and TM patterns occur at large angles. On a linear plot, the patterns would be indistinguishable; however, it is interesting to note that the intensity of the TM pattern is larger than that of the TE pattern. This is expected if one considers the reflection characteristics of the modes as discussed in Chapter 5. Considering the plane wave decomposition of the modes as discussed in Section 6.2, the transmission of waves with TM-like polarization increases at the Brewster angle (cf. Fig. 4.8.2), whereas the transmission of waves with TE-like polarization decreases.

6.6   Radiation from Two-Dimensional Waveguides

In Section 6.4, the pattern characteristics produced by one-dimensional modes were discussed. Frequently, the pattern characteristics of the two-dimensional modes can be analyzed in terms of the one-dimensional mode

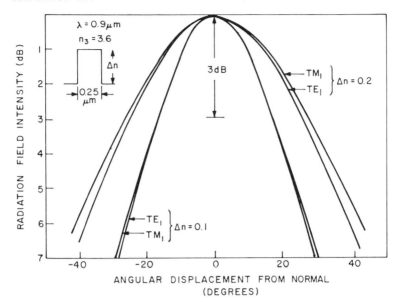

FIG. 6.5.1 The radiation patterns produced by the TE and TM modes radiating from a two-layer slab waveguide. The pattern produced by the TM mode has a half-power beam width $\theta_\perp$ slightly larger than that produced by the TE mode.

patterns. For example, in a laser structure in which $W \gg d^\circ$, W being the guide width in the plane of the junction and d° the width perpendicular to the junction, the radiation pattern will have $\theta_\perp \gg \theta_\parallel$. The half-power beam width $\theta_\perp$ can be determined by analyzing the radiation due to the slab waveguide modes.

The calculation of the radiation pattern can be made provided the facet fields are known. For example, the two-dimensional pattern given by (6.3.12) requires the two-dimensional Fourier transforms, e_x and e_y, of the x and y components of the facet field. Considering the E_{ms}^y modes discussed in Section 5.7, $e_y(k_x, k_y) \neq 0$ and $e_x(k_x, k_y) = 0$. The y component $E_y(x, y, z)$ in the waveguide satisfies

$$E_y(x, y, z) = \psi_{ms}(x, y) \exp(-i\beta_{ms}z) + \sum_{m', s'=1}^{\infty} \rho_{ms, m's'}\psi_{m's'}(x, y) \exp(i\beta_{m's'}z)$$

(6.6.1)

where we have assumed that mode E_{ms}^y is incident upon the laser facet. Note that (6.6.1) is similar to (6.4.1a), the field of the one-dimensional waveguide. The trapped modal wave functions are given by (5.7.4). The radiation modes of the dielectric rectangular waveguide must be determind by a different method from that used to find the trapped modes. In particular, the fields in the shaded regions of Fig. 5.7.1 were neglected for trapped mode calculations whereas the radiation modes have field extensions in all the shaded regions.

The magnetic field H_x can be determined approximately using (5.9.2):

$$k_0\eta_0 H_x(x, y, z) = -\beta_{ms}\psi_{ms}(x, y)\exp(-i\beta_{ms}z)$$
$$+ \sum_{m',s'} P_{ms,m's'}\beta_{m's'}\psi_{m's'}(x, y)\exp(i\beta_{m's'}z) \qquad (6.6.2)$$

At the facet, $z = 0$, so that (6.6.1) can be substituted into (6.3.8), yielding

$$e_y(k_x, k_x) = \bar{\psi}_{ms}(k_x, k_y) + \sum_{m',s'} P_{ms,m's'}\bar{\psi}_{m's'}(k_x, k_y) \qquad (6.6.3)$$

On the other hand, substituting (6.6.2) at $z = 0$ into (6.3.10) gives

$$\frac{k_y^2 + k_z^2}{k_z} e_y(k_x, k_y) = \beta_{ms}\bar{\psi}_{ms}(k_x, k_y) - \sum_{m',s'} P_{ms,m's'}\beta_{m's'}\bar{\psi}_{m's'}(k_x, k_y) \quad (6.6.4)$$

The transform e_y is obtained by performing a weighted average of (6.6.3) and (6.6.4) similar to the technique of Section 6.4. Multiplying (6.6.3) by $N(k_x, k_y)$ and adding to (6.6.4), we obtain

$$e_y(k_x,k_y) = \frac{(N + \beta_{ms})\,\bar{\psi}_{ms}(k_x,k_y) + \Delta}{N + (k_y^2 + k_z^2)/k_z} \qquad (6.6.5)$$

where

$$\Delta = N\sum_{m',s'} P_{ms,m's'}\bar{\psi}_{m's'}(k_x,k_y) - \sum_{m',s'} P_{ms,m's'}\beta_{m's'}\bar{\psi}_{m's'}(k_x, k_y) \qquad (6.6.6)$$

For the fundamental mode, $m = s = 1$, the transform e_y becomes

$$e_y(k_x, k_y) \simeq \frac{(N + \beta_{11})}{N + (k_y^2 + k_z^2)/k_z}\,\bar{\psi}_{11}(k_x, k_y) \qquad (6.6.7)$$

The parameter N is approximated similarly to that of Section 6.4. There are several types of radiation modes of the box waveguide of Fig. 5.7.1. Assume for the moment that β is decreasing. If the index step between regions 3 and 6 is small compared to that between regions 1 and 3, then the first set of radiation modes occurs along regions 6, 3, and 7. Next, the fields begin to leak into regions 1 and 5, and the shaded regions. (We assume here that the indices of the shaded regions are equal to the indices of regions 1 and 5.) As a first-order approximation, we assume

$$N \simeq (k_1^2 - k_x^2 - k_y^2)^{1/2} \qquad (6.6.8)$$

At the stationary phase point $k_x = k_0\cos\phi\sin\theta$, $k_y = k_0\sin\phi\sin\theta$, and $k_z = k_0\cos\theta$. Substituting (6.6.7) into (6.3.12), the far-field pattern is

$$E(\theta, \phi) = C(\hat{\phi}\cos\phi\cos\theta + \hat{\theta}\sin\phi)$$
$$\times \frac{(\kappa_1 - \sin^2\theta)^{1/2} + \beta_{11}/k_0}{(\kappa_1 - \sin^2\theta)^{1/2} + (\sin^2\phi\sin^2\theta + \cos^2\theta)/(\cos\theta)}$$
$$\times \bar{\psi}_{11}(k_0\cos\phi\sin\theta, k_0\sin\phi\sin\theta) \qquad (6.6.9)$$

In the xz plane, $\phi = 0$, so that $E_\phi(\theta, \phi = 0)$ is

$$E_\phi = C \frac{(\kappa_1 - \sin^2 \theta)^{1/2} + \beta_{11}/k_0}{(\kappa_1 - \sin^2 \theta)^{1/2} + \cos \theta} \cos \theta \bar{\psi}_{11}(k_0 \sin \theta, 0) \qquad (6.6.10)$$

whereas in the yz plane, where $\phi = \pi/2$, E is

$$E_\theta = C \frac{(\kappa_1 - \sin^2 \theta)^{1/2} + \beta_{11}/k_0}{\cos \theta(\kappa_1 - \sin^2 \theta)^{1/2} + 1} \cos \theta \bar{\psi}_{11}(0, k_0 \sin \theta) \qquad (6.6.11)$$

The half-power beam width $\theta_\perp$ is determined from (6.6.10) and $\theta_\parallel$ is found from (6.6.11). In passing, we mention the fact that the pattern characteristics of E_{ms}^x box modes are easily derived by simply following the procedure just demonstrated. However, according to the geometry discussed, with $W \gg d°$, the E_{ms}^y modes are dominant in contemporary laser structures.

6.6.1   Radiation Pattern of Box Modes

The radiation field produced by the fundamental mode incident on the laser facet can now be found using (6.6.9). The modal transform $\bar{\psi}_{11}(k_x, k_y)$ is made using (5.7.4). The results are rather complicated; however, no difficulties should be encountered in effecting the proper integration.

6.6.2   Radiation Pattern of Hermite–Gaussian Modes [14–16]

The transform functions of the Hermite–Gaussian modes, given by (5.7.20), are rather simple mathematically because Hermite polynomials transform onto themselves. Before considering the two-dimensional Fourier transform, consider the transformation of the function $X(\xi)$:

$$\bar{X}(p) = \frac{1}{2\pi} \int_{-\infty}^{\infty} X(\xi) \, e^{ip\xi} \, d\xi \qquad (6.6.12)$$

When $X(\xi)$ is given by (5.7.17), $\bar{X}(p)$ becomes [17]

$$\bar{X}(p) = 2^{-1/2}\pi^{-1/2} \exp(-p^2/2) H_{m-1}(p) \begin{cases} (-1)^{(m-1)/2}, & m = 1, 3, 5, \ldots \\ i(-1)^{(m-2)/2}, & m = 2, 4, 6, \ldots \end{cases}$$

$$(6.6.13)$$

Aside from the phase terms, the forms of the even and odd modes are identical. Consequently, the double Fourier transform becomes

$$\bar{\psi}_{ms}(k_x, k_y) = A_{ms} H_{m-1}(2^{-1/2}\bar{x}k_x) H_{s-1}(2^{-1/2}\bar{y}k_y) \times \exp\{-\tfrac{1}{4}[(\bar{x}k_x)^2 + (\bar{y}k_y)^2]\}$$

$$(6.6.14)$$

where A_{ms} contains the appropriate phase terms and other constants. Now substituting (6.6.14) into (6.6.9) we have the radiation pattern of the fundamental mode.

When $m = s = 1$, the Hermite polynomials (5.7.19) have unity values. From (6.6.10) the approximate pattern in the xz plane is

$$E_\phi = C' \cos\theta \exp\{-\frac{1}{4}(\bar{x}k_0 \sin\theta)^2\} \qquad (6.6.15)$$

and from (6.6.11) we estimate the pattern in the yz plane as

$$E_\theta = C' \cos\theta \exp\{-\frac{1}{4}(\bar{y}k_0 \sin\theta)^2\} \qquad (6.6.16)$$

The above expressions apply to large dielectric constant values since we have dropped $[(\kappa_1 - \sin^2\theta)^{1/2} + \beta_{11}/k_0]/[(\kappa_1 - \sin^2\theta)^{1/2} + \cos\theta]$ and $[(\kappa_1 - \sin^2\theta)^{1/2} + \beta_{11}/k_0]/[\cos\theta(\kappa_1 - \sin^2\theta)^{1/2} + 1]$. The A_{11} coefficient is included in C'. From (5.7.20) it is seen that the values of $\bar{x}$ and $\bar{y}$ represent the "spot widths" in the x and y directions at the laser facet. Neglecting the $\cos\theta$ term in (6.6.16) we find that the half-power beamwidth $\theta_{\parallel}$ satisfies

$$\exp\{-\frac{1}{4}[\bar{y}k_0 \sin(\theta_{\parallel}/2)] = 2^{-1/2}$$

giving

$$\theta_{\parallel} = 2\sin^{-1}(0.59(\lambda/\pi)\bar{y}) \qquad (6.6.17)$$

Similarly,

$$\theta_{\perp} = 2\sin^{-1}(0.59(\lambda/\pi)\bar{x}) \qquad (6.6.18)$$

The last two equations are applicable only to narrow beams. Take for example a planar stripe geometry laser with stripe width $S_t = 13~\mu m$. Assuming $\bar{y} \simeq 6~\mu m$ ($\bar{y}$ is generally smaller than S_t) and $\lambda = 0.9~\mu m$, we find from (6.6.17) that $\theta_{\parallel} = 3.2°$.

REFERENCES

1. G. E. Fenner and J. D. Kingsley, *J. Appl. Phys.* **43**, 3204 (1963).
2. R. F. Kazarinov, O. V. Konstantinov, V. I. Perel, and A. L. Efros, *Sov. Phys. Solid State* **7**, 1210 (1965).
3. N. E. Byer and J. K. Butler, *IEEE J. Quantum Electron.* **6**, 291 (1970).
4. M. J. Adams and M. Cross, *Solid-State Electron.* **14**, 865 (1971).
5. H. C. Casey Jr., M. B. Panish, and J. L. Merz, *J. Appl. Phys.* **44**, 5470 (1973).
6. T. Ikegami, *IEEE J. Quantum Electron.* **8**, 470 (1972).
7. H. S. Sommers, Jr., *J. Appl. Phys.* **44**, 3601 (1973).
8. J. K. Butler and J. Zorrofchi, *IEEE J. Quantum Electron.* **10**, 809 (1974).
9. S. Silver, *Microwave Antenna Theory and Design.* McGraw-Hill, New York, 1949.
10. R. E. Collin and F. J. Zucker, *Antenna Theory.* McGraw-Hill, New York, 1969.
11. G. H. Hockham, *Electron. Lett.* **9**, 389 (1973).
12. L. Lewin, *Electron. Lett.* **10**, 134 (1974).
13. L. Lewin, *IEEE Trans. Microwave Th. and Tech.* **23**, 576 (1975).
14. J. C. Dyment, *Appl. Phys. Lett.* **10**, 84 (1967).

15. T. H. Zachos, *Appl. Phys. Lett.* **12**, 318 (1968).
16. T. H. Zachos and J. E. Ripper, *IEEE J. Quantum Electron.* **5**, 29 (1969).
17. A. Erdelyi, W. Magnus, F. Oberhettinger, and F. G. Tricomi, *Table of Integral Transforms.* McGraw-Hill, New York, 1954.

Chapter 7

Modes in Laser Structures: Mainly Experimental

7.1 Introduction

Chapters 5 and 6 discussed the theory of cavity modes in laser diodes using simple dielectric waveguide models. In this chapter we focus on some of the key results relevant to the operation of practical structures, and present comparisons between theory and experiment. In particular, we are concerned with the observed transverse (m) and lateral mode (s) content of laser diodes and the means of controlling them.* Furthermore, we provide design curves which allow the key heterojunction laser parameters such as the far-field beam width and the degree of radiation confinement within the recombination region to be determined.

In Chapter 5, we outlined the major laser diode configurations in the order of their historical development. Figure 5.1.3 shows sketches useful in summarizing the key relationships between the position of the recombination region and that of the optical field in each of the structures.

The common feature of all heterojunction structures is the use of higher bandgap regions adjoining either one or both of the two sides of the active region. Although (AlGa)As alloy devices are the most widely studied and the most important of these structures, other materials can be used and the basic operating principles remain similar. Chapter 13 reviews work which has been done using compounds other than AlAs–GaAs. However, in this chapter, we

---

*A specific mode number is denoted s or m; the highest possible mode number capable of propagating is denoted S or M, respectively.

will use illustrations from the literature concerned with (AlGa)As devices since these provide the maximum degree of control over the laser properties resulting from the ease of constructing lattice-matched (i.e., ideal) hetero-junction structures.

In this chapter we focus on the transverse and lateral modes of laser diodes. The control of longitudinal modes is not usually possible in Fabry–Perot structures, and the distributed-feedback laser (Chapter 15) is specifically de-signed for the purpose of reducing the longitudinal mode content of laser diodes. We had occasion in Chapter 5 to discuss longitudinal modes in laser diodes and their relationship to the refractive index variation with wavelength and cavity length L.

7.2   Double-Heterojunction Lasers

The simplest laser structure to describe is the double-heterojunction laser. The highest order transverse mode which can propagate in the device depends on the thickness of the waveguide region and on the index steps at its bound-aries. Figures 7.2.1a and 7.2.1b show, for example, the field intensity distribu-tion for the fundamental mode (denoted mode $m = 1$) with a single high intensity maximum in the field intensity, and mode 2 (two high intensity maxima) and the corresponding far-field distribution. Figure 7.2.1c shows a microphotograph of a laser operating in the third mode, as indicated by the three maxima in intensity.

Information concerning the dominant transverse mode can be deduced from either near- or far-field measurements, but experimental considerations make the far field the more reliable source. The order of the dominant mode of the cavity can be deduced from the number of lobes in the beam profile. The fundamental mode gives rise to a single major lobe while higher order modes give rise to other lobes; the mode number for $m > 1$ is given by

$$m = 2 + \text{(number of low intensity lobes}$$
$$\text{between the two major lobes)}$$

Other useful data deduced from the radiation pattern are the angular sepa-ration between the two large lobes and the angular width of the lobe. The angular separation between the lobes depends mainly on the dielectric step at the heterojunctions (see Section 12.2.1) whereas the lobe widths are re-lated to the width of the waveguide region [1].

The simplest case to understand is the symmetrical DH laser. Figure 7.2.2 illustrates the change in the preferred transverse mode with increasing hetero-junction spacing d_3 of a DH laser keeping the refractive index steps $\Delta n \approx$ 0.08 [2]. With $d_3 = 0.7 \ \mu$m, only the fundamental mode is excited, as seen in the far-field pattern. Increasing d_3 to 1.1 μm results in a dominant second-order mode, whereas with $d_3 = 2.8 \ \mu$m, the third-order mode is dominant with admixture of the fourth order. Note in Fig. 7.2.2 that the width of the

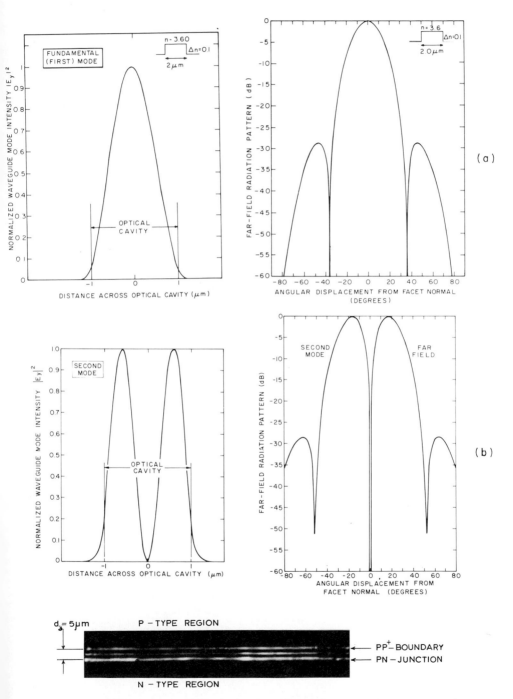

FIG. 7.2.1 Laser near- and far-field patterns of the (a) fundamental transverse mode, and (b) second mode and (c) a microphotograph of a single-heterojunction laser operating in the third mode.

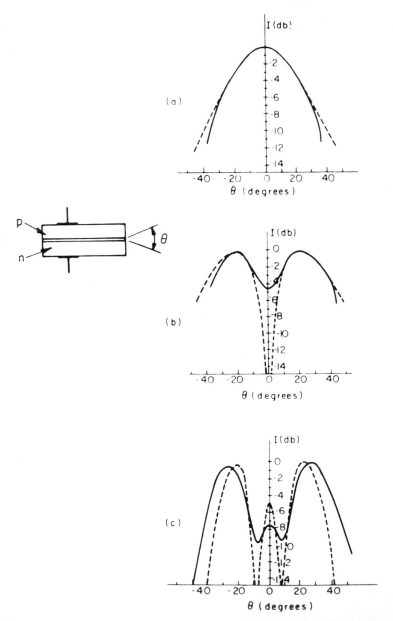

FIG. 7.2.2 Comparison of the experimental (solid lives) and theoretical (broken lives) far-field patterns for double-heterojunction lasers with varying thickness of optical cavity: (a) 0.7 μm, fundamental mode only; (b) 1.1 μm, second mode only; (c) 2.8 μm, third mode with small admixture of the fourth mode. [2].

major lobes decreases with increasing active region width, consistent with the increase in the thickness of the waveguide region (i.e., source size).

It is evident from this that simply increasing the width of the waveguiding region to reduce beam width is not practical. Arbitrarily increasing the width of the waveguiding region not only increases the threshold current density (see Chapter 8) but as we have seen, it results in the propagation of high order transverse modes, and consequently "rabbit ear" far-field patterns. Conversely, decreasing the heterojunction spacing (while keeping the radiation confinement constant) can decrease the threshold current density but at the expense of a broad beam.

A practical compromise between low threshold and moderate beam width is found by using the configuration of the double heterojunction found in Fig. 5.1.3 in which the recombination region (either n-type or p-type) is very narrow and the refractive index steps are moderate, producing optical tails spreading into the adjoining higher bandgap regions [3]. This thin DH structure yields a very practical device for efficient room temperature CW operation.

In the following, we present a series of theoretical plots which show the relationship between the internal device configuration and the near- and far-field distributions. Figure 7.2.3 shows the optical intensity distribution for various heterojunction spacings d_3 and with $\Delta n = 0.1$. Since the total optical power carried is the same in each curve, the increase in the peak intensity reflects the increase of field confinement as d_3 is *increased*. Conversely, as d_3 is *decreased*, an increasing fraction of the power propagates outside the region between the heterojunctions. This near-field intensity distribution is reflected in the breadth of the transverse profile of the beam as shown in Fig. 7.2.3. The beam width *narrows* as d_3 is decreased because this radiation spreading beyond the heterojunction boundaries increases the source size. In Fig. 7.2.4 we show the field intensity plots for various Δn values when $d_3 = 0.2$ μm. The peak field for the structure with $\Delta n = 0.22$ is larger than that for the structure with $\Delta n = 0.06$ since the total mode energy for each structure is identical. Figure 7.2.5 summarizes the change in the peak field intensity within the recombination region as a function of cavity dimension and Δn.

The peak field strength E_0 in the laser cavity can be estimated from the curves in Fig. 7.2.5 in terms of the total radiation power. The fundamental waveguide mode field in a two-dimensional slab waveguide is

$$E(x, z) = E_0 \psi(x) \exp(-i\beta z) \tag{7.2.1}$$

where the fields are normalized in Figs. 7.3.2–7.2.5 as

$$k_0 \int_{-\infty}^{\infty} \psi^2(x)\, dx = 1 \tag{7.2.2}$$

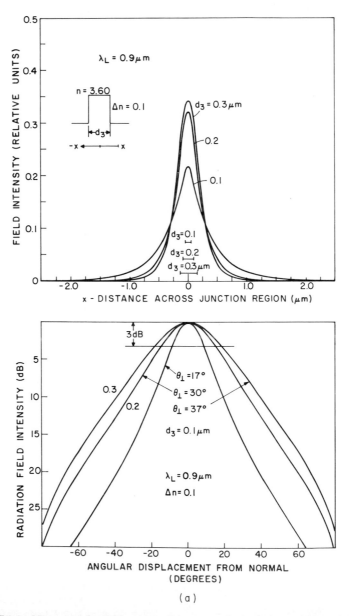

FIG. 7.2.3 Near- and far-field patterns for symmetrical DH lasers with various heter-ojunction spacings d_3 and refractive index step $\Delta n = 0.1$. The lasing wavelength is 0.9 μm. The near-field patterns are normalized in each figure to equal area under the curve, which implies constant power. (a) $d_3 = 0.1$, 0.2, 0.3 μm.

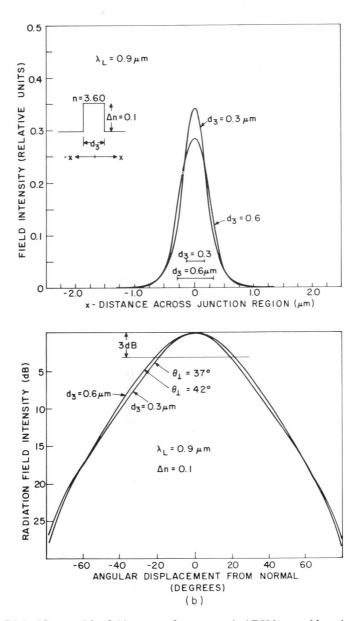

FIG. 7.2.3   Near- and far-field patterns for symmetrical DH lasers with various hetero-junction spacings d_3 and refractive index step $\Delta n = 0.1$. The lasing wavelength is 0.9 μm. The near-field patterns are normalized in each figure to equal area under the curve, which implies constant power. (b) $d_3 = 0.3$, 0.6 μm.

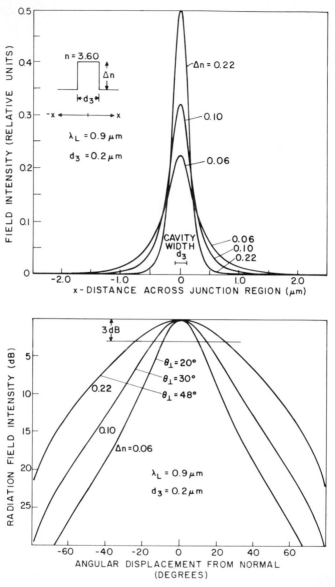

FIG. 7.2.4 Near- and far-field patterns for symmetrical DH lasers with heterojunction spacing $d_3 = 0.2$ μm and various refractive index steps. The near-field patterns are normalized for constant power.

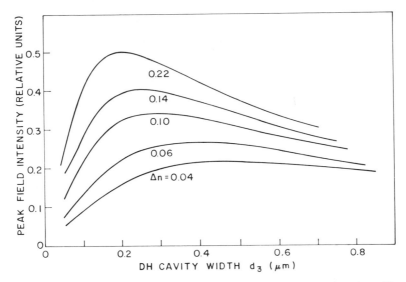

FIG. 7.2.5 The peak field intensities for the fundamental mode as a function of heterojunction spacing d_3. The modal power is equal for each condition. A reduction in the peak intensity results from a change of the spatial distribution.

In these symmetric double-heterojunction lasers, the peak field in the lateral direction occurs at $x = 0$ so that

$$E_{max} = E_0 \psi_{max} \tag{7.2.3}$$

The maximum field occurring at the laser facet can be written in terms of the radiation power per unit length along the facet. The incident power P_i is

$$P_i = P_\theta/(1 - R) \tag{7.2.4}$$

where P_θ is the radiation power and R the facet reflectivity. The field strength E_0 is

$$E_0 \approx \left| \frac{k_0 \eta_0 P_\theta}{(1 - R)n_3} \right|^{1/2} 10^4 \quad \text{V/cm} \tag{7.2.5}$$

where P_θ is dimensioned in watts per micrometer (power per unit length) and k_0 is in reciprocal micrometers. Assume, for example, that the total power radiated from a 50-μm stripe laser operating continuously is 5 mW; then $P_\theta = 10^{-4}$ W/μm. With $\lambda_0 = 0.9$ μm, $E_0 \sim 3.06$ kV/cm. From Fig. 7.2.5 we find for $\Delta n = 0.22$, $d_3 = 0.2$ μm, $\psi^2_{max} = 0.5$. Consequently, the maximum field at the laser facet is $E_{max} = (3.06)(0.707) = 2.16$ kV/cm.*

These examples were chosen to illustrate the main features of the dependence of the radiation pattern on Δn and d_3 for small d_3. Useful theoretical summary plots covering a broad range of Δn and d_3 values of practical interest

*This is well below the electric field intensity estimated at facet damage in Section 16.1.

for DH lasers are shown in Figs. 7.2.6 and 7.2.7. Figure 7.2.6 shows the dependence of $\theta_\perp$ on the waveguide region width (adjusted for the lasing wavelength) for Δn ranging from 0.04 to 0.62 [which encompasses the complete range in the (AlGa)As alloy system; cf. Section 12.2.1].

The effect of changing the laser parameters on the optical confinement within the two heterojunction spacings is directly shown in Fig. 7.2.7. The confinement factor Γ, representing the fraction of the radiation within the recombination region, is given as a function of Δn and d_3. The relation of Γ to the threshold current density and to the differential quantum efficiency is discussed in Chapter 8.

Although the curves of Figs. 7.2.6 and 7.2.7 provide the required information for device design, it is sometimes useful to have an analytical expression. An expression derived by Dumke [5] for $\theta_\perp$ can be used for small d_3 values ($\lesssim 0.1 \ \mu m$),

$$\theta_\perp \cong \frac{A d_3/\lambda}{1 + [A/1.2][d_3/\lambda]^2} \qquad \text{(radians)} \qquad (7.2.6)$$

where $A = 4.05(n_1{}^2 - n_3{}^2)$ with n_1 and n_3 the index values within and outside the recombination region, respectively, at wavelength λ. For a relatively wide cavity operating in the fundamental mode, (7.2.6) reduces to the familiar approximation $\theta_\perp \approx 1.2\lambda/d_3$.

Equation (7.2.6) is plotted in Fig. 7.2.6 where it is compared to the actual

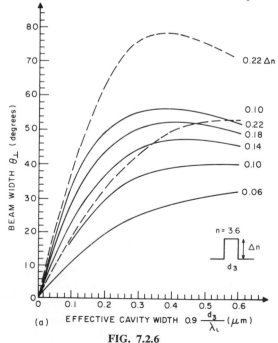

(a)   EFFECTIVE CAVITY WIDTH $0.9 \ \dfrac{d_3}{\lambda_L} (\mu m)$

FIG. 7.2.6

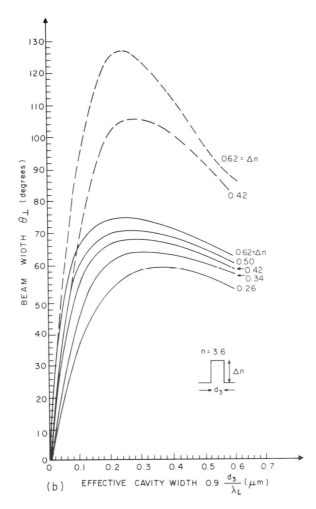

FIG. 7.2.6 Half-power radiation beam width $\theta_\perp$ as a function of normalized double-heterojunction spacing width (which accounts for changes in the lasing wavelength). (a) The refractive index treated as a parameter varies from 0.06 to 0.22, whereas in (b) the refractive index steps are larger. The dashed curves are numerical approximations [Eq. (7.2.6)] ($\lambda = 0.88\ \mu$m); the solid curves are calculated.

computer solutions. It is evident that the $\theta_\perp$ values obtained with (7.2.6) are far too large when d_3 is substantially greater than 0.1 μm, particularly with large Δn values.

An analytical expression also relates the beam width to the confinement factor in the range where (7.2.6) is valid,

$$\Gamma \cong \theta_\perp d_3/0.205\lambda \qquad (7.2.7)$$

where $\theta_\perp$ is in radians.

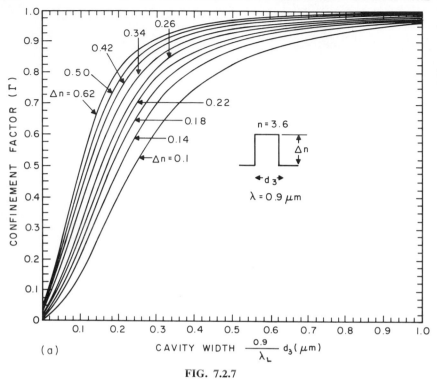

FIG. 7.2.7

We note that good agreement is obtained between the theoretical curve of Fig. 7.2.6 and experiment [6] as shown in Fig. 7.2.8 for a group of (AlGa)As/GaAs DH lasers. For lasers operating in the higher order modes, an extension of the theory is needed to calculate the beam divergence between the major lobes (see below). Our next concern, however, is obtaining the waveguide parameters that determine the maximum mode number which can propagate.

We now illustrate the effect of waveguide geometry on the cutoff conditions of the transverse modes. In Fig. 7.2.9, we plot three curves defining cutoff for the first four slab waveguide modes. These curves, obtained from (5.5.6), apply to a *lossless* waveguide with $n_3 = 3.6$. The ordinate gives Δn and the abscissa gives d_3/λ, the waveguide width normalized to the free-space wavelength.* A waveguide defined by a point lying to the right of each curve implies that that particular mode can propagate in the cavity. However, Fig. 7.2.9 only provides an approximate guide to the modes actually seen.

It is important to note that when the cavity region contains both a positive gain and lossy regions and when the surrounding layers are lossy (as is the

*The curves of Figs. 7.2.9–7.2.12 are general and apply to a slab waveguide bound by heterojunctions with index steps Δn. For the double-heterojunction laser $d_3 = d^\circ$, but the curves can be used for symmetrical LOC configurations as well where the heterojunction spacing is d°.

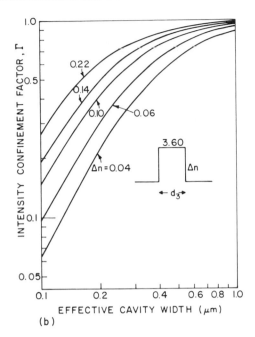

FIG. 7.2.7 The radiation confinement factor Γ within the recombination region of width d_3 of a symmetrical double-heterojunction laser diode as a function of the refractive index step Δn. In (a) the refractive index step varies from 0.1 to 0.62 and (b) applies to the lower confinement factors obtained for small index steps. The recombination region width is found by normalization for various lasing wavelength values [4].

case in diodes) the cutoff curves will be slightly changed. For example, the circled point of Fig. 7.2.9 represents the waveguide of Fig. 7.2.2a, which indicates the possibility of a second-order mode existing in the cavity although only the fundamental mode was seen. However, previous calculations using a complex dielectric constant indicated that there could *not* be a propagating second-order mode. The triangled point in Fig. 7.2.9 applies to the structure of Fig. 7.2.2b, which operated in the second mode. Note that the triangled point is well removed from the cutoff curve for the second-order mode whereas the circled point is not. Since the second-order mode is near cutoff, its optical fields extend deeply into the lossy passive layers, whereas the fundamental mode will be confined largely to the active gain region. Consequently, the second-order mode in the 0.7 μm waveguide is unlikely to reach threshold.

Finally, we discuss some of the characteristics of high order transverse modes. We have presented in Fig. 7.2.6 curves which relate the radiation half-power beam width of the *fundamental* mode to the cavity dimensions. The high order modes produce radiation patterns with two major lobes such as that shown in Fig. 7.2.1b. Thus, the high order modes are characterized by the major lobe separations and major lobe beam widths. In Figs. 7.2.10–7.2.12,

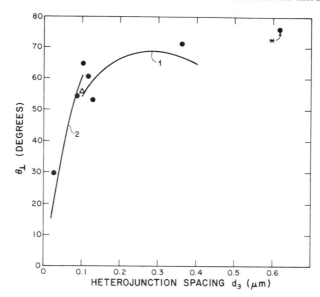

FIG. 7.2.8   Comparison of experimental beam width $\theta_\perp$ with theory for well-charac-terized $Al_xGa_{1-x}As/GaAs$ DH lasers [6]. Curve 1 is the theoretical curve, identical to that from Fig. 7.2.6, and curve 2 is obtained from Eq. (7.2.6). $\Delta x = 0.65 \pm 0.05$, $\Delta n = 0.4$.

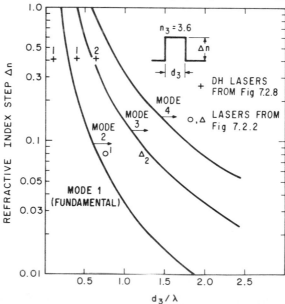

FIG. 7.2.9   Modal cutoff characteristics for symmetrical double-heterojunction lasers. The fundamental mode can propagate for all values of Δn and d_3/λ whereas for waveguides defined by points lying to the right of each curve high order mode propagation is possible. The $\bigcirc$, $\triangle$ points are for DH lasers from Fig. 7.2.2 and + points for DH lasers from Fig. 7.2.8.

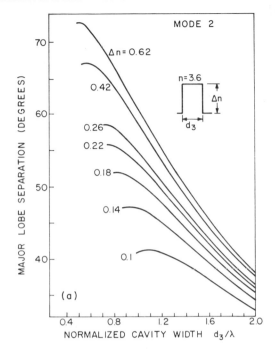

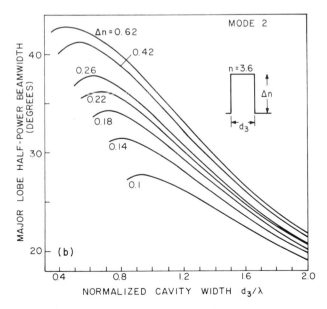

FIG. 7.2.10   Mode 2 characteristics for double-heterojunction lasers. Beam separation between major lobes is given as a function of normalized cavity width d_3/λ; and (b) half-power beam width of each of the major lobes.

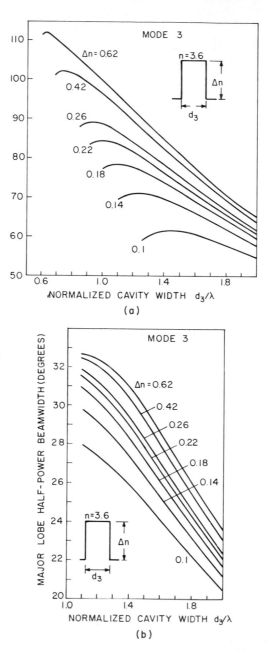

FIG. 7.2.11 Mode 3 characteristics for double-heterojunction lasers. (a) Beam separation between major lobes is given as a function of normalized cavity width d_3/λ; and (b) half-power beam width of each of the major lobes.

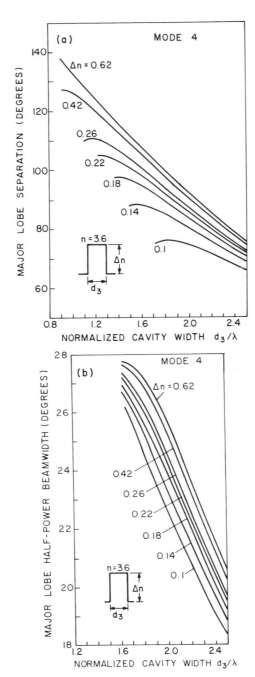

FIG. 7.2.12 Mode 4 characteristics for double-heterojunction lasers. (a) Beam separation between major lobes is given as a function of normalized cavity width d_3/λ; and (b) half-power beam width of each of the major lobes.

we relate the radiation characteristics of the high order modes to the cavity dimensions. The beam separation between the two major lobes and the half-power beam width of each lobe is given as a function of cavity width where the index step is treated as a parameter. For example, for $\Delta n = 0.18$, $d^\circ = 1 \ \mu m$, and $\lambda = 0.9 \ \mu m$, mode 2 ($m = 2$) would produce a radiation pattern with a 51° separation between major lobes. However, if the cavity operated in the third mode $m = 3$ the beam separation between the two major lobes would be approximately 75°, the beam separation increasing proportionately to the mode number m for a given cavity.

7.3   Four-Heterojunction Lasers

As discussed in the preceding section, the double-heterojunction configuration can be adjusted to yield a desired beam pattern. Addition of two more heterojunctions makes the control of the device properties more precise, but at the expense of additional fabrication complexity.

A possible advantage of using the FH structure is that the coupling of power from the active region to a mode is related to the modal field intensity. The fundamental mode has one antinode in the optical waveguide and consequently couples well to the active region when it is located in the center of the optical cavity. By positioning the recombination region at the center of the waveguide, one enhances the coupling to the fundamental transverse mode because in a symmetrical structure the fundamental mode peaks at the center of the waveguide. Application of this very simple concept must be treated with caution because of other factors which control dominant mode selection. For example, we have seen in Section 5.9 that facet reflectivity tends to favor high order mode operation.

The wave properties of FH can be calculated using the five-layer model described in Chapter 5. In this section, we present the results of some important symmetrical dielectric configurations of the basic FH structure shown in schematic form in Fig. 7.3.1. In Figs. 7.3.2 and 7.3.3 we show plots of the fractional radiation confinement Γ within the recombination region 3, as well as $\theta_\perp$ for various values of the refractive index steps (refer to Fig. 7.3.1), recombination region width d_3, and total outer heterojunction spacing d°. Note that Γ increases with decreasing d° only when d° is not too large compared to d_3. With large d°, the optical confinement is little affected by the outer heterojunctions, and we are left with the basic confinement due to the inner two heterojunctions. The contribution of the inner heterojunctions depends, of course, on d_3 and on the size of the refractive index steps enclosing it relative to that of the outer heterojunctions.

Figure 7.3.4 summarized the beam width for fixed $d^\circ = 2 \ \mu m$ as a function of the recombination region width for selected values of the refractive index

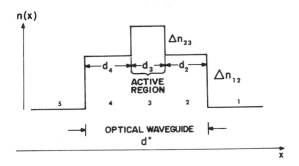

FIG. 7.3.1   Vertical geometry of symmetrical four-heterojunction laser diode.

steps. As the recombination region widens, the confinement factor increases and the far-field pattern broadens.

In this, the recombination region was centered within the outer heterojunctions. In the FH structure, off-center placement of the recombination region need not affect the preferred transverse mode, as shown in the example of Fig. 7.3.5a, which gives the internal dimensions of a four-heterojunction diode with a GaAs:Si recombination region $d_3 = 0.5$ μm [7]. The adjacent regions 2 and 4 consist of $Al_{0.03}Ga_{0.97}As$, while regions 1 and 5 consist of $Al_{0.15}$ $Ga_{0.85}As$. The separation between the outer heterojunctions $d° = 3.7$ μm. The radiation pattern of this laser, which operates in the fundamental mode, is shown on the left side of Fig. 7.3.5a. It consists of a single lobe in the direction perpendicular to the junction with $\theta_\perp = 17°$, which corresponds to the diffraction limit of a 3-μm aperture. Both the inner and outer sets of heterojunctions contribute to the radiation confinement, with the inner ones tending to peak the field in the recombination region and promote fundamental transverse mode operation.

A theoretical analysis of the gain for the various transverse modes of the FH laser shown in Fig. 7.3.5a is presented in Fig. 7.3.6. It is evident that the fundamental mode is theoretically preferred since it reaches threshold before the higher order modes. Furthermore, Fig. 7.3.6 shows that the position of the recombination region within the waveguide region of the specific FH structures studied is not critical, as experimentally confirmed. For example, it was found [7] that similar structures, except for the recombination region being placed either 1.2 or 2.5 μm from the p–p interface, had radiation patterns identical to those of the structure shown in Fig. 7.3.6. However, the radiation pattern is sensitive to the barrier height of the inner heterojunctions. For example, a structure similar to this but with higher Al content in regions 2 and 4 ($x_2 = x_4 = 0.006$), has $\theta_\perp \sim 35°$, indicative of much stronger peaking of the radiation near the recombination region.

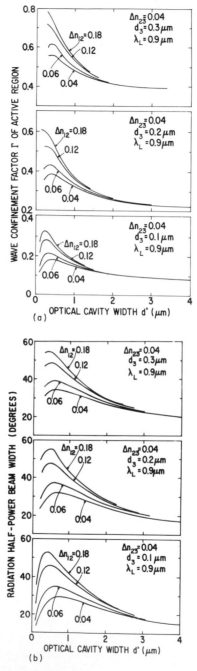

FIG. 7.3.2 Summary of FH device performance in fundamental mode operation. (a) The radiation confinement factor within d_3 as a function of device geometry; and (b) the radiation half-power beam width corresponding to the structural parameters of (a). Refer to Fig. 7.3.1 for the nomenclature.

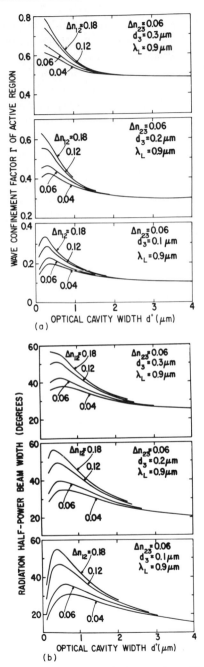

FIG. 7.3.3 Calculations for FH laser are similar to those illustrated in Fig. 7.3.2 but with different device parameters.

The insensitivity of the position of the recombination region with regard to the preferred mode of this structure results from the fact that the inner two heterojunctions provide substantial radiation guiding. However, if the inner heterojunctions are removed, then the mode pattern is affected by changing the recombination region position. Figures 7.3.5b and 7.3.5c show two examples in which the GaAs:Si recombination region is placed differently within the waveguide region (without inner heterojunctions). In Fig. 7.3.5b, the recombination region is near the p–p interface; whereas in Fig. 7.3.5c, the recombination region is nearer the center of the waveguide region, thus similar to the FH structure of Fig. 7.3.5a but without the inner heterojunctions. In contrast to the laser in Fig. 7.3.5a, the far-field radiation patterns of Figs. 7.3.5b and 7.3.5c contain high order transverse modes, and displacing the position of the recombination region changes the far-field pattern. With the recombination region centered as in Fig. 7.3.5c, a relatively pure fourth-order mode is seen, but with the recombination region near the edge of the waveguide as in Fig. 7.3.5b, several modes share the power. This behavior is qualitatively consistent with the change of coupling of the field to the recombination region, which itself provides only very weak mode guiding.

It is important to keep in mind the requirement for carrier confinement

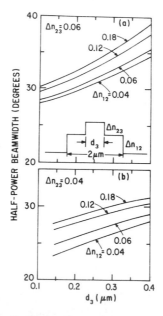

FIG. 7.3.4 Summary data plot for FH laser operating in the fundamental mode showing the far-field beam width for a fixed outer heterojunction spacing $d^0 = 2\,\mu$m as a function of the recombination width d_3 for selected values of the refractive index steps. Refer to Fig. 7.3.1 for the nomenclature.

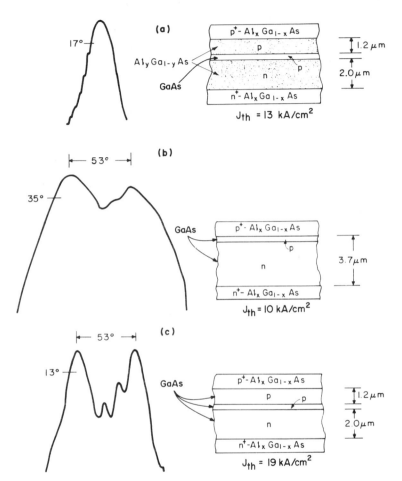

FIG. 7.3.5 Structures, far-field patterns, and threshold current densities of five-layer lasers with different internal placement and composition of heterojunctions [7].

within the recombination region of FH structures. If the heterojunction barrier is too low, carrier loss occurs, which raises the threshold current density. This is illustrated by the devices of Fig. 7.3.5 which shows the threshold current density for each structure. In Figs. 7.3.5a and 7.3.5b J_{th} is under 4 kA/ cm² μm^{-1} of optical cavity thickness, but it is much higher for Fig. 7.3.5c. The reason for the difference is the poor carrier confinement in Fig. 7.3.5c resulting from the absence of the inner heterojunctions. In fact, the *spontaneous* spectra reflect the emission from both the GaAs:Si and the GaAs:Ge regions in Fig. 7.3.5c, as can be seen in Fig. 7.3.7. Since the stimulated emission

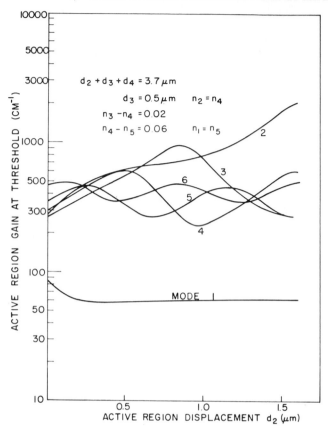

FIG. 7.3.6 Threshold gain curves for four-heterojunction structure of Fig. 7.3.5a as a function of the displacement of the recombination region from the p-side edge of the waveguide region. Each curve is labeled with a specific mode number; 1 is the fundamental mode.

occurs in the GaAs:Si region, the carriers diffusing beyond that region are wasted.

Note that the impact of the lost carriers on the threshold current density must be calculated as described in Section 8.1. If the carriers are confined to the narrow region 2 or 4 of Fig. 7.3.1, by the high potential barriers of the outer heterojunctions, then the J_{th} increase may not be excessive, depending on the thinness of these regions.

7.4 Asymmetrical Structures—Single-Heterojunction (Close-Confinement) Lasers

In the single-heterojunction (close-confinement) laser, the dielectric step on the p–p side of the waveguide is formed by a heterojunction, while the

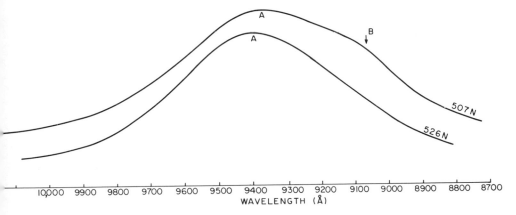

FIG. 7.3.7   Spontaneous spectra from lasers shown in Figs. 7.3.5a and 7.3.5c. The short wavelength emission (B) discernible in unit 507N is radiation from the GaAs:Ge passive region. Edge emission, 300 K, $I = 5$ mA. Both spectra are distorted on the high energy side due to selective internal absorption [7].

other dielectric boundary is the result of differences in doping level and carrier concentration between the p-type recombination region, generally formed by Zn diffusion, and the GaAs n-type substrate (2–4×10^{18} cm^{-3}) (see Section 12.2.1).

Guided wave propagation is impossible in an asymmetrical waveguide whose thickness is below a critical value set by the dielectric asymmetry and dielectric step values. Consider the asymmetrical waveguide of Fig. 7.4.1a in which the p-type recombination region is enclosed on one side with a large dielectric step Δn_{31} and a smaller step Δn_{35} on the other side. The dielectric asymmetry η is defined in (5.5.2).

Optical mode guiding within d_3 is only possible if the following conditions are satisfied [11]: For TE waves,

$$d_3 > \frac{\lambda_L}{2\pi (n_3{}^2 - n_5{}^2)^{1/2}} \tan^{-1}(\eta - 1)^{1/2} \qquad (7.4.1a)$$

and for TM waves,

$$d_3 > \frac{\lambda_L}{2\pi (n_3{}^2 - n_5{}^2)^{1/2}} \tan^{-1}\left[\frac{n_3{}^2}{n_1{}^2} (\eta - 1)^{1/2}\right] \qquad (7.4.1b)$$

where λ_L is the lasing wavelength (externally). Figure 7.4.1 shows a plot of Eqs. (7.4.1) for TE waves assuming an asymmetry $\eta = 5$, which is appropriate for single-heterojunction laser diodes [8]. The loss of mode propagation with decreasing d_3 because of the reduction in the radiation confinement within the recombination region is reflected in the increase in the threshold current density. Figure 7.4.2 shows experimental values of J_{th} as a function of the recombination region width; it shows that the lowest J_{th} is obtained with $d_3 \cong$

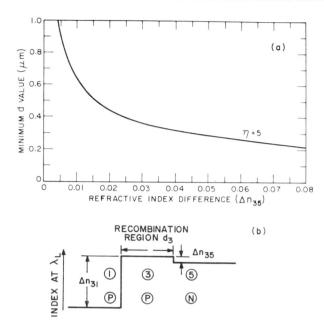

FIG. 7.4.1   (a) The asymmetrical waveguide of the single-heterojunction type and (b) the cutoff condition for the fundamental TE mode [8].

2 μm, and no lasing below 1 μm. Since these experimental devices had an estimated $\Delta n_{35} \approx 0.01$ at the p–n homojunction, the calculated cutoff value for d_3 should be 0.6 μm, which can be considered close agreement in view of the approximations made. Because of this small Δn, the properties of the device can be very temperature sensitive, as discussed in Section 8.3, since Δn can change with temperature.

Single-heterojunction lasers usually operate in the fundamental mode, but higher order modes can be excited if the diffused (confinement) region is widened to beyond 2.5 μm [12] (see, e.g., Fig. 7.2.1c, where $d_3 = 5$ μm). For the typical good quality single-heterojunction laser, d_3 is between 2 and 2.5 μm, and $\theta_\perp \approx 20°$; reasonable agreement between the calculated and experimental far-field radiation patterns has been obtained [12].

7.5   Large Optical Cavity Lasers—Symmetrical and Asymmetrical Structures

In the large optical cavity (LOC) laser the recombination region is placed at one edge of the waveguide region defined by two outer heterojunctions spaced a distance $d°$ apart. Figure 7.5.1 shows the symmetrical LOC with equal refractive indices in the outer regions, the three-heterojunction version

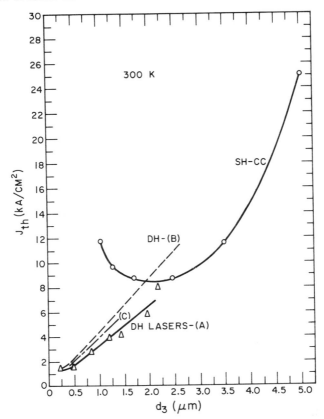

FIG. 7.4.2 Threshold current density as a function of region width d_3 for typical single- and double-heterojunction lasers. Curve A, from Kressel *et al.* [8]; curve B, Hayashi *et al.* [9]; curve C, Alferov *et al.* [10].

of the device with the p–n inner homojunction replaced by a low barrier hetero-junction, and the asymmetrical LOC configuration. The choice of LOC struc-ture is based on the desired radiation pattern. Fundamental mode operation with the smallest possible beam width is favored by (1) moderate (under 1 μm) heterojunction spacing, (2) three heterojunctions, and (3) dielectric asym-metry.

A detailed study of the preferred mode as a function of device parameters has been presented by Butler and Kressel [1]. We consider the examples in Fig. 7.5.2 where the relative threshold current density for various modes is plotted as a function of the waveguide thickness d°. Note that for the chosen sym-metrical index discontinuity $\Delta n = 0.06$,* the second mode is the first to reach

*These calculations neglect the small index step at the internal junction.

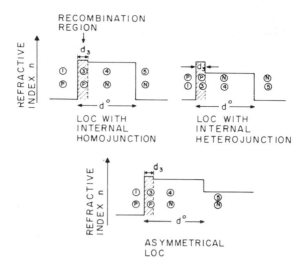

FIG. 7.5.1 Schematic cross sections of three variations of the large optical cavity structures: symmetrical LOC with p–n homojunction, LOC with p–n heterojunction and symmetrical LOC. Shading indicates the recombination region.

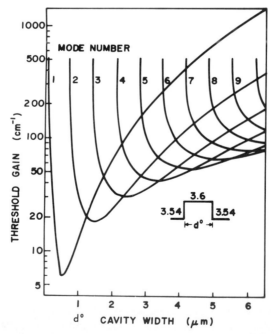

FIG. 7.5.2 Threshold gain (G_{th}) curves for the different cavity modes of a symmetrical LOC structure. The pertinent cavity parameters are $d_1 = 0, n_1 = n_5 = 3.54, n_3 = n_4 = 3.6$, $\alpha_1 = 20$ cm^{-1} and $\alpha_4 = \alpha_5 = 10$ cm^{-1}. For $d° < 0.5$ μm, d$° \simeq d_3$, and for d$° > 0.5$ μm, $d_3 = 0.5$ μm. (Refer to Fig. 7.5.1 for the nomenclature.)

threshold in a 2-μm cavity, the third mode reaches threshold first in a 3-μm cavity, and so on, facts observed experimentally [1]. Also, for large waveguide widths, the modal selection between the high order modes becomes less pronounced and end losses are important as competing factors in modal selection as discussed in Section 5.9.

It is clear from Fig. 7.5.2 that the threshold gain coefficient for mode 1 becomes extremely large in symmetrical wide optical cavities. The fact that the threshold for a particular mode is infinite below a certain cavity width simply indicates that the mode cannot propagate in the cavity.

Asymmetrical LOC structures can be designed [7] to propagate only the fundamental transverse mode, as illustrated in Fig. 7.5.3, which shows the profile of a device having $\theta_\perp = 14°$. In this particular cavity we estimate that only the fundamental waveguide mode can propagate as follows: Since the optical cavity is composed of p- and n-GaAs with only slightly differing indices of refraction, we assume that the index of the cavity is 3.6. Now define the p-(AlGa)As as region 5 and the n-(AlGa)As as region 1 with the optical cavity being region 3($d_2 = d_4 = 0$). We thus have a three-layer waveguide so that the modal cutoff conditions of Section 5.5.2 are applicable here. The indices $n_3 = 3.6$ for GaAs and $n_1 = 3.59$ for $Al_{0.02}Ga_{0.98}As$, $d_3 = 1.8$ μm, and $\lambda = 0.9$ μm. In this example, the asymmetry factor $\eta = x/y = 0.2/0.02 = 10$. Using (5.5.9), we find $d_3 < 2.35$ μm. Since $d_3 = 1.8$ μm, there will be *no* high order transverse mode propagation.

In this device, there is a homojunction between the two heterojunctions. The use of a triple-heterojunction structure (Fig. 7.5.1) in which the bandgap energy of the n-type region within the outer heterojunctions is about 40 meV

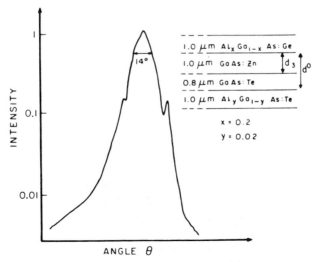

FIG. 7.5.3   Far-field pattern of asymmetric LOC structure operating in fundamental transverse mode.

higher than in the p-type recombination region, is another way of promoting fundamental mode operation [13] (see Section 14.1). Also, an undesired mode can be suppressed by a suitable angle-selective antireflection coating designed for low reflection of that mode. Hakki and Hwang [14] used a coating consisting of Al_2O_3/ZnS to obtain maximum transmission loss at 30° to extend the range of fundamental operation to higher power.

7.6 Experimental/Theoretical Radiation Patterns (Transverse Modes)

In this section we compare in detail the experimental and theoretical radiation patterns of several laser structures and show that good agreement is obtained [15]. The lasers had sawed sidewalls and all devices had electric fields polarized along the y direction (TE modes). The theoretical patterns were obtained using (6.2.11). The lasers, fabricated by liquid phase exitaxial growth, have a cross section shown schematically in Fig. 5.1.2. Also, since the lasers were grown as basically four-layer devices, we have taken $d_2 = 0$. The confining p- and n-$Al_xGa_{1-x}As$ layers are doped with Te and Ge, respectively, and have a carrier concentration of approximately 5×10^{17} cm^{-3}. The heterojunctions are made symmetric, i.e., the percentage of Al in the p- and n-type $Al_x Ga_{1-x}As$ layers is almost the same ($x \simeq 0.36$ for A, $x < 0.2$ for B, and $x \simeq 0.2$ for C). The LOC lasers B and C (see Fig. 7.5.1) have Ge and Si, respectively, in the compensated p-type GaAs (recombination) region 3. Each diode has an n-type GaAs layer region 4 doped with Te with a carrier concentration of 3–5 $\times 10^{17}$ cm^{-3}. There is a very small amount of Al ($x < 0.03$) intentionally added to the n-type GaAs region of diode B. The diodes have small cavity widths ($d° = 0.25 \pm 0.1$ μm for A, $d° = 2 \pm 0.1$ μm for B, and $d° = 1.84 \pm 0.1$ μm for C). The recombination regions for both B and C are rather thin ($d_3 = 0.4 \pm 0.1$ μm for B and $d_3 \simeq 0.5 \pm 0.1$ μm for C). Black wax is used on the back facet of A and B to reduce distortion of the far-field pattern by scattered radiation from the back facet.

The far-field radiation patterns for the lasers, measured in the plane perpendicular to the junction, are shown in Figs. 7.6.1–7.6.3. The propagating modes for lasers A, B, and C are the first second, and third modes, respectively. The effect of back-scattered radiation is shown by the distortion of Fig. 7.6.2 for angles less than $-45°$; for positive angles, the mounting block intercepts the scattered light. The black wax has absorbed the back light in Figs. 7.6.1 and 7.6.3.

The theoretical far-field radiation patterns for the lasers are also shown in Figs. 7.6.1–7.6.3. To match the theoretical curves to the experimental patterns, we have to estimate the propagation parameters in the different regions. Absorption coefficients of 20 and 10 cm^{-1} are taken for the p- and n-type regions, respectively. The refractive indices for p- and n-type GaAs are chosen to be 3.6 (except for the n-type GaAs region of B where the small amount of Al

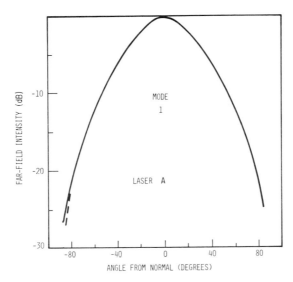

FIG. 7.6.1 Experimental (solid line) and theoretical (broken line) patterns for laser A, a DH structure. TE polarization. [15].

reduces the index to about 3.588). Choice of the cavity widths and the refractive indices of (AlGa)As regions comprises the most critical considerations for the theoretical curves. The index of refraction of the (AlGa)As region and hence the index discontinuity at the heterojunction, Δn, can be estimated from the percentage of Al present in the region. For example, for 20% Al in the p- and n-Al_xGa_{1-x}As regions of C ($x = 0.2$), we find a corresponding estimated $\Delta n - 0.62\Delta x = 0.12$ (see Section 12.2.1). The best matched theoretical curve to the experimental pattern for C is obtained however, with $\Delta n = 0.09$ (Fig. 7.6.3)—a probable result of the uncertain experimental Al fraction.

The following procedure is used to fit the experimental data. For the first approximation in the calculations, the measured values of d° and d_2 and the approximate value of Δn are used to obtain a theoretical far-field radiation pattern. First, the index of refraction step Δn is varied to get the desired angular separation between the two principal beams; then the cavity thickness d° is varied to fit the beam width. The experimental and theoretical curves are plotted simultaneously, using a computer and the parameters d° and Δn varied to minimize the difference between the two curves. For a fine curve fitting, Δn and d° can be varied at the same time. The values of the absorption coefficients, given in the preceding paragraph, are kept constant since their effect on the radiation pattern is minor. A summary of the best fit and the experimental parameters for the diodes is given in Table 7.6.1.

The parameters Δn and d° can be determined very accurately in the case

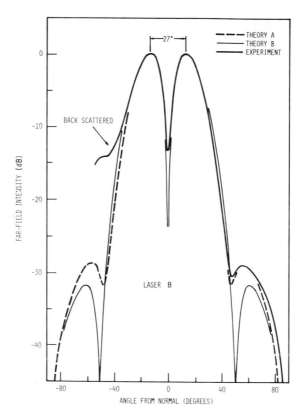

FIG. 7.6.2 Experimental and theoretical patterns for laser B. The back-scattered light occurs at negative angles less than 40° in this device because of light radiating from the rear facet and reflecting from the mounting block. Theories A and B apply to different cavity geometries. TE polarization [15].

when both a deep minimum and defined side lobes are present (Fig. 7.6.2). The index discontinuity at the heterojunctions and especially the cavity thickness have appreciable effects in the position of the "null" and the amplitude of the side lobe. For example, the theoretical curve B (Fig. 7.6.2) is obtained with $d° = 1.93\ \mu m$ and $\Delta n = 0.05$ where the radiation pattern null occurs at 47°. Decreasing the total cavity width by 0.02 μm (from 1.93 to 1.91 μm) shifts the null point by approximately 2° (from 47 to ~49°), and reduces the amplitude of the side lobe. Increasing Δn, by reducing n_1 and n_5, increases the amplitude of the side lobe, but does not have a significant effect on the position of the null. Moreover, curve fitting shows that removal of the small amount of Al from the n-type region 3 in B has a similar effect on the position of the null and the amplitude of the side lobe as decreasing the cavity width. The difference between the two theoretical curves of Fig. 7.6.2 is the refractive index of the n-type GaAs, which is 3.600 for case A and 3.588 for case B.

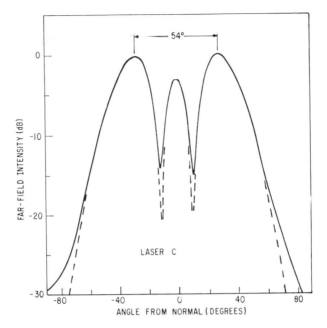

FIG. 7.6.3 Experimental (solid line) and theoretical (broken line) patterns for laser C. TE polarization [15].

TABLE 7.6.1
Experimental and Theoretical Laser Parameters[a]

Laser	Diode No.	Δn[b]	$d^0 (\mu m)$	$d_3 (\mu m)$	$\lambda (\mu m)$	$\theta_\perp{}^c$ (deg)	Observed dominant mode No.
			Measured Characteristics				
A (DH)	10/72–44/17	0.22	0.25 ± 0.1	0.25 ± 0.1	0.9	—	1
B (LOC)	8/72–29/5	0.06	2 ± 0.1	0.4 ± 0.1	0.89	27	2
C (LOC)	8/72–31/2	0.12	1.84 ± 0.1	0.5 ± 0.1	0.94	54	3
			From Fit to Radiation Data				
							Highest possible transverse mode No.[d]
A (DH)		0.21	0.25	0.25			1
B (LOC)		0.05	1.93	0.4			3
C (LOC)		0.09	1.85	0.4			4

[a]From Butler and Zoroofchi [15].
[b]Estimated from Al content x in material using $\Delta n = 0.62\, \Delta x$. The Al content was not measured directly in the diodes, but estimated from the melt composition used to grow the layers.
[c]Angular separation between two major lobes.
[d]From numerical results based on the theoretical parameters Δn, d^0, and d_3.

It is evident from these examples that the task of precisely fitting experimental radiation data with the theory is limited by the precision of the experimental device description. Nevertheless, starting with only "ballpark" estimates of the index steps but accurate dimensional data, good agreement is obtained by small adjustments of the index values.

7.7 Lateral "s" Modes

The lateral field and the corresponding radiation profiles of injection lasers are more complicated than the corresponding vertical field profiles, although the basic analysis is similar. The structure of the vertical modes is related to the dielectric waveguides, which have well-pronounced boundaries. Also, with greatly improved technology for fabricating layered devices, the grown boundaries are reasonably free of surface inhomogeneities. On the other hand, the boundaries along the *lateral* junction directions are more complicated. Basically, there are two types of lasers which have distinct boundaries for the optical fields in the plane of the junction: (1) stripe-geometry lasers and (2) lasers with sawed or etched sidewalls. The lateral field confinement of stripe-geometry lasers (see Chapter 12) is dependent on the width of the stripe contact and the method of construction. In general, the number of propagating lateral modes increases with the active area width and dielectric steps at the two sidewalls. Because sawed-sidewall lasers are usually very wide (100 μm) and the semiconductor–air index step very large, the number of modes can be extremely large, whereas for narrow planar stripe lasers (≤ 10 μm), the number of lateral modes is small.

Following along the simple concept of a mode guiding region in the plane of the junction of width W (in an ideal stripe-geometry laser the stripe width $S_t = W$), a fundamental lateral mode will radiate a beam in the plane of the junction with a full width at half-intensity $\theta_\parallel \approx \lambda/W$. Therefore, for very narrow lasers in the lateral plane, it is possible to visualize devices in which the beam width is the same in the plane of the junction as in the direction perpendicular to it. For example, assuming a confined lateral mode guiding region $W = 1$ μm, and $\lambda = 0.8$ μm, the fundamental mode beam width would be $\theta_\parallel \approx 0.8$ radian $\approx 45°$. This value is comparable to the typical beam width in the direction perpendicular to the junction plane of a device designed for room temperature CW operation.

If higher order modes are excited, then two principal lobes will be seen, with the subsidiary lobes increasing with the mode number, analogous to the discussion in Section 7.2 for the transverse modes. As discussed in Section 7.8, the maximum number of allowed lateral modes can be simply computed, being based on the internal critical angle at the sidewalls.* In the simplest

---

*Figure 7.2.9 can be used to predict the index step required for fundamental mode operation for a given W/λ.

case of lateral confinement by two dielectric steps, the separation between the two dominant lobes for high order modes can be computed from Figs. 7.2.10–7.2.12, where we substitute W for d_3.

7.7.1 Planar Stripe-Geometry Lasers

The active region width of double-heterojunction lasers is typically made small enough to ensure that only one transverse (perpendicular to the junction plane) mode can propagate. However, more than one lateral mode generally can oscillate, the number depending on the contact width, refractive index steps at the sidewalls, and the drive level. Multilateral mode operation is much more common in wide lasers than in narrow ones, as shown in Figs. 7.7.1 and 7.7.2. Figure 7.7.1 shows the distribution of optical intensity over the emitting facet for two lasers, one with a 13-μm stripe-contact width (oxide defined) and one with a 50-μm contact width. Multimode behavior is obvious

FIG. 7.7.1 Magnified photographs of the emitting facet of two oxide-isolated stripe-contact lasers, taken in laser light. The widths of the two stripe contacts are indicated below the photographs.

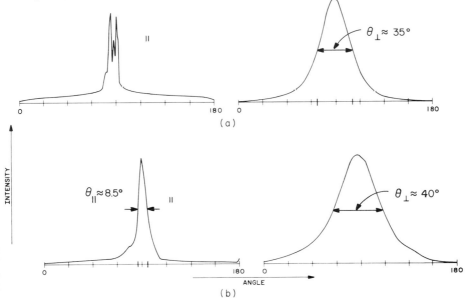

FIG. 7.7.2 Far-field emission patterns of the two lasers of Fig. 7.7.1. The emission patterns are scanned in the plane (||) and perpendicular ($\perp$) to the junction: (a) for the 50 μm laser and (b) 13 μm laser.

in the broader laser. Figure 7.7.2 shows corresponding far-field patterns, where again the wider laser shows strong multimoding. (There is evidence of a weak second-mode oscillation even in the narrower laser.)

These examples were selected from *planar* stripe-contact lasers where oxide isolation was used, thus providing a minimum of lateral radiation confinement. However, narrow *nonplanar* stripe lasers can also be made using strong boundaries, such as mesas formed by etching or by buried heterojunctions (Chapter 12) in which case the lateral mode content can be much higher for a given active area width because of the high dielectric steps at the lateral boundaries.

Figure 7.7.3 shows the order "s" of mode operation as a function of stripe width S_t near threshold [16]. Experimentally when $S_t < 10\ \mu$m, the stripe lasers operate in the fundamental $s = 1$ mode. When $S_t > 10\ \mu$m, "s" increases with width and with drive current above threshold. Presumably, full gain saturation does not occur at threshold (Chapter 17) in these planar devices.

There are no dielectric walls grown along the lateral direction for the *planar* stripe-geometry lasers. Basically, lateral confinement can be due to variation with respect to lateral position (relative to the stripe contact) of (1) the index of refraction which relates to the real part of the dielectric constant and (2) the optical field gain/absorption which relates predominately to the imaginary part of the dielectric constant. Since the lateral modes show approximate Hermite–Gaussian behavior, it is natural to assume that the refractive index, which is related in some manner to the current distribution, decreases quadratically from a point below the center of the stripe toward the outside region. The precise contributions to confinement are in question. Cook and Nash [17] suggested that the variation of the gain along the lateral direction is mainly responsible for lateral mode confinement, providing a net "step" $\Delta n \approx$

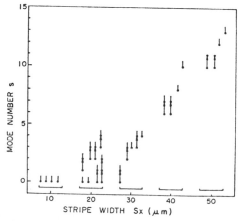

FIG. 7.7.3   The lateral mode number s as a function of the planar stripe width S_t near threshold. The arrows and lines denote mode transitions with increasing drive current [16].

0.001 (approximate). This index profile can change with current, providing for differing lateral mode propagation.

7.7.2 Sawed-Sidewall Lasers

In this section we compare theory and experiment concerning the lateral modes in sawed-sidewall lasers where the analysis is relatively simple. The "box modes" discussed in Section 5.7.1 are used to model the sawed-sidewall lasers. These lasers generally operate in a large number of lateral modes, but can be analyzed by considering the simple box waveguide structure. The lateral modes also directly relate to the lateral beam profile. One of the main complications to the lateral beam profile in wide lasers is due to the proliferation of lateral modes with increasing current density.* Figure 7.7.4 shows in detail

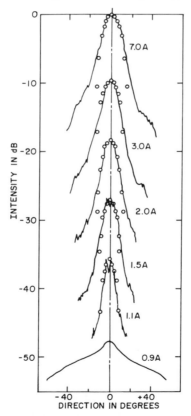

FIG. 7.7.4 The lateral beam profile for a sawed-sidewall laser for different drive levels. Relative intensities are preserved between the curves [20].

*Appendix B discusses the observation that more lateral modes are excited with increasing drive, an effect believed related to the fact that the gain coefficient does not remain exactly constant above threshold in practical lasers.

the lateral beam profiles of a laser from below threshold to 1.8 W output. The solid curves are experimental recordings with relative powers between curves reproduced. To better understand the lateral cavity modes, we summarize some rather sophisticated experiments reported by Sommers [18–20].

The modes of lasers with sawed sidewalls were described mathematically by the "box" modes of a rectangular waveguide, W wide and L long. The resonant condition satisfied by the modes is given by (5.7.5b). Place $\gamma^2 = -\beta^2 = -(q\pi/L)^2$. The transverse propagation constants h_{x3} and h_{y3} can be approximated by $(m\pi/d_3)$ and $(s\pi/W)$, respectively. Equation (5.7.5b) becomes

$$[2n_3/\lambda]^2 = [q/L]^2 + [s/W]^2 + [m/d_3]^2 \tag{7.7.1}$$

where n_3 is the refractive index of the cavity. The dispersion relation becomes

$$\lambda_{msq} - \lambda_0 = \frac{\lambda_0 n_3}{n_e}\left[\frac{q - q_0}{n_3 L}\lambda_0 + \frac{(s^2 - 1)\lambda_0^2}{(2n_3 W)^2} + \frac{(m^2 - 1)\lambda_0^2}{(2n_3 d_3)^2}\right] \tag{7.7.2}$$

where $\lambda_0 = \lambda_{1, 1, q_0}$ is the fiduciary wavelength near the center of resonance and n_e is the effective index (5.5.14). The lateral index integer s can be replaced by the lateral angle θ measured from the normal, of the principal radiation lobe of the lateral mode s,

$$\sin^2 \theta = [s\lambda_0/2W]^2 \tag{7.7.3}$$

Note that when $s = 1$, the fundamental mode, the major lobe occurs at $\theta = 0$ so that (7.7.3) holds only for large values of s, and therefore $s^2 - 1 \simeq s^2$.

For narrow recombination region heterojunction lasers, the maximum transverse mode number $m = 1$ (fundamental mode) so that only different q and s modes will be present in the cavity. For a constant θ value, we find the separation between the axial (longitudinal) modes is given by

$$\delta\lambda_{1, s, q}\bigg|_{s=\text{const}} = -\frac{\lambda_0^2}{2n_e L}\delta q \tag{7.7.4}$$

On the other hand, if we assume $q = $ const, then

$$\delta\lambda_{1, s, q}\bigg|_{q=\text{const}} = -\frac{\lambda_0}{2n_3 n_e}\delta(\sin^2 \theta) \tag{7.7.5}$$

Now since s assumes only integer values, θ will be discrete; however, because of the finite width of the cavity, the radiation lobes of the different s modes will have a finite width.

The lateral dispersion of a sawed double-heterojunction laser can be determined by a recording such as that in Fig. 7.7.5. The spectrometer resolution is around 1 Å, although the lateral resolution, determined by the spectrometer slit, is very high. The assignment of the q number in the figure can be followed from one trace to the next, shifting steadily to shorter wavelengths with in-

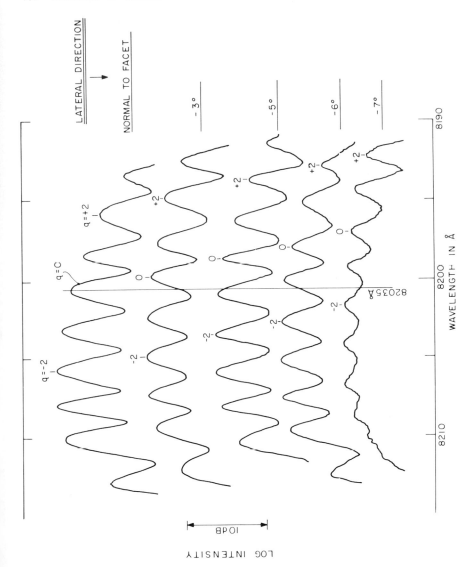

FIG. 7.7.5 Lateral dispersion characteristics. There is a shift of longitudinal mode groups with angle. The q numbers for the axial modes are given relative to $q = 0$ for 8203 Å viewed along the facet normal [20].

crease in viewing angle. Figure 7.7.6 compares the dispersion from the spectrum with (7.7.5) by a plot of the position of the peak of a selected longitudinal group against $\sin^2 \theta$. The value $n_3 n_e \simeq 16$.

As mentioned previously, the growth of the lateral beam profile with current is an indication that more high order modes are beginning to lase. Figure 7.7.7a is the optical spectrum at the two lateral angles of 6° and 9° from the facet normal of a device $L = 122 \ \mu m$ by $W = 71 \ \mu m$. Note that at 8924 Å, the lateral pattern (Fig. 7.7.7b) has a peak field at the facet normal which behaves as a fundamental lateral mode. On the other hand, at 8922 Å, the field has a null at the facet normal which is indicative of a high order mode.

Figure 7.7.8 is the linear plot of the peak of the longitudinal groups against $\sin^2 \theta$. A lateral scan at constant wavelength $\lambda = 8925.4$ Å is shown in Fig. 7.7.9. The lobes in Fig. 7.7.9 can be interpreted in Fig. 7.7.8 (the two parallel lines define the spectrometer resolution and setting). The lobes are predicted as the coincidence of the scan path with the slanted lines (the locus of the modes with fixed q). The position of the center of each rectangle is shown in Fig. 7.7.9 by a solid vertical line whereas the integers show the q value.

7.8 Summary

Most of the theory and understanding of the modal characteristics of semiconductor lasers has been applied to the transverse modes (mode number m). The outgrowth of this understanding is due to the fact that the geometry along the *vertical* direction is well defined because of the various grown heterojunc-

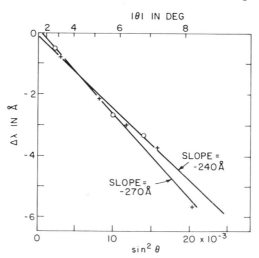

FIG. 7.7.6 Lateral dispersion data for laser spectrum of Fig. 7.7.5: ○ for $\theta < 0$; + for $\theta > 0$ [20].

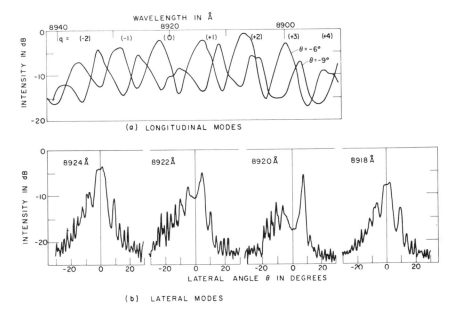

FIG. 7.7.7 Laser output with simultaneous spectral and spatial resolution. (a) Wavelength spectrum in different lateral directions and (b) lateral profiles at different wavelengths [19].

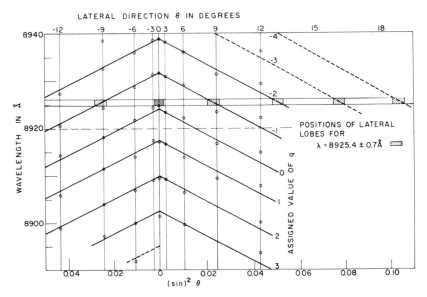

FIG. 7.7.8 Angular dependence of wavelength of different longitudinal mode groups [19].

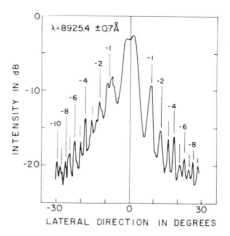

FIG. 7.7.9 Assignment of longitudinal mode numbers to lobes in spectrally resolved lateral profile [19].

tions. Consequently, the application of multilayered waveguide structures to the grown layered devices has been relatively successful.

On the other hand, the *lateral* modal characteristics of laser devices are rather complicated. For example, the sawed-sidewall devices tend to operate in an enormous number of lateral modes. The mesa-type lasers, which have strong lateral field confinement because of grown sidewalls, also operate in multilateral modes. Stripe-geometry devices of the planar type tend to operate in low order lateral modes and in fact go to the fundamental mode for narrow stripes, $S_t \leq 10 \ \mu m$, at least near threshold.

Basically, the models most applicable to the study of lateral modes are the buried rectangular dielectric slab and the parabolic varying index. The buried rectangular slab gives sinusoidal field solutions in the slab whereas the parabolically varying index gives the Hermite–Gaussian modes. Although the parabolically varying index can give useful results for field profiles, it cannot predict waveguide modal content; the cavity modal content is related to a cavity width and index step and the parabolically varying index model fails to define either.

Through the development of the multilayered slab waveguides, we defined the appropriate equations giving the modal content along the vertical direction. These same equations can be applied to the maximum number of allowed propagating lateral modes. The theory developed for the box modes treats the lateral and vertical modes as being independent. Consequently, it follows that the lateral modal content can be found in an identical manner as that used to find the vertical modal numbers. For example, in Fig. 5.7.1, if Δn_{36}

is the index step between regions 3 and 5, and 3 and 7, then the maximum number of lateral s modes S is given by

$$S = \text{In}[1 + (2W/\lambda)(n_3^2 - n_6^2)^{1/2}]$$

which is identical to (5.5.7).

REFERENCES

1. J. K. Butler and H. Kressel, *J. Appl. Phys.* **43**, 3403 (1972).
2. J. K. Butler, H. S. Sommers, Jr., and H. Kressel, *Appl. Phys. Lett.* **17**, 403 (1970).
3. H. Kressel, J. K. Butler, F. Z. Hawrylo, H. F. Lockwood, and M. Ettenberg, *RCA Rev.* **32**, 393 (1971).
4. J. K. Butler, H. Kressel, and I. Ladany, *IEEE J. Quantum Electron.* **11**, 402 (1975).
5. W. P. Dumke, *IEEE J. Quantum Electron.* **11**, 400 (1975).
6. H. Kressel and M. Ettenberg, *J. Appl. Phys.* **47**, 3533 (1976).
7. H. F. Lockwood and H. Kressel, *J. Crystal Growth* **27**, 97 (1974).
8. H. Kressel, H. F. Lockwood, and F. Z. Hawrylo, *J. Appl. Phys.* **43**, 561 (1972).
9. I. Hayashi, M. B. Panish, and F. K. Reinhart, *J. Appl. Phys.* **42**, 1929 (1971).
10. Zh. I. Alferov et al., *Sov. Phys.—Semicond.* **8**, 826 (1975).
11. W. W. Anderson, *IEEE J. Quantum Electron.* **1**, 228 (1965).
12. N. E. Byer and J. K. Butler, *IEEE J. Quantum Electron.* **6**, 291 (1970).
13. B. W. Hakki, *IEEE J. Quantum Electron.* **11**, 149 (1975).
14. B. W. Hakki and C. J. Hwang, *J. Appl. Phys.* **45**, 2168 (1974).
15. J. K. Butler and J. Zoroofchi, *IEEE J. Quantum Electron.* **10**, 809 (1974).
16. H. Yonezu, I. Sakuma, K. Kobayashi, T. Kamejima, M. Veno, and Y. Nannichi, *Jpn. J. Appl. Phys.* **12**, 1585 (1973).
17. D. D. Cook and F. R. Nash, *J. Appl. Phys.* **46**, 1660 (1975).
18. H. S. Sommers, Jr., *J. Appl. Phys.* **44**, 1263 (1973).
19. H. S. Sommers, Jr., *J. Appl. Phys.* **44**, 3601 (1973).
20. H. S. Sommers, Jr., and D. O. North, *Solid State Electron.* **8**, 675 (1976).

Chapter 8

Relation between Electrical and Optical Properties of Laser Diodes

In this chapter we analyze the relationships among the vertical device geometry, threshold current density, and differential quantum efficiency using the results of Chapters 3, 5, and 6. In Section 8.1 we consider the relationship among the current density, the injected carrier density, and the gain coefficient. In Section 8.2 we discuss the threshold current density and differential quantum efficiency of various laser structures. Section 8.3 is concerned with the temperature dependence of the threshold current density. In Section 8.4 we discuss lasers which exhibit unusually large changes of threshold with temperature as a result of changes in the refractive index step at one boundary of the waveguide region. Such lasers are also shown to be prone to anomalous pulse distortion effects.

8.1 Carrier Confinement and Injected Carrier Utilization

8.1.1 Carrier Confinement

The recombination region of a heterojunction laser can be n-type or p-type since injection can be provided by either type of heterojunction, as explained in Chapter 2. In this section, we concern ourselves with two major aspects of the problem: (1) carrier confinement assuming an ideal heterojunction with sufficient grading to eliminate the interfacial spikes, and (2) the effect of a finite interfacial recombination velocity on the carrier utilization in radiative recombination.

In the simplest case of low injected minority carrier density in the low band-gap energy side and equal initial majority carrier densities on both sides of the heterojunction, the illustration of Fig. 8.1.1a for a p–p heterojunction is appropriate. The potential barrier confining electrons $\varphi \cong E_{g2} - E_{g3} \cong \Delta E_g$ [1]. The situation is more complex when the doping levels differ on the two sides of the heterojunction, and the quasi-Fermi level shift in the low bandgap side is substantial because of high injection [2, 3]. The illustration Fig. 8.1.1b is appropriate for this case, where the effective barrier height is now reduced as indicated to reflect the relative positions of Fermi and quasi-Fermi levels with respect to the band edges. A low hole concentration in the high bandgap side shifts the Fermi level into the gap in that region which reduces φ. Furthermore, the effect of a high electron concentration on φ in the low bandgap p-region is not negligible because the upward shift of the quasi-Fermi level with injection will reduce the effective bandgap energy step. The quasi-Fermi level displacement into the parabolic conduction band with ΔN electrons in p-type material is given at $T = 0$ K by

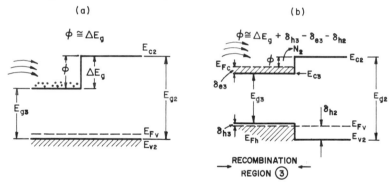

FIG. 8.1.1   Electron confinement at an idealized p–p heterojunction. (a) Low electron concentration injected into the low bandgap side; (b) high electron injection, with substantial filling of conduction band states.

$$E_{Fc} - E_c = \delta_e = 3.64 \times 10^{-15}(m_0/m_c^*)(\Delta N)^{2/3} \quad \text{(eV)} \qquad (8.1.1)$$

At finite temperatures, the method of Section 1.4 must, of course, be used to calculate δ_e.

The effect of carrier confinement loss on the threshold current density of laser diodes may be calculated with simplifying assumptions. We assume an ideal isotype heterojunction, neglecting interfacial spikes. (The subscript 3 denotes parameters for the active region.) As shown in Fig. 8.1.1, the carrier concentrations in the p-type active and passive regions are $P_0 + \Delta N$ and P_2, respectively. The quasi-Fermi levels E_{Fc} and E_{Fv} in the active region are indicated. Energy separation between the passive region conduction band edge E_{c2} and the active region edge E_{c3} is $\varphi = E_{c2} - E_{c3}$.

Our immediate interest is in determining the threshold current density in the case in which carrier leakage from the recombination region occurs. From Section 3.4 we know that a carrier pair density in the recombination region $(\varDelta N)_{th}$ is needed at threshold, and the minimum threshold current density, which we denote J_{th1}, is

$$J_{th1} = e(\varDelta N)_{th}d_3/\tau \qquad (8.1.2a)$$

where τ is the average carrier lifetime at threshold. The loss of electrons, from the p-type recombination region, gives rise to an excess diffusion current (Chapter 2)

$$J_2 = (eD_{e2}/L_{e2})N_2 \qquad (8.1.2b)$$

where N_2 is the electron density at the edge of the high bandgap side of the isotype heterojunction, and D_{e2} and L_{e2} denote the diffusion constant and diffusion length of electrons in the high bandgap p-side of the junction. (If hole injection into the n-side can occur as well, then an additional hole current flow can be added. For the moment we neglect this effect which is typically small relative to the electron loss.) Then the observed J_{th} value is

$$J_{th} = J_{th1} + J_2 = \frac{e(\varDelta N)_{th}d_3}{\tau} + \frac{eD_{e2}}{L_{e2}}N_2 \qquad (8.1.2c)$$

Continuing our illustration of a p-type recombination region, in order to calculate the carrier density at the edge of the high bandgap p-type region N_2, we need to establish first the position of the quasi-Fermi level in the conduction band of the recombination region 3 when it contains a carrier density $\varDelta N$, or more specifically $(\varDelta N)_{th}$, and then determine the population within the higher energy conduction band of the high bandgap region 2.

From Section 1.4, we recall that the electron quasi-Fermi level position for $\varDelta N$ injected electrons is found from

$$\varDelta N = 6.55 \times 10^{21}(m_{c3}^*)^{3/2} \int_{E_{c3}}^{\infty} \frac{(E - E_{c3})^{1/2}\, dE}{1 + \exp[(E - E_{Fc})/kT)]} \qquad (8.1.3a)$$

while the value of N_2 is

$$N_2 = M(6.55 \times 10^{21})(m_{c2}^*)^{3/2} \int_{E_{c2}}^{\infty} \frac{(E - E_{c2})^{1/2}\, dE}{1 + \exp[(E - E_{Fc})/kT]} \qquad (8.1.3b)$$

where M is the multiplicity of equivalent valleys.

Equation (8.1.3b) can be simplified under typical conditions where the energy separation between the electron quasi-Fermi level in the active region and the conduction band minimum of the higher bandgap region is substantially in excess of kT.

If $E_{c2} - E_{Fc} \gtrsim 4kT$, then $N_2 = N_{c2} \exp[-(E_{c2} - E_{Fc})/kT]$, and from (8.1.2b),

$$J_2 = \frac{eD_{e2}N_{c2}}{L_{e2}} \exp\left(\frac{-\varphi}{kT}\right) \qquad (8.1.4a)$$

where $\varphi = \Delta E_g - \delta_{h2} + \delta_{h3} - \delta_{e3}$.

Under high injection conditions, $\delta_{h3} \approx 0$; from (1.4.14) with $\delta_{h2} \gtrsim 4kT$, $\delta_{h2} \cong kT \ln(P_2/N_{v2})$. Hence,

$$J_2 = \frac{eD_{e2}}{L_{e3}} \left(\frac{N_{v2}}{P_2}\right) N_{c2} \exp\left[\frac{-(\Delta E_g - \delta_{e3})}{kT}\right] \qquad (8.1.4b)$$

The *total* threshold current density is, from (8.1.2c),

$$J_{th} = \frac{e(\Delta N)_{th}d_3}{\tau} + \left(\frac{eD_{e2}}{L_{e2}}\right)\left(\frac{N_{v2}N_{c2}}{P_2}\right)\exp\left[\frac{-(\Delta E_g - \delta_{e3})}{kT}\right] \qquad (8.1.5)$$

If we consider an n–n heterojunction, with hole confinement in region 3, then a similar analysis yields for hole leakage over the barrier into region 2,

$$N_2 = N_{v2} \exp(-\varphi/kT)$$

and hence

$$J_2 = \frac{eD_{h2}N_{v2}}{L_{h2}} \exp\left(\frac{-\phi}{kT}\right) \qquad (8.1.4c)$$

If more than one conduction band valley is within a reasonable energy range from the edge of the Γ minimum in the active region, then the population of these valleys will have to be taken into account in calculating the leakage current [Eq. (8.1.3b)].

Because of the lower mobility of holes compared to electrons, hole leakage effects will generally be smaller than electron leakage for a given heterojunction barrier.

A numerical estimate of J_2 can be made assuming the following reasonable parameter values for a double-heterojunction laser where the active region consists of GaAs, and the passive p-type region is (direct bandgap) $Al_{0.2}Ga_{0.8}As$ (hence $\Delta E_g \cong 0.2$ eV):

$L_{e2} = 1 \ \mu m$ (the width of the high bandgap region)

$D_{e2} = 50 \ cm^2/V\text{-}s$, $N_{c2} = 6 \times 10^{17} \ cm^{-3}$, $N_{v2} = 9 \times 10^{18} \ cm^{-3}$

$P_2 = 5 \times 10^{17} \ cm^{-3}$, $\delta_{e3} = 0.03$ cV

Then, from (8.1.4b)

$$J_2 = 8.6 \times 10^5 \exp[-(\Delta E_g - \delta_{e3})/kT]$$

and

$$J_2 = 1240 \ A/cm^2 \qquad (300 \ K)$$

This is a significant quantity. However, even a modest increase in ΔE_g reduces the electron leakage. For example, when $\Delta E_g - \delta_{e3} = 0.25$ eV, $J_2 \cong 60$ A/cm², a negligible quantity.

The use of high doping in the high bandgap region such that $\delta_{v2} \approx 0$, has a similar effect on reducing the leakage. Thus

$$J_2 = \frac{e D_{e2}}{L_{e2}} N_{c2} \exp\left[\frac{-(\Delta E_g - \delta_{e3})}{kT}\right] \tag{8.1.6}$$

With these values the leakage is reduced to only $J_2 \approx 7$ A/cm².

Note that the temperature dependence of (8.1.6) is of the form (since $N_c \propto T^{3/2}$)

$$J_2 \propto T^{3/2} \exp[-(\Delta E_g - \delta_{e3})/kT] \tag{8.1.7}$$

Although the numerical values calculated for the excess current are very much dependent on the numerical approximations, the important device-relevant results of the preceding are as follows:

1. The current "loss" is exponentially temperature dependent. In fact, luminescence from the high bandgap region has been experimentally observed by viewing the radiation emitted from the high bandgap region of a double-heterojunction laser [1]. This contributes to the temperature dependence of the threshold current density (Section 8.3).

2. The barrier height is a function of the Fermi level position and band structure of the high bandgap region. A particularly large effect on reducing the barrier height is expected when the bandgap energy of the p-type confining region is indirect, because the density of effective conduction band states is then increased by a factor of 50 to 60. In addition, the valence band density of states N_{c2} is also generally increased, resulting in a shift of the Fermi level into the gap for a constant hole density in that region. In fact, this analysis suggests that the hole concentration in that region should be maintained as high as possible consistent with other device requirements. A change in the hole concentration by a factor of 10, for example, reduces the barrier height by ~0.06 eV at room temperature. This is insignificant if the bandgap energy difference is 0.3 eV, but significant in terms of carrier confinement for low barriers of 0.1–0.2 eV, and becomes increasingly important with increasing temperature and reduced recombination region width.

3. The excess current density depends on the properties of the layer between the edge of the recombination region and the minority carrier sink. In the case of a four-heterojunction laser the presence of a second heterojunction a small distance beyond the one bounding the active region results in a low leakage current, even if the barrier height of the active region is relatively low. Thus, recombination region barrier heights of only 0.1 eV are quite acceptable, whereas they would result in a rather large temperature dependence of J_{th} for a double-heterojunction laser.

8.1.2   *Interfacial Recombination and Carrier Utilization*

So far in this chapter we have assumed that the heterojunction acts as an ideal barrier, i.e., a barrier without nonradiative carrier recombination. In practice, interfacial recombination centers do exist, and this assumption is only justified under certain conditions which depend on the width of the recombination region relative to the diffusion length. Burnham *et al.* [4] and Eliseev [5] have calculated the fraction of injected carriers which recombine radiatively for various conditions for an abrupt heterojunction, and James [6] has analyzed the problem for a graded heterojunction.

Assuming a p-type recombination region with a high potential barrier ($\varphi = 0.2$ eV or $\gg kT$) which repels electrons placed a distance d_3 from the injecting junction, the fraction of the injected electrons which recombine radiatively, γ^*, is given by [5]

$$\gamma^* = 1 - \frac{2(SL_e/D_e)}{(1 + SL_e/D_e)\exp(d_3/L_e) - (1 - SL_e/D_e)\exp(-d_3/L_e)} \quad (8.1.8)$$

where S is the interfacial surface recombination velocity (nonradiative centers are assumed), and L_e is the electron diffusion length as limited by the bulk material minority carrier lifetime τ and minority carrier diffusion constant D_e [$L_e = (D_e\tau)^{1/2}$]. (A similar expression holds for an n-type recombination region with appropriate L_h and D_h.)

Figure 8.1.2 shows γ^* as a function of SL_e/D_e for various values of d_3/L_e at room temperature. Since L_e is typically 2–5 μm in GaAs, it is evident that SL_e/D_e must be less than 10^{-2} for devices with the narrow recombination regions ($d_3/L_e = 0.1$) required for the lowest threshold laser diodes. For example, 90% utilization of the injected carriers in the case of $d_3/L_e = 0.1$ (assuming $L_e = 5$ μm and $D_e = 50$ cm²/s) requires $S \approx 10^3$ cm/s. This S value compares to $S \cong 10^6$ cm/s for a free GaAs surface.

Chapter 9 discusses epitaxial problems and misfit dislocations. Here we simply need to consider that the lattice misfit, and consequent misfit dislocation density at the heterojunction interface, can be theoretically related to the interfacial recombination velocity as follows. For small differences between the lattice parameter values a_1 and a_2, an adequate linear dislocation density estimate for {100} planes is obtained using the expression (assuming a $\langle 100 \rangle$ type Burgers vector)

$$\rho_{dl} \approx \sqrt{2}\,(\Delta a_0/\tilde{a}_0{}^2)\ \text{cm}^{-1} \quad (8.1.9)$$

where $\tilde{a}_0 = (a_1 + a_2)/2 \approx a_0$.

Experimental dislocation densities are commonly found to be within a factor of 3 of the value calculated from (8.1.9) for $\Delta a_0/a_0 \lesssim 1\%$.

The density of recombination centers N_{ss} introduced by dislocations lying

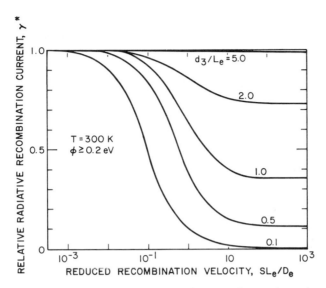

FIG. 8.1.2   The effect of interfacial recombination at an isotype heterojunction on the radiative efficiency is determined from the fractional radiative recombination current γ^* as a function of the reduced recombination velocity. $\phi \approx \Delta E_g$ is the confining potential barrier at the heterojunction [4].

in the interfacial plane can be calculated by assuming that each atom terminating an edge dislocation constitutes a recombination center. The calculated value of N_{ss} depends on the crystal structure and orientation. For a sphalerite structure on the (100) interfacial plane [7]

$$N_{ss} = 4\frac{a_1^2 - a_2^2}{a_1^2 a_2^2} \approx \frac{8\,\Delta a_0}{a_0^3}\ cm^{-2} \tag{8.1.10}$$

and for the (111) plane,

$$N_{ss} = \frac{4}{\sqrt{3}}\frac{a_1^2 - a_1^2}{a_1^2 a_1^2} \approx \frac{8}{\sqrt{3}}\frac{\Delta a_0}{a_0^3}\ cm^{-2} \tag{8.1.11}$$

The recombination velocity at the heterojunction interface can be estimated from the N_{ss} values:

$$S = v_{th}N_{ss}\sigma_t \tag{8.1.12}$$

where v_{th} is the thermal electron velocity and σ_t is the capture cross section for the center. A value of $\sigma_t \approx 10^{-15}\ cm^2$ is likely to be of the correct order of magnitude.

These expressions assume a simple model for the abrupt metallurgical interface between the two materials. In practice, matters are considerably more complicated, as discussed in Chapter 9, because the interface does not contain a simple array of misfit dislocations, particularly if the misfit becomes substantial. For the moment, we note that a low interfacial recombination velocity is obtained with $Al_xGa_{1-x}As/GaAs$ heterojunctions. The experimentally determined values are $S \cong 4 \times 10^3$ cm/s for $x = 0.25$ and 8×10^3 cm/s for $x = 0.5$ [8]. Since no misfit dislocations are usually noted in this alloy system where the lattice parameter is matched at the growth temperature, the origin of the interfacial recombination centers must be other than dislocations. No theoretical model is yet available.

There are few data correlating the lattice mismatch at heterojunctions of other III–V compounds to the surface recombination velocity. Studies of (InGa)P–GaAs interfaces show that for $\Delta a_0/a_0 \lesssim 0.1\%$, $S \lesssim 10^4$ cm/s, consistent with (8.1.10) and (8.1.12) with $v_{th} = 10^7$ cm/s and $\sigma_t = 10^{-15}$ cm^2. However, with $\Delta a_0/a_0 \approx 1\%$, $S \gtrsim 8 \times 10^5$ cm/s [9], approaching, in effect, the value $S \approx 10^6$ cm/s found at a free GaAs surface.

Ettenberg and Kressel [8] reported the important observation that for thin ($d \lesssim 1$ μm) double-heterojunction structures (with symmetrical heterojunction barrier heights), the apparent interfacial recombination velocity effectively decreases with decreasing heterojunction spacing. This means that, practically speaking, the recombination region width of DH lasers can be reduced below the value which would be theoretically limiting the internal quantum efficiency on the basis of the discussion following Eq. (8.1.8). This makes it possible to construct very low threshold current density lasers as described in Section 8.2.

We now turn our attention to the relationship among the current density, the injected carrier density, the width of the recombination region, and the carrier lifetime. This will allow us to relate these parameters to the gain coefficient at threshold and produce general relationships for the threshold current density as a function of basic parameters.

The injected carrier pair density ΔN within a recombination region d_3 wide changes with time according to the relationship

$$\partial(\Delta N)/\partial t = J/ed_3 - (\Delta N)/\tau \tag{8.1.13}$$

where the lifetime τ may depend on the injected carrier density if the background concentration is relatively low, as discussed in Section 1.5.2 and now analyzed for the case of a diode. For the moment, we assume that τ represents the *average* lifetime of the carriers in the recombination region in the vicinity of the threshold current density when the injected carrier pair density is $(\Delta N)_{th}$. In steady state, $\partial(\Delta N)/\partial t = 0$ and from (8.1.13) we obtain the familiar expression

$$(\Delta N)_{th} = J_{th}\tau/ed_3 \tag{8.1.14}$$

Because of the finite lifetime, a period of time denoted t_d is needed to establish equilibrium within the recombination region when a current pulse is applied to the diode. The delay is a function of the amplitude of the drive current density relative to the threshold current density. From (8.1.13) and neglecting the dependence of τ on ΔN,

$$t_d \cong \int_0^{(\Delta N)_{th}} \frac{d(\Delta N)}{[J/ed_3 - (\Delta N)/\tau]} = -\tau \ln\left(\frac{J}{ed_3} - \frac{(\Delta N)}{\tau}\right)\Bigg|_0^{(\Delta N)_{th}} \quad (8.1.15)$$

Using (8.1.14) [10],

$$t_d \cong \tau \ln[J/(J - J_{th})] \cong \tau \ln[I/(I - I_{th})] \quad (8.1.16)$$

Equation (8.1.16) has been shown [11] to be reasonably valid even when the lifetime decreases with injection level; it therefore provides one means of estimating the average spontaneous recombination carrier lifetime at threshold. An important consequence of (8.1.16) is that the *threshold current density depends on the pulse width* for pulse lengths on the order of the spontaneous lifetime. This places a limitation on the pulse modulation when the diode is taken through threshold. To overcome this limitation, devices capable of CW operation are dc-biased at the lasing threshold current, and the laser is modulated only in the operating region above threshold where the carrier lifetime is now the shorter *stimulated* lifetime (Section 14.3).

Below threshold, the average carrier lifetime can be estimated by measuring the radiation decay time as a function of the current amplitude. In Section 1.5.2 we showed that the lifetime is related to the sum of the initial carrier concentration $N_0 + P_0$ and the injected pair density ΔN:

$$\tau = [B_r(N_0 + P_0 + \Delta N)]^{-1} \quad (8.1.17)$$

Hence,

$$1/\tau = B_r(P_0 + N_0) + B_r \Delta N, \quad 0 = B_r(P_0 + N_0)\tau + B_r J\tau^2/ed_3 - 1 \quad (8.1.18)$$

Solving for τ,

$$\tau = \frac{ed_3(P_0 + N_0)}{2J}\left[\left(1 + \frac{4J}{eB_r d_3(P_0 + N_0)^2}\right)^{1/2} - 1\right] \quad (8.1.19)$$

In n-type material $N_0 \gg P_0$, whereas in p-type material $P_0 \gg N_0$. For *low* injection compared to the background concentration, (8.1.17) reduces to a constant lifetime independent of J:

$$\tau \cong [B_r(N_0 + P_0)]^{-1} \quad (8.1.20)$$

For *high* injection levels, $\Delta N \gg N_0 + P_0$, we obtain a reduction of the lifetime with current density. From (8.1.19),

$$\tau \cong (ed_3/B_r)^{1/2} J^{-1/2} \quad (8.1.21)$$

From the slope of the curve of lifetime versus current density in the "full" bimolecular regime, it is therefore possible to estimate B_r:

$$B_r = (ed_3)\left[\frac{\partial \tau}{\partial(1/J)^{1/2}}\right]^{-2} \quad (8.1.22)$$

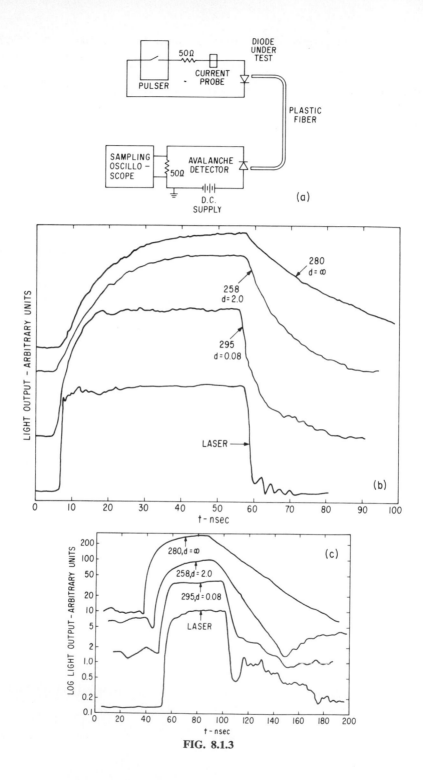

FIG. 8.1.3

The carrier lifetime is estimated from the decay of the luminescent pulse, which is usually exponential with time. Figure 8.1.3 shows the measurement apparatus used and pulsed information obtained [8]. (The plastic fiber is used to minimize the noise in the measurement by providing the highest possible degree of electrical isolation.) A relay type of pulser is used to obtain very short rise and fall times of the current through the diode, and a Si avalanche diode detector is used for the optical measurements. Rise or fall times of about 1 ns can be measured with such equipment. The diode lifetime is defined from measurement of the time required for the light pulse to decay to e^{-1} of its initial value.

An example of the measurement made on a $Al_{0.5}Ga_{0.5}As/GaAs$ DH laser (p-type, 8×10^{17} cm^{-3}, recombination region $d_3 = 0.1$ μm) is shown in Fig. 8.1.4 where the lifetime was deduced as a function of increasing diode current density J. Figure 8.1.5 shows the lifetime value $\tau = 2.3$ ns as deduced at threshold from the same laser using Eq. (8.1.16). As indicated in Fig. 8.1.4, this τ fits reasonably at the appropriate current density value of ~ 1000 A/cm^2, and both methods of determining τ therefore produce comparable values. In Fig. 8.1.4, the lifetime at high J values is proportional to $J^{-1/2}$. The curve in Fig. 8.1.4 is Eq. (8.1.19) plotted with $P_0 + N_0 = 10^{18}$ cm^{-3} and $B_r = 0.9 \times 10^{-10}$ cm^3/s. The fit to the experimental data is reasonable, considering that the estimated experimental accuracy in measuring τ is about 1 ns. We recall from Section 1.5.2 that a value of B_r in the vicinity of 10^{-10} cm^3/s is found from other experimental measurements.

Note that the injected carrier density at threshold can be deduced from these measurements using Eq. (8.1.14). With $\tau \cong 3$ ns, $d_3 = 0.1$ μm, and $J_{th} = 1000$ A/cm^2, we estimate $(\varDelta N)_{th} = 1.9 \times 10^{18}$ cm^{-3}, which is consistent with the 1.8×10^{18} cm^{-3} value theoretically estimated in Section 3.4. (However, the present material, is somewhat more highly doped than called for in the calculation of an "undoped" recombination region which was considered as an example in Section 3.4.)

It is evident from (8.1.14) that a low τ value at threshold results in an undesirable reduction in $\varDelta N$ for a given diode current density (i.e., J_{th} is increased). Hwang and Dyment [13] have studied the effect of increasing (by

---

FIG. 8.1.3   (a) Schematic diagram of apparatus for diode rise and fall time measurements. (b) Detected optical pulses from an injection laser above threshold and from three diodes of varying heterojunction spacings operating below lasing threshold. (c) The same data obtained using a logarithmic amplifier to illustrate the exponential nature of the fall time [8].

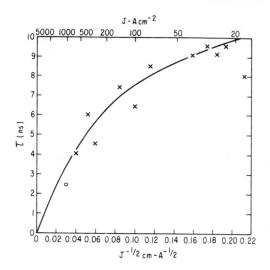

FIG. 8.1.4 Carrier lifetime as a function of the inverse square root of the current density of a double-heterojunction $Al_{0.5}Ga_{0.5}As/GaAs$:Ge diode with a background hole concentration $P_0 = 10^{18}$ cm^{-3}. The curve is Eq. (8.1.19) with $B_r = 0.9 \times 10^{-10}$ cm^3/s. The circle point lifetime was obtained using Eq. (8.1.16) [26].

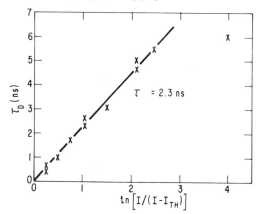

FIG. 8.1.5 Lasing delay as a function of the current overdrive. The lifetime at threshold is deduced from (8.1.16) to be 2.3 ns. Same diode as in Fig. 8.1.4 [8].

doping) the hole concentration of the p-type GaAs:Ge recombination region of double-heterojunction lasers. A correlation was established between the reduction in the minority carrier lifetime (with increasing hole concentration) and the increase in threshold current density, as shown in Fig. 8.1.6. Hence, it is desirable to minimize the initial free carrier concentration in the recombination region; this is also desirable because of the reduced free carrier absorption, as discussed in Section 8.2. In fact, the increased free carrier absorption within the recombination region with increasing doping certainly contributes

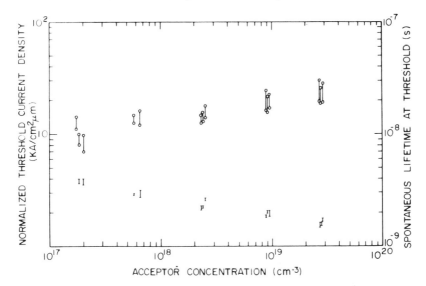

FIG. 8.1.6 Dependence of the normalized threshold current density (○) and of the spontaneous recombination lifetime (–) of electrons on the Ge acceptor concentration in the recombination region of a double-heterojunction (AlGa)As/GaAs laser [13].

to the increasing J_{th} values seen in Fig. 8.1.6. However, this requirement of low free carrier concentration is not incompatible with the use of high donor and acceptor concentrations if close compensation is maintained. For example, in GaAs grown by LPE the simultaneous doping with Si and Zn is one means of obtaining such highly doped, closely compensated, recombination regions.

8.2   Threshold Current Density and Differential Quantum Efficiency

To make the laser design curves as general as possible, we introduce certain parameters relating only to the internal geometry of the diode perpendicular to the junction plane. As noted previously, in the multilayer structure used to model the lasers, one layer is designated the "gain region" (or "active" region) in which stimulated emission occurs. We assume that this region is fully inverted with only free carrier absorption occurring within it. The other regions surrounding the gain region are "passive" and only absorb the stimulated radiation.

Following Section 5.6, the term *absorption coefficient* is used here in two ways. In the first instance, it refers to a bulk parameter of the material in a passive region of the laser. (This value is determined from conventionally measured absorption coefficient data using bulk samples.) In the second instance, the absorption coefficient is the value seen by a guided mode propagating in the plane of the junction. Here, to determine the absorption coefficient of the mode we must know its intensity distribution in the direction transverse to the junction plane. Each region of the laser, including the gain region, now makes a prorated contribution to the modal absorption coefficient dependent on the fraction of the radiation in that region.

The material in various regions of the laser is characterized by its complex relative dielectric constant κ. The imaginary part of κ is related to the absorption coefficient whereas the real part is related to the index of refraction. The contributions to the effective absorption coefficient include free carrier absorption within the recombination region, α_{fc}, a *weighted* absorption coefficient $\bar{\alpha}_0$ from all *passive* regions which takes into account the fraction of the radiation in each region, and the cavity end loss α_{end} (see Chapter 5).

We consider now the waveguide modal field as the medium for transferring energy from the gain region to the passive regions, ignoring for the moment the radiation losses at the end facets. The fraction of the save power confined to the active region is defined as Γ. We now define a quantity G such that ΓG is proportional to the power from the active region going into the waveguide mode, while $\bar{\alpha}_0$ is proportional to the power drained from the waveguide mode by the passive regions. For a mode to propagate without magnitude change, the gain and loss must be balanced. From this condition, G_{th} is defined as

$$\Gamma G_{th} = \bar{\alpha}_0 \tag{8.2.1}$$

As shown in Section 5.6, this expression can be simplified if each of the passive regions has the same bulk absorption coefficient α_i*

$$G_{th} = \alpha_i (1 - \Gamma)/\Gamma \tag{8.2.2}$$

Therefore, G_{th} represents the recombination region gain coefficient at the threshold for a laser with *no free carrier absorption* within the recombination region ($\alpha_{fc} = 0$) and *no cavity end loss* ($\alpha_{end} = 0$). The calculation of G_{th} is very convenient since it allows us to isolate some key device properties, including inherent modal preference, without introducing confusing nonvarying factors which enter into the device performance. Once G_{th} is calculated, the active region gain coefficient g_{th} at threshold for a laser of *finite length* and known α_{fc} value is easily calculated as follows. Equating the net gain coefficient of the recombination region to the losses outside that region, we obtain

$$\Gamma(g_{th} - \alpha_{fc}) = \Gamma G_{th} + \alpha_{end} \tag{8.2.3}$$

Hence,

$$g_{th} = G_{th} + \alpha_{fc} + \Gamma^{-1}\alpha_{end} \tag{8.2.4}$$

*If the α_i values differ in the various passive regions, the absorption coefficient is determined from the fraction of the radiation in each region. In a symmetrical DH laser, equal wave spread into the two higher bandgap bounding layers can be assumed.

In terms of these quantities, the external differential quantum efficiency η_{ext} is given by

$$\eta_{\text{ext}} = \eta_i(\Gamma^{-1}\alpha_{\text{end}}/g_{\text{th}})$$

or

$$\eta_{\text{ext}} = \eta_i\{\alpha_{\text{end}}/[\alpha_{\text{end}} + (\alpha_{\text{fc}} + G_{\text{th}})\Gamma]\} \qquad (8.2.5)$$

where η_i is the internal quantum efficiency.*

A cavity of length L and facet reflectivities R_1 and R_2 has

$$\alpha_{\text{end}} = (2L)^{-1} \ln[(R_1 R_2)^{-1}] \qquad (8.2.6)$$

The free carrier absorption coefficient in the recombination region depends on the total density of carriers which includes the initial concentration N_0 or P_0, for an n-type or p-type region, respectively, and the injected carrier pair density ΔN. Hence the total free carrier density at threshold (for an n-type region) is

$$N + P = N_0 + 2\Delta N_{\text{th}} \qquad (8.2.7a)$$

and similarly for a p-type region,

$$P + N = P_0 + 2\Delta N_{\text{th}} \qquad (8.2.7b)$$

where we neglect the very small background minority carrier concentration.

The free carrier absorption associated with the initial carriers can be estimated from the experimental approximation, valid in the vicinity of the band-gap energy of GaAs at 300 K,

$$\alpha_{\text{fc}} = 0.5 \times 10^{-17}N \qquad (\text{or} \quad P) \qquad (8.2.8)$$

which is deduced from Fig. 8.2.1 [14] on the basis of absorption measurements made on bulk GaAs. (At 77 K, α_{fc} is about $0.2 \times 10^{-17}N$.)

For the contribution due to the injected carriers, we need to know ΔN_{th}. Since this quantity depends on the gain coefficient as well as the properties of the active region, a first-order determination with any degree of precision is difficult. However, as we have had occasion to discover (e.g., see Fig. 3.3.6), ΔN_{th} is likely to be in the 1–2×10^{18} cm^{-3} range at room temperature in typical laser diodes. Thus, on the basis of (8.2.8) we would expect the free carrier absorption due to these carriers to be in the 10–20 cm^{-1} range.

The experimentally determined values of the free carrier absorption coefficient (deduced from laser measurements following the procedure described

---

*The internal quantum efficiency is not a well-defined quantity in laser diodes. In the simple model of laser dynamics, η_i should be unity above the lasing threshold where the gain and carrier density are considered to be independent of current. In fact, most measurements show $\eta_i = 0.6$–0.7 at room temperature and η_i approaches unity only at very low temperatures. Inhomogeneities in the active region could contribute to the variable internal quantum efficiency seen. Chapter 17 discusses the simple model for the laser dynamics.

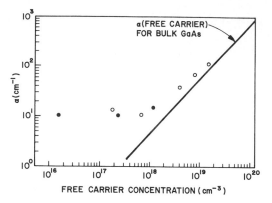

FIG. 8.2.1 Comparison of "bulk" free carrier absorption α and laser loss (α_{fc}) as a function of carrier concentration. The solid line is the "bulk" free carrier loss in GaAs just below the bandgap energy. The circles represent the laser loss at various background concentrations within the recombination region of a DH laser; $\bullet$ = n-type active layer, $\bigcirc$ = p-type active layer [14].

later in this section) for a series of (AlGa)As/GaAs DH lasers is shown in Fig. 8.2.1. Each of the data points represents a laser with a different initial carrier concentration in the recombination region. Note that for an initial concentration below 10^{18} cm^{-3}, the absorption coefficient is constant at about 10 cm^{-1}, but increases gradually as the doping level in the recombination region is increased above 10^{18} cm^{-3}. Thus, we can consider the α_{fc} value of 10 cm^{-1} a reasonable approximation for the contribution of the injected carriers in good quality lasers. This value is used in the subsequent J_{th} and differential quantum efficiency estimates. It is clear, however, that the injected carrier density can be substantially higher than the values of Fig. 8.2.1 for lossy devices—very short lasers, for example, or those containing a high flaw density, in which case an increased estimate of α_{fc} is called for. Note that free carrier absorption can be relatively large for highly doped recombination regions, a detrimental effect which reduces the device efficiency. For example, with $P_0 = 10^{19}$ cm^{-3}, $\alpha_{fc} \cong 50$ cm^{-1} due to the initially present carriers alone.

Higher values of α_{fc} are obtained in single-heterojunction lasers than in typical DH lasers since the recombination region is Zn doped to an average level in the 10^{18} cm^{-3} range. A detailed analysis [15] of such structures shows that $\alpha_{fc} \approx 30$ cm^{-1} at room temperature but decreases with temperature to ≈ 10 cm^{-1} at 77 K.

Once g_{th} is known, the threshold current density is determined by the thickness d_3 of the recombination region, the internal quantum efficiency, the carrier loss over the barrier (Section 8.1.1), and the relationship between the injected carrier density and the gain coefficient. As discussed in Section 3.4, the gain is related to the nominal current density J_{nom} by

$$g \propto J_{nom}^b \propto [(J/d_3)\eta_i]^b \tag{8.2.9}$$

a relationship valid only beyond some minimum J_{nom} value needed for population inversion. Hence at threshold,

$$J_{\text{th}} \propto (d_3/\eta_i)\, g_{\text{th}}^{1/b} \qquad (8.2.10)$$

The most direct method of predicting J_{th} from basic parameters is to calculate g_{th}, then determine J_{nom} from theoretical g vs. J_{nom} curves as given, for example, for GaAs in Section 3.3, and hence compute $J_{\text{th}} = (d_3/\eta_i)\, J_{\text{nom}}$. When an analytical g vs. J_{nom} relationship is available, the calculation is eased. For example, for undoped GaAs, it was noted in Section 3.3 that in a limited g range ($30 \leq g \leq 100$ cm^{-1}),

$$g = \beta_s^{-1}(J_{\text{nom}} - J_1) \quad (\text{cm}^{-1}) \qquad (8.2.11)$$

where β_s and J_1 have the values indicated in Table 3.3.1 at various temperatures. It can easily be shown that (Section 3.4)

$$J_{\text{th}} = \frac{d_3}{\eta_i}\left(\frac{g_{\text{th}}}{\beta_s} + J_1\right) \quad (\text{A/cm}^2) \qquad (8.2.12)$$

Figure 8.2.2 shows the calculated J_{th} using (8.2.12) compared to experimental values for Al$_x$Ga$_{1-x}$As/GaAs double-heterojunction lasers [16]. (A value of $\eta_i = 1$ is assumed.) As the refractive index step Δn is decreased, the degree of radiation confinement is decreased, resulting in an increase in J_{th} with decreasing d_3. For $d_3 \gtrsim 0.2$ μm, a linear relationship between J_{th} and d_3 is calculated,

$$J_{\text{th}}/d_3 = 4850 \text{ A/cm}^2\,\mu\text{m} \qquad (8.2.13)$$

Extensive experimental data [17] concerning DH lasers with various dopants in the recombination region indicate that for $d_3 \gtrsim 0.2$, the J_{th} values indeed fall in the range

$$J_{\text{th}}/d_3 = (4.0 \pm 1) \times 10^3 \text{ A/cm}^2\,\mu\text{m} \qquad (8.2.14)$$

For smaller d_3 values, the radiation confinement loss becomes significant. In addition, for relatively small heterojunction barrier heights, the loss of carrier confinement discussed in Section 8.1.1 can produce a significant excess leakage current which increases the observed threshold current density. Therefore, to predict the J_{th} dependence in detail for specific structures requires a determination of the confinement factor Γ and the absorption coefficients in the passive regions (i.e., G_{th}) which play an increasing role in determining the device performance as more of the radiation is outside the active region. The value G_{th} can be calculated for structures of varying complexity by appropriate solution of the wave equations as discussed in Chapter 5.

Particularly important diodes used for room temperature CW operation are thin DH structures with $d_3 \lesssim 0.3$ μm. As shown schematically in Fig. 8.2.3 (for an asymmetric structure), the field may extend through the thin p-type (AlGa)As region 1 into the p$^+$ GaAs contact layer (Section 12.1) at the

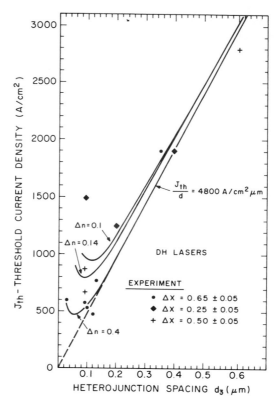

FIG. 8.2.2   Comparison of experimental and calculated (solid curves) threshold current density at room temperature of double-heterojunction $Al_xGa_{1-x}As/GaAs$ laser diodes with undoped (n-type) recombination regions. The width of the active region and the Al fraction were varied. The index step value Δn for each calculated curve is indicated. These curves were obtained from (8.2.12) assuming that the absorption coefficient α_i in each of the regions of the laser is 10 cm^{-1} and that the cavity end loss $\alpha_{end} = 23$ cm^{-1}. Hence, $g_{th} = 33/\Gamma$. The radiation confinement factor Γ was estimated from the calculations in Chapter 7. Unity internal quantum efficiency is assumed; a lower value increases the calculated J_{th} proportionately. Full carrier confinement is also assumed [16].

device surface which is highly absorbing at the lasing wavelength, particularly if the recombination region contains (AlGa)As instead of GaAs. The results of a series of theoretical calculations [18] for symmetrical structures are shown in Fig. 8.2.4 in which G_{th} is calculated for various Δn values and distances between the $Al_{0.1}Ga_{0.9}As$ recombination region ($\lambda_L \cong 0.8$ μm) and the GaAs surface "cap" region.

If the recombination region contains GaAs instead of $Al_{0.1}Ga_{0.9}As$, the effect of the absorption in the surface GaAs layer is also important because the high free carrier concentration in that region ($>10^{19}$ cm^{-3}) results

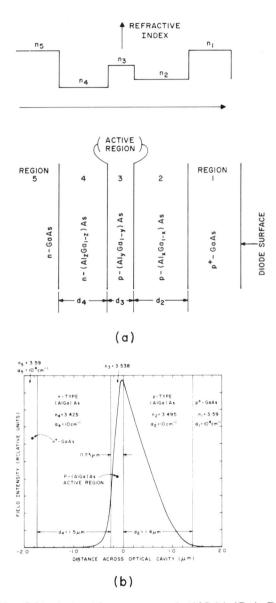

FIG. 8.2.3 Near field calculated for an asymmetric (AlGa)As/GaAs DH laser, schematic in (a), in which the radiation is preferentially spreading toward the surface of the structure. The index values are indicated as well as the thickness of each relevant region. The index values were first estimated from the (AlGa)As compositions in each region and then fine-tuned to match the experimental far-field pattern. The thicknesses were measured on the actual laser [18].

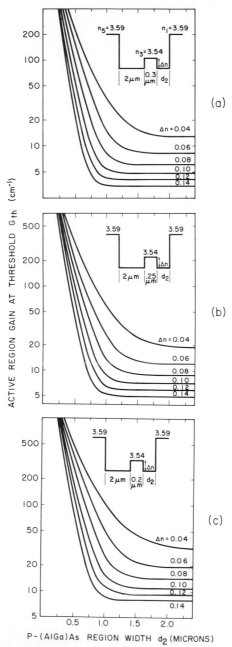

FIG. 8.2.4 The active region gain coefficient ($\lambda_L = 0.8$ μm) G_{th} at threshold (assuming infinitely long Fabry–Perot cavity, $L = \infty$), calculated for various device parameters with quantities noted in the insert sketch held constant. Both the refractive index step Δn and the width d_2 of the p-type (AlGa)As region 2 are varied [18].

in a high absorption coefficient, ≥ 50 cm^{-1}. Experimental data, in general agreement with this, show that a spacing of ≥ 0.8 μm between the recombination region and the surface "cap" layer is, in fact, needed to eliminate the deleterious effect of the surface GaAs layer [19].

The effect of changing the width of the recombination region on G_{th} can be seen from Fig. 8.2.5. As d_3 is decreased, more of the wave propagates outside the recombination region, and the device loss becomes more sensitive to the distance between the recombination region and the GaAs "cap" region.

A common approximation found in the literature is based on a linear relationship between J_{nom} and g. This results in a dependence of J_{th} of the form

$$J_{th} = \bar{\beta}^{-1}(\bar{\alpha} + L^{-1} \ln (R^{-1})) \qquad (8.2.15)$$

where $\bar{\alpha} = \Gamma(\alpha_{fc} + G_{th})$ and $\bar{\beta}$ is a constant appropriate to specific devices. For very strongly confined structures, $\Gamma \cong 1$ and $\bar{\alpha} \cong \alpha_{fc}$.

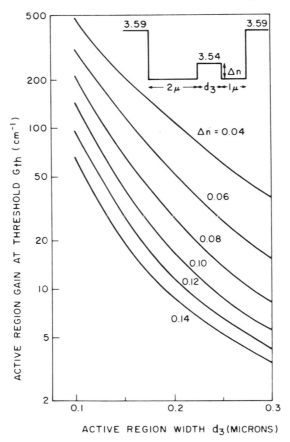

FIG. 8.2.5   The active region gain coefficient G_{th} ($\lambda_L = 0.8$ μm) at threshold as a function of the active region width d_3 for various Δn values [18].

Experimentally, one finds that (8.2.15) is well obeyed in single-heterojunction lasers [20] as well as in double-heterojunction lasers with heavily doped and compensated recombination regions [21]. For a given device structure, the traditional method of determining $\bar{\alpha}$ and $\bar{\beta}$ is to fabricate from one wafer a large number of diodes with varying lengths L and determine the dependence of J_{th} and η_{ext} on L. The better method is to use dielectric coatings [20] which change the facet reflectivity. Thus, a single diode gives η_{ext} and J_{th} data, a method which eliminates the generally unavoidable metallurgical variability among diodes. A linear g_{th} vs. J relationship yields a linear curve of the type shown in Fig. 8.2.6a for a DH laser having a heavily doped GaAs:Si recombination region, and $\bar{\beta}$ is seen to be 2.1×10^{-2} cm/A. The internal quantum efficiency $\eta_{\text{i}} = 0.55$ and $\bar{\alpha} = \Gamma(\alpha_{\text{fc}} + G_{\text{th}}) = 15$ cm^{-1} are deduced from Fig. 8.2.6b.

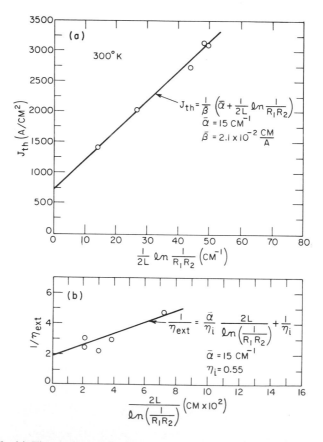

FIG. 8.2.6 (a) Threshold current density at 300 K as a function of the Fabry–Perot cavity end loss, $(1/L) \ln (1/R_1 R_2)$, of a thin DH laser. The facet reflectivity was varied with SiO coatings of various thicknesses. (b) Differential quantum efficiency as a function of the reciprocal cavity end loss of the same diode described in part (a). [21].

The reflectivity of one facet can be determined by comparing the power output from the coated and the uncoated facet, P_1 and P_2. With facet reflectivities R_1 and R_2, $P_1/P_2 = (R_2/R_1)^{1/2} [(1 - R_1)/(1 - R_2)]$.

For single-heterojunction lasers, a comparative analysis was made to determine whether a linear fit of the form (8.2.15) was appropriate by attempting superlinear plots as shown in Fig. 8.2.7. It is evident that the linear equation is indeed appropriate.

Caution must be exercised in analyzing laser data by changing the facet reflectivity or the diode length:

1. If different diodes are used, much scatter in the data may be observed owing to quality variations among diodes. In addition, in short lasers (i.e., where the Fabry–Perot cavity length becomes comparable to the diode width), total internal reflection is likely to occur. This produces the odd result that the differential quantum efficiency of *short* lasers is *higher* than that of long lasers because the radiation is internally trapped [20]. In addition, because of total internal reflection, the effective facet reflectivity $R \cong 1$, which reduces the threshold current density below the expected value for short lasers.

2. If the facet reflectivity is changed, be it by changing the dielectric coating or immersion of fluids, it is essential that the facet reflectivity be accurately determined. With dielectric coatings, one may leave one facet uncoated and measure the ratio of the emission from the two sides to determine the reflectivity of the coated facet. With fluids, it is essential to determine that the facet has not been damaged by the fluid by remeasuring the laser in air after the experiment. Finally, the problem of total internal reflection with dielectric facet coatings cannot be ignored when the facet reflectivity becomes very low.

We now briefly explore the implications of a superlinear gain dependence on the threshold current density of more complex structures. Considering the simplest case of an LOC or FH structure, in which the outer heterojunctions spaced d° apart confine the radiation, the fraction of the radiation within the *recombination region d_3* is approximately (see Section 7.3 for exact calculations)

$$\Gamma \cong d_3/d^\circ \tag{8.2.16}$$

where it is assumed that the field is weakly confined by the two inner heterojunctions. Hence rewriting the expression for g_{th},

$$g_{th} = \bar{\alpha}_0/\Gamma + \alpha_{fc} + \Gamma^{-1}\alpha_{end}$$

or

$$g_{th} = (d^\circ/d_3)(\bar{\alpha}_0 + (d_3/d^\circ)\alpha_{fc} + \alpha_{end}) \tag{8.2.17}$$

We then obtain

$$J_{th} = B_0' d_3^{(1-1/b)} d^{\circ\,(1/b)}(\bar{\alpha} + (d_3/d^\circ)\alpha_{fc} + \alpha_{end})^{1/b} \tag{8.2.18}$$

where B_0' is a constant.

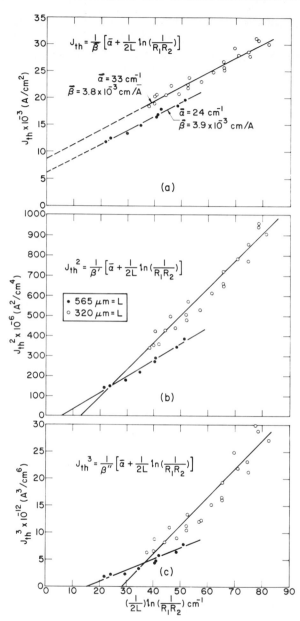

FIG. 8.2.7 Determination of the best fit of experimental data of J_{th} as a function of facet reflectivity for two lasers selected from a wafer of single-heterojunction laser diode material. The data are best fitted with the linear relationship in (a) with the $\bar{\alpha}$ and $\bar{\beta}$ parameters indicated [20].

It is evident from (8.2.18) that if $b > 1$ (and keeping $d°$ and $\bar{\alpha}_0$ constant), it is possible to reduce J_{th} by reducing the recombination region width d_3 as much as possible. This analysis implies that the recombination region is suitably placed for effective coupling to the optical field. In the case of the fundamental mode the recombination region should be placed at the center of the waveguide where the field intensity is a maximum (Chapter 7).

The four-heterojunction laser concept is well suited to optimize a laser structure with a very narrow recombination region within a wide cavity. In fact, among the lowest reported J_{th} values have been obtained with FH lasers in which $d_3 \lesssim 0.1$ μm, as summarized in Table 8.2.1 [22, 23]. The lowest J_{th} of $\sim$600 A/cm² compares to $J_{th} \approx 500$ A/cm² achieved with the simpler DH structures (Fig. 8.2.2).

Because of scatter in the data, it is difficult to judge quantitatively the superlinear dependence of gain on current in the FH devices. The results of Casey et al. [24] and Thompson et al. [22] indicate $1 < b < 3$ on the basis of plots of J_{th} as a function of the cavity end loss using groups of lasers from selected wafers.

In concluding this section, it is appropriate to consider some numerical examples to illustrate the calculation of J_{th} and η_{ext}. Consider the following double-heterojunction laser which we will use as an example.

1. *Recombination region* GaAs, n-type (10^{16} cm⁻³), width $d_3 = 0.2$ μm.
2. *Bounding layers* $Al_{0.2}Ga_{0.8}As$ ($E_g = 1.68$ eV), with 2×10^{18} cm⁻³ electrons and holes, respectively, each 1 μm thick. Therefore, the bandgap energy step at the heterojunctions (see Section 12.2) $\Delta E_g = 1.68 - 1.42$ eV $= 0.26$ eV; $\alpha_i = 10$ cm⁻¹ in each region.
3. *Laser length* $L = 500$ μm. Broad-area device. Facet reflectivity $R_1 = R_2 = 0.32$; $\alpha_{end} = L^{-1} \ln R^{-1} = 23$ cm⁻¹.

The refractive index step (see Section 12.2) $\Delta n = 0.62 \Delta x = 0.12$. Hence, from Fig. 7.2.7a the radiation confinement factor $\Gamma \cong 0.5$. From (8.2.2),

$$g_{th} = \frac{10(1 - 0.5)}{0.5} = 10 \text{ cm}^{-1}$$

Assume $\alpha_{fc} = 10$ cm⁻¹; then from (8.2.4)

$$g_{th} = 10 + 10 + 23/0.5 = 66 \text{ cm}^{-1}$$

Hence, from (8.2.12) and Table 3.3.1

$$J_{th} = \frac{0.2}{\eta_i} \left(\frac{66}{0.044} + 4100 \right) = \frac{1120}{\eta_i} \text{ A/cm}^2$$

The differential quantum efficiency is calculated from (8.2.5):

$$\eta_{ext} = \eta_i \frac{23}{23 + 0.5(10 + 10)} = 0.7\eta_i$$

TABLE 8.2.1

Low Threshold Four-Heterojunction Laser Data[a]

d_3 (μm)	$d°$ (μm)	x_3^b	Al concentrations[a]		L (μm)	J_{th}(A/cm^2)	$\theta_\perp$ (deg.)	η_{ext} (%)	Ref.
			$x_{2,4}$	$x_{1,5}$					
0.095	0.8	≈ 0	0.12	0.39	1030	650	51	33	c
0.04	0.8	≈ 0	0.12	0.30	670	900	41	20	d
0.04	0.45	≈ 0	0.13	0.42	527	575	55	26	d
0.065	0.35	≈ 0	0.12	0.32	625	720	52	30	d

[a]Refer to Fig. 7.3.1 for definition of layer numbers.

[b]Some small Al concentration ($x_3 \lesssim 0.03$) may exist in these layers judging from the emission wavelengths reported.

[c]M. B. Panish, H. C. Casey, Jr., S. Sumski, and P. W. Foy, *Appl. Phys. Lett.* **11**, 590 (1973).

[d]G. H. B. Thompson and P. A. Kirkby, *Electron. Lett.* **9**, 295 (1973).

For this device, the hole "leakage" from inadequate confinement to the active region is negligible, as can be seen as follows. The high electron concentration in the n-type $Al_{0.2}Ga_{0.8}As$ layer ensures that the Fermi level in that region is at the conduction band edge. Therefore, the potential barrier confining the holes to the active region is essentially the bandgap energy difference of 0.26 eV (neglecting the relatively small effect due to the quasi-Fermi levels within the recombination region). Hence, using (8.1.4c) with the hole diffusivity in n-type $Al_{0.2}Ga_{0.8}As$ estimated to be 5 cm^2/s, the diffusion length limited by the width of the region to 1 μm and a valence band effective density of states value of 9×10^{18} cm^{-3}, we obtain the negligible $J_2 = 2.8$ A/cm^2.

If we assume an internal quantum efficiency $\eta_i = 0.7$, the J_{th} value for this device would be 1600 A/cm^2 and the differential quantum efficiency $\eta_{ext} = 49\%$ (measured from both sides). Finally, the beam width in the direction perpendicular to the junction is estimated from Fig. 7.2.6a to be $\theta_{\perp} = 40°$. Referring to Fig. 8.3.1, such a laser can be expected to have a J_{th} increase by a factor of ~ 1.5 between 22 and 70°C.

Considering another illustration, assume now that the GaAs active region is n-type with $N_D - N_A = 3 \times 10^{18}$ cm^{-3} ($N_D = 6 \times 10^{18}$ cm^{-3}), with other device parameters as above. Then the total free carrier absorption coefficient α_{fc} in the active region is the sum of the contribution of the initial electrons, which from (8.2.8) is ~ 15 cm^{-1}, and the injected carrier contribution of about 10 cm^{-1}. Hence, $\alpha_{fc} = 25$ cm^{-1}. Thus, $g_{th} = 10 + 25 + 23/0.5 = 81$ cm^{-1}. From Fig. 3.3.3, we find that J_{nom} corresponding to this gain value is 5000 A/cm^2 μm, hence

$$J_{th} = \frac{d_3 J_{nom}}{\eta_i} \; A/cm^2 = \frac{1000}{\eta_i} \; A/cm^2$$

However, because of the higher free carrier absorption the differential quantum efficiency is lower than for the undoped recombination region,

$$\eta_{ext} = \eta_i \frac{23}{23 + 0.5(10 + 25)} = 0.57 \eta_i$$

The threshold current density can be similarly calculated from theoretical gain versus J_{nom} values at various temperatures and for different device dimensions.

8.3   Temperature Dependence of J_{th}

The threshold current density increases with temperature in all types of semiconductor lasers; but, because of the many factors which enter into determining J_{th}, no single expression is rigorously valid for all devices or temperature ranges. It is common to use an approximation $J_{th} \propto \exp(T/T_0)$ (where T_0 is usually 40–100 K in the vicinity of room temperature), but such an expression has no theoretical basis as will become evident when the factors which can affect J_{th} are considered:

1. The carrier confinement can change if the potential barrier at the heterojunction is too low compared to kT (Section 8.1).

2. The radiation confinement Γ can change for small Δn values (Section 8.4).

3. The internal quantum efficiency can decrease with increasing temperature, although this effect is usually small in good quality heterojunction lasers.

4. The minority carrier lifetime may change, affecting the relationship between the current density and the density of injected carriers in the recombination region.

5. The effective absorption coefficient may be temperature dependent, particularly if Γ is changing because the wave spreads beyond the recombination region.

6. Assuming that all these factors make minor contributions (e.g., in a *strongly* confined double-heterojunction laser because of high heterojunction walls), then the dominant temperature-related effect on J_{th} is the need for more injected carriers with increasing temperature to maintain inversion, i.e., more carriers are needed in the recombination region to maintain a given gain coefficient.

Assuming constant internal quantum efficiency and carrier confinement, the lowest possible J_{th} dependence is that limited by the increased injected carrier density needed to obtain a given threshold gain coefficient. For the undoped GaAs recombination region case, with **k** conservation, the injected pair density ΔN increases with temperature (80–400 K) as shown in Fig. 3.3.5 for a gain coefficient $g = 50$ cm^{-1}. The carrier density is seen to increase as $\sim T^{1.33}$. With other doping levels in the recombination region, this dependence will of course vary, as can be deduced from the g vs. J_{nom} plots shown in Section 3.3.

Experimentally, one generally observes a much steeper temperature dependence of J_{th} above 300 K than anticipated from the change in the required carrier density alone. Because the threshold gain coefficient may increase with temperature for the reasons enumerated, J_{th} vs. T can be predicted only from the sum of the variation of individual device parameters. In some cases, a J_{th} dependence quite close to the theoretical one is observed. Figure 3.3.5 shows such an example for an (AlGa)As/GaAs DH laser with an undoped recombination region where $J_{th} \propto T^{1.4}$ is observed to 300 K [25]. Above room temperature, however, which is generally the region of maximum practical interest, the loss of carrier confinement can become important for lasers with relatively low heterojunction barriers. In practice, one finds for DH lasers the results summarized in Fig. 8.3.1 where the ratio of the J_{th} at 22 and at 70°C

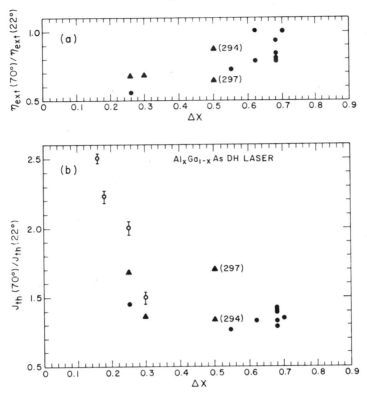

FIG. 8.3.1 Experimental data concerning the temperature dependence of (a) the differential quantum efficiency and (b) the threshold current density for double-heterojunction laser diodes having Al concentration differences Δx at the heterojunction barriers. The figure of merit is the ratio of the parameters at 22 and 70°C. Data are from Goodwin *et al.* [3] ($\bigcirc$) [$J_{\text{th}}(65°)/J_{\text{th}}(10°)$] and Kressel and Ettenberg [16] ($\bullet$ = undoped active region, $\blacktriangle$ = Ge-doped active region).

is plotted with the corresponding change in the external differential quantum efficiency. The important result is that the lowest J_{th} temperature dependence is reached when the difference in the Al concentration at the heterojunction barriers is $\geq 50\%$, corresponding to a bandgap energy difference of 0.4–0.5 eV. A detailed comparison of the theoretical and experimental J_{th} vs. T is shown in Fig. 8.3.2 for an $Al_{0.62}Ga_{0.38}As/GaAs$ DH laser with no change in the differential quantum efficiency. The experimental values are somewhat higher than the calculated values based on (8.2.11) with the parameters of Table 3.3.1, but the difference in the temperature interval indicated is relatively modest.

So far we have been mainly concerned with the laser properties *above* room temperature (more of which are discussed in Section 8.4). With regard to the

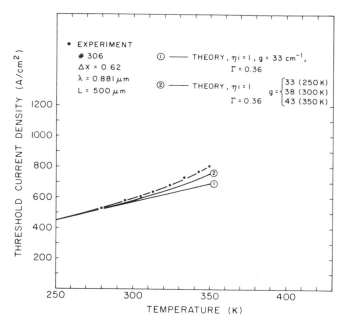

FIG. 8.3.2 Temperature dependence of the threshold current density of a double-heterojunction $Al_{0.62}Ga_{0.38}As/GaAs$ laser. The calculated curves use Eq. (8.2.12) with the parameters of Table 3.3.1 and those indicated in the figure. The differential quantum efficiency of this device was constant between 22 and 70°C [16].

temperature dependence of J_{th} *below 300 K*, it is generally found that most heterojunction devices of reasonable quality have a J_{th} increase of a factor of 6 to 10 between 77 and 300 K, whereas homojunctions change by a factor of about 40 to 60. Figure 8.3.3 illustrates this effect for typical (AlGa)As/GaAs double-heterojunction lasers, and single-heterojunction and homojunction lasers fabricated by liquid phase epitaxy. The J_{th} temperature dependence of the single-heterojunction laser is somewhat increased relative to that of the DH devices because of the higher free carrier absorption, which increases from about 10 to 30 cm^{-1} between 77 and 300 K [15].

The large increase in the homojunction laser J_{th} with temperature results from a large increase in absorption with temperature, compared to the hetero-junction devices, as well as a change in the degree of radiation confinement with temperature, the refractive index step being larger (at the lasing wave-length) at low temperatures than at higher temperatures. Figure 8.3.4 shows experimentally [15] determined plots of $\bar{\alpha}$ and $\bar{\beta}$ [Eq. (8.2.15)] as a function of temperature for a homojunction and single-heterojunction laser diode, both of which have similar 2-μm-wide active region and p$^+$ doping levels, except that the single-heterojunction laser contains (AlGa)As ($E_g = 1.67$ eV at 300

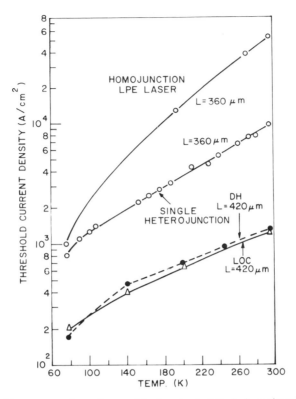

FIG. 8.3.3   Temperature dependence of J_{th} for a typical GaAs homojunction laser diode made by liquid phase epitaxy, compared to a single-heterojunction laser diode, a double-heterojunction diode with a recombination region about 0.5 μm wide, and a large optical cavity diode.

K) in the p$^+$ bounding layer. Note that the largest difference is observed in the change in the average absorption coefficient $\bar{\alpha}$ which, for the homojunction device, reaches 100 cm^{-1} at room temperature, a factor of 3 larger than $\bar{\alpha}$ of the single-heterojunction laser.

As discussed in detail by Kressel *et al.* [15], the effective absorption coefficient is higher at high temperatures in the homojunction laser because of the shift of the lasing energy relative to the absorption edge in the adjoining p$^+$ GaAs region. Lacking effective radiation confinement, much of the wave extends into that region, making the average absorption coefficient $\bar{\alpha}$ very sensitive to the absorption of the radiation in the p$^+$ GaAs region. The contribution of the *n-type* region to $\bar{\alpha}$ is relatively minor, since the absorption coefficient at the GaAs lasing energy of ∼1.37 eV (resulting from stimulated emission in a highly doped p-type region) is substantially below the absorption edge in n-type material.

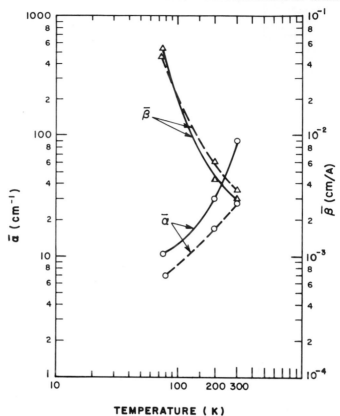

TEMPERATURE (K)

FIG. 8.3.4 Basic parameters $\bar{\alpha}$ and $\bar{\beta}$ of single-heterojunction (broken line, $E_{g2} = 1.67$ eV) and homojunction (solid line, $E_{g2} = 1.42$ eV) GaAs lasers used to describe its J_{th} variation with temperature based on Eq. (8.2.15). The largest difference is in the temperature dependence of the absorption coefficient $\bar{\alpha}$ [15].

In summary, Figs. 8.3.3 and 8.3.4 show that the J_{th} values of GaAs single-heterojunction and homojunction lasers are quite comparable at low temperatures, because the differences in radiation and carrier confinement for structures having recombination regions of about 2 μm do not play a dominant part in the 77 K performance.

8.4 Optical Anomalies and Radiation Confinement Loss in Asymmetrical Heterojunction Lasers

Early in the development of single-heterojunction laser diodes anomalous properties were observed at high temperatures in some diodes, including very large increases in threshold current density over temperature intervals as small as 5°C and low frequency oscillations in the optical emission. It was suspected that loss of radiation confinement was occurring due to a reduction in the index step at the p–n junction. The strong dielectric asymmetry of the single-heterojunction laser makes the mode guiding properties and the onset of "cut off" critically dependent on the index step at the p–n junction as discussed in Section 7.4. However, direct evidence of such loss of mode guiding is not easily obtained unless the far-field pattern changes noticeably. If in fact, mode guiding is changed, then we would expect to see a *narrowing* of the beam width $\theta_\perp$ with increasing temperature as more of the radiation is leaking from the p-type recombination region into the n-type passive region.

However, because of experimental difficulties in precisely controlling the index step at the p–n junction by the Zn diffusion step (Chapter 12), these experiments are best conducted with devices in which the individual regions are epitaxially grown. In the following we describe the results of such an experiment [27] designed to measure directly the radiation loss in an asymmetric laser consisting of the LOC configuration shown in Fig. 8.4.1. The low n–n boundary ($\Delta n \approx 0.01$) of the waveguide region $3 + 4$ is formed by a very slight difference in the Al concentration, and by a higher electron concentration in the passive region 5. (As described in Section 12.2.1 the index increases with increasing carrier concentration.)

Figure 8.4.1 shows the dramatic change in the far field perpendicular to the junction plane as measured at 22°C ($\theta_\perp = 20°$) and at 75°C ($\theta_\perp = 10°$). This beam width reduction results from an effective aperture doubling due to the field spreading into the n-type passive region 5. Of course, if the radiation confinement to the recombination region 3 is reduced with increasing temperature, we also expect to see a dramatic increase in the threshold current density. This is in fact observed as seen in Fig. 8.4.2. For comparison we also show J_{th} vs. T for a LOC device where the heterojunction barrier is symmetric at $\Delta n \cong 0.2$. Here J_{th} only doubles between 22 and 70°C compared to a factor of about 10 increase in J_{th} for the asymmetric suffering from loss of radiation confinement.

In addition to this anomalous behavior of the beam width and J_{th}, the strong reduction in optical confinement with temperature results in a deterioration of the optical pulse shape—an effect identical to that seen in some single-heterojunction lasers at elevated temperatures. Continuing with our strongly asymmetric LOC laser, we find that the optical pulse shape deteriorates markedly with evidence of instability in the output. In Fig. 8.4.3, we show the current and optical pulse shape at 22, 60, and 77.5°C of the device having the $\theta_\perp$ properties of Fig. 8.4.2. The pulse deterioration becomes particularly noticeable at 77.5°C, where there is also a marked increase in the threshold current. Similar pulse anomalies have been commonly seen in

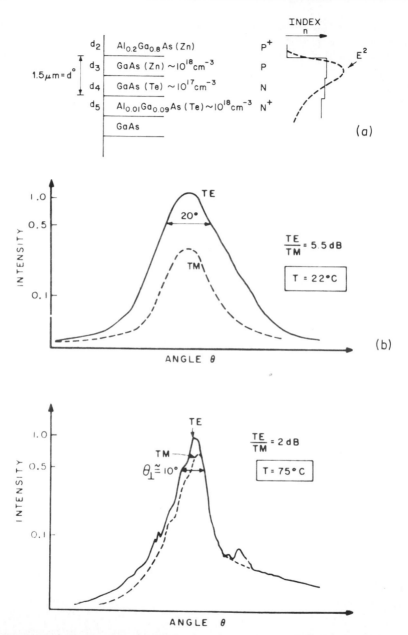

FIG. 8.4.1 (a) Profile of an asymmetric LOC laser. (b) Far-field pattern of this laser diode at 22 and 75°C showing the effect of a narrowing of the far-field pattern due to a reduction in the refractive index with increasing temperature. The index step at the n–n interface is about 0.01 [27].

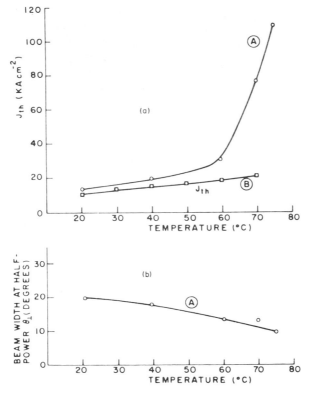

FIG. 8.4.2 (a) Change of the threshold current density with temperature of a LOC laser with temperature-dependent radiation pattern of Fig. 8.4.1 (curve Ⓐ), compared with LOC laser having temperature-independent radiation pattern (curve Ⓑ). (b) Angular divergence $\theta_\perp$ at half-power point corresponding to laser of curve Ⓐ [27].

single-heterojunction lasers; the effect is clearly connected with a fluctuating degree of optical confinement, which is lost and then partially restored during each pulse.

There have been attempts to explain the optical anomalies in terms of the interaction of saturable absorbers in the n-type region of the single-hetero-junction laser with the radiation "leaking" from the recombination region [28, 29]. At this time, these models are purely qualitative, particularly since there is no independent evidence for saturable absorbing centers in the n-type GaAs used for laser fabrication. The related problem of optical anomalies in other laser structures has been reviewed [30]. A general discussion of insta-bilities in laser diode output is presented in Chapter 17.

In summary, we find that asymmetrical laser diodes with marginal index steps at one boundary can show an anomalous increase in J_{th} and pulse

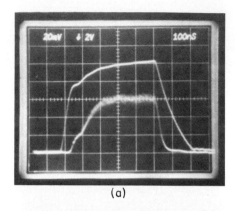

(a)

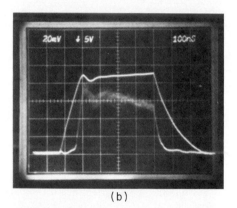

(b)

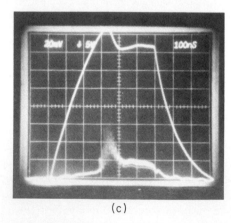

(c)

FIG. 8.4.3 Current and optical output pulse of a strongly asymmetric LOC laser with the properties shown in Fig. 8.4.2 as a function of temperature. The deterioration of the optical pulse shape is evident at high temperature. (a) T = 22°C, I (peak current) = 10 A; (b) $T = 60°C$, $I = 22$ A; (c) $T = 77.5°C$, $I = 37$ A.

deterioration effects quite comparable to those sometimes seen with single-heterojunction lasers. This results from the small index step at the p–n boundary of single-heterojunction lasers which can decrease with increasing temperature due to two factors: (1) the position of the lasing photon energy with respect to the band edges in the p-type recombination region and in the bounding n-type region; (2) the increase with temperature in the free carrier concentration in the recombination region needed to reach threshold temperature. This carrier density increase depresses the index within the recombination region, further decreasing, therefore, the difference Δn between the n-type and p-type regions. For example, the initial (room temperature) refractive index step, at a p–n junction diffused into heavily n-type GaAs (2–4×10^{18} cm^{-3}), is estimated (from analysis of single-heterojunction lasers) [15] to be only 0.01. A doubling of the threshold current density, with a consequent injection of an additional pair concentration of 2×10^{18} cm^{-3}, reduces Δn_{34} by ~ 0.003, or 30%.

Thus, it is clear that in order to maintain the high temperature properties of single-heterojunction lasers (and of all strongly asymmetric structures) it is essential to maintain the index difference substantially above a minimum value. This can be estimated on the basis of the calculated cutoff values of Section 7.4, which provides a bare minimum needed to maintain lasing for a given geometry. For the single-heterojunction laser, the use of very highly n-type substrate material is one means of providing for the required large index step at the p–n junction because this minimizes the refractive index of the n-type region. In double-heterojunction lasers, the problem is avoided by sufficiently increasing the bandgap step at the lower boundary of the asymmetrical structure (Section 12.2.1).

REFERENCES

1. H. Kressel, H. F. Lockwood, and J. K. Butler, *J. Appl. Phys.* **44**, 4095 (1973).
2. D. L. Rode, *J. Appl. Phys.* **45**, 3887 (1974).
3. A. R. Goodwin, J. R. Peters, M. Pion, G. H. B. Thompson, and J. E. A. Whiteaway, *J. Appl. Phys.* **46**, 3126 (1975).
4. R. D. Burnham, P. D. Dapkus, N. Holonyak, Jr., D. L. Keune, and H. R. Zwicker, *Solid State Electron.* **13**, 199 (1970).
5. P. G. Eliseev, *Sov. J. Quantum Electron.* **2**, 505 (1973).
6. L. W. James, *J. Appl. Phys.* **45**, 1326 (1974).
7. D. B. Holt, *J. Phys. Chem. Solids* **27**, 1053 (1966).
8. M. Ettenberg and H. Kressel, *J. Appl. Phys.* **47**, 1538 (1976).
9. R. U. Martinelli, private communication.
10. K. Konnerth and C. Lanza, *Appl. Phys. Lett.* **4**, 120 (1964).
11. J. E. Ripper, *J. Appl. Phys.* **43**, 1762 (1972).
12. H. Namizaki, H. Kan, M. Ishi, and A. Itoh, *Appl. Phys. Lett.* **24**, 486 (1974).
13. C. J. Hwang and J. C. Dyment, *J. Appl. Phys.* **44**, 3241 (1973).

14. E. Pinkas, B. I. Miller, I. Hayashi, and P. W. Foy, *IEEE J. Quantum Electron.* **9**, 281 (1973).

15. H. Kressel, H. Nelson, and F. Z. Hawrylo, *J. Appl. Phys.* **41**, 2019 (1970).

16. H. Kressel and M. Ettenberg, *J. Appl. Phys.* **47**, 3533 (1976).

17. P. G. Eliseev, *Sov. J. Quantum Electron.* **2**, 505 (1973); M. B. Panish and I. Hayashi, *Applied Solid State Science* (R. Wolfe, ed.), Vol. 4. Academic Press, New York, 1974.

18. J. K. Butler, H. Kressel, and I. Ladany, *IEEE J. Quantum Electron.* **11**, 402 (1975).

19. H. C. Casey, Jr., and M. B. Panish, *J. Appl. Phys.* **46**, 1393 (1975).

20. M. Ettenberg and H. Kressel, *J. Appl. Phys.* **43**, 1204 (1971).

21. H. Kressel, J. K. Butler, F. Z. Hawrylo, H. F. Lockwood, and M. Ettenberg, *RCA Rev.* **32**, 393 (1971).

22. G. H. B. Thompson and P. A. Kirkby, *Electron. Lett.* **9**, 295 (1973).

23. M. B. Panish, H. C. Casey, Jr., S. Sumski, and P. W. Foy, *Appl. Phys. Lett.* **11**, 590 (1973).

24. H. C. Casey, Jr., M. B. Panish, W. O. Schlosser, and T. L. Paoli, *J. Appl. Phys.* **45**, 322 (1974).

25. H. Kressel and H. F. Lockwood, *Appl. Phys. Lett.* **20**, 175 (1972).

26. J. P. Wittke, M. Ettenberg, and H. Kressel, *RCA Rev.* **37**, 159 (1976).

27. H. F. Lockwood and H. Kressel, *J. Crystal Growth* **27**, 97 (1974).

28. M. J. Adams, S. Gründorfer, B. Thomas, C. F. L. Davies, and D. Mistry, *IEEE J. Quantum Electron.* **9**, 325 (1973).

29. S. Gründorfer, M. J. Adams, and B. Thomas, *Electron. Lett.* **10**, 354 (1974).

30. J. E. Ripper and J. A. Rossi, *IEEE J. Quantum Electron.* **10**, 435 (1974).

Chapter 9

Epitaxial Technology

In this chapter we consider the epitaxial technology used to produce hetero-junction devices, which includes liquid phase epitaxy (LPE), vapor phase epitaxy (VPE), and molecular beam epitaxy (MBE). Of these, the LPE technology is the simplest for a wide variety of III–V compounds and has been most extensively used for heterojunction laser diodes. It is discussed in greatest detail here. Molecular beam epitaxy (basically an evaporation technique requiring high vacuum technology) offers potentially the broadest range of materials possibilities and best layer control on a nearly atomic thickness scale. It is also the most difficult from the point of view of equipment, instrumentation, and control and does not always produce the desired material quality. Vapor phase epitaxy is widely used for the commercial production of Ga(AsP) LEDs and offers a broad range of possibilities with equipment requirements that are simpler than those needed for MBE, but more complex than those for LPE. It is particularly useful for compositional grading.

Also included in this chapter is a discussion of the lattice parameter matching problem at heterointerfaces and methods used to minimize the dislocation density in the active region of the devices.

9.1 Liquid Phase Epitaxy

Beginning with the preparation of Ge for tunnel diodes [1], the deposition of semiconductor films by liquid phase epitaxy has been developed into a generally useful technique for the preparation of many III–V compounds

287

because it offers unique advantages in the preparation of certain materials, for example, GaAs and (AlGa)As for light-emitting diodes.

Basically, LPE involves the precipitation of material from a cooling solution onto an underlying substrate. The solution and the substrate are kept apart in the growth apparatus and the solution is saturated with the material to be grown until the desired growth temperature is reached. The solution is then brought into contact with the substrate surface and allowed to cool at a rate and during a time interval which are appropriate for the generation of the desired layer. When the substrate is single crystalline and the lattice constant of the precipitating material is the same or nearly the same as that of the substrate, the precipitating material forms an epitaxial layer on the substrate surface.

Since a solvent for the material to be deposited is needed in LPE, the usefulness of the process is limited to applications in which the solvent does not adversely affect the epitaxially deposited layer. Fortunately, this is not the problem in the case of III–V compound semiconductors because a normal constituent of the compound can be employed as solvent. For the deposition of III–V compound films, LPE has the following advantages over other epitaxial techniques:

1.   simplicity of equipment;
2.   generally higher deposition rates;
3.   elimination of hazards due to use of reactive gases and their reactive products, which are often highly toxic, explosive, or corrosive;
4.   larger selection of dopants that can be readily incorporated into the epitaxy; and
5.   the nonrequirement of vacuum equipment.

The LPE technique does, however, suffer from drawbacks compared to VPE. In particular, the reproducible preparation of ternary or quaternary alloys is difficult when the distribution coefficients of the constituent elements vary greatly. Furthermore, because LPE growth occurs over an extended temperature interval, the layer homogeneity in the direction of growth is sometimes difficult to control. Finally, because of the presence of the solvent in the solution, the stoichiometry of the material cannot be readily adjusted as is the case with VPE, nor is it easy to deposit polycrystalline films on grossly dissimilar substrates (e.g., GaAs on SiO_2). In comparison to MBE, LPE is less flexible in the layer thickness control and potential range of materials which can be prepared.

9.1.1   Growth Apparatus

The growth apparatus employed in liquid phase epitaxy are of three basic types: the "tipping" furnace, in which solution–substrate contact is achieved by tipping the furnace; the vertical furnace, in which the substrate is "dipped" into the solution; and the multibin system, in which layers are sequentially grown by bringing the substrate into contact with different solutions.

The original *tipping furnace* [1] is shown in Fig. 9.1.1. The substrate is held tightly against the flat bottom at the upper end of a graphite boat, and solution containing the material to be deposited is placed at the lower end. The graphite boat is fixed in position at the center of a constant temperature zone of the quartz furnace tube. With a flow of hydrogen through the furnace tube, the graphite boat is heated to an appropriate growth temperature. The heating power is then reduced and regulated to attain a suitable cooling rate and the furnace tipped to bring the solution into contact with the substrate. The composition of the solution is such that, at the time of tipping, it is saturated or nearly saturated with the growth material which during cooling precipitates from the solution and forms a film on the substrate surface. The solution remains in contact with the substrate for a defined temperature interval after which the tube is tipped to its original position. Remnants of the solution adhering to the film surface are removed by wiping and dissolution in a suitable solvent.

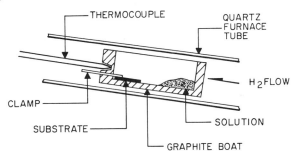

FIG. 9.1.1 Schematic showing the basic liquid phase epitaxial growth technique using a tipping furnace as originally developed by Nelson [1].

A growth apparatus employing the *dipping technique* is shown in Fig. 9.1.2. In this vertical growth system [2], a graphite or Al_2O_3 crucible is used as a reservoir for the solution. The substrate is positioned in a holder just above the solution while its temperature rises, and at the desired temperature the substrate is immersed in the solution. Growth is terminated by withdrawal of the substrate from the solution at an appropriate temperature. The dipping technique is useful when an oxide film forms on the solution during heating because the substrate is inserted through the "scum" and brought into contact with clean liquid. The vertical design also allows doping of the solution during the growth cycle to form a p–n junction within the grown film by the addition of another dopant through an exit port in the substrate holder.

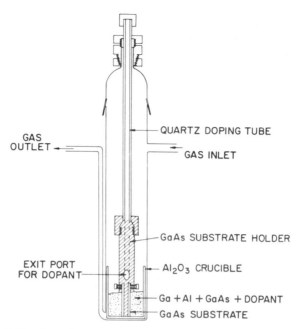

FIG. 9.1.2   Growth apparatus employing the dipping technique [2].

The third basic growth system uses a *multibin boat*, an important innovation in LPE technology because it allows sequential deposition of several semiconductor layers during one growth cycle and is used for device fabrication. The graphite boat [3] used in the first model of this apparatus is shown in Fig. 9.1.3. This graphite boat is provided with three reservoirs and a movable graphite slide, the upper surface of which constitutes the bottoms of the reservoirs. The substrate is placed in a recessed area of the slide and prior to growth is outside the reservoirs. The graphite boat, with the bins filled with appropriate solutions, is inserted into the quartz furnace tube of a furnace equipped similarly to that shown in Fig. 9.1.1. A long rod fitted into a sleeve at the end of the furnace is used to slide the substrate sequentially into the bottom of the various reservoirs. In this manner, by a choice of appropriate

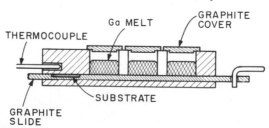

FIG. 9.1.3   Schematic showing the basic multiple-bin graphite boat for the sequential deposition of several layers during one growth cycle [3].

solutions and temperature schedules, different types of films can be deposited sequentially onto the substrate surface. Growth rates as high as $\sim 2 \, \mu$m/min can be obtained, although better layer control is obtained with slower growth rates obtained by a programmed slow cool of the furnace.

Instead of relying on the cooling of the furnace to produce the temperature transient for growing, another method has been described which uses Peltier cooling at the substrate–solution interface produced by an electric current flowing across the interface. In this method the furnace temperature can be held constant if desired. Considering a highly n-type substrate in contact with the solution, a current flow from the substrate into the solution produces a cooling effect which is the driving force for epitaxial growth. This technique was first applied to InSb growth by Kumagawa et al. [4], to GaAs/(AlGa)As growth by Daniels and Michel [5] (superimposed on furnace cooling), and then used by Lawrence and Eastman [6] without furnace cooling with direct current only. Current densities of 10–15 A/cm^2 produced GaAs layers at a growth rate of 0.6–1.2 μm/min at a constant furnace temperature of 800°C.

The quality of the materials and devices generated depends on a multitude of factors, such as the purity and inertness of the materials used in the construction of the growth apparatus, the purity of the gaseous ambient and solution materials, type of dopant additives, growth temperatures, and growth rate. The role played by these factors differs depending on the material deposited and the desired device; their effects are therefore discussed in later sections of this text.

9.1.2   Growth Kinetics

Growth from solutions has been widely used and studied, but prior to the introduction of the LPE technique, the interest was in the growth of spontaneously generated platelets. An introductory treatment of the factors which affect the nucleation of crystals from solutions can be found in the book by Cottrell [7]. The driving force for the nucleation is the supersaturation of the solution as the temperature is reduced (see Fig. 9.1.4 for some III–V compounds of interest) and the crystals formed are those in which the free energy, which includes the surface energy, is minimized. Thus, precipitation of new material will be favored where the lattice match is closest and/or the resultant change in the shape of the crystal results in the smallest increase in the surface energy. If a single-crystal substrate with a matching lattice parameter at an appropriate temperature is present, it becomes the favored site for nucleation and crystal growth.

A theoretical analysis of the growth rate of crystals from solution has been made using a number of simplifying assumptions [8,9]. Assuming that the growth rate is limited by the transport of the minor constituent to the surface (arsenic in the case of GaAs growth from gallium solution), and that no rate-limiting surface attachment kinetics are involved, the velocity at which the

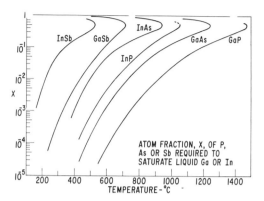

FIG. 9.1.4 Solubility of III–V compounds in Ga and In. The curves represent experimental data compiled by Hall [59].

material grows can be calculated as a function of the time elapsed after the introduction of the substrate into the solution. If the concentration of the minor constituent decreases exponentially with time as the crystal is cooled, the theoretical growth velocity curves of Fig. 9.1.5 are obtained [8] when the solution initially is either supersaturated, saturated, or undersaturated. In the latter case, a negative velocity simply means that some dissolution of the substrate occurs initially. Note that very rapid changes in the growth rate occur in the early growth stage which can lead to the formation of poor interfaces and solvent inclusions, particularly if the solution is highly supersaturated. Thus, the best growth occurs when the initial supersaturation or undersaturation is small.

The growth velocity V_s affects the morphology of the epitaxial layer because of the possibility of constitutional supercooling. A theoretical analysis of this phenomenon was made by Tiller [10] for solution growth. In general, constitutional supercooling will *not* occur for large temperature gradients and/or small growth velocity:

$$\frac{1}{V_s}\left(\frac{dT}{dx}\right) \geq M \quad (°C\text{-s}/cm^2) \qquad (9.1.1)$$

where dT/dx is the temperature gradient in the liquid at the interface. The constant M depends on the diffusion coefficient of the minor constituent, and its liquidus slope and initial concentration at the interface between the solution and the solid. The value of M was theoretically estimated by Tiller [10] for the solution growth of GaAs, GaP, SiC, ZnTe, and B_6P, and is in the range of 10^{-7} 10^{-9} °C-s/cm^2, depending on the material and the temperature. In the case of GaAs growth, for example, M decrease by an order of magnitude between 1000 and 700°C.

The specific case of GaAs LPE from Ga solutions was analyzed by Minden [11]. Although it is clear that the substrate must be cooler than the

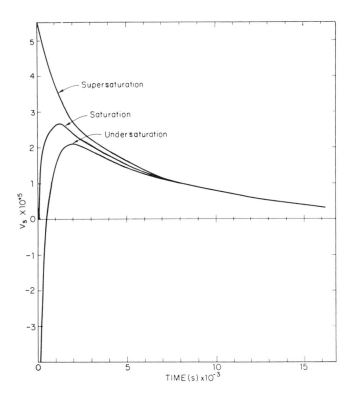

FIG. 9.1.5 Theoretical growth velocity curves for LPE GaAs for various degrees of saturation of the solution [8].

solution in order to prevent crystallization in the liquid in front of the substrate, the minimum temperature gradient is not easily calculated because many of the relevent parameters are not well known quantitatively. Typically, the estimated minimum temperature gradient ranges from 5 to 100°C/cm, depending on the thickness of the solution and the temperature of growth. As evident from the temperature dependence of M, the required temperature gradient increases with decreasing temperature with V_s constant. Therefore, layers grown over a large temperature interval may show a good region above the substrate interface but a region near the surface which is uneven and contains inclusions of Ga due to constitutional supercooling.

Few experimental studies comparing theory and experiment in the area of LPE growth kinetics have so far appeared. One study of the growth of GaAs from Sn solutions [12] shows that the depth of the material dissolved from the substrate when an unsaturated Sn solution is placed on GaAs can be reasonably well predicted based on solubility data and an empirical determination of some other parameters. The time dependence of the etchback process was measured. At 600°C, for example, equilibrium is reached at the end of approximately 60 min; the solution reaches 80–90% saturation in the first 25 min. Thus, a fair amount of time is necessary to establish equilibrium between the substrate and the solution, but this will, of course, depend on the temperature.

9.2   Vapor Phase Epitaxy

The most widely used vapor phase epitaxial technology uses open tube systems in which the primary source chemicals are predominantly gaseous at room temperature. This allows a high degree of flexibility in introducing dopants into the material as well as control of composition gradients by accurate flow metering. Zinc doping is performed using elemental Zn, whereas H_2Se is used for Se doping. Furthermore, multilayer n- and p-type structures can be grown by shifting from one gas flow to another with appropriate valves without removing the material from the reactor. Included in the III–V compounds prepared by VPE are [13] GaAs, GaP, GaSb, GaN, InAs, InP, AlAs, and AlN; and among the ternary alloys: Ga(AsP), Ga(AsSb), (GaIn)As, (InGa)P, and (InAs)P. However, the preparation of the Al containing alloys, (AlGa)As for example, is complicated by the reactivity of the gases which attack the walls of the reactor if standard equipment is used.

Figure 9.2.1 shows a schematic diagram of the apparatus used for growing III–V compounds where AsH_3, PH_3, or SbH_3 is used as the As, P, or Sb source and elemental Ga, In, or Al provides the other element of the compound. Detailed descriptions of the preparation and properties of various

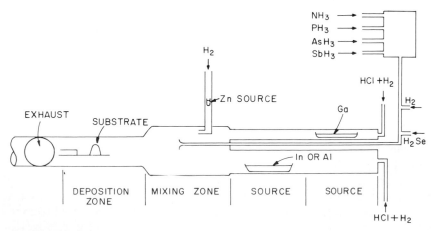

FIG. 9.2.1   Schematic diagram of apparatus used to grow various III–V compounds by vapor phase epitaxy [13].

compounds can be found in the cited references: GaAs, GaP, and Ga(AsP) [14]; InAs, InP, and (InAs)P [15]; GaSb and Ga(AsSb) [16] (these layers are usually p-type as grown, with hole concentrations in the low 10^{16} cm^{-3}); (InGa)As [17] and (InGa)P [18]; and AlAs. [19].

To illustrate [20] the technology used for ternary alloy growth, we consider (InGa)P grown using the apparatus of Fig. 9.2.1. The typical growth temperature is between 700 and 800°C, at growth rates of 12–30 μm/hr, depending on gas flow rates. The use of separate quartz tubes to contain the In and Ga source materials allows the independent control of the HCl concentrations over each of the metal sources. HCl reacts with Ga and In to form monochlorides of these metals:

$$yM(l) + HCl(g) = yMCl(g) + (1 - y)HCl(g) + \frac{y}{2}H_2(g) \qquad (9.2.1)$$

Here, M is In or Ga and y is the mole fraction of HCl consumed in the reaction. The metal monochlorides are carried in hydrogen into the mixing zone where they mix but do not react with gaseous phosphine, the source of phosphorus. In the reduced temperature of the deposition zone, where the substrate is positioned, (InGa)P is formed as an epitaxial film with HCl as the gaseous by-product according to the reaction

$$MHCl(g) + p^*(g) + H_2(g) = MP(s) + HCl(g) \qquad (9.2.2)$$

Here, p* denotes PH$_3$ and the products of the decomposition of PH$_3$ (P$_2$ and P$_4$). *In situ* doping with n- and p-type dopants is accomplished with H$_2$Se and Zn vapor, respectively, using sidearms as shown in Fig. 9.2.1. Junctions are formed by introducing the dopants sequentially during growth without removing the substrate.

This system allows the gradual changing of the alloy composition or more abrupt transitions if heterojunctions are desired. Grading is accomplished at a given temperature by changing the ratio of the HCl flow rates to the In and Ga sources (HCl$_{In}$/HCl$_{Ga}$) (see Fig. 9.2.2). Precision electronically activated gas flow controllers are used for each of the metal sources.

The appearance of the wafer surface is generally smooth; however, surface defects such as hillocks may occur whenever small leaks exist in the growth apparatus. The substrate wafer preparation prior to growth is also important in this regard. For GaAs substrates etching in Karo's acid of the (100) substrates was found satisfactory.

The undoped layers have a carrier concentration of 10^{15} to 10^{16} cm^{-3} and have always been n-type. Silicon is believed to be the major contaminant in the material. The hydrogen carrier gas is purified in a palladium diffuser. The HCl and phosphine gas used are the purest commercially available.

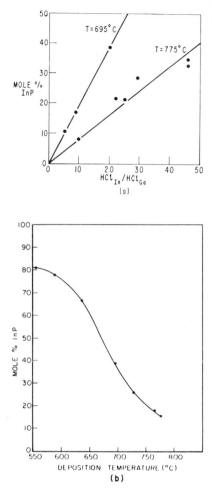

FIG. 9.2.2 The dependence of the mole fraction of InP in the $In_{1-x}Ga_xP$ alloy on (a) the ratio of the HCl flow rate over the In and Ga sources and (b) deposition temperature [20].

9.3 Molecular Beam Epitaxy

There is a relatively long history of preparation of semiconductor films by evaporation. For example, Schoolar and Zemel [21] grew PbS by this method in 1964. However, since the great emphasis on heterojunction optoelectronic structures starting in 1970, there has been increasing emphasis on evaporation methods (now usually denoted *molecular beam epitaxy*) as a means of preparing complex multilayer heterojunction structures with extreme control. Figure

9.3.1 shows an example of a vacuum apparatus ($\sim 10^{-10}$ Torr) used for the preparation of GaAs. The two ovens shown contain the compound (or its constituents) to be deposited. (Dopants require additional ovens.) Each source is provided with a shutter. The substrate on which the material is to be deposited is provided with a heater by which the desired temperature is obtained. The apparatus contains facilities for measuring the material deposited, including a spectral analyzer to monitor the environment under which the material is grown, as well as the vaporizing species from the ovens. The shutter operations can be automatically controlled depending on the measured properties of the gases in the system to allow accurate composition and thickness control of the epitaxial layer.

Reviews of the deposition technology for various materials have been published [22,23]. Consider, for example, GaAs, which is grown using at least the two ovens. One contains GaAs primarily as a source of As_4 (As is much more volatile than Ga), the second contains Ga. The substrate is held between 520 and 600° C. [To grow (AlGa)As, an additional oven containing Al is used.] The growth rate is relatively low, 60–600 Å/min. The rate of As_4 and Ga arrival at the substrate is controlled with the shutters to produce as stoichiometric a film composition as possible. The dopants used (from other ovens in the system) are Sn for donors and Ge for acceptors. Zinc is not as easily used because of its low sticking coefficient. The carrier mobility values obtained are comparable to those found in GaAs prepared by other methods. However,

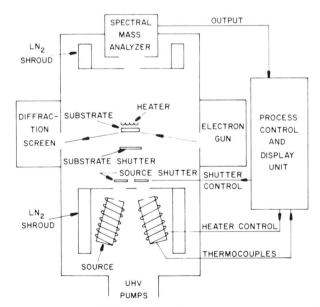

FIG. 9.3.1 Schematic diagram of molecular beam epitaxy system [23].

there is evidence that the radiative efficiency of the material, possibly because of native point defects, is typically not as high as in material prepared by liquid phase epitaxy.

9.4   Lattice Mismatch Effects

Epitaxial growth of one crystal on another is possible if they join along a plane boundary and possess in this plane a common two-dimensional cell, and differ only slightly in their cell dimension a_0 and/or angular orientation θ (for equal cell edge lengths) [24].

If we consider the (100) plane of the simplest cubic structures of Fig. 9.4.1a for illustration, it is clear that an approximate match of the two structures (with different lattice constants) on an atomic scale can only be achieved if the crystal is elastically strained, i.e., each atom of A and B is slightly displaced near the boundary from its original position. However, if this strain is relatively large, the strain energy stored in the crystal can be reduced by the formation of dislocations at the interface (see below). In the case of the simple structure shown in Fig. 9.4.1b, edge dislocations are formed which lie in the interfacial plane. In fact, two perpendicular sets of parallel edge dislocations forming a square grid are required to accommodate the lattice mismatch in two directions. Ideally, these dislocations will exit at the sides of

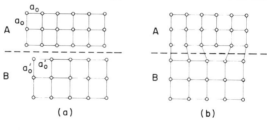

(a)   (b)

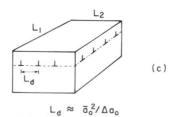

(c)

$$L_d \approx \bar{a}_0^2 / \Delta a_0$$

FIG. 9.4.1   Schematics showing the formation of an edge misfit dislocation in joining single cubic crystal A with lattice constant a_0 and substrate B with lattice constant a_0': (a) Separate crystals; (b) formation of edge dislocation when crystals are joined; (c) formation of dislocations at edge of crystal $L_1 \times L_2$. The distance between dislocations is L_d.

the crystal, assuming that a crystal of finite dimensions $L_1 \times L_2$ is grown (Fig. 9.4.1c), and accommodate the lattice mismatch such that at a distance significantly above the growth interface there is no appreciable strain and the material is dislocation-free.

Figure 9.4.2 shows a misfit dislocation in the zinc-blende III–V compounds [25]. The misfit dislocations of interest are mostly of the 60° type with {111} glide planes, and the Burger's vector makes a 60° angle with the dislocation axis along ⟨110⟩. The dangling bonds associated with the dislocation core determine to a large extent the electrical and optical properties of the dislocations. As we will illustrate further in this chapter, the centers constitute nonradiative recombination sites and also impact the interfacial recombination velocity at the heterojunction interface, an effect we explore in more

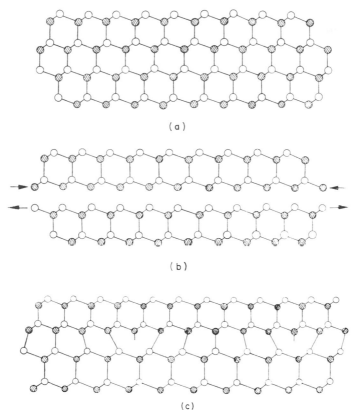

(a)

(b)

(c)

FIG. 9.4.2 Misfit dislocations in a {111} heterojunction in a zinc-blende cubic lattice seen in the (01$\bar{1}$) plane: (a) Perfect crystal; (b) crystal cut along the (111) plane and expanded on one side while contracted on the other; (c) the two materials bonded together showing edge dislocation and "dangling" bond [25].

detail in Chapter 8. Also associated with the dislocation is a strain field which decreases with distance r from the core as r^{-1}. Largely as a result of their strain field, considerable energy is needed to form dislocations.

Using simple arguments, it can be shown that epitaxial growth should occur only if $\Delta a_0/\tilde{a}_0 \lesssim 0.1$ or $\Delta\theta/\theta \lesssim 0.1$ [24]. In LPE, a lattice mismatch greater than about 2% commonly results in uneven nucleation on the substrate and polycrystalline growth. The reason is that the free energy of the crystal is increased by forcing a fit with the substrate. Thus, isolated nucleating islands will form with outward growth in the form of platelets or columns. When these meet material nucleating on adjoining regions, a polycrystalline epitaxial film is formed. However, there are significant differences in the case of growth which favor the {111} planes. Holt [25] has pointed out that the density of dangling bonds is lower by as much as a factor of ~ 2 at {111} heterojunction interfaces than for other planes. Furthermore, we note that dislocation movement is easier on the {111} planes, which are the slip planes in zinc-blende lattices. Thus, rearrangement of dislocations during growth with maximum effect to accommodate the misfit can occur. These theoretical speculations have been borne out in practice. With lattice mismatch, heteroepitaxy using LPE is easiest on the (111) growth plane, although it is not always obvious whether the (111)A or (111)B face is superior.

In view of the complexity of the nucleating process in the presence of a large lattice misfit, it is obviously unrealistic to expect that a simple analysis will yield quantitative defect density data. It is nevertheless instructive to use a simple analysis because the correct order of magnitude dislocation density can be calculated.

Assuming that each edge dislocation relieves an elastic strain equal to the Burger's vector $\mathbf{b}$ ($|\mathbf{b}| = a_0$ for the *simple cubic* structure) the spacing between edge dislocations is $L_d = b(\Delta a_0/\tilde{a}_0)^{-1} \approx \tilde{a}_0^2/\Delta a_0$ where $\tilde{a}_0$ is the median lattice constant* ($\tilde{a}_0 \approx a_0$), and the linear density of dislocations ρ_{dl} is

$$\rho_{dl} \approx \Delta a_0/a_0^2 \qquad (9.4.1a)$$

Equation (9.4.1a) must be modified for the crystal type and orientation to take into account the Burger's vector of the edge dislocations formed and its relationship with respect to the growth plane which determines the efficacy of the strain-relieving dislocations. In the sphalerite structure with $\frac{1}{2}\langle 110\rangle$ Burger's vectors, $\mathbf{b} = \frac{1}{2}\langle 110\rangle$, hence $b = a_0\sqrt{2}$ and the linear dislocation density is

$$\rho_{dl} \cong \sqrt{2}\,(\Delta a_0/a_0^2) \qquad (9.4.1b)$$

when the dislocation is in the plane of the interface, e.g., {100}, {110}, or {111}. This expression is adequate for $\Delta a_0/a_0 \lesssim 1\%$.

* The quantity $\Delta a_0/a_0$ will henceforth denote the misfit strain; the two lattice parameter values are assumed to be close in value.

With this as an introduction, we can consider in greater detail the conditions for the generation of misfit dislocations in the usual case where the epitaxial layer is much thinner than the substrate. If we ignore the possibility of plastic deformation of the substrate (which can occur as discussed in Section 9.5), then three possibilities remain for accommodating the strain $\Delta a_0/a_0$ due to the lattice misfit: (a) the film remains elastically strained; (b) dislocations are generated to relieve the strain fully; or (c) a combination of the two.

The prediction of when these possibilities are realized is, in principle, possible by considering the energy stored when the crystal is elastically strained compared to the energy needed to generate misfit dislocations. In equilibrium, the energy of the crystal will tend to be minimized by an appropriate combination of residual elastic strain and misfit dislocation formation. If we consider the first few atomic layers epitaxially deposited, it is intuitively obvious that they are easily elastically deformed without the need for forming dislocations. Only when the thickness of the epitaxial film increases, and the film becomes more rigid, should dislocations form. The important point is that the interfacial defect density is expected to depend on the thickness of the epitaxial layer for a given strain $\Delta a_0/a_0$. This has been experimentally confirmed (Sections 9.4.1 and 9.4.2). In the following we review the physical basis of the effect.

A comprehensive theoretical calculation of the effect has been presented by van der Merwe and co-workers [26]. For our present purpose, we review the simple analysis of Matthews [27] which provides an order of magnitude estimate of the maximum film thickness which can grow prior to misfit dislocation formation. Basically, this involves a calculation of the strain energy in the epitaxial layer, which is compared to the energy required to form misfit dislocations. We consider for simplicity {100}, {111}, or {110} planes which contain the misfit edge dislocations. It is easily shown for a plane strain system, such as the epitaxial layer, that the elastic energy for a strain ε_s, assuming an isotropic elastic system and a film height h, is

$$E_\varepsilon = B_1 h \varepsilon_s \qquad (9.4.2a)$$

where $B_1 = 2G_s(1 + \sigma)/(1 - \sigma)$ (G_s is the shear modulus* and σ is the Poisson ratio, ≈ 0.3).

The energy E_{dis} per unit length of an edge dislocation is shown in standard texts (see the Bibliography) to be approximately

$$E_{dis} \cong \tfrac{1}{2} B_2 b \ln(R/b) \qquad (9.4.2b)$$

where $B_2 = G_s b/2\pi(1 - \sigma)$, R is the extent of the strain field, and b is the magnitude of the Burger's vector. A common approximation in a crystal in which R is very much larger than the Burger's vector is $E_{dis} \cong G_s b^2$. For thin films, however, the retainment of the logarithmic term in (9.4.2b) may be jus-

* $G_s = Y/2(1 + \sigma)$, where, Y (Young's modulus) $= 10^{12}$ dynes/cm^2 for GaAs.

tified. [Note that (9.4.2b) neglects the core energy itself, a quantity which, while not well established, is probably about $\frac{1}{2} B_2 b$.] In the following, we also neglect the small difference in the shear modulus between the epitaxial layer and the substrate in discussing interfacial dislocations.

Let us now assume that the total misfit strain is accommodated by an elastic strain ε_s and the formation of misfit dislocations to accommodate the remainder δ; hence,

$$\Delta a_0/a_0 = \varepsilon_s + \delta \tag{9.4.3}$$

We assume that two sets of dislocations form to accommodate the two-dimensional misfit. The separation between dislocations uniformly spaced along a [110] direction is

$$L_{\text{dis}} = b/\delta \tag{9.4.4}$$

Therefore, the number of dislocations per unit length is $2L_{\text{dis}}^{-1} = 2\delta/b$. Assuming that the dislocations are noninteracting, we estimate the energy E_δ due to dislocations to be

$$E_\delta = 2\delta E_{\text{dis}}/b = B_2\delta \ln(R/b) = B_2(\Delta a_0/a_0 - \varepsilon_s) \ln(R/b) \tag{9.4.5}$$

Since the *total energy* E of the crystal is minimized with respect to the elastic strain ε when

$$\partial E/\partial \varepsilon_s = 0 = \partial E_\varepsilon/\partial \varepsilon_s + \partial E_\delta/\partial \varepsilon_s \tag{9.4.6}$$

we obtain the equality

$$2\varepsilon_s^* B_1 h = B_2 \ln(R/b) \qquad \text{or} \qquad \varepsilon_s^* = (B_2/2B_1 h) \ln(R/b) \tag{9.4.7}$$

where ε_s^* is the elastic strain value which minimizes the energy of the system. If $\varepsilon_s^* > \Delta a_0/a_0$, the layer remains elastically strained and *no misfit dislocations form*. On the other hand, if $\varepsilon_s^* < \Delta a_0/a_0$, then dislocations will form to relieve the strain $\delta = \Delta a_0/a_0 - \varepsilon_s^*$.

To determine the limit at which dislocations will be formed, Matthews [27] uses the condition $\varepsilon_s^* = \Delta a_0/a_0$. Thus we obtain the *critical layer thickness* h_c for dislocation formation:

$$h_c \cong \frac{B_2}{2B_1\Delta a_0/a_0} \ln\left(\frac{h_c}{b}\right) \tag{9.4.8a}$$

where we take the layer thickness to represent the outer limit of the strain field extent R.

Substituting for B_1 and B_2 from (9.4.2),

$$h_c \cong \frac{b \ln(h_c/b)}{8\pi(1 + \sigma)\Delta a_0/a_0} \tag{9.4.8b}$$

with h_c on the order of 10^{-4} cm, we can approximate (9.4.8b) by

$$h_c \approx \frac{b}{2\Delta a_0/a_0} \approx \frac{a_0}{2\sqrt{2}\,\Delta a_0/a_0} \tag{9.4.8c}$$

Determining the maximum film thickness prior to the formation of misfit dislocations is particularly important in structures in which a thin layer can be sandwiched between two layers of different lattice parameters. For example, in double-heterojunction structures, the width of the active region is usually below 1 μm, and conditions may exist whereby a dislocation-free active region is produced—a very desirable result indeed for the performance of the device (see Section 9.4.2).

Another consequence of this analysis is that dislocations prefer to lie in the interface whenever possible for maximum misfit relief, since the fewer dislocations introduced, the lower is the crystal energy. Thus, dislocations that are in the substrate at an angle to the interface tend toward a "bending over" configuration in order to accommodate the lattice misfit as much as possible, rather than simply propagate upward with unchanged direction. As we shall see in this section, such processes do indeed occur in some practical situations.

We now turn to a review of key experimental results concerning defect generation due to lattice mismatch. Although the experimental results have been obtained mostly in VPE, the major conclusions reached are believed relevant to LPE synthesis, for which extensive detailed experimental data are not yet available.

The analysis of the lattice misfit must consider two contributions:

1. the misfit at the growth temperature, and
2. the change in the lattice misfit with temperature as the crystal is cooled to room temperature.

The lattice misfit originates at a given temperature as a result of a difference in film and substrate doping as well as a result of a difference in lattice parameters for dissimilar materials.

9.4.1   Defect Generation Due to Doping Variations in Homoepitaxy

The generation of defects due to a lattice mismatch arising from doping differences between the substrate and the epitaxial layer has been exhaustively studied in silicon by Sugita *et al.* [28]. The substrate boron concentration was changed with respect to that of the epitaxial film deposited from the vapor phase with a resultant mismatch varying from $\sim 10^{-1}$ to $\sim 10^{-3}\%$. A key result of these experiments is that the defect density in thin films *does* depend on the layer thickness, as predicted [26] for small lattice misfit. It was found, for example, with a lattice misfit of 0.019% that the misfit dislocation density was negligible for film thicknesses up to 2.4–2.9 μm but that the density increased with thicker layers. When the misfit was as small as 0.003–0.006%, the density of misfit dislocations was negligible even with films $\sim 20\,\mu$m thick. With a lattice mismatch of 0.2%, the measured distance between dislocations was 13 μm, whereas it was 30–50 μm for a lattice mismatch of 0.011–0.016%. A comparison of these findings with a rigorous theory of the defect generation is difficult because autodoping occurs during epitaxial growth with the result that the lattice mismatch is not abrupt. Although a quantitative comparison of these Si epitaxy results with other materials and growth conditions is hazardous, it is clear that very small differences in lattice constant can give rise to dislocations which may significantly affect the electrical and optical properties of the epitaxial films. The lattice mismatch $\Delta a_0 / \Delta c$ due to a concentration c of impurities will depend on factors such as the difference between the tetrahedral radius of the dopant and the host atoms (Table 1.2.1).

Using the same simple arguments as these, the *linear* dislocation density in a simple cubic lattice due to a simple misfit plane is

$$\rho_{dl} = \Delta c \, (\Delta a_0 / \Delta c) \, (1/a_0)^2 \qquad (9.4.9)$$

Misfit edge dislocations due to doping differences in LPE GaAs p–n junctions grown on the (100) plane have been observed by Abrahams and Buiocchi [29]. The p-side of the junction contained 2×10^{19} Zn/cm^3, whereas the n-side contained 2×10^{18} Te/cm^3. The estimated lattice misfit was $\Delta a_0 / a_0 = 0.0005/5.65 = 9 \times 10^{-5}$ with a linear density of edge dislocations at a (100) plane of $\rho_{dl} = 4 \times 10^3$ cm^{-1} as revealed by etching the edge of the crystal. This compares to $\sim 2 \times 10^3$ cm^{-1}, predicted from Eq. (9.4.1).

9.4.2 Lattice Mismatch in Heteroepitaxy

Heteroepitaxy involving III–V and other semiconductor compounds has been the subject of extensive research in recent years. The work has been motivated by the need for heterojunction devices and also to enable the single-crystal growth of a variety of materials on available large-area substrates such as Si, Ge, GaAs, GaP, GaSb, InAs, and InSb. In this section we consider a system which has been exhaustively studied by electron microscopy: Ga(AsP) grown by VPE on GaAs. As shown in Table 9.4.1, the lattice misfit between GaAs and GaP is 3.6%. However, materials required for the fabrication of visible-light-emitting diodes have the composition GaAs$_{0.6}$ P$_{0.4}$, and the lattice misfit is 1.4% when GaAs substrates are used. In addition to the lattice misfit at the growth temperature, the thermal contraction of the layer and that of the substrate differ in this system (see Table 9.4.2).

Early experimental results [30] involving an abrupt discontinuity at the interface showed that the dislocation density was high (10^7–10^8 cm^{-2}) throughout the layer, in contradiction to the simple theory which predicts interfacial dislocations only close to the growth interface. In addition, the material is frequently bowed, indicative of a high degree of strain.

Such high dislocation densities in the active region of the LED are unacceptable, and thus much work has been done toward reducing the dislocation density. The earliest approach involved grading the composition. More recently, work has been done on using step compositional variations—a process

TABLE 9.4.1
Some Parameters of Interest in the Synthesis of Ternary Alloys[a]

Alloy system		Lattice parameter[b] a_0 (Å)		Difference (%)	Melting temperature T^m (K)		E_g (300 K)[c]	
a	b	a	b		a	b	a	b
InSb	GaSb	6.479	6.095	6.1	803	985	0.17[d]	0.73
InAs	GaAs	6.058	5.653	6.9	1210	1511	0.35[d]	1.42[d]
InP	GaP	5.869	5.451	7.3	1343	1738	1.34[d]	2.26
AlAs	GaAs	5.661	5.653	0.14	2013	1511	2.16	1.42[d]
InAs	InP	6.057	5.870	3.2	1210	1343	0.35[d]	1.34[d]
AlP	GaP	5.451	5.451	~0.01	2823	1738	2.4	2.26
GaSb	AlSb	6.095	6.135	0.65	985	1323	0.73[d]	1.65
InAs	AlAs	6.057	5.661	6.7	1210	2013	0.35[d]	2.16
InSb	AlSb	6.479	6.135	4.7	803	1323	0.17[d]	1.65
GaAs	GaP	5.653	5.451	3.6	1511	1738	1.42[d]	2.26
InP	AlP	6.057	5.451	10.5	1343	2823	1.34[d]	2.4
GaSb	GaAs	6.095	5.653	7.5	985	1511	0.73[d]	1.42[d]
InAs	InSb	6.057	6.479	6.8	1210	803	0.35[d]	0.17[d]
InSb	InP	6.479	5.869	10	803	1343	0.17[d]	1.34[d]
GaSb	GaP	6.095	5.451	11.1	985	1738	0.73[d]	2.26
AlSb	AlP	6.135	5.451	11.8	1323	2823	1.65	2.4
AlSb	AlAs	6.135	5.661	8	1323	2013	1.65	2.16
AlP	AlAs	5.451	5.661	3.8	2823	2013	2.4	2.16

[a]Note: Bulk-grown single-crystal substrates of InSb, InP, GaP, GaSb, and GaAs are available.
[b]The lattice parameters generally vary very nearly linearly with composition in the ternary alloys. However, this is rarely the case for the bandgap energy variation (see text).
[c]The bandgap energy values are within 10 meV.
[d]Denotes direct bandgap transition material.

TABLE 9.4.2

Thermal Expansion Coefficient of Selected Materials[a]

Alloy system	α_{th} (°C^{-1})	a_0 (27°C)	a_0 (~600°C)	Ref.
InP	$(4.75 \pm 0.1) \times 10^{-6}$	5.8697	5.8870	b
GaP	$(5.91 \pm 0.1) \times 10^{-6}$	5.4510	5.4742	c
GaAs	$(6.63 \pm 0.1) \times 10^{-6}$	5.6525	5.680	d,e
Ge	5.75×10^{-6}	5.6570	5.6603	f
AlAs	$(5.20 \pm 0.05) \times 10^{-6}$	5.6605	~5.6790	g
InAs	$(5.16 \pm 0.1) \times 10^{-6}$	6.057	6.080	e

[a]The thermal coefficient of expansion may be assumed to vary linearly with composition in ternary alloys.

[b]I. Kudman and R. J. Paff, J. Appl. Phys. 43, 3760 (1972).

[c]E. D. Pierron, D. L. Parker, and J. B. McNeely, J. Appl. Phys. 38, 4669 (1967).

[d]M. E. Stranmanis and J. P. Krumme, J. Electrochem. Soc. 114, 640 (1967).

[e]R. J. Paff, private communication.

[f]D. F. Gibbons, Phys. Rev. 112, 136 (1958).

[g]M. Ettenberg and R. J. Paff, J. Appl. Phys. 41, 3926 (1970).

which works under restricted conditions to reduce the dislocation density of the uppermost layer. We consider these two approaches now starting with grading.

Grading the composition does not eliminate the misfit dislocations since, after all, the lattice mismatch must be accommodated. However, grading distributes the dislocations over a larger volume such that the *average* density in a cross section of the film is reduced. The result is improved devices which utilize the surface of the layer. For example, using a 12-μm tapered transition (3.3% phosphorus/μm) region from GaAs to GaAs$_{0.6}$P$_{0.4}$, Stringfellow and Green [31] found that the dislocation density was reduced from $> 10^8$ cm^{-2} near the GaAs–taper region interface to 10^6 cm^{-2} in the Ga(AsP) region of constant composition. Although this value is still relatively high, the material obtained is useful for many electronic applications.

A detailed experimental study by Abrahams *et al.* [32] of the defect structure in graded Ga(AsP) on GaAs using electron microscopy has cleared up a number of earlier uncertainties concerning the origin and nature of the defects formed. The following are their major conclusions:

1. The formation of both abrupt and graded heterojunctions gives rise to $\langle 110 \rangle$ dislocations lying in the (100) growth plane and to *inclined* dislocations formed because the edge dislocations do not commonly terminate at the edge of the grown crystal. This is shown in schematic form in Fig. 9.4.3. The result is that *segmented* dislocations are observed in the top view of the growth plane (Fig. 9.4.4). The inclined dislocations will therefore propagate into the constant composition portion of the crystal which succeeds the graded composition region. This explains why the dislocation density is relatively high throughout the epitaxial layer despite a shallow concentration gradient.

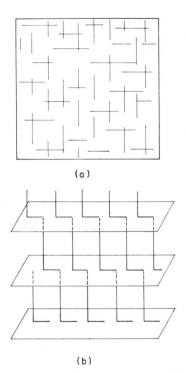

(a)

(b)

FIG. 9.4.3 (a) Schematic representation of segmented misfit dislocations formed in a plane of misfit due to a change in lattice parameter (top view of growth plane). (b) Simplified schematic illustration of the propagation of dislocations through multiple misfit planes. Initial dislocations weave in and out of successive misfit planes leading to a constant density of inclined dislocations with increasing layer thickness [32].

2.   The observed dislocation density can be surprisingly well predicted on the basis of the concentration gradient. If ρ_d denotes the average dislocation density (per square centimeter) due to the lattice parameter gradient emerging from the edge of the crystal per unit thickness, and $\Delta c/\Delta x$ is the phosphorus concentration gradient (% P/μm), then

$$\rho_d \cong (\Delta a_0/a_0^2)\,(\Delta c/\Delta x) \qquad (9.4.10)$$

The density of inclined dislocations ρ_I threading the area of constant composition is given by

$$\rho_I = 2n_A/m \cong (2/m)(\Delta a_0/a_0^2)(\Delta c/\Delta x) \qquad (9.4.11)$$

where m, the only adjustable parameter, is a multiple of the average length of the segmented dislocations in the growth plane. Figure 9.4.5a shows the experimental dependence of ρ_d on $\Delta c/\Delta x$, and Fig. 9.4.5b shows ρ_I as a function of $\Delta c/\Delta x$ ($m \approx 8$).

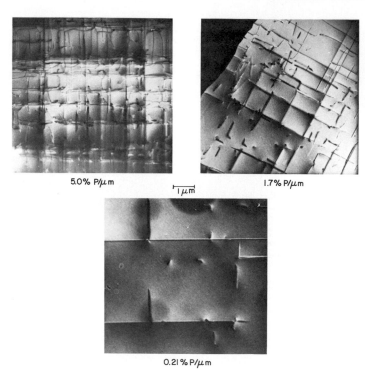

5.0% P/μm   1.7% P/μm

0.21% P/μm

FIG. 9.4.4 Lattice misfit dislocation networks in GaAs$_{1-x}$P$_x$ layers, which were vapor-deposited with different compositional grading rates on GaAs substrates. The density of misfit dislocations decreases with decreasing compositional gradient. The gradients are given in units of mole percent GaP per micrometer of growth [32].

There has been some debate in the literature concerning the origin of the bowing observed in epitaxial layers and the role in defect formation of the thermal contraction difference between layer and substrate. A detailed study by Abrahams *et al.* [33] shows that the inclined dislocations just discussed are responsible for the net bending moment in the epitaxial layer (Fig. 9.4.6a) when the lattice mismatch is small and the inclined dislocations form an ordered array (Fig. 9.4.6b). However, when the lattice mismatch is large, the inclined dislocations are randomly arranged (Fig. 9.4.6c) and no net bending moment exists (i.e., no wafer bowing) despite the very large localized stresses in the layer. These authors concluded that since the calculated local stresses due to the differential thermal mismatch are smaller than those due to the lattice mismatch at the growth temperature, the lattice mismatch is mainly responsible for defect generation in Ga(AsP). Other authors [30,31] have also concluded that the lattice mismatch at the growth temperature was the dominant factor in dislocation formation in Ga(AsP) for the following reason:

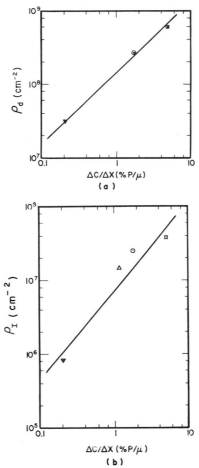

FIG. 9.4.5 Dislocation density in graded composition Ga(AsP) prepared by vapor phase epitaxy as a function of the phosphorus gradient $\Delta c / \Delta x$: (a) Dependence of the misfit dislocation density ρ_d (defined as the number per square centimeter emerging from the *edge* of a crystal) on $\Delta c / \Delta x$; (b) dependence of the inclined dislocation density ρ_I (defined as the dislocation density at the *top* of the crystal) as a function of $\Delta c / \Delta x$ [32].

1.   Dislocations moving under thermal stress would tend to form tangled networks, while the observed dislocations are mostly straight.

2.   The generation of dislocations by thermal stress requires sources, such as Frank–Read sources, which were not observed.

3.   The dislocations are decorated by impurities which suggests that they are formed during growth when the impurities are highly mobile. Saul [34], on the other hand, concluded from a study of the VPE growth of GaP on GaAs that defects were formed during the cooling process following growth.

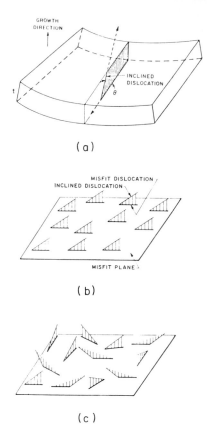

FIG. 9.4.6 Ordering of inclined dislocations associated with misfit dislocations: (a) Schematic representation of inclined dislocation and its associated half-plane: (b) ordered array of inclined dislocations; (c) disordered array. The shaded regions are the extra half-planes of the dislocations [33].

He presented a theoretical analysis relating these effects with the width of the graded transition region [35].

We now turn our attention to heteroepitaxial structures with *abrupt composition changes*, producing step changes in lattice parameter. We find that significant differences exist depending on whether the film has a smaller or larger lattice parameter than the substrate.

Historically, the first well-studied system was Ge/GaAs, which can be grown epitaxially both ways: Ge on GaAs or GaAs on Ge. The lattice misfit is only $\sim 0.08\%$ in the usual growth temperature range. Misfit dislocations with spacings of about 4 μm and inclined dislocations were observed following VPE deposition at 800°C of Ge on (100) GaAs [36]. When GaAs was grown on Ge, Meieran [37] found misfit dislocations only if the epitaxial film thickness exceeded 2 μm, which is only qualititatively consistent with our earlier analysis. [The predicted h_c value is ~0.3 μm for (9.4.8c).] However, other data concerning the epitaxial growth of Ge on GaAs are in better agreement with theory [27]. There is debate concerning the role of the differential thermal contraction and of the lattice mismatch at the growth temperature [38, 39] on dislocation formation. It is probable that the relative importance of the two effects depends on the material and the growth temperature. If the material can be easily plastically deformed during a significant portion of the cooling cycles, such as Ge grown at 800°C, slip occurs and defects are generated as a result of differential thermal contraction. Thus, Meieran [37] did observe dislocations presumably due to plastic flow to a depth of 15 μm (the approximate epitaxial GaAs layer thickness) in the *Ge substrate*. See Section 9.5 for further discussion of the subject of dislocation formation in the substrate in heteroepitaxy. On the other hand, if the material is grown at very low temperatures, then only the misfit dislocations introduced at the growth temperature will be observed.

Turning to another material, dramatic illustration of the increasing dislocation density at the interface with increasing misfit is shown in Fig. 9.4.7 where we see the interface as examined by transmission electron microscopy [40]. The layers consist of $In_xGa_{1-x}P$ grown by VPE on GaAs. Starting with the perfectly matched lattice at the growth temperature ($x = 0.49$), where no dislocations are observed, we see a gradual dislocation increase as the misfit increases. For a misfit of about 1% the epitaxial layer is grossly defect-ridden with a single step growth of this magnitude. Note that close examination of the samples shows that even for moderate misfit values the misfit dislocations are not confined in step growth to a single plane, but rather extend over an interfacial region as wide as 1000 Å.

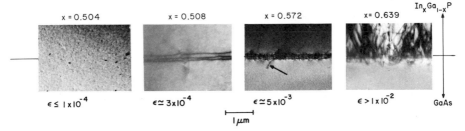

FIG. 9.4.7 Transmission electron micrographs of $In_xGa_{1-x}P$ epitaxial layers, deposited by vapor phase epitaxy on GaAs, showing the progressively increasing misfit dislocation density as the misfit increases. The section at the left shows a lattice-matched structure with no interfacial dislocations [40].

It is noteworthy that misfit dislocation networks in III–V compounds are not always produced in two directions in the growth plane because of asymmetry effects which produce preferential dislocation formation in one crystal direction, an effect particularly noted when the misfit dislocation density is low.

The crystal structure of III–V compounds consists of two interpenetrating face-centered cubic (fcc) lattices of different species. Thus, if the (111) plane in GaAs consists of Ga atoms, the ($\bar{1}\bar{1}\bar{1}$) plane is made up of As atoms. This asymmetry is further manifested along $\langle 110 \rangle$ directions (i.e., the atomic distribution along a [110] direction in a III–V compound differs from that along a [1$\bar{1}$0] direction). Therefore, there is no reason to expect mechanical properties along these two directions to be the same, and indeed this fact has been borne out by several experiments, of which surface etching is one [41]. Abrahams *et al.* [42] have directly observed by transmission electron microscopy asymmetric dislocation arrays along $\langle 110 \rangle$ directions of (001) foils of (InGa)P and Ga(AsP) with the density along one direction being greater than the other. This suggests that dislocation formation and propagation are easier along one direction, a fact related to the difference in core structure of dislocations along the two $\langle 110 \rangle$ directions.

This asymmetry affects the heterojunction defect morphology. Investigations [43, 44] of (100) heteroepitaxial III–V alloys with small ($< 10^{-4}$) strains have shown that misfit dislocations are introduced initially along one {110} direction only and that greater strains (or film thicknesses) must be incurred in order for the orthogonal (1$\bar{1}$0) set to form. Olsen *et al.* [41] have also observed asymmetric cracking in lattice mismatched deposits of several III–V compounds (by vapor phase epitaxy) and found that if growth occurred on both sides of a (100) substrate, the unidirectional cracks on the top side were rotated 90° from those on the bottom. Asymmetric cracking was readily observed in layers that were under tension (e.g., $In_xGa_{1-x}P/GaAs$ for $x < 0.49$), but rarely in those under compression (e.g., $In_xGa_{1-x}P/GaAs$ for $x > 0.49$). Tensile cracks were found to form at strains of $\sim 0.15\%$, which corresponds to a critical stress of $\sim 5 \times 10^9$ dynes/cm² for cracking. Asymmetric cracking can be explained by introducing asymmetric dislocations into the Cottrell fracture mechanism [41]. The surface "crosshatch" pattern, which is observed on compositionally graded VPE III–V compounds, also has an asymmetric appearance, much the same as that of the misfit dislocations in electron micrographs.

Nagai [45] observed asymmetric bending in (InGa)As and Ga(AsP) alloys grown on (100) GaAs substrates, and has shown that if growth occurs on both sides of the substrate, a "saddlelike" curvature is observed, i.e., convex about one [110] direction but concave about the other. These observations are entirely consistent with the concept of asymmetric dislocations.

Although the misfit strain is *applied* equally along $\langle 110 \rangle$ directions, *relief* occurs more easily in one direction, and the other direction exhibits greater bending due to elastic strain. On the other side of the substrate, symmetry rotates by 90° and the axis of greater bending is perpendicular to the one on the top side. Thus, the bending is applied along perpendicular axes but from opposite sides, so "saddlelike" bending occurs.

The impact of misfit dislocations on the radiative efficiency of the material is of major concern in optoelectronic applications. The negative effect of dislocations in this regard is illustrated in Fig. 9.4.8 [46], which shows an epitaxial layer of $In_{0.01}Ga_{0.99}As/GaAs$ grown by VPE. The optical micrograph

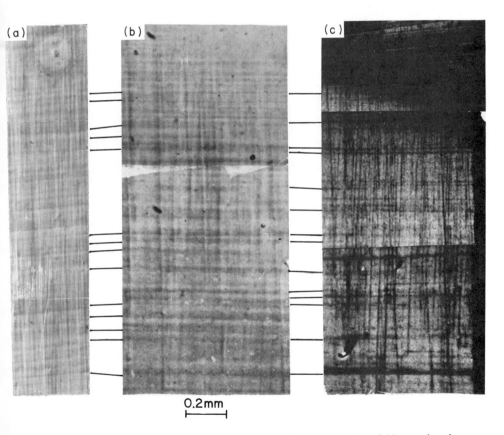

0.2mm

FIG. 9.4.8 (a) Optical photograph, (b) x-ray reflection topograph, and (c) scanning electron microscope cathodoluminescence photograph of the same region of $In_{0.01}Ga_{0.99}As/GaAs$ VPE sample. The optical photograph was taken on the original sample. The wafer was then angle-lapped, and (b) and (c) were taken from the same region. The black lines indicate where a one-to-one correspondence can be obtained between the figures [46].

shows the dislocation network (crosshatching) which gives rise to the lines clearly visible. The x-ray topograph of the angle-lapped sample reveals the dislocation network. The scanning electron microscope cathodoluminescence scan photograph on the right shows the radiation emitted from the material. Note that the dislocations are dark, evidence of their nonradiative nature.

For moderate lattice misfit, *epitaxial layers grown by LPE* show basically a similar tendency to the formation of networks of misfit dislocations as described for VPE. However, the dislocation distribution in LPE material grown on substrates with a relatively large ($>1\%$) lattice mismatch does not appear to yield a well-defined dislocation distribution as found in VPE Ga (AsP). Figure 9.4.9 shows an x-ray topograph of an $In_{1-x}Ga_xP$ layer ($x \cong 0.7$) grown by LPE on a (111) GaAs substrate. The approximate lattice parameter mismatch is 1.4%. Note in Fig. 9.4.9 the cellular structure formed by dislocations arranged in low angle grain boundaries with a misorientation between

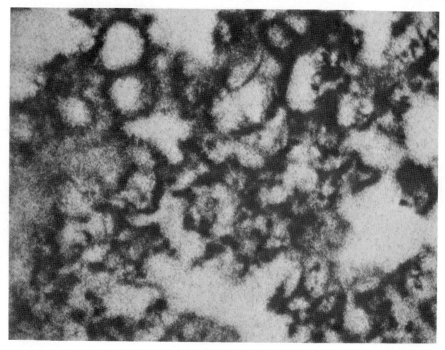

FIG. 9.4.9   X-ray topograph of $In_{0.3}Ga_{0.7}P$ layers deposited on GaAs substrate by LPE showing a cellular dislocation morphology. The low angle grain boundaries are misoriented by $\sim 0.3°$.

"cells" of ~0.3°. This distribution pattern may arise from dislocation redistribution to a lower energy configuration in the growth cycle or from the action of Frank–Read dislocation sources active at high temperatures, whereby resultant dislocations expand until they meet dislocations formed from adjacent sources, thus giving rise to the cellular structure seen. In any case, the result is the familiar "polygonization" pattern seen in plastically deformed metals following annealing.

Turning our attention to the means of reducing the dislocation density by *step compositional changes*, we find the following experimental observations:

1. The dislocation density in the epitaxial layer grown by LPE is generally lower than in the substrate if both have the same lattice parameter. In LPE growth of GaAs on GaAs, for example, the dislocation density in the epitaxial layer is typically lower by a factor of 3 to 10 (although orientation-dependent effects are no doubt a variable) because many of the dislocations tend to bend into the interfacial plane. This effect is not generally observed in III–V compound homoepitaxial VPE growth where dislocations do propagate into the layer.

2. If a lattice mismatch has to be accommodated, it is found that the dislocation density of the surface layer in liquid phase heteroepitaxy can be reduced by growing several thin distinct layers sequentially rather than a single thick one. This has been demonstrated, for example, in the case of GaAs grown on GaP, [47], and is a consequence of the fact that not all dislocations propagate upward when an interface between two epitaxial layers is formed because of their bending into the interfacial plane.

3. Dislocations tend to bend into the interfacial plane in heteroepitaxial layers if the layer is in compression, thus minimizing the density of inclined dislocations. This effect is discussed in detail below.

We mentioned earlier with respect to Ga(AsP) grown on GaAs *without* grading that the dislocation density is very high, and that inclined dislocations propagate throughout the layer. In view of these observations is it possible to produce step-graded structures which are close to the ideal of having the misfit dislocations mostly confined to the interfacial plane? The answer is yes, if the lattice parameter of the epitaxial layer is *larger* than that of the substrate [opposite to the Ga(AsP) on GaAs case], and the misfit is modest. Olsen *et al.* [48] have made a careful study using the $In_xGa_{1-x}P/GaAs$ system where, by adjusting x in VPE, it is possible to produce epitaxial layers on GaAs with a lattice parameter which is either smaller or larger than that of GaAs. The conclusion of this study is that with the epitaxial layer in *compression* (i.e., larger lattice parameter than the substrate) the dislocations tend to lie in the interfacial plane and the inclined dislocation density is minimized. However, if the epitaxial layer is in *tension*, then one notes a high inclined dislocation density, with evidence of microcracks in the layer for large mismatch values.

To illustrate this we turn to Fig. 9.4.10 where we compare the dislocation density as initially viewed at the surface of the substrate (left) and the epitaxial layer (right). Starting at the top, with the epitaxial layer in *compression* ($\Delta a_0/a_0 = 3 \times 10^{-3}$), we note that the dislocation density in the epitaxial layer is actually *lower than that in the substrate*, since initially present dislocations in the substrate have bent over in the interfacial plane, where they help to relieve the misfit strain. Continuing to the case in which the epitaxial layer *matches* the lattice parameter of the substrate (0 strain), the dislocation density is seen to be approximately the same as in the substrate. However, when the epitaxial layer is in *tension* (misfit 3×10^{-3}), a very high dislocation density is seen in the lower illustration of Fig. 9.4.10.

To explain these observations, the model of Jesser and Matthews [49] may be appropriate. These authors suggested that the stress in the epitaxial layer would tend to bend the inclined dislocations propagating from the substrate into the substrate–epitaxial layer interface. If these dislocations reach the edge of the crystal, then they will terminate without the need for inclined dislocations to propagate into the epitaxial layer. This is evidently the case, since we see in Fig. 9.4.10 (top) that the inclined dislocation density in the epitaxial layer, despite the mismatch, is actually lower than that in the substrate. The high dislocation density of the layer in tension is believed to be related to the tendency to form microcracks in such layers with associated high dislocation densities [48].

To summarize these observations, it is evident that a fundamental mechanism exists, helpful in producing quality heteroepitaxial structures, where the inclined dislocation density is minimized by using multiple step growth either in VPE or LPE. The available evidence suggests that for step grading it is preferable to work with epitaxial layers which are in compression rather than in tension.

The use of very thin epitaxial layers is another method for obtaining dislocation-free interfaces as mentioned earlier. An interesting example of this effect in a double-heterojunction configuration of (AlGa)As/AlGaAsP/(AlGa)As, where the misfit at the growth temperature was about 10^{-4}, was obtained by Rozgonyi *et al.* [50], who grew the structure by LPE. They found that dislocation-free interfaces were obtained when the thickness of the middle layer of AlGaAsP was about 1 μm or less. Turning to Eq. (9.4.8c), the computed value of $h_c \cong 2$ μm is in good agreement considering the approximations.

Finally, we note that an interesting effect occurs in *LPE growth* which tends to produce precisely lattice-matched layers even if the solution composition is only *near* that needed to produce such a layer. It is found that the grown layer composition will be "pulled" toward the lattice-matched composition at the growth temperature. For example, if $In_xGa_{1-x}P$ is grown on

SUBSTRATE   Epi LAYAR

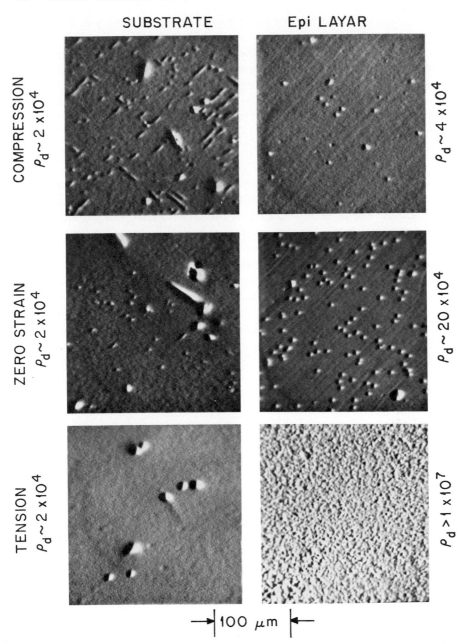

FIG. 9.4.10 Dislocation density emerging through the surface of the substrate GaAs (left) and of the In$_x$Ga$_{1-x}$P epitaxial layer grown by VPE. The misfit strain for the top and bottom samples is the same (about 3×10^{-3}). However, in the top layer the lattice parameter is greater than that of GaAs, whereas the reverse is true for the bottom sample. In the middle sample the lattice parameter is matched at the growth temperature (i.e., $x = 0.49$) [40].

GaAs, there is a tendency for the material grown to have $x \cong 0.5$, which matches the GaAs substrate lattice parameter (see Section 11.3.4). The presumed reason for this effect is the minimization of the free energy of the system by reducing misfit dislocations. This very useful phenomenon is unique to LPE growth (as far as determined to date), and greatly simplifies the growth of layers using quaternary alloys where a range of composition exists which matches the substrate lattice parameter (Section 11.4).

9.5 Substrate Considerations

As discussed in the preceding sections, epitaxial deposits are adversely affected when the lattice constant of the substrate and that of the layer differ significantly. The crystalline quality of the grown material is also influenced by the condition of the substrate surface and by the presence in the substrate of a high density of such crystalline defects as dislocation clusters, doping nonuniformities, strains and inclusions. Although systematic work dealing with effects of substrate flaws is scarce, observations concerned with such effects are scattered throughout the literature. Surface preparation prior to epitaxial growth is generally known to be important to minimize defect density. In many applications, however, when the LPE process is associated with "meltback," surface damage and contamination are removed along with substrate material to a depth of several microns before deposition occurs. In these instances the solution is brought into contact with the substrate surface at a temperature higher than that at which the solution is saturated with the material to be deposited. As cooling proceeds, material is dissolved from the substrate surface until the saturation temperature is reached and film deposit is initiated. Unless perturbed by a high defect density, the meltback tends to occur along a well-defined crystallographic plane leaving an extremely flat film–substrate interface, even when the initial substrate is marred by minor surface irregularities.

The most common substrate in laser work, GaAs, is subjected to chemical polishing before epitaxial growth. The surface damage is first removed by mechanical lapping with 5 μm Al_2O_3 powder, after which final polishing is carried out under a rotating polishing pad kept moistened with a chemical etch, usually 0.05% bromine in methanol or dilute sodium hypochlorite (Clorox). For detailed descriptions of procedures and results the reader is referred to articles by Sullivan and Kolb [51] and Oldham [52]. In considering the effects of substrate conditions, it is also worth noting that it is one of the advantages of the LPE process is that the solution in contact with the substrate surface can serve as a leaching agent [53] to render innocuous contamination present on or in the surface of the substrate.

As noted in Section 9.4.2, it is a common observation that the LPE layer has a lower dislocation density than the substrate (factors of 3 to 10 being common). However, when the substrate dislocation density is excessive, LPE growth can be affected. In this case, the growth of an intermediate layer is helpful. Figure 9.5.1a shows an etched cross section of an epitaxial structure obtained by the growth of a highly Zn-doped ($N_A \approx 2 \times 10^{19}$ cm^{-3}) GaAs film on a Te-doped ($N_D \approx 2 \times 10^{18}$ cm^{-3}) GaAs substrate with a dislocation density of about 2×10^3 cm^{-2}. The dislocations in this substrate are depicted in the anomalous x-ray topograph shown in Fig. 9.5.2. The irregularity of the interface in the cross section is believed due to the substrate dislocations; the small black spots are Zn-decorated dislocations [29]. Fig. 9.5.1b shows the same substrate, but here an intermediate n-type layer with the same doping density as that of the substrate was first grown followed by a Zn-doped layer. In this case, the interface is smooth and shows no evidence of precipitation at dislocation sites.

In general, the presence of inclusions in the substrate will have harmful effects on the properties of the films. In the case of the VPE deposition of silicon, for example, it is known that stacking faults nucleate at precipitate sites of fast diffusing impurities [54]. Similarly in GaAs, stacking faults may nucleate at inclusions present in substrates highly doped with Te and Si ($N_D \approx 3 \times 10^{18}$ cm^{-3}) [55]. In Fig. 9.5.3, inclusions present in Te- and Si-doped GaAs substrates are shown in (a) and (b), respectively. In the Te-doped substrate,

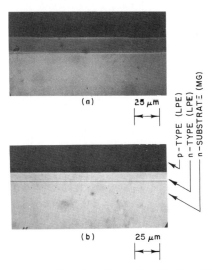

FIG. 9.5.1 (a) Cross section of junction formed by Zn-doped LPE layer of GaAs ($N_A \approx 2 \times 10^{19}$ cm^{-3}) deposited on the poor quality GaAs substrate shown in Fig. 9.5.2. Note irregularities at the interface. The small spots are due to Zn-decorated dislocations. (b) Cross section of improved junction formed by double epitaxy using a multiple bin on the same substrate. The intermediate layer is GaAs:Te ($N_D \approx 10^{18}$ cm^{-3}).

GaAs, (220)

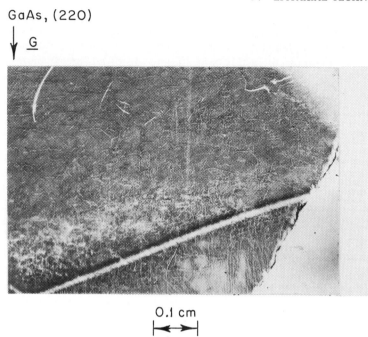

0.1 cm

FIG. 9.5.2 Anomalous x-ray transmission topograph of mediocre-quality melt-grown GaAs substrate.

the inclusions are small Ga_2Te_3 precipitates, whereas those in the Si-doped material are unidentified but may involve oxygen [56].

Other flaws such as doping, nonuniformity, and strains present in substrates have harmful effects. The x-ray topograph in Fig. 9.5.4 shows the presence of doping nonuniformities and strains in a substrate which yielded inferior epitaxial laser material. Topographic methods using x-rays are a powerful means of determining defect densities in epitaxial layers and substrates, as well as determining strains. A comprehensive review of the methods is given by Rozgonyi and Miller [57].

Various chemical etchants are also useful in determining defect densities in substrates. An extensive review of GaAs etchants, procedures, and results is given by Stirland and Straughan [58].

In the discussion so far we have emphasized the process of dislocation formation within the epitaxial layer to relieve the strain arising from the lattice misfit. In fact, dislocations can also form in the *substrate* if the strain is sufficiently high and growth occurs in a temperature interval where dislocation formation or multiplication is probable in the substrate for the stress resulting from the strain. Thus, the strain due to the lattice misfit is accommodated by plastic flow in the substrate and dislocation formation in the

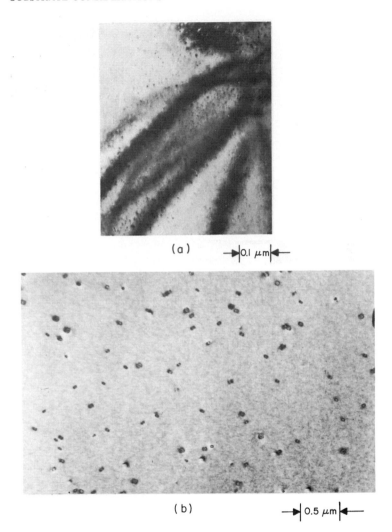

(a) →|0.1 μm|←

(b) →|0.5 μm|←

FIG. 9.5.3 Electron transmission micrographs showing (a) Ga_2Te_3 precipitates in a GaAs:Te substrate and (b) unidentified precipitates in a GaAs:Si substrate [56].

epitaxial layer, with residual elastic strain remaining when the wafer is cooled to room temperature.

An example of dislocation formation in the substrate in the source of growing an epitaxial layer of $GaAs_{0.91}Sb_{0.09}$ by liquid phase epitaxy on (100) GaAs is shown in Fig. 9.5.5. The surface of the epitaxial layer is shown in Figs. 9.5.5a and 9.5.5b at two different magnification levels to illustrate the "crosshatch" due to misfit dislocations in the epitaxial layer (which has a

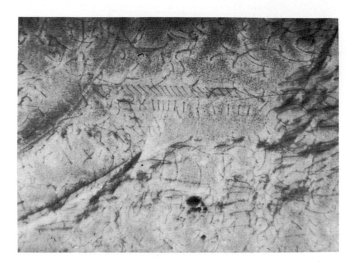

125 μm
|←→|

FIG. 9.5.4 X-ray topograph showing nonuniform doping and strains in a GaAs:Te substrate [56].

larger lattice parameter than the substrate). In Fig. 9.5.5c is presented a cathodoluminescence scan of the angled sample which clearly shows the dislocations in the substrate [as well as in the very thin GaAs intermediate layer grown prior to the Ga(AsSb) layer]. The total misfit strain is 0.69% and the maximum stress in the substrate is estimated to have reached a value of the order of 10^8 dynes/cm^2. This is apparently sufficient in the growth temperature range of 760–740°C to either nucleate dislocations at the interface, or produce these by multiplication in GaAs from existing dislocations. However, the latter is less likely, in view of the low ($\lesssim 10^3$ cm^{-2}) dislocation density initially present in the substrate.

REFERENCES

1. H. Nelson, *RCA Rev.* **24**, 603 (1963).
2. J. M. Woodall., H. Rupprecht, and W. Reuter, *J. Electrochem. Soc.* **116**, 899 (1969).
3. H. Nelson, U.S. Patent No. 3,565,702 (1971), filed February 14, 1969.
4. M. Kumagawa, A. F. Witt, M. Lichtensteiger, and H. C. Gates, *J. Electrochem. Soc.* **120**, 583 (1973).

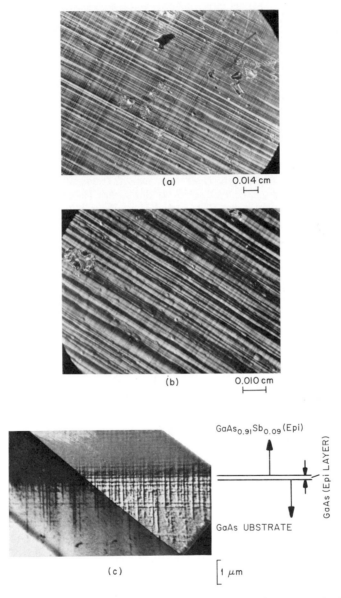

(a)   0.014 cm

(b)   0.010 cm

GaAs$_{0.91}$Sb$_{0.09}$ (Epi)

GaAs (Epi LAYER)

GaAs SUBSTRATE

(c)   1 μm

FIG. 9.5.5 Appearance of epitaxial layer surface, GaAs$_{0.91}$Sb$_{0.09}$ grown by LPE on a (100) GaAs substrate (with a thin intermediate GaAs epitaxial layer); $\Delta a_0/a_0 = 0.69\%$. (a) and (b) structure associated with misfit dislocations in the epitaxial layer as revealed by the A/B etch. (c) Cathodoluminescence scan (E. R. Levin, unpublished) of sample angled to 1° showing the dislocations in the substrate resulting from the epitaxial layer growth. The growth temperature interval was 760–740°C and the thickness of the substrate was 350 μm.

5. J. J. Daniels and C. Michel, *Proc. 1974 Symp. GaAs Related Compounds*. Inst. Phys. and Phys. Soc., London, 1975.
6. D. J. Lawrence and L. F. Eastman, *J. Crystal Growth* **30**, 267 (1975).
7. A. H. Cottrell, *Theoretical Structural Metallurgy*, p. 210. St. Martin's, New York, 1962.
8. W. A. Tiller and C. Kang, *J. Crystal Growth* **2**, 345 (1968).
9. I. Crossley and M. B. Small, *J. Crystal Growth* **11**, 157 (1971).
10. W. A. Tiller, *J. Crystal Growth* **2**, 69 (1968).
11. H. T. Minden, *J. Crystal Growth* **6**, 228 (1970).
12. T. Mitsuhata, *Jp. J. Appl. Phys.* **9**, 90 (1970).
13. J. J. Tietjen, R. E. Enstrom, and D. Richman, *RCA Rev.* **31**, 635 (1970).
14. J. J. Tietjen and J. A. Amick, *J. Electrochem. Soc.* **113**, 7241 (1966).
15. J. J. Tietjen, H. P. Maruska, and R. B. Clough, *J. Electrochem. Soc.* **116**, 492 (1969).
16. R. B. Clough and J. J. Tietjen, *Trans. Met. Soc. AIME* **245**, 583 (1969).
17. R. E. Enstrom *et al.*, *Proc. Int. Conf. GaAs, 3rd Aachen, Germany* (1970).
18. C. J. Nuese, D. Richman, and R. B. Clough, *Met. Trans.* **2**, 789 (1971).
19. M. Ettenberg, A. G. Sigai, S. Gilbert, and A. Dreeben, *J. Electrochem. Soc.* **118**, 1355 (1971).
20. A. G. Sigai, C. J. Nuese, R. E. Enstrom, and T. Zamerowski, *J. Electrochem. Soc.* **120**, 936 (1973).
21. R. B. Schoolar and Z. N. Zemel, *J. Appl. Phys.* **35**, 1848 (1971).
22. A. Y. Cho, *J. Vac. Sci. Technol.* **8**, 531 (1971).
23. L. J. Chang and R. Ludeke, "Molecular beam epitaxy," *in Epitaxial Growth* (J. W. Mathews, ed.). Academic Press, New York, 1975.
24. An introductory treatment of the subject can be found in J. Friedel, *Dislocations*. Addison-Wesley, Reading, Massachusetts, 1964.
25. D. B. Holt, *J. Phys. Chem. Solids* **27**, 1053 (1966).
26. J. H. van der Merwe, *Single Crystal Films* (M. H. Francombe and H. Sato, eds.), p. 139. Pergamon, Oxford, 1964.
27. J. W. Matthews, Coherent interfaces and misfit dislocations, *in Epitaxial Growth* (J. W. Matthews, ed.), Part B, p. 562. Academic Press, New York, 1975.
28. Y. Sugita, M. Tamura, and K. Sugawara, *J. Appl. Phys.* **40**, 3089 (1969).
29. M. S. Abrahams and C. J. Buiocchi, *J. Appl. Phys.* **37**, 1973 (1966).
30. D. A. Grenning and A. H. Herzog, *J. Appl. Phys.* **39**, 2783 (1968).
31. G. B. Stringfellow and P. E. Greene, *J. Appl. Phys.* **40**, 502 (1969).
32. M. S. Abrahams, L. R. Weisberg, C. J. Buiocchi, and J. Blanc, *J. Mater. Sci.* **4**, 223 (1969).
33. M. S. Abrahams, L. R. Weisberg, and J. J. Tietjen, *J. Appl. Phys.* **40**, 3758 (1969).
34. R. H. Saul, *J. Electrochem. Soc.* **115**, 1184 (1968).
35. R. H. Saul, *J. Appl. Phys.* **40**, 3273 (1969).
36. G. O. Krause and E. C. Teague, *Appl. Phys. Lett.* **10**, 251 (1967).
37. E. S. Meieran, *J. Electrochem. Soc.* **114**, 292 (1967).
38. H. Holloway and L. C. Bobb, *J. Appl. Phys.* **39**, 2467 (1968).
39. R. Feder and T. B. Light, *J. Appl. Phys.* **43**, 3114 (1972).
40. G. H. Olsen and M. Ettenberg, to be published.
41. G. H. Olsen, M. S. Abrahams, and T. J. Zamerowski, *J. Electrochem. Soc.* **121**, 1650 (1974).
42. M. S. Abrahams, J. Blanc, and C. J. Buiocchi, *Appl. Phys. Lett.* **21**, 185 (1972).
43. G. A. Rozgonyi, P. M. Petroff, and M. B. Panish, *Appl. Phys. Lett.* **24**, 251 (1974).
44. M. S. Abrahams, J. Blanc, and C. J. Buiocchi, *J. Appl. Phys.* **45**, 3277 (1974).

45. H. Nagai, *J. Appl. Phys.* **43**, 4254 (1972).
46. G. H. Olsen, *J. Crystal Growth* **31**, 223 (1975).
47. M. Ettenberg, S. H. McFarlane, III, and S. L. Gilbert, *Proc. Int. Symp. Gallium Arsenide Related Compounds, 4th, Sept. 25–27, 1972, Boulder, Colorado.*
48. G. H. Olsen, M. S. Abrahams, C. J. Buiocchi, and T. J. Zamerowski, *J. Appl. Phys.* **46**, 1643 (1975).
49. W. A. Jesser and J. W. Matthews, *Phil. Mag.* **15**, 1097 (1967).
50. G. A. Rozgonyi, P. M. Petroff, and M. B. Panish, *J. Crystal Growth* **27**, 106 (1974).
51. M. V. Sullivan and G. A. Kolb, *J. Electrochem. Soc.* **110**, 585 (1963).
52. W. G. Oldham, *Electrochem. Technol.* **3**, 57 (1965).
53. H. Kroemer, *Transistor I*, p. 132. RCA Laboratories, Princeton, New Jersey, 1956.
54. D. Pomerantz, *J. Appl. Phys.* **38**, 5020 (1967).
55. H. Kressel, M. S. Abrahams, F. Z. Hawrylo, and C. J. Buiocchi, *J. Appl. Phys.* **39**, 5139 (1968).
56. H. Kressel, H. Nelson, S. H. McFarlane, M. S. Abrahams, P. LeFur, and C. J. Buiocchi, *J. Appl. Phys.* **40**, 3587 (1969).
57. G. A. Rozgonyi and D. C. Miller, *Thin Solid Films* **31**, 185 (1976).
58. D. J. Stirland and B. W. Straughan, *Thin Solid Films* **31**, 139 (1976).
59. R. N. Hall, *J. Electrochem. Soc.* **110**, 385 (1963).

BIBLIOGRAPHY

Special Issue, Vapor growth and epitaxy, *J. Crystal Growth* **31** (1975).

W. T. Read, *Dislocations in Crystals.* McGraw-Hill, New York, 1953.

R. G. Rhodes, *Imperfections and Active Centers in Semiconductors.* Macmillan, New York, 1964.

Chapter 10

Binary III-V Compounds

In this chapter we describe some of the major properties of the binary compounds of interest in the preparation of luminescent devices. Since GaAs has been the most extensively studied, a major share of the chapter is devoted to it. It is important to note, however, that many of the results obtained with GaAs are applicable to other materials and can provide guidelines for their preparation.

10.1 Gallium Arsenide

10.1.1 Crystal Stoichiometry

Many important differences between the properties of GaAs prepared by vapor phase epitaxy, melt growth or liquid phase epitaxy, or molecular beam epitaxy are due to stoichiometric differences. Figure 10.1.1 shows an expanded and idealized GaAs phase diagram [1] which can serve as the basis for a discussion of the dependence of the crystal stochiometry on the growth conditions. To begin with, note that GaAs grown at its melting temperature T^m from an As-Ga solution has a deficiency of Ga atoms, thus incorporating a significant concentration δ of Ga vacancies (V_{Ga}), indirectly estimated to be as high 10^{17}–10^{19} cm^{-3} [2]. Since the growth temperature may deviate slightly from T^m, variations in the V_{Ga} concentration occur with corresponding inhomogeneity throughout a Bridgman or Czochralski grown ingot. Although the vacancy concentration is reduced during the cooling of the crystal, a significant density remains, particularly vacancies associated with impurity atoms.

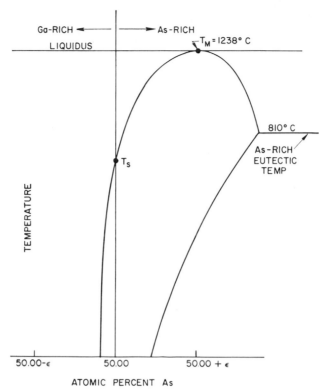

FIG. 10.1.1 The idealized solidus region of the GaAs binary phase diagram. T_s is the only temperature at which the solid in equilibrium with either an As- or Ga-rich melt is stoichiometric [1].

It is clear from Fig. 10.1.1 that the Ga deficiency can be reduced by growing the crystal below T^m from a Ga–As solution. At a growth temperature T_s (estimated in the 700–850° C range) [1] $\delta = 0$; and while at this temperature some Ga and As vacancies are, of course, formed in equal amounts as required by thermodynamic considerations, the concentration is relatively low. Thus, the temperature range used for LPE growth (700–900° C) is the most desirable from the point of view of stoichiometry. Below T_s, an excess of arsenic vacancies forms.

Vapor phase epitaxial growth is also generally carried out in the same low temperature range. It differs from LPE, however, in that the crystal stoichiometry is very sensitive to the relative pressures of the gaseous constituents. Although it is possible to grow GaAs over a relatively wide range of pressures, the effect on stoichiometry of the crystal can be significant. Thus, to obtain material of quality equal to that obtained by LPE, a close control of the gas constituents and growth conditions is required; but the proper conditions for obtaining stoichiometric crystals are not always easy to determine *a priori*.

Some additional observations can be made from Fig. 10.1.1 relevant to the incorporation of impurities, which is discussed in Section 10.1.3. If LPE material is grown over a wide temperature interval from an initial temperature above T_s by slowly cooling the Ga solution, the V_{Ga} concentration will predominate in the material grown above T_s whereas the V_{As} concentration will predominate in that grown below T_s. Thus, we may expect that amphoteric dopants, which can readily replace either Ga or As in the crystal lattice, will be incorporated differently in the crystal as the growth temperature decreases. This is the case with Si, for example, which is predominantly a donor in material grown at high temperatures but an acceptor in LPE material grown below about 800–850°C [3], although simple thermodynamic arguments based on a single donor and acceptor are inadequate (see Section 10.1.3).

The vacancy concentration can be changed after growth by appropriate thermal treatment followed by rapid cooling. A general theoretical discussion of this subject is given by Kröger [4]. A detailed analysis with discussion of published experimental results has been made by Logan and Hurle [2]. The formation of vacancies may also occur in LPE material during the warm-up and cooling period of the furnace [1]. At 600°C, for example, the diffusivity of As vacancies was quoted as $\sim 10^{-11}$ cm^2/s (1.3 eV activation energy), and a 1-hr anneal under vacuum or flowing H$_2$ will generate a significant density of As vacancies to a depth of about 2 μm. These vacancies can form acceptor centers, combine with impurities, or promote the switching of amphoteric impurities from Ga to As sites. As a result, in Zn-doped material, the hole concentration near the surface is increased, whereas in n-type material the electron concentration is reduced [5].

10.1.2 Major Dopants

Table 10.1.1 lists the ionization energies of various dopants in GaAs divided into three major categories: simple donors, simple acceptors, complex levels involving the group IV atoms, and transition metals. Although most dopants affect the electrical and optical properties of GaAs equally whatever the method of growth, notable exceptions occur, as now discussed.

The group IV dopant *germanium* is predominantly a shallow acceptor in LPE GaAs [6], predominantly a donor in VPE GaAs [7], but a donor or acceptor to almost equal extent in MG GaAs. A relatively deep (0.08 eV) acceptor level [6] is prominent in MG [8,9] n- and p-type GaAs:Ge but is generally negligible in p-type LPE material [6,10]. This level may be due to a complex of some type, possibly involving an As vacancy [11], but this identification is still uncertain. A still deeper level involving Ge and possibly a Ga vacancy is

TABLE 10.1.1a
Ionization Energy of Transition Metals in GaAs[a]

Element	Ionization energy		
	From photoluminescence at 20 and 4 K[b]	From electroluminescence at 77 K[c]	From electrical measurements[d]
Cr	0.85	—	0.79
Mn (acceptor)	0.114, 0.112[e]		0.094
Fe	~0.2 and 0.5	0.36	0.52, 0.37[f]
Co	0.58	0.345	0.16
Ni	—	0.35	0.21
Cu	0.170, 0.155[g] 0.165[h]	—	0.145[g]
Ag	0.239[i]	—	0.235[i]

TABLE 10.1.1b
Impurity Ionization Energies in GaAs

Type	Element	E_i (eV)	Remarks	Ref.
Simple donors	S_{As}	0.00610		a
	Se_{As}	0.00589		a
	Te_{As}	0.0058		b
	Sn_{Ga}	0.006		b
	C_{Ga}	Similar to Sn		c
	Ge_{Ga}	0.00608		a
	Si_{Ga}	0.00581		a
	Cr	Shallow	LPE material	d
	O	Similar to Sn	LPE material only[e]	f
	Pb_{Ga}	Shallow	LPE material	g
Simple acceptors	Cd_{Ga}	0.0345		h,i
	Zn_{Ga}	0.029		j
		0.032		k
		0.030		l
		0.034		m
	Mg_{Ga}	0.030		n
		0.028		i
	Be_{Ga}	0.030		n
		0.028		i
	C_{As}	0.026		i
		0.025		m
	Sn	0.2 ± 0.02 ⎱ Believed to be Sn_{As}		g
		0.171 ⎰		o
	Pb	~0.12		g
	Ge_{As}	0.038		p,q
	Si_{As}	0.035		i
Complex centers	Ge (acceptor)	~0.08	LPE and MG material	p,r
	Si (acceptor)	~0.1	LPE material	s
	Si (acceptor)	~0.22	LPE material	s
		0.23	Si ion-implanted GaAs	t

References for Table 10.1.1a

[a]Data compiled by E. W. Williams, and H. B. Bebb, "Semiconductor and Semimetals" (R. K. Willardson and A. C. Beer, eds.), Vol. 8, p. 321. Academic Press, New York, 1972. Reported for materials *not* prepared by LPE.

[b]E. W. Williams and D. M. Blacknall, *Trans. AIME* **239**, 387 (1967).

[c]H. Strack, *Trans. AIME* **239**, 381 (1967).

[d]R. W. Haisty and G. R. Cronin, *Proc. Int. Conf. Phys. Semicond., 7th, Paris,* p. 1161 (1964).

[e]T. C. Lee and W. W. Anderson, *Solid State Commun.* **2**, 265 (1964).

[f]F. A. Cunnell, J. T. Edward, and W. R. Harding, *Solid State Electron.* **1**, 97 (1960).

[g]H. J. Queisser and C. S. Fuller, *J. Appl. Phys.* **37**, 4895 (1966).

[h]C. J. Hwang, *J. Appl. Phys.* **39**, 4307 (1968).

[i]M. Blatte, W. Schairer, and F. Willman, *Solid State Commun.* **8**, 1265 (1970).

References for Table 10.1.1b

[a]C. J. Summers, R. Dingle, and D. E. Hill, *Phys. Rev. B* **1**, 1603 (1970).

[b]Estimate by R. Dingle, quoted by H. C. Casey, Jr., and F. A. Trumbore, *Mater. Sci. Eng.* **6**, 69 (1970).

[c]E. W. Williams, *Phys. Rev.* **168**, 922 (1968).

[d]E. Andre and J. M. LeDuc, *Mater. Res. Bull.* **4**, 149 (1969).

[e]A deep donor level at ~ 0.75 eV was found in melt-grown GaAs by R. W. Haisty, E. W. Mehal, and R. Stratton, *J. Phys. Chem. Solids* **23**, 829 (1962).

[f]R. Solomon, *Proc. Int. Symp. Gallium Arsenide, 2nd.* Inst. Phys., Phys. Soc. Conf. Ser. No. 7, p. 11 (1968).

[g]H. Kressel, H. Nelson, and F. Z. Hawrylo, *J. Appl. Phys.* **39**, 5647 (1968).

[h]E. W. Williams and H. B. Bebb, *J. Phys. Chem. Solids* **30**, 1289 (1969).

[i]D. J. Ashen, P. J. Dean, P. D. Greene, D. T. J. Hurle, J. B. Mullin, and A. M. White, *J. Phys. Chem. Solids* **36**, 1041 (1975).

[j]D. E. Hill, *J. Appl. Phys.* **41**, 1815 (1970).

[k]C. J. Hwang, *J. Appl. Phys.* **38**, 4811 (1967).

[l]E. W. Williams and D. M. Blacknall, *Trans. AIME* **239**, 387 (1967).

[m]E. W. Williams, "Semiconductor and Semimetals" (R. K. Willardson and A. C. Beer, eds.), Vol. 8, p. 321. Academic Press, New York, 1971.

[n]H. Kressel and F. Z. Hawrylo, *J. Appl. Phys.* **41**, 1865 (1970).

[o]W. Schairer and E. Grobe, *Solid State Commun.* **8**, 2017 (1970).

[p]H. Kressel, F. Z. Hawrylo, and P. LeFur, *J. Appl. Phys.* **39**, 4059 (1968). The value quoted is $E_i \sim 0.03$ eV. However, from the experimental data $E_g - hv = 0.038$ eV, which sets an upper limit to E_i.

[q]F. E. Rosztoczy, F. Ermanis, I. Hayashi, and B. Schwartz, *J. Appl. Phys.* **41**, 264 (1970).

[r]E. W. Williams and C. T. Elliott, *Brit. J. Appl. Phys. D* **2**, 1657 (1969).

[s]H. Kressel, J. U. Dunse, H. Nelson, and F. Z. Hawrylo [*J. Appl. Phys.* **39**, 2006 (1968)] suggested that the level involved [V_{As} + Si].

[t]An acceptor level with $E_i = 0.23$ eV was observed following Si ion implantation in MG GaAs by T. Itoh and Y. Kushiro [*J. Appl. Phys.* **42**, 5120 (1971)], who suggested that this center identification was consistent with a [V_{As} + Si] complex.

commonly observed in MG GaAs but not in LPE GaAs. This center gives rise to a broad emission at 77 K centered at 1.20–1.25 eV [12]. Further, in highly Ge-doped LPE GaAs ($>5 \times 10^{18}$ cm^{-3}) another recombination band appears at about 1.35 eV [6,10,13], the intensity of which increases with increasing Ge concentration and thus appears to form a compensating or neutral complex center.

It should be mentioned that because of its relatively low vapor pressure and diffusion rate in GaAs, Ge is often advantageously used as an acceptor instead of Zn in GaAs LPE. In the growth of multilayer films, for instance, unwanted acceptor contamination of n-type layers which occurs with Zn is avoided by the use of Ge.

The mobility of GaAs:Ge prepared by LPE at 760°C has been studied as a function of hole concentration at room temperature (Fig. 10.1.2) [14]. A ratio $N_A/N_D = 10$ was deduced on the basis of Hall measurements. (However, this ratio must depend on the growth conditions; the data in Fig. 10.1.5, for example, show a smaller N_A/N_D ratio.) Figure 10.1.2 also shows that the measured and theoretical mobility values agree reasonably well in the concentration range ($P \sim 10^{17}$ cm^{-3}) below which impurity band conduction becomes a significant factor.

Tin is predominantly a donor in material prepared by all techniques, and there is no report of p-type Sn-doped GaAs. In addition to the shallow donor, Sn gives rise to an acceptor center in LPE GaAs with $E_i \cong 0.18$ eV [15] which appears to be due to Sn_{As} [16] (Sn on an As site), but this is still somewhat

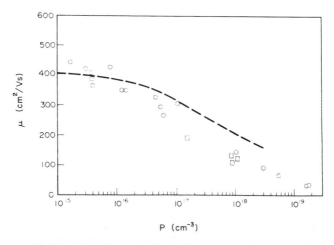

FIG. 10.1.2 Mobility of LPE p-type GaAs: Ge grown at 760°C, (100) plane, versus hole density at 300 K. Data points are experimental values; dashed line from theory, assuming $E_A = 35$ meV, g (spin degeneracy) $= 4$, and $N_D/N_A = 0.1$ [14].

uncertain. The degree of compensation depends on the LPE growth temperature, but few data are available. For material grown at 700°C, $N_D/N_A = 3.6$ [14] and the 300 K mobility data shown in Fig. 10.1.3a, are in good agreement with theory. The minority carrier (hole) diffusion length has been determined [18] as a function of electron concentration as shown in Fig. 10.1.3b.

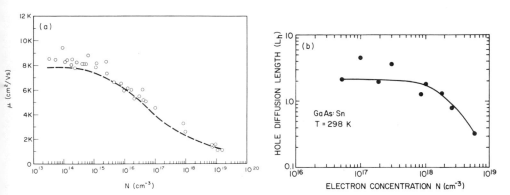

FIG. 10.1.3 (a) Mobility at 300 K of LPE n-type GaAs: Sn grown at 700°C, (100) plane, versus electron density. ○, Experimental values; – – –, theory [17], assuming $N_A = 2 \times 10^{14}$ cm^{-3} + $N_D/3.6$ [14]. (b) Hole diffusion length in microns as a function of the electron concentration in GaAs: Sn grown by liquid phase epitaxy [18].

Lead, predominantly a donor in GaAs, also gives rise to an acceptor level with $E_i \cong 0.12$ eV [6]. Because of its very low segregation coefficient, there is no practical advantage in the use of Pb as a dopant.

Silicon is one of the most extensively studied dopants in GaAs because of its advantageous use in light-emitting devices (Section 14.6.1). GaAs:Si grown by MG or VPE is always n-type [19]; in LPE material, the conductivity type, the net carrier concentration and the degree of compensation depend on the growth conditions, which are now discussed.

Radiative recombination involving an acceptor level with $E_i \cong 0.1$ eV is very prominent in LPE GaAs:Si in addition to that involving the shallow $E_i \sim 0.03$ eV level, which is seen in MG and VPE material [19]. Measurements by Spitzer and Panish [21] of the absorption bands associated with localized vibrational modes of point defects on various atomic sites show that Si occupies Ga sites and As sites, and also forms [$Si_{As} + Si_{Ga}$] pairs. The sum of Si $Si_{As} + Si_{Ga} + 2[Si_{As} + Si_{Ga}]$ accounts quite well for the total Si in the material. The interesting fact is that for all the materials studied, $Si_{Ga} > Si_{Ga}$. Thus, it is not possible to account for the p-type GaAs obtained by LPE by assuming that the only acceptors are the Si_{As} ones.

Tellurium, selenium, and *sulfur* are shallow donors with ionization energies 5–6 meV. However, in GaAs prepared by all techniques, these impurities also form complex centers, which quite definitely include one or more Ga vacancies. These deep centers, which give rise to a well-known broad radiative emission band at $\sim$ 1.2 eV (77 K) [12], shown in Fig. 10.1.4, are harmful to luminescent device performance. The formation of such complexes is qualitatively explained by the fact that the strain energy of the crystal is reduced when a vacancy moves next to a relatively large impurity atom, such as Se or Te. Furthermore, if the centers are neutral, as should be the case when Ga vacancies are next to group VI atoms on As sites, there is an additional free energy reduction due to the reduced Coulombic interaction. It has been proposed by Vieland and Kudman [23] that in GaAs:Se the complex formed is $[V_{Ga} + 3Se]$; in GaAs: Te the center may consist of $[V_{Ga} + 3Te]$. These are the incipient forms of Ga_2Se_3 and Ga_2Te_3, respectively, and at sufficiently high Se or Te concentrations, inclusions of these compounds in the doped material are therefore to be expected. Gallium telluride precipitates have in fact been identified in LPE GaAs with Te concentrations in excess of 2–4 $\times 10^{18}cm^{-3}$ [22].

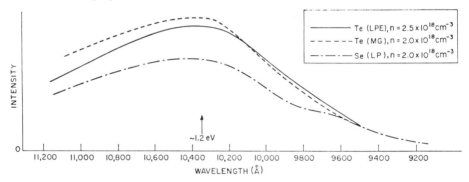

FIG. 10.1.4   Deep-level luminescence at 77 K believed due to a Ga vacancy–impurity complex in Te- and Se-doped GaAs [22].

As we noted previously for Ge and Sn, the broad 77 K luminescent bands in the 1.20–1.25 eV range associated with complexes of the group IV dopants in MG and VPE material are either very weak or absent in LPE material. Although these centers may also be associated with Ga vacancies, as is the case with the group VI dopants, it is possible that oxygen plays a dominant role in their formation. This has been suggested in the case of VPE GaAs:Si as a result of observations made of the intensity of this band as a function of the gas used to prepare the material [19].

10.1.3   Impurity Incorporation in LPE

Assuming growth from a dilute solution and equilibrium between the bulk of the solid and the solution, the equilibrium constant K describing the relationship between the dopant concentration in the solid N^s (in cubic centimeters) and the dopant atomic fraction in the liquid N^l is [24].

$$K = PN^s/N^l V_{Ga} \qquad (10.1.1)$$

were we have assumed that the dopant is an acceptor on Ga sites, and P is the hole concentration at the growth temperature. A similar treatment can be made for single donors. If the dopant is fully and singly ionized, then

$$N^s = P - N \qquad (10.1.2)$$

where N is the free electron concentration, which is related to the intrinsic carrier concentration N_i by

$$N_i{}^2 = PN \qquad (10.1.3)$$

We now consider two limiting conditions. If the material is intrinsic (i.e., relatively low dopant concentration), then $N^s \ll N_i$ and $N = P = N_i$. Equation (10.1.1) then simplifies to

$$K = N^s N_i/N^l V_{Ga} \qquad (10.1.4)$$

Hence

$$N^s = k_s(T)N^l \qquad (10.1.5)$$

and the distribution constant $k_s(T)$ is given by

$$k_s(T) = KV_{Ga}/N_i \qquad (10.1.6)$$

On the other hand, when the dopant concentration exceeds the intrinsic carrier concentration, $N^s \cong P \gg N_i$, and Eq. (10.1.1) reduces to

$$K = (N^s)^2/N^l V_{Ga} \qquad (10.1.7)$$

or

$$N^s = (KV_{Ga})^{1/2}(N^l)^{1/2} \qquad (10.1.8)$$

On the basis of this discussion, we would expect that at *low concentration*, $N^s \propto N^l$, whereas at *high concentrations* $N^s \propto (N^l)^{1/2}$. Since in GaAs $N_i = 10^{16}$–10^{17} cm^{-3} at the usual LPE growth temperatures of 800–900°C, the extrinsic approximation is the appropriate one for the usual doping range of interest. Experimentally, it is found, however, that $N^s \propto N^l$ (even for N^s exceeding 10^{18} cm^{-3}) for most of the impurities studied so far in GaAs with the exception of Zn and probably Be. This means that in general, the assumption of equilibrium between the liquid and the bulk of the solid is incorrect and the Fermi level position at the surface of the solid differs from that further in the bulk of the solid. The explanation proposed by Merten and Hatcher [25] is that a surface barrier exists due to electrostatic forces with a width on the order of the Debye screening length L_D

$$L_D = (\varepsilon k T/4\pi Ne^2)^{1/2} \qquad (10.1.9)$$

where e is the electronic charge, ε the dielectric constant, k the Boltzmann constant, and N the electron concentration at the growth temperature.* In effect, the solution–solid interface behaves as a Schottky barrier and this basic model has been used to explain the incorporation of impurities in solution growth [26,27].

In essence, the argument is that the impurity concentration at the solid–liquid interface is "frozen" to an extent which depends on the growth velocity, the impurity diffusion coefficient in the solid D_i, and on L_D. On the basis of a simple analysis which compares the dopant flux through the distance L_D at a growth velocity V_s, it can be shown that equilibrium is established between the bulk of the solid and the liquid only if $D_i/L_D \gg V_s$ [25]. This means that for fast diffusing impurities or sufficiently small growth rates, $N^s \propto (N^l)^{1/2}$ (if no complications exist such as complex formation, precipitation, or the incorporation of the dopant as a neutral species). If, on the other hand, $D_i/L_D \ll V_s$, then the incorporation of impurities is controlled by the carrier concentration in the band-bent region at the surface of the solid, and hence $N^s \propto N^l$. The distribution coefficient is then given by the following expressions [26]:

For donors,

$$k_s(T) = k_0(T) \exp(-\phi_B/kT) \qquad (10.1.10a)$$

whereas for acceptors,

$$k_s(T) = k_0'(T) \exp(-\phi_B/kT) \qquad (10.1.10b)$$

Here $k_0(T)$ and $k_0'(T)$ are concentration-independent terms, and ϕ_B is the Schottky barrier height (0.6–1 eV in GaAs) [28].

This model predicts a low acceptor segregation coefficient if the diffusion coefficient is low. Furthermore, this model explains the variation of the distribution coefficient with growth plane by differences in the barrier height. For example, since ϕ_B is greater on the (111) As face than on the (111) Ga face, [29], k_s should be greater on the (111) As face than on the (111) Ga face for donors, and vice versa for acceptors. There is some experimental evidence in agreement with this prediction.

We now consider quantitatively whether the equilibrium criteria are satisfied under normal LPE growth velocities $V_s = 10^{-4}$–10^{-7} cm/s. Considering Sn, for example, at about 900°C, $D_{Sn} \approx 10^{-14}$ cm^2/s [30]; with $L_D \approx 10^{-5}$ cm, $D_{Sn}/L_D \approx 10^{-9}$ cm/s, which is usually much smaller than V_s. Hence, equilibrium between the bulk of the solid and the solution is *not* established. On the other hand, in the case of a fast diffusing dopant such as Zn, $D_{Zn} \approx 10^{-11}$ cm^2/s, $D_{Zn}/L_D \approx 10^{-6}$ cm/s, and equilibrium is established for moderate growth rates. Beryllium should behave similarly since its diffusivity is

*If the material is intrinsic at the growth temperature, $N = N_i$ in Eq. (10.1.9) and the Debye length is the "intrinsic" one.

also high, whereas sulfur may represent an intermediate case. A mathematical analysis for the dependence of the effective distribution coefficient as a function of $D_i/L_D V_s$ is given by Zschauer and Vogel [26].

The most commonly used dopants in GaAs are the group IV elements Ge, Si, and Sn, the group II element Zn, and the group VI elements Te and Se. With the exception of Zn, the incorporation of these impurities in GaAs can be described by a temperature-dependent distribution coefficient, which relates the linear dependence of the atomic concentration in the solid to that in the liquid.

Table 10.1.2 lists distribution coefficients reported for LPE growth at various temperatures and growth planes. Although the spread in the values reported in some cases is considerable, the results are still of practical interest. Some of these differences are due to varying growth rates or accuracy in the measurement of the dopant concentration in the solid. We have indicated in Table 10.1.2 the method used to deduce the dopant concentration in the solid. Radioactive tracer methods are expected to give the most accurate results but have been used by only a few investigators. In many cases, it is assumed that a one-to-one correspondence exists between the carrier concentration and the dopant concentration. This is a reasonable assumption for Te and Se for concentrations $\leq 2 \times 10^{18}$ cm^{-3}, but not for the group IV dopants, which are amphoteric. Note in Table 10.1.2 that no data are given for Te, Se, or S concerning the growth plane dependence of k_s. The only comment in the literature is that k_s is higher on the (111) As than on the (111) Ga plane [31].

Figure 10.1.5 shows the variation of the total Ge density in $GaAs:Ge$ and the hole concentration as a function of the Ge concentration in the Ga solution at a growth temperature range of 800–875°C. The hole concentration is significantly lower than the total Ge concentration particularly at high doping levels because of the formation of donors and complex centers.

Because of the formation of Sn acceptors, the electron concentration is also lower than the total Sn concentration in $GaAs:Sn$, with the compensation ratio dependent on the growth temperature and possibly the Sn density. It has been reported that k_{Sn} is significantly higher on the (111) As plane than on the (100) and (111) Ga planes [32]. However, since only the electron density was measured, it is possible that the degree of compensation was changing.

In $GaAs:Si$, the carrier concentration is a function of the growth temperature for a given growth plane, as shown in Fig. 10.1.6 for materials growth at two temperatures [33]. The growth plane also strongly affects the incorporation of Si in GaAs [34] with the closer compensation being observed on the (100) than on the (111) As face. The temperature at which p-type instead of n-type materials is grown is highest on the (111) As face and lowest on the (100) face, as shown in Fig. 10.1.7 [35], indicating that the incorporation of Si acceptors is favored on the (100) face as compared to the (111) As

TABLE 10.1.2   Distribution Coefficient k_s of Some Dopants in GaAs (LPE Growth)

Element	Type	k_s	Atom conc. range (cm⁻³)	Growth face	Approx. growth T(°C)	Method	Ref.
Tin	Donor	1×10^{-4}	3×10^{14}–4×10^{16}	(100)	860	Conductivity	a
		0.4×10^{-4}	$\sim 10^{14}$–10^{18}	(100)	700	Conductivity	b
		1.1×10^{-4}	$\sim 5 \times 10^{14}$–10^{16}	(100)	700	Conductivity	c
		20×10^{-4}	$\sim 10^{18}$–10^{19}	(100)	910	Mass spectrometry	d
Tellurium	Donor	0.35	2×10^{17}–4×10^{19}	(111) As	1000	Radioactive tracer	e
		0.67 ± 0.3	4×10^{17}–2×10^{18}	(100)	890	Mass spectrometry	f
		1	5×10^{14}–10^{17}	(100)	800	Conductivity	g
Selenium	Donor	~1	5×10^{14}–10^{17}	(100)	1000	Conductivity	h
		5	5×10^{14}–10^{17}	(100)	800	Conductivity	h
Chromium	Donor	$\sim 10^{-5}$	5×10^{15}–2×10^{18}	(111) Ga; (100)	700–850	Conductivity	i
		5–10×10^{-5}	Not given	(111) As	700–850	Conductivity	i
Germanium	Acceptor	8.3×10^{-3}	$\sim 10^{16}$–5×10^{18}	(111) As	875–900	Radioactive tracer	j
						Mass spectrometry	
Oxygen	Donor	$\sim 3 \times 10^{-4}$	10^{15}–6×10^{16}	(100)	600–750	Conductivity	k
Silicon	Amphoteric	6.2×10^{-2}	10^{16}–10^{17}	(100)	680–730	Hall measurements $(N_D + N_A)$	l
	Amphoteric	8.3×10^{-2}	10^{16}–10^{17}	(100)	800–815	Hall measurements $(N_D + N_A)$	l

[a] J. S. Harris and W. L. Snyder, *Solid State Electron.* **12**, 337 (1969).

[b] R. Solomon, *Proc. Int. Symp. Gallium Arsenide, 2nd, 1968* Inst. Phys. Phys. Soc. Conf. Ser. No. 7, p. 2 (1969).

[c] J. Vilms and J. P. Garrett, *Solid State Electron.* **15**, 443 (1972).

[d] H. Kressel, H. Nelson, and F. Z. Hawrylo, *J. Appl. Phys.* **39**, 5647 (1968). The distribution coefficient depends on the growth conditions and Sn concentration. At high Sn concentrations, the electrically active part is much smaller than the total concentration. For comprehensive data and analysis see M. B. Panish, *J. Appl. Phys.* **44**, 2676 (1973).

[e] H. C. Casey, Jr., M. B. Panish, and K. B. Wolfstirn, *J. Phys. Chem. Solids* **32**, 571 (1971).

[f] H. Kressel, F. Z. Hawrylo, M. S. Abrahams, and C. J. Buiocchi, *J. Appl. Phys.* **39**, 5139 (1968).

[g] C. S. Kang and P. E. Greene, *Proc. Int. Symp. Gallium Arsenide, 2nd, 1968* Inst. Phys. Phys. Soc. Conf. Ser. No. 7, p. 18 (1969).

[h] P. D. Greene, *Solid State Commun.* **9**, 1209 (1971).   [i] E. Andre and J. M. LeDue, *Mater. Res. Bull.* **4**, 149 (1969).

[j] F. E. Rosztoczy and K. B. Wolfstirn, *J. Appl. Phys.* **42**, 426 (1971).

[k] R. Solomon, *Proc. Int. Symp. Gallium Arsenide, 2nd, 1968* Inst. Phys. Phys. Soc. Conf. Ser. No. 7, p. 11 (1969).

[l] H. G. B. Hicks and P. D. Greene, *Proc. Int. Symp. Gallium Arsenide, 3rd, 1970* Inst. Phys. Phys. Soc. Conf. Ser. No. 9, p. 92 (1971).

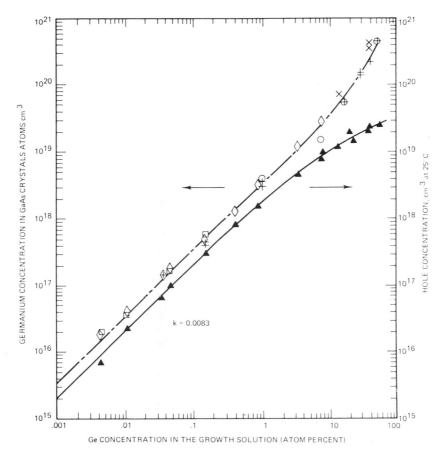

FIG. 10.1.5 Germanium and hole concentrations in LPE GaAs versus Ge concentration in the growth solutions. The formation of the donors and complex centers results in a lower hole than Ge concentration in the grown material. The material was grown in the 900–875°C range [17].

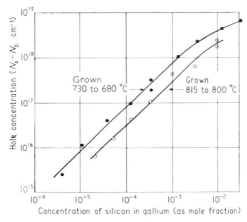

FIG. 10.1.6 Relationship between Si concentration in the solution and hole concentration in LPE GaAs grown in two temperature ranges [33].

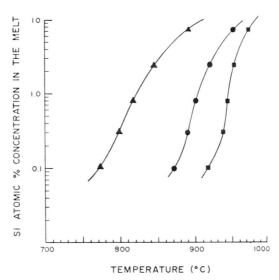

FIG. 10.1.7 The temperature at which the transition from n- to p-type material occurs in the growth of GaAs: Si as a function of the Si concentration in the Ga solution. The three curves denote growth on the (100) (●), (111)A (■), and (111)B (▲) planes [35].

face. This observation is consistent with the Schottky barrier model discussed earlier.

The incorporation of *Zn in GaAs* has been studied experimentally at 1000°C in material grown from Ga- and As-rich solutions in sealed ampules [36]. The Zn concentration in the solid increases as the square root of the concentration in the liquid (Fig. 10.1.8), which indicates that equilibrium is established between the liquid and the bulk of the solid, as expected for a fast diffusing impurity. It should be noted that the Zn solubility is higher for a given concentration in the liquid when the material is grown from an As-rich than when grown from a Ga-rich solution [33]. The difference is due to the higher V_{Ga} concentration in GaAs when grown from As-rich solutions. With regard to the growth plane dependence of Zn incorporation, N^s appears to be higher for a given N^l in material grown on the (111) Ga face than when grown on the (111) As face, although detailed data are not available.

The *temperature dependence* of the distribution coefficient has been studied for some dopants. Figure 10.1.9 shows that k_{Te} and k_{Se} increase with decreasing temperature, whereas k_{Sn} decreases with decreasing temperature. The incorporation of Zn should also decrease with decreasing temperature (Fig. 10.1.8). With regard to Ge, the distribution coefficient appears to increase with decreasing temperature, but extensive data are lacking [41].

At this time it is not possible to determine whether the observed temperature-dependent distribution coefficients of various dopants reflect the true

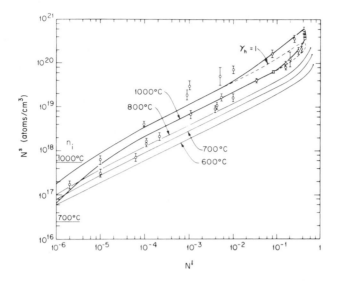

FIG. 10.1.8 Zinc concentration in GaAs versus the Zn atomic fraction in the Ga solution N^l along the 600, 700, 800, and 1000°C liquidus isotherms in the Ga–As–Zn system [37]. The isotherms at 800°C and below are terminated at the approximate liquid compositions where Zn_3As_2, a secondary solid phase, appears. The experimental data, at 1000°C, are from (○) Casey *et al.* [38] and (□) Chang and Pearson [39].

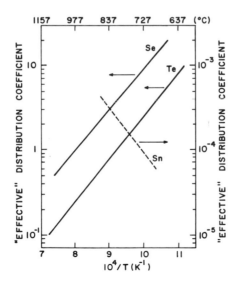

FIG. 10.1.9 The relationship between the "effective" distribution coefficients and LPE growth temperature for Se, Te, and Sn in GaAs. Se data from P. D. Greene [40]; Te and Sn data from Kang and Greene [32].

incorporation rate or are simply artifacts due to differences in the growth rate with changing temperature. In particular, note that in the Schottky barrier model, the distribution coefficient of donors should increase with decreasing temperature [Eq. (10.1.10)]. Experimentally, this is the case with Te and Se but not with Sn. Thus, this simple model does not entirely explain the observations, and it is possible that the differences arise due to the fact that Te and Se fill As sites while Sn fills mainly Ga sites, and that the concentrations of As and Ga vacancies vary differently with temperature.

10.1.4   Luminescent Efficiency

In view of the importance of GaAs in many luminescent device applications, it is appropriate to consider the radiative efficiency of the material as an individual parameter. The discussion in this section is quite general in that a similar behavior is expected in other materials. We use GaAs for illustration since well-documented data are available.

As discussed in Chapter 1, minority carriers injected into a material (using a p–n junction, electron beam, or optical excitation) can recombine by band-to-band transitions or via impurity states. The energy may be given off as a photon, in which case the recombination is called radiative, or it may be dissipated in the form of phonons (i.e., heating of the lattice), in which case the recombination is nonradiative. The nonradiative processes include recombination at a free surface or at inclusions within the crystal, recombination via impurity–vacancy complex centers, or recombination via individual vacancies. In addition, Auger processes (Chapter 1) may occur in highly doped materials in which the energy released by the electron–hole recombination is transferred in the form of kinetic energy to a third electron or hole. We recall that the radiative efficiency is expressed as

$$\eta_i = (1 + \tau_r/\tau_{nr})^{-1} \tag{10.1.11}$$

where τ_r and τ_{nr} are the minority carrier lifetime for radiative and nonradiative recombination, respectively, with no distinction made in the nature of the processes. Furthermore, for low injection levels, and assuming band-to-band recombination

$$\tau_r \cong B_r/N \quad \text{(n-type material)}, \qquad \tau_r \cong B_r/P \quad \text{(p-type material)} \tag{10.1.12}$$

where B_r is the recombination coefficient. Therefore, if the nonradiative lifetime is constant, the radiative efficiency will increase with increasing electron or hole concentration in n- or p-type material, respectively.

Experimentally, we find that η_i, as measured by photoluminescence or cathodoluminescence in GaAs, does indeed increase but only until $N \approx 2 \times 10^{18}$ cm^{-3} in n-type material [42], and $P \approx 10^{19}$ cm^{-3} in Zn [43] and Ge-

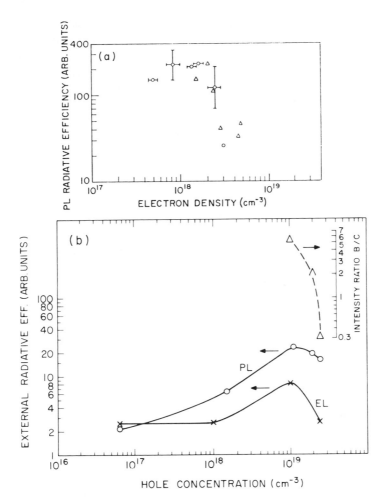

FIG. 10.1.10 (a) Photoluminescent radiative efficiency at 77 K versus electron density in Te-doped (○) and Se-doped (△) LPE GaAs [22]. (b) External radiative efficiency at room temperature (arbitrary units) as a function of hole concentration as determined by photoluminescence (○) and electroluminescence (×) of p–n junctions where the p-side is GaAs:Ge and the n-side of fixed composition ($N = 2 \times 10^{18}$ cm^{-3}), melt grown. The upper portion of the figure (△) shows the decrease in the ratio of the intensity of bands B and C at 77 K with increasing hole concentration. Band C was not detectable for $P < 10^{19}$ cm^{-3} and not seen at 300 K [44].

doped p-type material [44]. Figure 10.1.10a shows the relative dependence of η_i on N in n-type GaAs:Te and GaAs:Se prepared by LPE. The maximum η_i occurs at $N \cong 2\text{--}3 \times 10^{18}$ cm^{-3}, and the formation of complex centers and precipitates is probably a dominant reason for the eventual η_i decrease [22].

In p-type GaAs, on the other hand, it is believed that Auger recombination processes can become important in the 10^{19} cm^{-3} range [45,46].

Figure 10.1.10b shows the relative radiative efficiency of GaAs:Ge as a function of the hole concentration, and the maximum in efficiency occurs at about $P \approx 10^{19}$ cm^{-3} [44]. The role of defects, such as precipitates or impurity–vacancy complexes, in the decrease in the radiative efficiency in highly p-type GaAs is difficult to assess. Indeed, precipitates of Zn_3As_2 have been observed by transmission electron microscopy [47] in VPE GaAs, and similar precipitates may be present in p-type GaAs prepared by various methods, which represent a limiting factor on the radiative efficiency. With regard to defects, nonradiative recombination centers involving Ga vacancies have been shown to degrade the radiative efficiency. For example, GaAs:Zn grown from Ga-rich solutions has a higher radiative efficiency than material grown from As-rich solutions [48]. This observation is consistent with the fact that melt-grown materials commonly have lower efficiencies than similarly doped LPE materials [49]. Annealing studies with n-type MG GaAs in which additional vacancies are generated have shown a similar correlation between V_{Ga}-related centers and reduced photoluminescent efficiency [50].

Because of the sensitivity of the radiative efficiency to the density of defects difficult to measure by other techniques, photoluminescence or cathodoluminescence measurements are widely used for the selection and study of materials and the determination of their relative quality. In addition, these measurements are also useful in selecting materials with the best possible diffusion length (Section 10.1.5), because the radiative efficiency can be correlated with the diffusion length, both being decreased by a high density of flaws.

10.1.5   Minority Carrier Diffusion Length

The minority carrier diffusion length, L_e or L_h, is related to the minority carrier mobility, μ_e or μ_h, and the lifetime τ ($\tau^{-1} = \tau_r^{-1} + \tau_{nr}^{-1}$) by

$$L_{e,h} = [\tau\mu_{e,h}(e/kT)]^{1/2} \qquad (10.1.13)$$

Since τ may be limited by crystalline defects and contaminants the diffusion length is an important measure of the quality of the material for a given doping level. A convenient and direct method of measuring the diffusion length consists of measuring the current in a p–n junction as a function of the distance from a small region of minority carrier generation using either an electron beam or finely focused light beam [51–53] (Fig. 10.1.11). Because corrections have to be made for surface recombination and the depth and spread of the penetrating electron beam, the results are subject to some uncertainty. The diffusion length can also be deduced from photoyield experi-

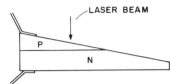
LASER BEAM

FIG. 10.1.11 Arrangement for the determination of the electron diffusion length by measuring the current through a p–n junction as a function of its distance from the locus of carrier generation using a laser beam.

TABLE 10.1.3
Minority Carrier Diffusion Length in LPE GaAs

Type	Dopant	Carrier concentration (cm^{-3})	Diffusion length (μm)	Ref.
p	Ge	5×10^{17}	6–7	a
p	Ge	6×10^{16}	20	b
p	Ge	2.0×10^{18}	10.5	b
p	Ge	8×10^{18}	2.5	c
p	Ge	1.1 ± 10^{19}	5.5	b
p	Si	Not stated	6–7	d
p	Zn	5×10^{18}	6	e
p	Si	7×10^{18}	~3	f
p	Si	5×10^{17}	~2–3.6	g
p	Zn	5×10^{16}	5	g
p	Cd	5×10^{16}	3	g
n	Sn	7×10^{17}–5×10^{18}	2.8–2.5	g
n	Undoped	5×10^{15}	5–11	g
n	Sn	5×10^{16}–10^{19}	8–1	h

[a] H. Schade, H. Nelson, and H. Kressel, *Appl. Phys. Lett.* **18**, 121 (1971).

[b] M. Ettenberg, H. Kressel, and S. L. Gilbert, *J. Appl. Phys.* **44**, 827 (1973).

[c] G. A. Acket, W. Nijman, and Ht. Lam, Jr., *Appl. Phys.* **45**, 3033 (1974).

[d] K. L. Ashley and F. H. Doerbeck, *J. Appl. Phys.* **42**, 4493 (1971).

[e] L. W. James, G. A. Antypas, J. Edgecumbe, R. L. Moon, and R. L. Bell, *J. Appl. Phys.* **42**, 2976 (1971).

[f] S. Garbe and G. Frank, *Proc. Int. Symp. on Gallium Arsenide, 3rd, London,* Inst. Phys. Phys. Soc. Conf. Ser. No. 9, p. 208 (1970).

[g] Zh. I. Alferov, V. M. Andreev, V. I. Murygin, and V. I. Strenin, *Sov Phys. Semicond.* **3**, 1234 (1970).

[h] H. C. Casey, Jr., B. I. Miller, and E. Pinkas, *J. Appl. Phys.* **44**, 1281 (1973).

ments using negative electron affinity surfaces [54]. We list in Table 10.1.3 the diffusion length values reported for LPE GaAs by various investigators. It is of interest that LPE materials appear to have longer diffusion lengths than GaAs prepared by other methods with the same carrier concentration, suggesting fewer unwanted recombination centers probably related to stoichiometric differences. For example, in p-type GaAs, the diffusion length reported for MG and VPE [55] material is generally below 3 μm.

10.2 Gallium Phosphide

The major interest in GaP has been centered on its use for red- and green-emitting electroluminescent diodes, and its incorporation in ternary or quaternary alloys. In this section we review some basic material properties, including ionization energies of impurities, distribution coefficients in solution growth, and transport properties.

TABLE 10.2.1
Impurity Ionization Energies in GaP

Type	Element	E_i (eV)	Ref.
Simple donors	S_P	0.104	[a]
	Se_P	0.102	[a]
	Te_P	0.090	[a]
	Si_{Ga}	0.082	[a]
	Sn_{Ga}	0.065	[b]
	O_P	0.896	[c]
	Ge_{Ga}	$\sim$0.3	[d]
Simple acceptors	C_{Ga}	0.041	[e]
	Co	0.41	[f]
	Cd_{Ga}	0.097	[a]
	Zn_{Ga}	0.064	[a]
	Mg_{Ga}	0.054	[g]
	Be_{Ga}	0.056	[h]
	Si_P	0.203	[a]
Isoelectronic traps	N	$\sim$0.008	[i]
	Bi	$\sim$0.038	[j]
	Zn–O	0.30	[k]
	Cd–O	0.40	[k]
	Mg–O	0.15	[l]

[a] P. J. Dean (unpublished) quoted by H. C. Casey, Jr. and F. A. Trumbore, *Mater. Sci. Eng.* **6**, 69 (1970).

[b] P. J. Dean, R. A. Faulkner, S. Kimura, and M. Ilegems, *Phys. Rev. B* **4**, 1926 (1971).

[c] P. J. Dean and C. H. Henry, *Phys. Rev.* **176**, 928 (1968).

[d] K. K. Shih, G. D. Pettit, and M. R. Lorenz, *J. Appl. Phys.* **39**, 1557 (1968). Rough approximation from Ge–Zn pair recombination spectra.

[e] D. B. Bortfeld, B. J. Curtis, and H. Meier, *J. Appl. Phys.* **43**, 1293 (1972).

[f] D. H. Loescher, J. W. Allen, and G. L. Pearson, *J. Phys. Soc. Jpn. Suppl.* **21**, 239 (1966).

[g] P. J. Dean, E. A. Schönherr, and R. B. Zetterstrom, *J. Appl. Phys.* **41**, 3475 (1970).

[h] E. G. Dierschke and G. L. Pearson, *J. Appl. Phys.* **41**, 321 (1970).

[i] R. A. Faulkner (unpublished), quoted in Ref. a.

[j] P. J. Dean, J. D. Cuthbert, and R. T. Lynch, *Phys. Rev.* **179**, 754 (1969).

[k] J. D. Cuthbert, C. H. Henry, and P. J. Dean, *Phys. Rev.* **170**, 739 (1968).

[l] R. N. Bhargava, C. Michel, W. L. Lupatkin, R. L. Bronner, and S. K. Kurtz, *Appl. Phys. Lett.* **20**, 227 (1972); P. J. Dean and M. Ilegems, *J. Luminescence* **4**, 201 (1971).

10.2.1   Major Dopants

Table 10.2.1 shows the ionization energies of the principal dopants in GaP. The values shown for the simple donors and acceptors were obtained by optical or Hall measurements of relatively pure samples. As is generally the case, the ionization energies decrease with increasing dopant concentration. This is illustrated in Fig. 10.2.1 in GaP:Te, where E_i decreases as the average spacing between the Te atoms [56]

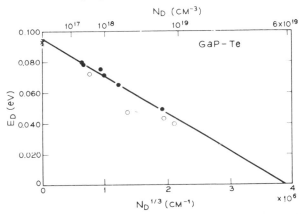

FIG. 10.2.1   Tellurium donor ionization energy in GaP plotted as a function of the donor concentration; $\times = E_D$ value deduced from luminescence spectra; ● = solution-grown crystals; ○ = vapor transport needles or blades [56].

$$E_D = E_D{}^0 - 2.3 \times 10^{-8} N_D{}^{1/3} \tag{10.2.1a}$$

Similarly for GaP:Zn [57]

$$E_A = E_A{}^0 - 3 \times 10^{-8}(N_A - N_D)^{1/3} \tag{10.2.1b}$$

Silicon and germanium are amphoteric dopants in GaP, but the material grown from Ga solutions is always n-type, indicating a predominance of donors. No evidence has yet been reported for the existence of an acceptor level due to Sn.

The trapping levels introduced by the isoelectronic centers are listed separately in Table 10.2.1. These traps [58] in GaP are of great technological importance since they determine the radiative efficiency of the material for red emission (Zn–O pair) and green emission (N) as described is Section 1.7.

Owing to the strong phonon–electron interaction and large effective electron mass ($m_c{}^* = 0.35\, m_0$) [59], the mobility in GaP is low compared to that in GaAs. Figure 10.2.2 shows μ_e at 300 K as a function of doping in n-type material prepared by VPE, solution growth, and LPE. No significant μ_e difference has been noted in GaP prepared by different techniques. The anal-

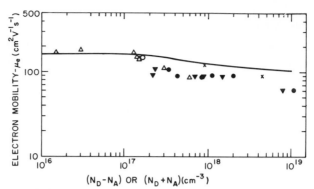

FIG. 10.2.2 Relationship between electron mobility in n-type GaP at 300 K and $N_D - N_A$ or $N_D + N_A$. The solid curve is the theoretical curve of μ_e vs. $(N_D + N_A)$ from Hara and Akasaki [60]. The experimental data are from the following sources: ○, Undoped solution-grown material $N_D - N_A$, from Plaskett *et al.* [61]. Solution-grown, Te-doped material: $N_D - N_A$, from Plaskett *et al.* [61]. Solution-grown, Te-doped material: ●, $(N_D - N_A)$; ▼, $(N_D + N_A)$, from Montgomery [56]. △, Sulfur- and selenium-doped-material prepared by VPE $(N_D - N_A)$, from Woods and Lorenz [62]. × Sulfur-doped material prepared by VPE, $(N_D + N_A)$, from Hara and Akasaki [60].

ysis of Epstein [63] indicates a maximum μ_e of 150–174 cm²/V-s at 300 K, and the calculations of Hara and Akasaki [60] show that μ_e is almost independent of the ionized impurity concentration up to $N_D + N_A \cong 10^{18}$ cm^{-3} because of the overwhelming effect of polar scattering compared to ionized impurity scattering. This is not true, of course, at low temperatures.

The most commonly used acceptor in GaP in Zn. Figure 10.2.3 shows the

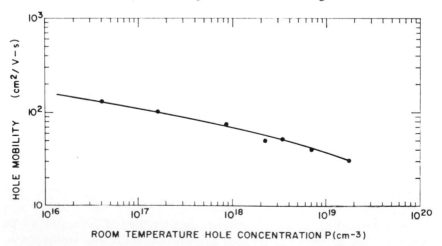

FIG. 10.2.3 The dependence of hole mobility at 300 K on hole concentration in GaP: Zn prepared by VPE [57].

dependence of the mobility at room temperature on the hole concentration. These values are applicable both to VPE and solution-grown material [57]. Note that μ_e and μ_h are quite comparable in GaP.

10.2.2 Impurity Incorporation by LPE

The distribution coefficients of S, Se, and Te have been determined by Trumbore et al. [24] in GaP grown from Ga solution at 1040°C. Figures 10.2.4–10.2.6 show that the donor concentration in the solid is a linear function of the concentration in the liquid when $N_D < 2 \times 10^{18}$ cm^{-3} (slope $m =$ 1), whereas $m = 1/2$ above this value. As discussed earlier (Section 10.1) the linear slope is consistent with the band bending model for impurity incorpora-

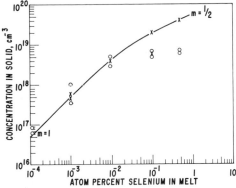

FIG. 10.2.4 Selenium and electron concentration in GaP as a function of the Se concentration in the Ga solution at a growth temperature of 1040°C: ×, Se concentration; ○, $(N_D - N_A)$ [24].

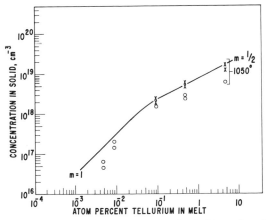

FIG. 10.2.5 Tellurium and electron concentration in GaP as a function of the Te concentration in the Ga solution at a growth temperature of 1040°C: ×, Te concentration; ○, $(N_D - N_A)$ [24].

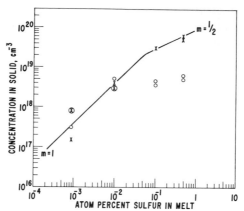

FIG. 10.2.6   Sulfur and electron concentration in GaP as a function of the concentration of sulfur in the Ga solution at a growth temperature of 1040°C: ×, S concentration; ○, $(N_D - N_A)$ [24].

tion. The deviation from linearity at high concentrations may be indicative of "wash out" of the band bending region when it becomes very thin and/or the formation of impurity complexes [64].

In the case of Zn-doped material, Fig. 10.2.7 [57] shows $m = 1/2$ over a significant range of doping values (similar to the behavior observed in GaAs). This is consistent with the fact that the Zn incorporation behavior is essentially ideal because of its high diffusion coefficient. Figure 10.2.7 also shows that the distribution coefficient for Zn should theoretically decrease with decreasing temperature, as is indeed the case experimentally (see the following text). On the other hand, the Te distribution coefficient increases with decreasing temperature. However, it is important to note that the distribution coefficient of volatile impurities is difficult to determine in the open flow growth systems commonly used in LPE because some of the dopant may be lost during growth or during the equilibration period prior to growth.

In view of the possible dependence of the distribution coefficient on the growth rate, it is not obvious that the observed temperature dependence in all cases reflects the incorporation of the impurity under equilibrium conditions. Sudlow *et al.* [66] have shown that the incorporation of Zn is not kinetically controlled because of its high diffusion coefficient, and hence is growth rate independent over a rather wide range. However, for S and Te, a strong effect of the crystal orientation on the incorporation of these dopants was noted. Sudlow *et al.* [66] suggested that only when growth occurs from stirred solutions at slow cooling rates is the true temperature dependence of the S and Te distribution coefficients observed.

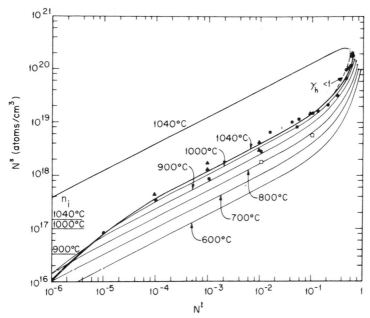

FIG. 10.2.7 Zn concentration in GaP versus the Zn concentration in the solution N^l along the 600, 700, 800, 900, 1000, and 1040°C liquidus isotherms [37]. All but the 1040°C curves are terminated at the approximate liquid compositions where Zn_3P_2, a secondary solid phase, appears. The experimental data are from Trumbore et al. [24] ▲, Panish and Casey [65] (●), and Chang and Pearson [39] (□).

It is difficult to grow very pure, uncompensated GaP by any technique. Typically, undoped LPE layers are n-type with $N_D - N_A \cong 10^{15}–10^{16}$ cm^{-3}. The most common residual impurities are S and Si. Using VPE, n-type layers with $N_D - N_A$ values in the 10^{15} cm^{-3} range with $\mu_e = 168–178$ cm^2/V-s have been obtained. The compensating acceptor density in these layers was found to be relatively low ($N_A = 1.28 - 7.8 \times 10^{14}$ cm^{-3}) [67].

10.3 Gallium Antimonide

Liquid phase epitaxy was used by Burns [68] to grow n-type GaSb from Ga solutions and p-type GaSb from Sn solutions (Sn is an acceptor in GaSb). Blom [69] studied the luminescent properties of GaSb p–n junctions and found that layers free from Ga inclusions could best be prepared by growing on the (111) Sb face of GaSb substrates. Two acceptor centers with $E_A = 25$

and 45 meV were found which were attributed to native defects; they are also present in GaSb grown from the melt [70].

10.4   Indium Arsenide

Indium arsenide LPE layers grown on InAs substrates from In solutions were used by Brown and Porteous [71] for the fabrication of laser diodes. The (100) and (111) As faces gave useful results but growth on the (110) face was poor because of poor wetting of the surface (at a growth temperature starting at 470°C). Growth on the (111) In face was also disappointing because of the formation of nonplanar junctions. With Sn as a dopant at a concentration of 10^{-2} wt % in the solution, the electron concentrations did not exceed 10^{18} cm^{-3}. With Te, however, the same concentration in the solution yielded $N_D - N_A \cong 10^{19}$ cm^{-3}. In p-type material, $N_A - N_D \approx 10^{19}$ cm^{-3} was obtained with 0.03 wt % Zn concentration in the solution. It should be noted that pre-cipitates may appear in n-type MG InAs:Te at concentrations in excess of 3×10^{19} cm^{-3} [72]. Similar precipitation is very probable in LPE material as well.

Indium arsenide layers have been grown on the (111) As face of InAs sub-strates from undoped In solutions between 600 and 570°C. These n-type layers have electron concentrations of $\sim 10^{16}$ cm^{-3} and room temperature mobility values of 32,000 cm^2/V-s [73], comparable to values obtained by VPE [74,75].

10.5   Indium Phosphide

Studies have been reported of spontaneously generated platelets of InP formed by slowly cooling InP–In solutions from 850°C, [74,77], and data have been obtained which should be applicable to LPE materials. Undoped InP platelets ($N_D - N_A \approx 10^{16}$ cm^{-3}), like VPE layers [75], have μ_e values at 300 K as high as 4450 cm^2/V-s [76] whereas Te-doped materials with elec-tron concentrations between 10^{17} and 10^{19} cm^{-3} have mobilities between 300 and 1000 cm^2/V-s. Similar mobility values were reported for LPE InP layers doped with Sn and Te [78], as shown in Fig. 10.5.1. InP:Ge was found to be compensated n-type, with corresponding lower mobilities (Fig. 10.5.1). The following impurity distribution coefficient values were determined in the 650–600°C range for growth on the (111) P plane of InP substrates: $k_{Sn} = 0.0022$, $k_{Te} = 0.4$, and $k_{Ge} = 0.011$ [78].

The luminescent properties of these materials were studied, particularly at low temperatures, and various near-bandgap radiative transitions identi-fied. The Te donor ionization energy was found to be 8 meV [76] and the Si acceptor ionization energy was deduced to be ≈ 31 meV. The ionization

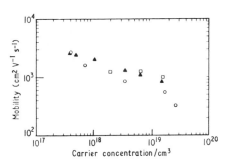

FIG. 10.5.1   Variation of mobility at 300 K with carrier concentration in LPE layers of InP doped with ▲, Sn; ○, Ge; and □, Te [78].

energies of Zn and Cd were calculated to be 47.6 and 56.1 meV, respectively [79].

10.6   Aluminum Arsenide and Aluminum Phosphide

Both AlAs and AlP are hygroscopic, and the data available concerning their properties are mostly from absorption [80] and refractive index studies [81]. Single crystals of n-type ($N = 3 \times 10^{17}$ cm^{-3}) AlAs have been prepared by VPE with mobilities as high as 280 cm^2/V-s [82]. Silicon is the dominant residual donor ($E_D \cong 0.07$ eV) [83]. The preparation of n-type AlP has been accomplished by vapor phase epitaxy [84] as well as by solution growth [85]. In the latter technique, an Al-rich AlP solution was used enclosed in a sealed tube with a graphite crucible. The platelets were obtained by slow cooling from 1350°C. The growth platelets could be stored in xylene. In a normal atmosphere, however, the crystals decompose into Al_2O_3:H_2O and phosphine (PH$_3$).

REFERENCES

1. J. S. Harris, Y. Nannichi, G. L. Pearson, and G. F. Day, *J. Appl. Phys.* **40**, 4575 (1969).
2. R. M. Logan and D. T. J. Hurle, *J. Phys. Chem. Solids* **32**, 1739 (1971).
3. H. Rupprecht, J. M. Woodall, K. Konnerth, and D. G. Pettit, *Appl. Phys. Lett.* **9**, 221 (1966).
4. F. A. Kröger, "The Chemistry of Imperfect Crystals." North-Holland Pub., Amsterdam, 1964.
5. E. Munoz, W. L. Snyder, and J. L. Moll, *Appl. Phys. Lett.* **16**, 262 (1970).
6. H. Kressel, F. Z. Hawrylo, and P. LeFur, *J. Appl. Phys.* **39**, 4059 (1968).
7. E. W. Williams, *Solid State Commun.* **4**, 585 (1966).
8. D. E. Hill, *Phys. Rev.* **133**, A866 (1964).
9. H. Kressel, *J. Appl. Phys.* **38**, 4383 (1967).
10. F. E. Rosztoczy, F. Ermanis, I. Hayashi, and B. Schwartz, *J. Appl. Phys.* **41**, 264 (1970).

11. E. W. Williams and L. T. Elliott, *Brit. J. Appl. Phys.* (*D*) **2**, 1657 (1969).
12. E. W. Williams and D. M. Blacknall, *Trans. AIME* **239**, 387 (1967).
13. R. Romano-Moran and K. L. Ashley, *J. Appl. Phys.* **43**, 1301 (1972).
14. J. Vilms and J. P. Garrett, *Solid State Electron.* **15**, 443 (1972).
15. H. Kressel, H. Nelson, and F. Z. Hawrylo, *J. Appl. Phys.* **39**, 5647 (1968).
16. W. Schairer and E. Grobe, *Solid State Commun.* **8**, 2017 (1970).
17. F. E. Rosztoczy and K. B. Wolfstirn, *J. Appl. Phys.* **42**, 426 (1971).
18. H. C. Casey, Jr., B. I. Miller, and E. Pinkas, *J. Appl. Phys.* **44**, 1281 (1973).
19. H. Kressel and H. von Philipsborn, *J. Appl. Phys.* **41**, 2244 (1970).
20. H. Kressel, J. U. Dunse, H. Nelson, and F. Z. Hawrylo, *J. Appl. Phys.* **39**, 2006 (1968).
21. W. G. Spitzer and M. B. Panish, *J. Appl. Phys.* **40**, 4200 (1969).
22. H. Kressel, M. S. Abrahams, F. Z. Hawrylo, and C. J. Buiocchi, *J. Appl. Phys.* **39**, 5139 (1968).
23. L. J. Vieland and I. Kudman, *J. Phys. Chem. Solids* **24**, 437 (1963).
24. F. A. Trumbore, H. G. White, M. Kowalchik, R. A. Logan, and C. L. Luke, *J. Electrochem. Soc.* **112**, 782 (1965).
25. U. Merten and A. P. Hatcher, *J. Phys. Chem. Solids* **23**, 533 (1962).
26. K. H. Zschauer and A. Vogel, *Proc. Int. Symp. Gallium Arsenide,* *3rd* Inst. Phys., Phys. Soc. Conf., Ser. No. 9, p. 100 (1970).
27. H. C. Casey, Jr., M. B. Panish, and K. B. Wolfstirn, *J. Phys. Chem. Solids* **32**, 571 (1971).
28. These values are tentative since the condition of the interface plays an important role in the barrier height.
29. D. Kahng, *Bell Syst. Tech. J.* **43**, 215 (1964).
30. O. Madelung, "Physics of III–V Compounds." Wiley, New York, 1964.
31. H. Beneking and W. Vits, *Proc. Int. Symp. on Gallium Arsenide,* *2nd.* Inst. Phys., Phys. Soc. Conf., Ser. No. 7, p. 96 (1968).
32. C. S. Kang and P. D. Greene, *Proc. Inst. Symp. on Gallium Arsenide,* *2nd* Inst. Phys., Phys. Soc. Conf., Ser. No. 7, p. 18 (1968).
33. H. G. B. Hicks and P. D. Greene, *Proc. Int. Symp. Gallium Arsenide,* *3rd* Inst. Phys., Phys. Soc. Conf., Ser. No. 9, p. 92 (1970).
34. H. Kressel and H. Nelson, *J. Appl. Phys.* **40**, 3720 (1969).
35. B. H. Ahn, R. R. Shurtz, and C. W. Trussell, *J. Appl. Phys.* **42**, 4512 (1971).
36. M. B. Panish and H. C. Casey, Jr., *J. Phys. Chem. Solids* **28**, 1673 (1967). ,
37. A. S. Jordan, *J. Electrochem. Soc.* **119**, 123 (1972).
38. H. C. Casey, Jr., M. B. Panish, and L. L. Chang, *Phys. Rev.* **162**, 660 (1967).
39. L. L. Chang and G. L. Pearson, *J. Phys. Chem. Solids* **25**, 23 (1964).
40. P. D. Greene, *Solid State Commun.* **9**, 1299 (1971).
41. Zh. I. Alferov, D. Z. Garbuzov, E. P. Morozov, and D. N. Tretyakov, *Sov. Phys. Semicond.* **3**, 600 (1969).
42. E. W. Williams and H. B. Bebb, Photoluminescence II: GaAs, *in* "Semiconductors and Semimetals" (R. K. Willardson and A. C. Beer, eds.), Vol. 8, p. 321. Academic Press, New York, 1972.
43. H. J. Queisser and M. B. Panish, *J. Phys. Chem. Solids* **28**, 1177 (1967).
44. H. Kressel and M. Ettenberg, *Appl. Phys. Lett.* **23**, 511 (1973).
45. K. H. Zschauer, *Solid State Commun.* **7**, 1709 (1969).
46. L. R. Weisberg, *J. Appl. Phys.* **39**, 5149 (1968).
47. M. S. Abrahams, Private communication, (1970).
48. M. B. Panish, *J. Phys. Chem. Solids* **29**, 409 (1968).

49. M. B. Panish, H. J. Queisser, L. Derick, and S. Sumski, *Solid State Electron.* **9**, 311 (1966).
50. C. J. Hwang, *J. Appl. Phys.* **40**, 1983 (1969).
51. See, for example, C. J. Hwang, S. E. Haszko, and A. A. Bergh, *J. Appl. Phys.* **42**, 5117 (1971).
52. K. Maeda, A. Kasami, M. Toyama, and N. Wakamatsu, *Jpn. J. Appl. Phys.* **8**, 65 (1969).
53. K. L. Ashley and J. R. Biard, *IEEE Trans. Electron. Dev.* **14**, 429 (1967).
54. H. Schade, H. Nelson, and H. Kressel, *Appl. Phys. Lett.* **18**, 121 (1971).
55. T. S. Rao-Sahib and D. B. Wittry, *J. Appl. Phys.* **40**, 3745 (1969), and references cited therein.
56. H. C. Montgomery, *J. Appl. Phys.* **39**, 2002 (1968).
57. H. C. Casey, Jr., F. Ermanis, and K. B. Wolfstirn, *J. Appl. Phys.* **40**, 2945 (1969).
58. A review is given by W. Czaja, Isoelectronic impurities in semiconductors, *Festkorperproblema* **XI**, 65 (1971).
59. M. Hashimoto and I. Akasaki, *Phys. Lett.* **25A**, 38 (1967).
60. T. Hara and I. Akasaki, *J. Appl. Phys.* **39**, 285 (1968).
61. T. S. Plaskett, S. E. Blum, and L. M. Foster, *J. Electrochem. Soc.* **114**, 1303 (1967).
62. J. F. Woods and M. R. Lorenz, *J. Appl. Phys.* **39**, 5404 (1968).
63. A. S. Epstein, *J. Phys. Chem. Solids* **27**, 1611 (1966).
64. H. Kressel and I. Ladany, *Solid State Electron.* **11**, 647 (1968).
65. M. B. Panish and H. C. Casey, Jr., *J. Phys. Chem. Solids* **29**, 1719 (1968).
66. P. D. Sudlow, A. Mottram, and A. R. Peaker, *J. Mater. Sci.* **7**, 168 (1972).
67. M. G. Craford, W. O. Groves, A. H. Herzog, and D. E. Hill, *J. Appl. Phys.* **42**, 2751 (1971).
68. J. W. Burns, *Trans. AIME* **242**, 432 (1968).
69. G. M. Blom, *J. Appl. Phys.* **42**, 1057 (1971).
70. R. D. Baxter, F. J. Reid, and A. C. Beer, *Phys. Rev.* **162**, 718 (1967).
71. M. A. C. S. Brown and P. Porteous, *Brit. J. Appl. Phys.* **18**, 1527 (1967).
72. B. P. Kotrubenko and V. N. Lange, *Sov. Phys.-Semicond.* **4**, 521 (1970).
73. V. L. Dalal and W. Hicinbothem (unpublished).
74. J. J. Tietjen, H. P. Maruska, and R. B. Clough, *J. Electrochem. Soc.* **116**, 492 (1969).
75. M. C. Hales, J. R. Knight, and C. W. Wilkins, *Proc. Int. Symp. Gallium Arsenide, 3rd.* Inst. Phys., Phys. Soc. Conf., Ser. No. 9, p. 50 (1970).
76. U. Heim, O. Roder, H. G. Queisser, and M. Pilkuhn, *J. Luminescence* **1,2**, 542 (1970).
77. O. Röder, U. Heim, and M. H. Pilkuhn, *J. Phys. Chem. Solids* **31**, 2625 (1970).
78. F. E. Rosztoczy, G. A. Antypas, and C. J. Casan, *Proc. Int. Symp. Gallium Arsenide, 3rd* Inst. Phys., Phys. Soc. Conf., Ser. No. 9, p. 86 (1970).
79. A. M. White, P. J. Dean, K. M. Fairhurst, W. Bardsley, E. W. Williams, and B. Day, *Solid State Commun.* **11**, 1099 (1872).
80. M. R. Lorenz, R. J. Chicotka, G. D. Pettit, and P. J. Dean, *Solid State Commun.* **8**, 693 (1970).
81. H. G. Grimmeiss and B. Monemar, *Phys. Status Solidi (a)* **5**, 109 (1971).
82. M. Ettenberg, A. G. Sigai, S. Gilbert, and A. Dreeben, *J. Electrochem. Soc.* **118**, 1355 (1971).
83. H. Kressel, F. H. Nicoll, M. Ettenberg, W. M. Yim, and A. G. Sigai, *Solid State Commun.* **8**, 1407 (1970).
84. D. Richman, *J. Electrochem. Soc.* **115**, 945 (1968).
85. H. Sonomura and T. Miyanchi, *Jpn. J. Appl. Phys.* **8**, 1263 (1969).

Chapter 11

Ternary and Quaternary III–V Compounds

11.1 General Considerations

Table 9.4.1 shows some key properties of interest in the growth of the 18 ternary alloys consisting of combinations of GaAs, GaP, GaSb, InSb, InAs, InP, AlAs, AlP, and AlSb. Only some of these ternaries are useful for a particular application since the same parameters can sometimes be obtained with more than one ternary system. For example, In(AsP) and (InGa)As are very similar except that the lattice parameter mismatch between the two end binaries is smaller in In(AsP) than in (InGa)As. This makes In(AsP) potentially more desirable in some applications. Figure 11.1.1 contains the lattice parameter versus E_g of various compounds and shows the wide variations possible.

The bandgap energy is generally not a linear function of the composition in alloys. It has been found empirically [1] that the bandgap energy $E_g(x)$ of a ternary compound varies with composition x as follows:

$$E_g(x) = E_{g1} + bx + cx^2 \tag{11.1.1}$$

where E_{g1} is the bandgap energy of the lower bandgap binary and b and c are constants with $E_{g2} = E_{g1} + b + c$; E_{g2} is the bandgap energy of the higher bandgap binary.

Table 11.1.1 lists the $E_g(x)$ values experimentally determined for a number of the better known ternary systems where the bandgap transition remains direct throughout. Figures 11.1.2–11.1.10 show the bandgap energy as a function of composition of various ternary alloys. It has long been assumed

357

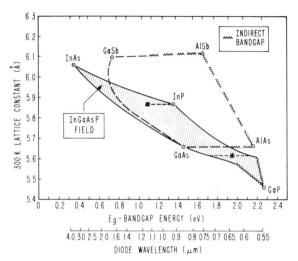

FIG. 11.1.1 Lattice constant versus bandgap energy and diode emission wavelength at room temperature. The shaded region encompasses an important quaternary alloy, InGaAsP, which is seen to encompass a broad bandgap energy and lattice constant range. A lattice-matched heterojunction configuration is obtained by choosing a lattice constant and two material compositions with different bandgap energies. For illustration, we show a lattice-matched heterojunction to InP ($E_g = 1.34$ eV) with (■) $In_{0.8}Ga_{0.2}As_{0.35}P_{0.65}$ ($E_g \cong$ 1.1 eV), and (∗) one matched to $In_{0.34}Ga_{0.66}P$ ($E_g \cong 2.17$ eV) with $In_{0.3}Ga_{0.7}As_{0.1}P_{0.9}$ ($E_g \cong 1.95$ eV). [This structure can be grown on Ga(AsP)].

TABLE 11.1.1

300 K Bandgap Variation for Several Ternary Alloys with Direct Gaps Throughout

Ternary	$E_g(x)$ (eV)	Ref.
$In_{1-x}Ga_xAs$	$0.35 + 0.63x + 0.45x^2$	a
$InAs_{1-x}Sb_x$	$0.35 - 0.771x + 0.596x^2$	b
$InAs_{1-x}P_x$	$0.35 + 0.891x + 0.101x^2$	c
$GaAs_xSb_{1-x}$	$0.725 - 0.32x + (1.005)x^2$	d

[a] Empirical fit to data (Fig. 11.1.3) with Eq. (11.1.1).
[b] G. B. Stringfellow and P. E. Greene, *J. Electrochem. Soc.* **118**, 805 (1971).
[c] G. A. Antypas and T. O. Yep, *J. Appl. Phys.* **42**, 3201 (1971).
[d] G. A. Antypas and L. W. James, *J. Appl. Phys.* **41**, 2165 (1970).

that the X minima in GaAs are *below* the L minima, with $E_{gX} \cong 1.81$–1.86 eV, but more recent work [2] indicates that the X minima are *higher* than the L minima by 0.1 to 0.2 eV, which places E_{gL} near 1.7 eV. Figure 11.1.6 shows for (AlGa)As the estimated E_{gL} variation assuming that E_{gL} in AlAs is $\sim$ 2.4 eV. Note that the crossover from a direct to indirect bandgap in (AlGa)As and Ga(AsP) is unchanged because the X minima are lower than the L minima in AlAs and GaP.

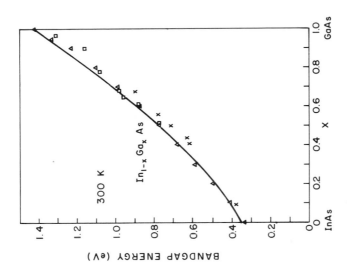

FIG. 11.1.3   The bandgap energy as a function of composition for $In_{1-x}Ga_xAs$ as determined by different investigations: $\triangle$, Wu and Pearson [3]. $\square$, Woolley et al. [4]; and $\times$, Hockings et al. [5].

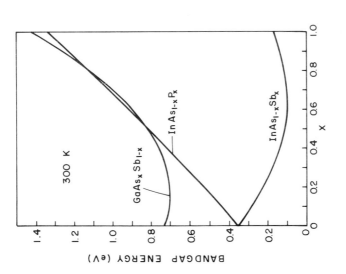

FIG. 11.1.2   The bandgap energy as a function of composition for GaAs–GaSb, InAs–InP, InAs–InSb, and GaSb–InSb. The curves are plotted from the equations in Table 11.1.1.

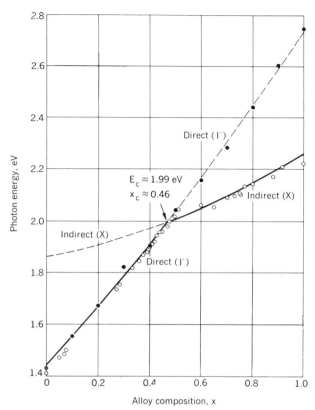

FIG. 11.1.4   Direct and indirect conduction band minima at 300 K for $GaAs_{1-x}P_x$ as a function of x: ●, Electroreflectance data [6]; ○, electroluminescence data [7]. The L conduction band minima are not shown. In GaAs, $E_{gL} \approx 1.7$ eV, and $E_{gX} = E_{gL}$ at $x \cong 0.3$.

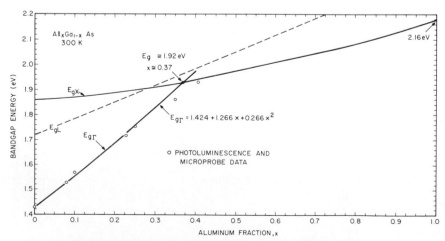

FIG. 11.1.5   Direct bandgap energy of $Al_xGa_{1-x}As$ as determined by (○) microprobe measurements and photoluminescence (I. Ladany and H. Kressel, unpublished). These values agree with those deduced from electroreflectance data [8].

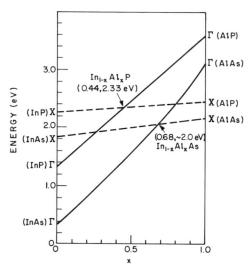

FIG. 11.1.6 The 300 K bandgap energy as a function of composition for alloys of InP–AlP and InAs–AlAs. The compositions where the crossover from direct to indirect bandgap occurs are indicated [9].

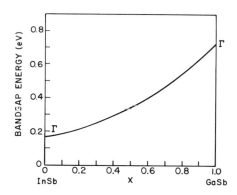

FIG. 11.1.7 Bandgap energy of $Ga_xIn_{1-x}Sb$ versus x at 300 K [10].

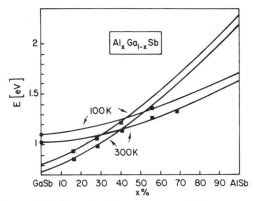

FIG. 11.1.8 Direct and indirect bandgap energy variation with composition. Experimental points: ■, Mathieu *et al.* [11]; ●, Kosichi *et al.* [12].

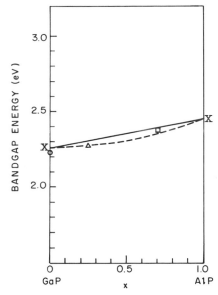

FIG. 11.1.9 The 300 K bandgap energy as a function of composition for $Al_xGa_{1-x}P$ at 300 K. The experimental electroluminescence data are from (△) Kressel and Ladany [13] and (□) Chicokta *et al.* [14]; (○) A-line GaP.

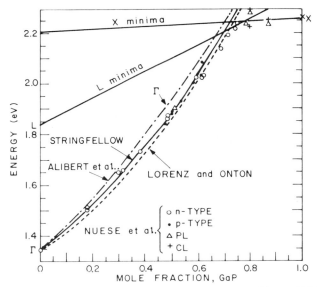

FIG. 11.1.10 Variation of the bandgap energy of $In_{1-x}Ga_xP$ with x at 300 K as deduced from various measurements. The curve of Alibert *et al.* [15], is deduced from electro-reflectance data. The other data are based on electroluminescence, photoluminescence (PL), or cathaodoluminescence (CL). Data from Lorenz and Onton [16], Stringfellow [17], and Nuese *et al.* [18]. The variation of the X and L minima are based on Pitt *et al.* [19].

We show in Fig. 11.1.11 the variation of the lattice parameter of several ternaries as a function of composition. Vegard's law is quite well obeyed in all the III–V ternary alloys discussed here. The thermal coefficient of expansion is also important and values are given in Table 9.4.2 for binaries. In the case of ternaries, the thermal coefficient of expansion varies quite linearly with composition as shown in Fig. 11.1.12 for (InGa)P [20].

11.2 Phase Diagrams—Introduction

In LPE growth of ternary compound films, it is obviously desirable to be able to predict theoretically the dependence of the ternary crystal composition on the liquid composition at various temperatures on the basis of limited experimental data. In principle, this is possible, and much work has been reported concerning the phase diagrams of various III–V compound ternary alloys. Although a full discussion of these results is beyond the scope of this chapter, we will review the major considerations and problems which enter into the phase diagram calculations. As will become evident in this summary, practical phase diagrams can be formulated, but "first principle" calculations

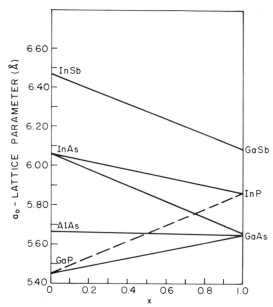

FIG. 11.1.11   Lattice parameter at 300 K as a function of composition for several III–V materials.

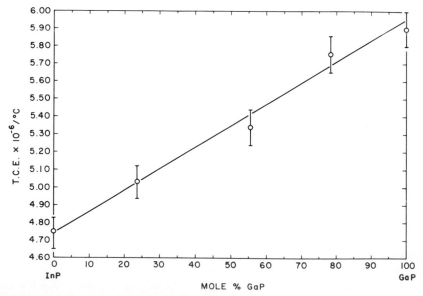

FIG. 11.1.12   Thermal coefficient of expansion of $In_xGa_{1-x}P$ as a function of x. Note the linear relationship [20].

rarely yield useful results. Thus, a great deal of experimental data are required for the majority of systems to make up for the fact that most solutions are far from ideal.

We begin by formulating general relationships in which no assumptions are made concerning the nature of the solutions [21,22]. Consider A, B, and C which combine to form compounds (AC) and (BC), independently, and the ternary $(AC)_{1-x}(BC)_x$. The chemical potential of each constituent at temperature T in the *liquid* solution (superscript l) is given by

$$\mu_A{}^l(T) = \mu_A^{0l} + RT \ln \gamma_A N_A{}^l, \qquad \mu_B{}^l(T) = \mu_B^{0l} + RT \ln \gamma_B N_B{}^l$$
$$\mu_C{}^l(T) = \mu_C^{0l} + RT \ln \gamma_C N_C{}^l, \qquad N_A{}^l + N_B{}^l + N_C{}^l = 1 \qquad (11.2.1)$$

where γ_i is the activity coefficient of element i in the solution. In the *solid* solution (superscript s),

$$\mu_{AC}^s(T) = \mu_{AC}^{0s}(T) + RT \ln[\gamma_{AC}(1 - x)],$$
$$\mu_{BC}^s(T) = \mu_{BC}^{0s}(T) + RT \ln(\gamma_{BC} x) \qquad (11.2.2)$$

$N_A{}^l$, $N_B{}^l$, and $N_C{}^l$ denote the atomic fractions of A, B, and C in the liquid, respectively, and 0 in the superscript denotes the pure (or unmixed) state of the constituent in question.

At the growth temperature T the chemical potential equalities are

$$\mu_{AC}^s(T) = \mu_A{}^l(T) + \mu_C{}^l(T), \qquad \mu_{BC}^s(T) = \mu_B{}^l(T) + \mu_C{}^l(T) \qquad (11.2.3)$$

Combining Eqs. (11.2.1), (11.2.2), and (11.2.3), we obtain

$$RT \ln[\gamma_{AC}(1 - x)] = \mu_A^{0l}(T) + \mu_C^{0l}(T) + RT \ln(\gamma_A \gamma_C N_A{}^l N_C{}^l)$$
$$RT \ln(\gamma_{BC} x) = \mu_B^{0l}(T) + \mu_C^{0l}(T) - \mu_{BC}^{0s} + RT \ln(\gamma_B \gamma_C N_B{}^l N_C{}^l) \qquad (11.2.4)$$

Using an analysis by Vieland [23], $\mu_i^{0l}(T)$ and $\mu_i^{0s}(T)$ can be related to binary information as follows:

$$\mu_{AC}^{0s}(T) = \mu_A^{Sl}(T) + \mu_C^{Sl}(T) - \Delta S_{AC}^F(T_{AC}^m - T)$$
$$\mu_{BC}^{0s}(T) = \mu_B^{Sl}(T) + \mu_C^{Sl}(T) - \Delta S_{BC}^F(T_{BC}^m - T) \qquad (11.2.5)$$

where T_{AC}^m and T_{BC}^m are the melting points of (AC) and (BC), respectively; S_{AC}^F and S_{BC}^F are the entropy of formation of AC and BC, respectively; and the superscript Sl denotes the stoichiometric liquids ($N_A{}^l = N_C{}^l = \frac{1}{2}$ and $N_B{}^l = N_C{}^l = \frac{1}{2}$). Equations (11.2.5.) neglect small terms including the specific heat differences between liquid and solid at T.

From Eq. (11.2.1) it follows that

$$\mu_A^{Sl}(T) = \mu_A^{0l}(T) + RT \ln(\gamma_A^{Sl}/2)$$
$$\mu_B^{Sl}(T) = \mu_B^{0l}(T) + RT \ln(\gamma_B^{Sl}/2) \qquad (11.2.6)$$
$$\mu_C^{Sl}(T) = \mu_C^{0l}(T) + RT \ln(\gamma_C^{Sl}/2)$$

Substituting Eqs. (11.2.6) into Eqs. (11.2.5),

$$\mu_{AC}^{0s}(T) = \mu_A^{0l}(T) + \mu_C^{0l}(T) + RT \ln(\gamma_A^{Sl}\gamma_C^{Sl}/4) - \Delta S_{AC}^F(T_{AC}^m - T)$$
$$\mu_{BC}^{0s}(T) = \mu_B^{0l}(T) + \mu_C^{0l}(T) + RT \ln(\gamma_B^{Sl}\gamma_C^{Sl}/4) - \Delta S_{BC}^F(T_{AC}^m - T)$$

(11.2.7)

Combining Eqs. (11.2.4) and (11.2.7)

$$\gamma_{AC}(1 - x) = \left[\left(\frac{4\gamma_A\gamma_C}{\gamma_A^{Sl}\gamma_C^{Sl}}\right)N_A{}^lN_C{}^l\right]\left[\exp\frac{\Delta S_{AC}^F}{RT}(T_{AC}^m - T)\right]$$

$$\gamma_{BC}x = \left[\left(\frac{\gamma_B\gamma_C}{\gamma_B^{Sl}\gamma_C^{Sl}}\right)N_B{}^lN_C{}^l\right]\left[\exp\frac{\Delta S_{BC}^F}{RT}(T_{BC}^m - T)\right]$$

(11.2.8)

Equations (11.2.8) define the basic relationship between the composition of the solid and that of the liquid. Of the terms involved, ΔS_{AC}^F, ΔS_{BC}^F, T_{AC}^m, and T_{BC}^m can be measured; values for many III–V compounds are available, although the accuracy of the entropy data is frequently uncertain [24]. The real problem is the determination of the activity coefficients in the liquid and the solid. Of course, in ideal solutions the activity coefficient is unity and matters are simple. But this is not the case when the constituents of the solutions interact.

Three methods have been used to estimate the activity coefficients in the ternary solutions of III–V compounds. We discuss first the *quasi-regular* solution approximation [22,25]. Considering first a binary solution of A and C, the activity coefficients are defined in terms of a temperature-dependent interaction coefficient α_{AC},

$$RT \ln \gamma_A = \alpha_{AC}N_C^{l2}, \qquad RT \ln \gamma_C = \alpha_{AC}N_A^{l2} \qquad (11.2.9)$$

and similarly for a solution of B and C. To determine experimentally α_{AC} and α_{BC}, the following equation derived by Vieland [23] is used which follows from Eqs. (11.2.8) when $\gamma_{AC}(1 - x) = 1$, as appropriate to a binary solution:

$$\alpha_{AC} = \frac{-RT}{2(0.5 - N_A{}^l)^2}\left[\ln 4N_A{}^l(1 - N_A{}^l) + \frac{\Delta S_{AC}^F}{RT}(T_{AC}^m - T)\right] \quad (11.2.10)$$

and similarly for BC.

Values of α_{AC} and α_{BC} are deduced as a function of temperature from experimental data of the liquidus curves of (AC) and (BC) solutions in a solvent of the type shown in Fig. 9.1.4 [23,26]. It turns out that for many of the III–V binary solutions the interaction coefficient is of the form

$$\alpha_{AC} = -(const)T + const \qquad (11.2.11)$$

Thus, γ_A and γ_C can be computed as a function of temperature and solution composition. The term quasi-regular solution model is used because this analysis is not appropriate to a regular solution, which by definition has a temperature-independent and concentration-independent interaction coefficient which follows from the assumption that the atoms are randomly distributed.

Having determined the empirical activity coefficients in the binary liquid solutions it now remains to determine those in the ternary solution. One approach [21,25] is to use the relations [27]

$$RT \ln \gamma_A = \alpha_{AC} N_C'^2 + \alpha_{AB} N_B'^2 + (\alpha_{AC} + \alpha_{AB} - \alpha_{BC}) N_B' N_C'$$

$$RT \ln \gamma_B = \alpha_{BC} N_C'^2 + \alpha_{AB} N_A'^2 + (\alpha_{BC} + \alpha_{AB} - \alpha_{AC}) N_A' N_C' \qquad (11.2.12)$$

$$RT \ln \gamma_C = \alpha_{AC} N_A'^2 + \alpha_{BC} N_B'^2 + (\alpha_{AC} + \alpha_{BC} - \alpha_{AB}) N_A' N_B'$$

The right-hand side of Eqs. (11.2.8) is now fully defined in terms of interaction parameters determined from binary solutions which, in principle, is a great convenience in predicting the properties of the ternary phase diagram. The remaining difficulty lies in determining the activity coefficients γ_{AC} and γ_{BC} of (AC) and (BC), respectively, in the *solid ternary* solution. The simplest assumption consists of an expression similar to those for the activity coefficient in the liquid;

$$RT \ln \gamma_{AC} = \beta x^2, \qquad RT \ln \gamma_{BC} = \beta(1 - x)^2 \qquad (11.2.13)$$

where β is an interaction coefficient that must be empirically determined by an analysis of experimental ternary alloy data.

A second method of describing the ternary liquid solution activity coefficients [28] uses the formalism of Darken [29]. Although more satisfying from the consistency point of view than the quasi-regular solution representation, the additional term in the definition of the activity coefficient does not materially affect Eqs. (11.2.8). Thus, the calculated phase diagram with this formalism does not differ from that obtained using the quasi-regular model [30].

The third method of determining the activity coefficients is the "quasi-chemical" method [21] based on an analysis by Guggenheim [31]. Here, the interaction coefficients in the liquid and solid solutions are calculated on the basis of assumed interaction energies between the different nearest neighbor atoms. For a solution of A and C, for example,

$$\alpha'_{AC} = Z[E_{AC} - \tfrac{1}{2}(E_{AA} + E_{CC})] \qquad (11.2.14)$$

when E_{ij} represents the interaction energy of an ij nearest neighbor pair and Z is the number of nearest neighbors to each atom.

The ternary solution activity coefficient calculation by this method is rather complex, but to illustrate the technique we simply consider the expressions for γ_A and γ_C in a binary solution [21]:

$$\gamma_A = \left(\frac{z - 1 + 2N_A'}{N_A'(z + 1)} \right)^{z/2}, \qquad \gamma_C = \left(\frac{z + 1 - 2N_A'}{(1 - N_A')(z + 1)} \right)^{z/2} \qquad (11.2.15)$$

Here,

$$z = [1 + 4N_A{}^l(1 - N_A{}^l)][(\exp \alpha'_{AC}/ZRT) - 1]^{1/2}$$

Although the quasi-chemical analysis does represent an attempt to deal with the fundamental interaction between atoms, it does not avoid the need to calculate the interaction coefficients empirically since the interaction energy in (11.2.15) cannot be accurately calculated from first principles. Thus, in the final analysis, one must generally resort to empirical curve fitting to obtain the activity coefficients. This is not to say, however, that the various parameters do not fit an overall pattern. An analysis by Stringfellow [32] is of interest in this regard. Starting with the melting temperature and entropy of fusion of the pure III–V compounds and the electronegativity, molar volume, and energy of sublimation of the constituent elements, he deduced parameters from which a phase diagram can be calculated. Although such a calculated diagram is unlikely to be accurate, it does provide a starting point for the synthesis of a given ternary alloy.

Before proceeding with a review of experimental results in a number of systems, some general observations are in order.

1.   It is evident from the number of adjustable parameters in these equations that any set of reasonably consistent ternary data can be fitted to curves representing these equations. Thus, such curve fitting does not prove the fundamental validity of the assumptions made concerning the nonideal behavior of the solid and liquid. Nevertheless, the curves obtained constitute useful aids in LPE if the adjustable parameters used fit a useful range of solution concentrations and temperatures. This is fortunately the case for a number of the systems discussed herein.

2.   If the interaction parameters do strongly depend on the composition of the liquid and solid solutions, any generalizations based on limited data would be hopeless. However, Foster and Woods [33] have concluded from an analysis of the available data for InSb–GaSb, InAs–GaAs, and InP–GaP that although the interaction coefficients do depend on the concentration to varying degrees, the variations need not be excessive.

3.   The degree of deviation from ideality of the solutions is related to the excess free energy of solution formation. Foster and Woods [33] have shown that the excess free energy of formation of $(AC)_{1-x}(BC)_x$ increases with increasing lattice parameter difference between (AC) and (BC). This is reasonable since the lattice strain is increased. For this reason, the construction of reliable phase diagrams on the basis of limited experimental data is simplified when, as in the case of GaAs–AlAs or AlP–GaP, the lattice parameter difference is very small.

4.   Experimental data used to construct phase diagrams are generally obtained under equilibrium growth conditions. However, in LPE growth,

which may be quite fast, the composition of the solution adjacent to the solid being formed may change because of the depletion of a constituent with a high distribution coefficient, or the loss of a constituent by oxidation or evaporation in open systems. Thus, great care must be exercised in using phase diagram data to predict crystal compositions quantitatively.

5.   In the formation of a ternary compound (AB)C, the relative values of the distribution coefficient of A and B will depend on the difference in the energy of formation of AC and BC, which is reflected in the relative values of the melting temperatures of AC and BC. Thus, in the growth of (AlGa)As, for example, the distribution coefficient of Al is much greater than that of Ga since $T_{AlAs}^m > T_{GaAs}^m$. Similarly, in the growth of (InGa)As, the distribution coefficient of Ga is much greater than that of In since $T_{GaAs}^m > T_{InAs}^m$. Therefore, the greater the difference in T^m of the two endpoint binaries, the more difficult it is to control the concentration of the ternary alloy accurately.

11.3   Principal Ternary Alloys

11.3.1   AlAs–GaAs

Because of the small lattice parameter difference between AlAs and GaAs, their ternary solutions are the closest in the III–V systems to being ideal and the alloys are among the easiest to prepare by LPE, as first shown by Rupprecht *et al.* [34]. Of particular importance in device fabrication is that the lattice parameters of AlAs and GaAs are equal at about 900°C, but not at room temperature where $a_0 = 5.661$ (AlAs) and 5.653 Å (GaAs), because of different thermal expansion coefficients (Table 9.4.2). (a_0 can be assumed linear in Al composition in this alloy system.) The expected elastic strains in heterojunction structures have been observed [35]. However, misfit dislocations are rarely seen.

The use of quaternary alloys allows an additional degree of freedom to help match both the lattice parameter and the thermal coefficient of expansion for any bandgap (Section 11.4). For example, by adding small amounts of phosphorus to the outer (AlGa)As layers of a double-heterojunction laser with GaAs in the recombination region, it is possible to obtain a matching thermal coefficient of expansion of the outer and inner layers of the device [36, 37]. However, this is accomplished by having a lattice mismatch at the growth temperature, and misfit dislocations can easily be formed (Section 9.4). The presence of such dislocations may be more detrimental to device performance than the elastic strain of the active region.

An accurate determination of the direct bandgap energy $E_{g\Gamma}$ as a function of alloy composition (made by electroreflectance measurements) can be analytically expressed by (Fig. 11.1.5) [8]

$$E_{g\Gamma} = 1.424 + 1.266x + 0.266x^2 \qquad (11.3.1)$$

The dependence of the X minima on composition is not well known, except for the endpoint values of ~ 1.86 eV in GaAs and 2.16 eV in AlAs [38]. As shown in Fig. 11.1.5, the Γ–X crossover energy $E_{gc} = 1.92$ eV at $x = 0.37$ is consistent with other data [39–41]. Note that the effective Γ–X energy separation is reduced by the upward shift of the Fermi level into the conduction band of n-type material, as discussed in Section 12.2.3, when the material is highly doped.

With regard to the phase diagram, the solid solution can be assumed to be ideal [$\gamma_{GaAs} = \gamma_{AlAs} = 1$ in (11.2.13)], which implies that the Ga and Al atoms are randomly arranged in the crystal with no strain energy introduced by replacing Ga by Al atoms. For the liquid solutions, the quasi-regular solution approximation was used [22, 25] to fit experimental ternary data (Fig. 11.3.1) with the parameters shown in Table 11.3.1.

The usual growth temperature range is 800–900°C. Figure 11.3.2 shows that the distribution coefficient of Al is very high compared to that of Ga and that it increases with decreasing temperature. However, because of depletion of Al from the solution near the interface at high growth rates, the *effective* distribution coefficient in LPE growth may be much lower than the equilibrium value. An additional problem in this system is the oxidation of Al if traces of oxygen remain in the gas stream. This will also reduce the "effective" Al concentration in the liquid. Careful hydrogen purification is essential for reproducible epitaxial growth to reduce the oxygen content to <1 ppm in the H_2 gas stream.

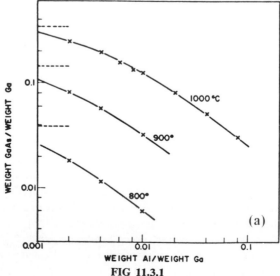

FIG 11.3.1

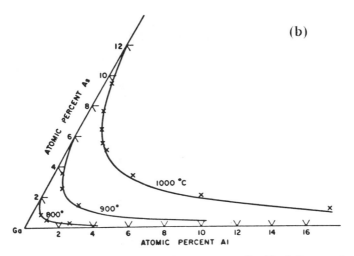

(b)

ATOMIC PERCENT As

1000 °C

900°

800°

Ga

ATOMIC PERCENT Al

FIG. 11.3.1 (a) Weight of GaAs required to saturate a Ga–Al solution as a function of the Al/Ga ratio at 1000, 900, and 800°C. The dashed lines correspond to the solubility values measured in pure Ga. (b) The solubility of As as a function of the Al concentration in the solution at 1000, 900, and 800°C using the data points of (a). The solid lines are theoretically calculated values [22].

TABLE 11.3.1

Parameters Used to Calculate Ga–Al–As Phase Diagram[a]

	GaAs	AlAs	
T^m (K)[b]	1511	2013	
ΔS^F (eu/mole)	16.64	22.8	
	Ga–As	Al–As	Ga–Al
α (cal/mole)	$-9.16T + 5160$	$-9.16T + 9040$	104
	$\beta = 0$ (ideal solution)		

[a]M. Ilegems and G. L. Pearson, *Proc. Int. Symp. Gallium Arsenide, 2nd.* Inst. Phys., Phys. Soc. Conf. Ser. No. 7, p. 3 (1968).

[b]The melting temperatures used by various authors may differ slightly (e.g., see Table 11.3.3).

The Al content of the grown ternary layer typically decreases with increasing distance from the substrate unless special precautions are taken to prevent the depletion of Al from the liquid [42]. Very thick (~500 μm) layers of quite uniform composition have been grown by maintaining a small thermal gradient across the solution which contained, in addition to the GaAs substrate, an (AlGa)As source wafer to replenish the Al in the solution. Also, to further homogeneity, large solutions can be used as well as very low growth rates [43].

As for GaAs, the preferred dopants for (AlGa)As are Sn, Te, Zn, Ge, and

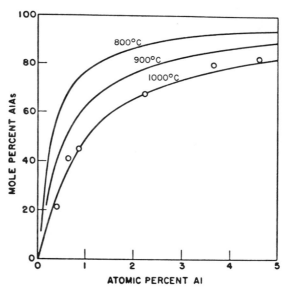

FIG. 11.3.2   Alloy composition of $Al_xGa_{1-x}As$, as measured by electron beam probing, as a function of the Al concentration in the solution for material grown at 1000°C. The solid lines are theoretically calculated solidus isotherms [22].

Si. However, as shown in Fig. 11.3.3, the "effective" LPE distribution coefficient (i.e., measured in terms of carrier concentration at room temperature) decreases with x [44]. The effect for Ge is particularly marked because of an increasing ionization energy (and therefore fewer free carriers at 300 K), and probable compensation effects. As evident from these data, Zn* and Te are particularly important dopants because carrier densities $\gtrsim 10^{18}$ cm^{-3} are easily achieved with small dopant concentrations in LPE solution. Silicon in $Al_xGa_{1-x}As$ is particularly complex because of its amphoteric behavior; detailed studies have appeared [45–48].

The mobility values of electrons in $Al_xGa_{1-x}As$ remain relatively constant, as shown in Fig. 11.3.4 in the direct bandgap region of alloy composition [49], decreasing steeply, however, for $x \gtrsim 0.3$ because of the much lower effective mass in the X minima. This phenomenon is, of course, quite general, and is observed in all similar alloys.

Some measurements have been reported of the minority carrier diffusion

---

*However, because of the volatility of Zn, problems may be encountered in preventing cross contamination of the solutions in multiple-bin growth of heterostructures. Fast growth rates with minimum exposure to high temperatures during growth are helpful in this regard.

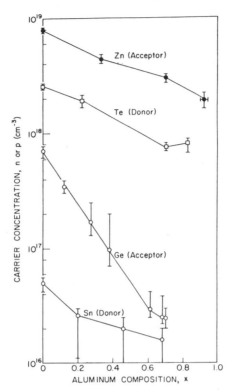

FIG. 11.3.3 Carrier concentration at 300 K in $Al_xGa_{1-x}As$ for four dopants. The dopant mole percent in the solution used to grow the layers by LPE was 0.5 % for each point. The layers were grown on (100) GaAs at temperatures of 840–810°C [44].

length in (AlGa)As [50]. In $Al_{0.05}Ga_{0.95}As$:Ge, $L_e = 3.5$ μm ($P = 1 \times 10^{18}$ cm^{-3}) and in $Al_{0.2}Ga_{0.8}As$:Ge $L_e = 2$ μm ($P = 3 \times 10^{18}$ cm^{-3}). There are insufficient data to determine whether differences in the ternary crystal properties significantly change the diffusion length.

In the direct bandgap energy portion of the alloy ($x \lesssim 0.37$), where the donors are "tied" to the Γ conduction band minimum, the ionization energy of Sn, Te, or other shallow donors remains similar to that in GaAs ($\sim$5 meV). In the indirect bandgap portion of the alloy, however, the donors are considerably deeper (Table 11.3.2), as deduced from photoluminescence and cathodoluminescence studies [51], reflecting the higher electron mass in the X conduction band minima of AlAs. The ionization energy of the shallow acceptor Zn remains essentially constant in the direct bandgap material, while that of the shallow acceptor Ge increases from $\sim$0.04 eV in GaAs to $\sim$0.06

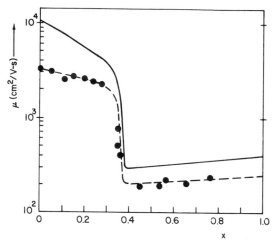

FIG. 11.3.4   Experimental and theoretical variation of the mobility of n-type Al_xGa_{1-x}-As at 300 K. The solid curve is the theoretically limited mobility due to lattice scattering; the dashed curve is the total mobility including impurity and disorder scattering; $N_D - N_A = 2 \times 10^{17}$ cm^{-3}; $N_D + N_A = 6 \times 10^{17}$ cm^{-3} [49].

TABLE 11.3.2

Ionization Energy of Common Dopants in $Al_xGa_{1-x}As$

Bandgap energy (eV)	x	Dopant	E_i (meV)	Ref.
1.42–1.8	0–0.3	Zn	~30	a
1.42–1.8	0–0.3	Ge	~35–60	b
2.09	0.8	Zn	56 ± 5	c
2.14	0.95	Te	62 ± 5	c
2.11	0.85	Sn	59 ± 5	c
2.16	1.0	Si	~70	d

[a] Zh. I. Alferov and O. A. Ninua, *Sov. Phys.-Semicond.* **4**, 519 (1970).

[b] Zh. I. Alferov, D. Z. Garbuzov, O. A. Ninua, and V. G. Trofim, *Sov. Phys.-Semicond.* **5**, 987 (1971).

[c] H. Kressel, F. H. Nicoll, F. Z. Hawrylo, and H. F. Lockwood, *J. Appl. Phys.* **41**, 4692 (1970).

[d] H. Kressel, F. H. Nicoll, M. Ettenberg, W. M. Yim, and A. G. Sigai, *Solid State Commun.* **8**, 1407 (1970). A value as low as $E_D = 52$ meV has been reported for Si, for $x = 0.8$, by T. Hänsel *et al.*, *Phys. Status Solidi(a)* **16**, K31 (1973).

eV at $x \cong 0.3$ [52, 53], and continues to increase as shown in Fig. 11.3.5. (Note that the ionization energy will depend on the dopant concentration as discussed in Section 1.3.)

The luminescence from indirect bandgap (AlGa)As commonly exhibits a complex structure of the type seen in AlAs and GaP and other indirect bandgap semiconductors [51]. Recombination processes involving deep centers

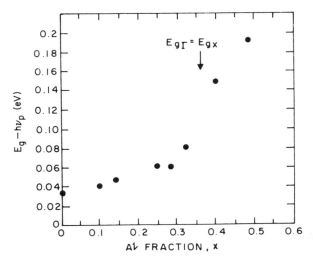

FIG. 11.3.5   Ionization energy of Ge in Al$_x$Ga$_{1-x}$As at 77 K. The Ge concentration is about 5×10^{17} cm^{-3} (H. Kressel and I. Ladany, unpublished).

are observed in both direct and indirect bandgap (AlGa)As, some of which appear similar to those in GaAs [54]. For example, in heavily Te-doped material a broad photoluminescence band centered at $h\nu = E_g - \Delta E$ eV appears at 77 K (similar to that attributed in GaAs to the V_{Ga} complex discussed in Section 10.1) where ΔE increases from 0.3 to 0.5 eV as x increases from 0 to 0.4. In Si-doped material, the characteristic emission band due to the complex level $\sim$0.1 eV above the valence band deepens with increasing Al content [45]. In Ge-doped material, a deep level is seen in addition to the shallow acceptor level which results in a broad $\sim$1.55 eV emission band at 77 K [52, 54]. The origin of this band is as yet unknown, but probably involves a point-defect-related complex.

Certain chemical features of (AlGa)As are worth noting because of their role in device preparation. At low and high Al contents, the chemical properties of the alloy are essentially those of GaAs and AlAs, respectively. Thus, as in the case of AlAs, the hygroscopic nature of high Al content Al$_x$Ga$_{1-x}$As impairs its usefulness in devices. Although the hygroscopic effect is not troublesome for values of x lower than about 0.6, an *abrupt* change in the reaction of the alloy with hot HCl and HF has been found to occur at $x \approx 0.3$. At lower values of x essentially no reaction occurs, but at values only slightly higher rapid solution of the alloy takes place. This characteristic of the alloy can be advantageously utilized in device preparation. In the LPE generation of multilayer films, for instance, difficulties concerned with the precise control of doping and surface features of the final layer can be avoided by the growth of an additional high Al content layer which can readily be removed in hot HF without disturbing the underlying GaAs layer [55].

A doped, high Al content film can also be used as a source for impurity diffusion into the underlying substrate, leaving a planar, undisturbed, diffused surface after removal of the source layer in hot HF. Figure 11.3.6 shows a typical epitaxial layer before and after the removal of the high Al content (AlGa)As layer, leaving behind a smooth and flat surface ready for metallization or other device processes.

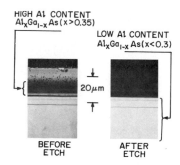

HIGH Al CONTENT
$Al_xGa_{1-x}As(x>0.35)$

LOW Al CONTENT
$Al_xGa_{1-x}As(x<0.3)$

$20\mu m$

BEFORE
ETCH

AFTER
ETCH

FIG. 11.3.6   Cross sections showing typical (AlGa)As multilayer films before and after removal of the high Al content (AlGa)-As surface layer by etching in hot HF [56].

11.3.2   InAs–GaAs

The $In_xGa_{1-x}As$ phase diagram has been calculated by Stringfellow and Greene [21] using the quasi-chemical model, by Antypas [57] using Darken's formalism for the liquid solutions, and by Wu and Pearson [3] using the quasi-regular model. In the latter study, α_{InGa} was empirically found to depend on the In–Ga ratio as shown in Table 11.3.3, in contrast to the single (regular solution) value of $\alpha_{InGa} = 1066$ cal/mole used by Stringfellow and Greene [21], and 2000 cal/mole used by Antypas [57]. Each investigator is apparently

TABLE 11.3.3

Parameters Used to Calculate In–Ga–As Phase Diagram[a]

	GaAs	InAs	
$T^m(K)$	1515	1210	
ΔS^F (eu/mole)	$16.64^{a,b}$	$14.52^{a,b}$	

	Ga–As	In–As	In–Ga
α (cal/mole)	$5900 - 9.9T^a$ $-3.7T^b$	$4030 - 10.16T^a$ $4300 - 9.16T^b$	$\begin{cases} 1100 + 0.16T + 9.8TN^l_{Ga}; \ N^l_{In} > 0.65 \\ 1100 + 0.07T + 4.5\ TN^l_{Ga};\ 0.4 < N^l_{In} \\ \quad < 0.65 \\ 1100;\quad N^l_{In} < 0.4 \\ 1000^b \end{cases}^a$

β(cal/mole) $= 2.83T - 1130^a$; 2000^b

[a]Quasi-regular solution approximation. T. Y. Wu, Preparation and Properties of In_xGa_{1-x}-As with Application to Electroluminescent Devices. Tech. Rep. 5111–5, Stanford Electron. Lab. (August 1971).

[b]G. A. Antypas, *J. Electrochem. Soc.* **117**, 1393 (1970).

able to fit a limited portion of the data with the various chosen approximations. As an illustration, we show in Fig. 11.3.7a a corner of the ternary phase
diagram of interest in growing (InGa)As on GaAs substrates [3]. Figure
11.3.7b shows the crystal composition as a function of the Ga concentration

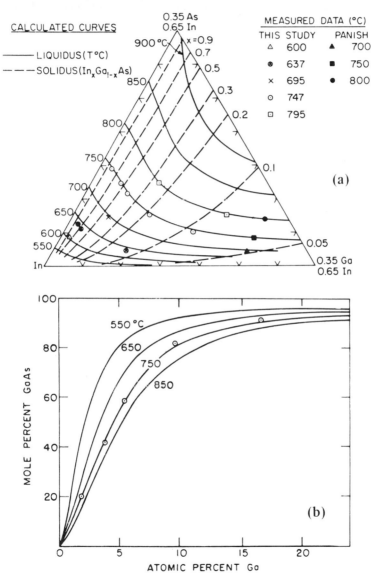

FIG. 11.3.7 (a) The In-rich corner of the InAs–GaAs ternary phase diagram; (b) mole
percent GaAs versus Ga concentration in the In–Ga solution [3]. Solid lines are calculated
solidus isotherms. Experimental data were obtained at a growth temperature of 747°C.
The experimental data in (a) are from Wu and Pearson [3] and Panish [59].

in the liquid for growth between 550 and 850°C. In using these curves to enable the generation of material of one particular composition, the requisite Ga concentration in the liquid is derived from Fig. 11.3.7a and the In concentration from Fig. 11.3.7b.

In LPE growth of $In_xGa_{1-x}As$, the best crystal morphology in the Ga-rich composition range was obtained by growth on the (111) Ga face of GaAs substrates at $\approx 800°C$ and at a cooling rate which did not exceed 0.25°C/min [3]. In a single epitaxially deposited layer, single-crystal growth is generally obtained only with $x \leq 0.2$ on the (111) Ga face. But good growth is difficult on the (100), (110), or (112) As faces with $x > 0.05$. With regard to growth on InAs substrates, the {111} planes also gave the best results but the growth temperature should not exceed 600°C [57].

In LPE growth of $In_xGa_{1-x}As$ devices reported so far [60,61], Te was generally used as the donor and Zn as the acceptor. Germanium was found to act amphoterically, giving n-type material at high temperatures but p-type material at low temperatures, a behavior similar to that of Si in GaAs [60].

Undoped n-type samples with $0 \leq x \leq 0.2$ ($N \approx 10^{17}$ cm^{-3}) have room temperature mobilities of 4000–5000 cm^2/V-s [60]. Sulfur is a possible residual contaminant in alloys grown from In solutions, since even high purity commercially available In sometimes contains a significant residue of this element; the sulfur, however, can be removed by appropriate treatment [58]. Much of the interest in this alloy has been centered on the composition range for ~ 1.1 μm emission (Chapter 13).

11.3.3 InAs–InP

The InAs–InP alloy is of particular interest because much the same bandgap range is covered as with (InGa)As but with a smaller lattice parameter change with composition, and a smaller melting temperature difference between endpoint binaries.

The phase diagram for $In_xAs_{1-x}P$ has been calculated by Antypas and Yep [62] using the parameters shown in Table 11.3.4, with Darken's formalism for

TABLE 11.3.4

Parameters Used to Calculate In–As–P Phase Diagram[a]

	InAs	InP	
$T^m(K)$	1215	1335	
ΔS^F (eu/mole)	14.52	13	
	In–As	In–P	As–P
α (cal/mole)	$4300 - 9.16T$	$9700 - 9.7T$	2000
	$\beta = 1000$ cal/mole		

[a]G. A. Antypas and T. O. Yep, *J. Appl. Phys.* **42**, 3201 (1971).

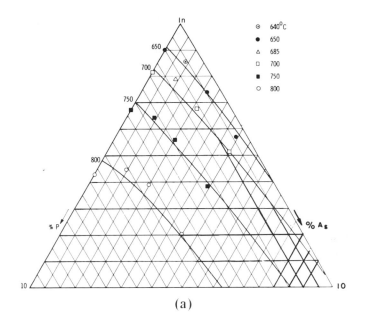

(a)

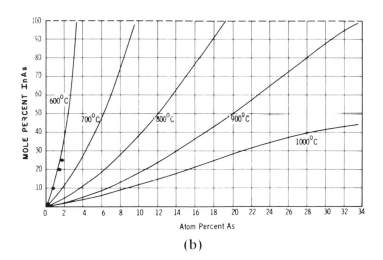

(b)

FIG. 11.3.8 (a) Calculated liquidus isotherms (solid lines) with experimental data in the In-rich corner of the InAs–InP ternary phase diagram. (b) Mole percent InAs in material grown at 600°C compared to experimental data [62].

the liquid solution activity coefficients. A portion of their ternary plot is shown in Fig. 11.3.8a. Because of lack of data, it has not been possible to compare experimental and calculated values over an extensive composition and growth temperature range. Good agreement with the calculated liquidus isotherm curves, however, was obtained in the 600–800°C growth temperature range, which is of practical interest for obtaining useful epitaxial layers (Fig. 11.3.8b).

Indium phosphide crystals grown by the liquid encapsulation technique [63] provide useful large-area substrates for LPE growth. Best results are obtained by growth on the (111) P face. The LPE films not deliberately doped have background concentrations $N_D - N_A = 4 \times 10^{16}$ to 4×10^{17} cm^{-3} and exhibit room temperature mobility values of 2000–3000 cm^2/V-s in the P-rich portion of the alloy system [62]. Photoluminescent spectra at 77 K of the undoped samples show a deep level recombination of unknown origin with $h\nu = E_g - \Delta E$, ΔE decreasing from 0.25 eV in pure InP to 0.1 eV in In$_{0.74}$ As$_{0.26}$P. This level is not seen in Zn-doped material.

11.3.4   InP–GaP

These alloys were first prepared by the growth from the melt in polycrystalline form [64], later by growth from solution [65–67], by LPE [68, 69], and by VPE [70, 71].

The In$_{1-x}$Ga$_x$P phase diagram has been calculated by the quasi-regular solution approximation [30, 72] (but with different thermodynamic parameters; see Table 11.3.5) and by the quasi-chemical analysis [73]. These calculations have yielded only modest agreement with experiment over a large range of values. The difficulty in the calculations arises from the high degree of nonideality of the solid solution due to the large lattice parameter mis-

TABLE 11.3.5

Parameters Used to Calculate In–Ga–P Phase Diagrams

	InP	GaP	
T^m(K)	1333	1813	
ΔS^F (eu/mole)	14.76[a]; 14[b]	12.85[a]; 16.8[b]	
	In–P	Ga–P	In–Ga
α (cal/mole)	$9030 - 9.75T$[a]	$14{,}690 - 13.15T$[a]	1066[a]; 1070[b]
	$4500 - 4T$[b]	$2800 - 4.8T$[b]	
	$\beta = 0$[a]; $\beta = 3500$ cal/mole[b]		

[a]A. W. Mabbitt, *J. Mater. Sci.* **5**, 1043 (1970).

[b]M. B. Panish and M. Ilegems, *Proc. Int. Symp. Gallium Arsenide, 3rd.* Inst. Phys., Phys. Soc. Conf. Ser. No. 9, p. 67 (1970).

match of InP and GaP, and possibly also from the choice of a constant α_{InGa}. Note that various values of α_{InAs} had to be empirically determined in the In–Ga–As system for different In concentrations (Table 11.3.3), whereas the In–Ga–P calculations assumed a regular In–Ga solution behavior through-out.

There has been much discussion in the literature regarding the $In_xGa_{1-x}P$ composition at which the lowest bandgap transition becomes indirect. A crossover bandgap energy of 2.26 eV at $x = 0.73$ (300 K) has been quoted [74], while others reported values of $E_{gc} = 2.17$ eV at $x = 0.63$ [75–77]. The difference is quite significant with regard to possible applications of this alloy for laser diode fabrication. The best current estimate, based on pressure experiments of Pitt et al. [19], is shown in Fig. 11.1.10. It appears that the L minima are lower than the X minima in InP, and that the reverse is true in GaP. As shown in Fig. 11.1.10, the L minima cross the Γ minimum at $x \cong$ 0.63 and $E_{gc} \cong 2.17$, whereas the X minima cross the Γ minimum at $E_{gc} \cong$ 2.26 and $x \cong 0.74$. On the basis of these results, it appears that the alloy has an indirect lowest energy bandgap for $E_g \gtrsim 2.2$ eV at room temperature, although some uncertainty still remains concerning the limits for laser opera-tion.

Gallium arsenide substrates match the lattice parameter of $In_{0.49}Ga_{0.51}P$ ($E_g \cong 1.9$ eV). However, the value of x must be very closely controlled in order to avoid the formation of a high density of dislocations with the as-sociated formation of a cellular (polycrystalline) morphology (Section 9.4) in LPE growth. Stringfellow et al. [78] found that really good epitaxial layers could be prepared only in the composition range $0.48 \lesssim x \lesssim 0.53$ where the lattice mismatch with the substrate does not exceed 0.2–0.3%. The major interest in this alloy lies in its use in the bounding regions of heterojunction lasers where the lattice-matched recombination region consists of appro-priate composition In(GaAs), InGaAsP, or Ga(AsP) (Chapter 13 and Section 14.5).

An interesting and very useful observation reported by Stringfellow and co-workers [78] is that the material deposited has a tendancy toward the lattice-matched composition for solution compositions designed to produce slightly mismatched layers. This "pulling" effect is probably a quite general phenomenon in LPE growth, and is useful in decreasing the difficulty of growing lattice-matched heterojunction structures since nature provides the "fine tuning" not easily accomplished by precise control of the solution com-position and growth temperature.

The distribution and diffusion coefficients of impurities in (InGa)P are not yet known in detail. However, results [68] indicate that for Te, Sn, and Se, $N_D - N_A = 3 \times 10^{21} N^l$, where N^l is the atom fraction of the dopant in the liquid. Silicon is amphoteric, but predominantly a donor.

A detailed study of the optical properties of Zn- ($E_A \approx 60$ meV) and Si-doped LPE $In_{1-x}Ga_xP$ has been made in the vicinity of the crossover composition region by Bachrach and Hakki [79], and Cd has been studied in VPE $InGa_{0.5}P_{0.5}$. An ionization energy of about 60 meV is deduced for Cd (decreasing with concentration, Section 1.7.1) [80]. Lightly doped material has been studied by Chevallier and Laugier [81] who found that the direct bandgap material luminescence was similar to that of InP. Qualitatively similar conclusions were reached by Onton and Chicotka [82] who studied the low temperature luminescence of Te-doped material in the direct and indirect bandgap composition range. These results suggest that the shallow donor ionization energy is essentially determined by the lowest conduction band minimum (or minima in the indirect bandgap material). This is also the case in (AlGa)As (Section 11.3.1) and is probably a general phenomenon in the III–V ternaries.

11.3.5   GaAs–GaSb

The ternary $GaAs_xSb_{1-x}$ phase diagram was calculated by Antypas and James [83] using the parameters shown in Table 11.3.6, with Darken's formalism for the liquid solution activity coefficients. The experimental studies were limited to the As-rich side of the alloys ($x > 0.75$) with layers grown on the (111) As face of GaAs substrates. Figure 11.3.9 shows the calculated phase diagram and Fig. 11.3.10 shows the observed dependence of crystal composition on the Sb concentration in the solution at a 720°C growth temperature. The values are in agreement, but the available data are too limited to determine the range of validity of the calculated phase diagram.

There is growing interest in this alloy because it can be used to produce lattice-matched heterojunctions in conjunction with AlGaAsSb (Section 11.4 and Chapter 13). Because of the large lattice parameter change with composition (7.5% across the full composition range), a miscibility gap may exist for intermediate composition values. However, excellent devices have been

TABLE 11.3.6
Parameters Used to Calculate Ga–As–Sb Phase Diagram[a]

	GaAs	GaSb	
T^m(K)	1511	985	
ΔS^F(eu/mole)	16.64	12.3	
	Ga–As	Ga–Sb	As–Sb
a (cal/mole)	$-3.7T$	$11{,}500 - 13T$	2400
	$\beta = 4500$ cal/mole		

[a]G. A. Antypas and L. W. James, *J. Appl. Phys.* **41**, 2165 (1970).

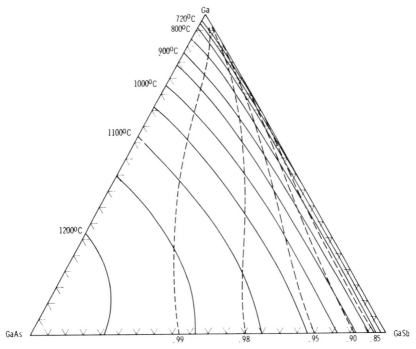

FIG. 11.3.9 Calculated GaAs–GaSb ternary phase diagram showing liquidus isotherms (———) and GaAs isoconcentration curves (– – –) [83].

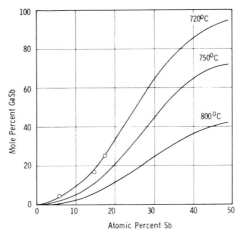

FIG. 11.3.10 Mole percent GaSb in epitaxial layer (———), computed from Fig. 11.3.9, compared with experimental data (○) for material grown at 720°C [83].

prepared in the 1.1 eV bandgap energy range in the As-rich composition range.

11.3.6   GaAs–GaP

Ga(AsP) is widely used for light-emitting diodes. Vapor phase epitaxy is the favored method for preparing this material primarily because composition grading is required in order to obtain good quality material on GaAs (Chapter 9). This is difficult to accomplish under controlled conditions in LPE. Furthermore, the more convenient (AlGa)As alloys cover very nearly the same bandgap region, except for a somewhat higher maximum direct bandgap in $GaAs_{0.54}P_{0.46}$ at $E_{gc} = 1.99$ eV compared to ~ 1.92 eV in (AlGa)As. LPE Ga(AsP) has been prepared by Panish [84] with a tipping furnace and by Shih [85] with a vertical furnace, both using GaP substrates. The phase diagram was calculated using the regular solution approximation [86], whereas Osamura et al. [87] compared the quasi-chemical equilibrium and the regular solution models. There appeared to be relatively little difference when the calculated values (using either model) were compared with experimental data.

11.3.7   InAs–InSb

$InAs_{1-x}Sb_x$ alloys cover a bandgap range of 0.35 to ~ 0.1 eV, and are therefore suitable for infrared light-emitting diodes and detectors. They are also of interest because of their potential for mobilities that are higher than those in any other known semiconductor. Stringfellow and Greene have studied LPE growth of this alloy system using a steady state growth technique [88]. A calculated In–As–Sb phase diagram [21] was verified experimentally in the course of this work and liquid isotherms were calculated. The isotherms and experimental data obtained by measurement of the solubility of InAs in InSb liquids are shown in Fig. 11.3.11. Figure 11.3.12a compares the calculated and measured concentration lines. The shape of the pseudobinary curves (Fig. 11.3.12b) is responsible for many problems encountered in the LPE growth of $InAs_{1-x}Sb_x$: The solid composition is strongly temperature dependent, the growth temperatures are low, and the As distribution coefficient is very large. In the work of Stringfellow and Greene [88], these growth problems were alleviated by the use of apparatus (Fig. 11.3.13) allowing steady state LPE growth. In this apparatus the growth temperature is held constant, a temperature gradient between substrate and source wafer furnishing the driving force for epitaxial growth and its control. Conditions for successful growth are summarized in Table 11.3.7. Because of a 7% difference in the lattice parameters of InAs and InSb, high quality growth of $InAs_{1-x}Sb_x$ on InAs and InSb substrates is obtained only at values of $x < 0.15$ and $x >$

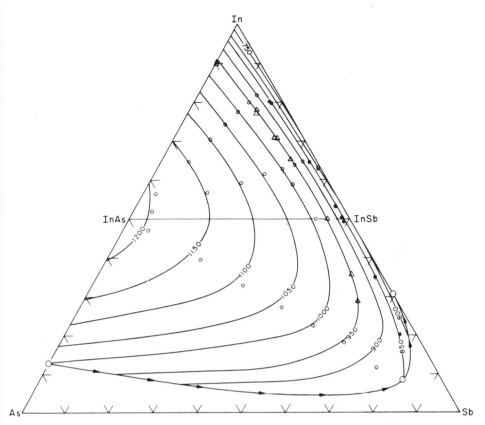

FIG. 11.3.11 Calculated liquidus isotherms for the InAs–InSb ternary system compared with the data of Shih and Peretti [89] (○), and data obtained from solubility measurements of InAs in In–Sb solutions (●, △, □) [88].

0.9, respectively. Successful growth at other values of x requires suitable alloy substrates. With regard to electrical properties, electron mobility values of 30,000 cm²/V-s were obtained at 300 K when $x < 0.35$ and $N = 2 \times 10^{16}$ cm^{-3}. At $x = 0.89$ an electron mobility of 67,000 cm²/V-s at 300 K is typical.

11.3.8 AlP–GaP

This alloy system offers only modest advantages in that the highest bandgap (indirect) obtainable with the alloy is only slightly higher than that of GaP, 2.45 versus 2.26 eV at room temperature (Fig. 11.1.9). However, because of the good lattice parameter match, this ternary system is of potential interest for the fabrication of heterojunctions with GaP. The material was first prepared in platelet form from Ga solution by Merz and Lynch [92] and by

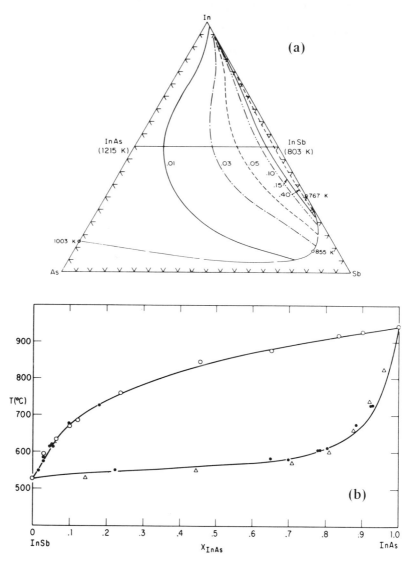

FIG. 11.3.12 (a) Calculated solidus isoconcentration curves for the InAs–InSb system; (b) calculated pseudobinary phase diagram for the InAs–InSb system [88]. Liquidus data points obtained by solubility measurements of InAs in In–Sb solutions (●), and from the results of Shih and Peretti [90] (○). The solidus points were obtained by the growth of crystals at near-equilibrium conditions (●) and from Woolley and Smith [91] (△).

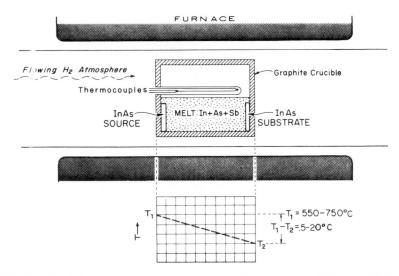

FIG. 11.3.13 Schematic diagram of apparatus used to grow epitaxial layers of In(AsSb) alloys by a steady state LPE technique [88].

TABLE 11.3.7

Conditions for the Growth of $InAs_{1-x}Sb_x{}^a$

x	$T\,(°C)$	Liquid composition	$T\,(°C)$	Growth rate $(\mu m/min)$	Substrate
0.04	720	$N_{In}^l = 0.690$ $N_{Sb}^l = 0.220$ $N_{As}^l = 0.090$	6.8	15	InAs (111) B
0.08	719.5	$N_{In}^l = 0.500$ $N_{Sb}^l = 0.416$ $N_{As}^l = 0.084$	8	1	InAs (111) B
0.15	670	$N_{In}^l = 0.500$ $N_{Sb}^l = 0.450$ $N_{As}^l = 0.050$	7.2	0.67	InAs (111) B
0.20	610	$N_{In}^l = 0.500$ $N_{Sb}^l = 0.475$ $N_{As}^l = 0.025$	7.6	0.3	$InAs_{0.92}Sb_{0.08}$ (111) B
0.31	579	$N_{In}^l = 0.500$ $N_{Sb}^l = 0.484$ $N_{As}^l = 0.016$	14.1	0.17	$InAs_{0.85}Sb_{0.15}$
0.89	520	$N_{In}^l = 0.630$ $N_{Sb}^l = 0.366$ $N_{As}^l = 0.004$	1.5	0.7	InSb (111) B

^{a}G. B. Stringfellow and P. E. Greene, *J. Electrochem. Soc.* **118**, 805 (1971).

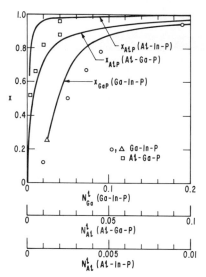

FIG. 11.3.14 The calculated relationship between the solid and liquid composition for $Al_xGa_{1-x}P$, $Al_xIn_{1-x}P$, and $In_{1-x}Ga_xP$ at 1100°C [30]. The experimental data are from (○) Panish [65]; (△) Foster and Scardefield [94]; and (□) Panish et al. [93].

LPE by Kressel and Ladany [13]. The ternary is stable in normal ambient when the Al concentration is below 30–40%.

Some of the thermodynamic properties of the ternary were determined by Panish et al. [93]. A calculation has been made of the phase diagram using the regular solution approximation and the assumption of an ideal solid solution [30]. Figure 11.3.14 compares the calculated dependence of the Al content of the ternary as a function of the Al content of the solution to experimental values. Note the large distribution coefficient of Al, which makes control of the crystal composition difficult.

Chicotka et al. [14] found that the volatility of the usual dopants at the temperature needed to grow $Al_xGa_{1-x}P$ layers of uniform composition was too high for convenient doping of the layers when grown in the typical open flow LPE system. A sealed system was used, maintained at a constant temperature to prevent the condensation of the dopant on the cooler portions of the pyrolytic BN crucible. Growing in the 1070–970°C temperature interval, the "effective" distribution coefficients for S, Te, and Zn were found to be 4.0, 0.033, and 0.006, respectively, for the approximate composition $0.7 \leq x \leq 0.9$.

One of the reasons for the initial interest in (AlGa)P was the possibility of shifting the efficient red Zn–O recombination band of GaP into a shorter wavelength range, thus improving its brightness. It was found that the band does shift as expected with increasing bandgap energy [13, 92]. However, because of the difficulty of incorporating oxygen in the ternary in the presence of the Al in the Ga solution, the density of Zn–O pairs was found to be too low to be effective in producing efficient luminescence.

11.3.9 Other Ternary Systems

The *InP–AlP* offers potentially the highest direct bandgap energy of the III–V ternary systems (Fig. 11.1.6). Although polycrystalline material has been prepared from the melt [95], LPE growth is very difficult because of the great difference in the melting temperatures of InP and AlP with a consequent very large distribution coefficient for Al, as shown in the calculated curves of Fig. 11.3.14. Thus, this ternary is more difficult to grow than (AlGa)P or (InGa)P. In addition, the lattice parameter mismatch between InP and AlP is quite large (Table 9.4.1), adding further complexity to the growth.

The *InAs–AlAs system* is in the same class of difficulty (or worse) as InP–AlP and has so far been prepared only in polycrystalline form from the melt [95].

Of the remaining systems listed in Table 9.4.1, some offer no apparent useful properties (such as *AlAs–AlP*) and have not been prepared. Others, such as *InSb–GaSb* and *InSb–AlSb* [96] have been prepared in polycrystalline form. We refer to the book by Madelung [97] for a review of some of the major properties of these ternaries. Interaction parameters and other data useful in calculating the phase diagram for all the III–V ternary systems on the basis of the binary compound data can be found in the paper by Stringfellow [32].

The $Al_xGa_{1-x}Sb$ alloys are interesting because of the small change in lattice parameter with composition. The crossover from direct to indirect minimum bandgap energy occurs at $x = 0.4$ (300 K) at ~ 1.1 eV [11] (Fig. 11.1.8). The calculated Ga–Al–Sb ternary phase diagram is shown in Fig. 11.3.15 [22]. The regular solution approximation used the parameters in Table 11.3.8.

11.4 Quaternary Compounds

The interest in quaternary alloys has centered on their use in conjunction with binary and ternary compounds to form lattice-matching heterojunction structures in bandgap energy regions outside the (AlGa)As range. Chapter 13 reviews the device results obtained.

Three classes of quaternary alloys have received particular attention:

1. Alloys in which Al is substituted for Ga to increase the bandgap energy with minimal change in lattice parameter;

2. alloys which match the lattice parameter of commonly available melt-grown substrates such as InAs, GaAs, GaSb, and InP; and

3. alloys lattice-matched to Ga(AsP) to produce visible emission lasers.

Alloys of III–V compounds which have been studied, or are of potential

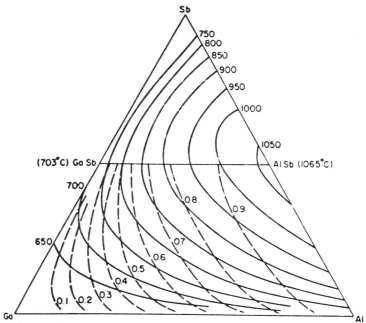

FIG. 11.3.15   Liquidus and solidus curves in the GaSb–AlSb ternary phase diagram. The solid lines are the liquidus isotherms calculated at fixed temperatures between 650 and 1050°C. The dashed lines are the solidus isoconcentration lines and give the composition of the $Al_xGa_{1-x}Sb$ in equilibrium with the solution. The isoconcentration lines have been drawn for solid compositions ranging from $x = 0.1$ to 0.9 [22].

TABLE 11.3.8

Parameters Used to Calculate Ga–Al–Sb Phase Diagram[a]

	GaSb	AlSb	
T^m (K)	976	1338	
ΔS^F(eu/mole)	12.3	10.4	
	Ga–Sb	Al–Sb	Ga–Al
α (cal/mole)	$-13T + 11,500$	$-13T + 18,000$	104

[a]M. Ilegems and G. L. Pearson, *Proc. Int. Symp. Gallium Arsenide, 2nd.* Inst. Phys., Phys. Soc. Conf. Ser. No. 7, p. 3 (1968).

interest, include InGaAsSb, AlGaAsSb, InGaAsP, and AlGaAsP. Of these, the Al-containing alloys are most easily prepared by LPE. The phase diagram can be calculated using interaction parameters for the atoms on the two sublattices of the generalized system $A_xB_{1-x}C_yD_{1-y}$ in which the A and B atoms are on the group III sublattice and the C and D atoms on the group V sublattice.

Ilegems and Panish [98] calculated quaternary phase diagrams with the solid decomposed into ternary alloys: ABC, ACD, ABD, and BCD. Jordan and Ilegems [99] obtained equivalent formulations considering the solid as a mixture of binary alloys: AC, AD, BC, and BD, with restrictions set by the structure of the solid. The large number of variables needed to match experimental data precludes attempts to match fully the theoretical phase diagrams to experimental values over broad composition ranges. Besides, the interesting composition range tends to be limited by the lattice-matching device requirements noted.

A key virtue of some of the quaternary alloys is that a rather broad composition range (hence bandgap energy) can be obtained with a constant lattice parameter. This is directly seen in Fig. 11.1.1 where InGaAsP, for example, is observed to encompass a broad field, each constant a_0 value corresponding to the bandgap energy range subtended by the two outer lines. Of course, the fact that some portion of the alloy has an indirect bandgap composition sets a restriction with regard to the luminescent properties. However, the quaternary alloy can be advantageously used in the passive region of heterojunction devices where only the bandgap energy magnitude and refractive index are important.

Assuming a linear dependence on composition of the lattice parameter a_{AC} for the binary AC (and similarly for the other lattice parameters), the lattice parameter of the alloy $A_xB_{1-x}C_yD_{1-y}$ is

$$a_0 = xya_{AC} + x(1-y)a_{AD} + (1-x)ya_{BC} + (1-x)(1-y)a_{BD} \quad (11.4.1)$$

The bandgap energy determination is a more complicated process because of possible multiple conduction band minima crossover and bowing parameters. However, for compositions of common interest which are quite near one of the binaries, the bowing parameter can be neglected and the bandgap energy may be approximated from the bandgaps of the binaries $E_{AC}, \ldots,$ assuming linear variations:

$$E_g \cong xyE_{AC} + x(1-y)E_{AD} + (1-x)yE_{BC} + (1-x)(1-y)E_{BD}$$
$$(11.4.2)$$

If we focus on those quaternary alloy compositions which match various available melt-grown single crystals, we see from Table 11.4.1 that a substantial bandgap energy range is covered by keeping the lattice parameter constant and changing the constituents of the alloys.

The alloy system of particular practical interest in Table 11.4.1 is the one which yields a heterojunction laser on InP substrates in which the recombination region has a bandgap energy of 0.75–1.2 eV (allowing for a minimum 0.15 eV bandgap energy step at the heterojunctions). The growth of InGaAsP on InP has been studied by Antypas and Moon [100], in the growth temperature range of 625–650°C, on (100), (111) A, and (111) B substrates.

TABLE 11.4.1

Quaternary III–V Alloys Lattice-Matched to Binary Compounds at 300 K[a]

Substrate	Epitaxial layer composition	Lattice parameter (Å)	Bandgap energy E_g (eV)
InAs	$In_xGa_{1-x}As_ySb_{1-y}$ $(1-y) = 0.916(1-x)$	6.058	0.35–0.70
InP	$In_xGa_{1-x}As_yP_{1-y}$ $y = 2.16(1-x)$	5.869	0.75–1.34[b]
GaAs	$In_xGa_{1-x}As_yP_{1-y}$ $(1-y) = 2.04x$	5.653	1.42–1.90[b]

[a] R. Sankaran, G. A. Antypas, R. L. Moon, J. S. Esher, and L. W. James, *J. Vac. Soc.* **13**, 932 (1976).

[b] Can be directly seen in Fig. 11.1.1.

The use of lattice-matched GaAs substrates is of lesser interest since the attainable bandgap energy range is comparable to that achievable with (AlGa)As. However, it is possible to produce devices with a higher direct bandgap energy by using a somewhat smaller lattice parameter material as a substrate, for example Ga(AsP). As seen from Fig. 11.1.1, by drawing a horizontal line, it then becomes possible to lattice-match InGaAsP bounding regions to a Ga(AsP) recombination region in a double-heterojunction configuration. It is evident, therefore, that the InGaAsP quaternary alloys offer an interesting range of possibilities in producing visible emission lasers (Section 14.5). No experimental work has been reported using InGaAsSb alloys grown on InAs, although single-crystal layers on GaAs substrates have been studied [101].

The alloys using Al-for-Ga substitutions have been experimentally studied with the AlGaAsSb/Ga(AsSb) heterojunction system of interest as a means of achieving lasing emission in the 1.1 eV range. However, unless precautions are taken (Chapter 9), the use of GaAs substrates leads to a rather severe lattice parameter mismatch and a resultant high ($>10^5$ cm^{-2}) dislocation density in the diode recombination region. The advantageous feature of the AlGaAsSb/Ga(AsSb) system is that lattice matching *at the heterojunction interface* is readily achieved when the material is grown by LPE. Antypas and Moon [102] studied growth on (100) GaAs substrates between 760 and 720°C. Since the distribution coefficient of Sb is practically independent of the Al concentration, the solution constituents are easily adjusted to produce a lattice-matched heterojunction. Table 11.4.2 shows the solution compositions and resultant solid compositions.

Epitaxial layers of AlGaAsP were studied by Ilegems and Panish [103], and heterojunction structures by Burnham *et al.* [104]. Epitaxial layers of In GaAsP on Ga(AsP) were studied by Hitchens *et al.* [105].

It is worth noting that the growth of lattice-matched quaternary layers is probably not as difficult as anticipated on the basis of the required solution

TABLE 11.4.2

Growth and Characterization Parameters for AlGaAsSb Liquid Phase Epitaxial Layers[a]

Growth temperature (°C)	Melt composition[b] (g)			Solid composition (atom %)		Lattice parameter (Å)	Bandgap (eV)
	Ga	Sb	Al	x_{Sb}	x_{Al}		
720–700	4.00	1.25	0	6.5	0	5.701	1.18
720–700	4.00	1.25	0.0015	5.8	4.7	5.691	1.31
720–700	4.00	1.25	0.0035	5.4	10.7	5.690	1.47
720–700	4.00	1.25	0.0055	4.8	14.7	5.690	1.58
760–740	4.00	1.25	0	4.3	0	5.684	1.23
760–740	4.00	1.25	0.0015	4.1	2.4	5.684	1.30
760–740	4.00	1.25	0.0035	4.0	4.4	5.686	1.35

[a]G. A. Antypas and R. L. Moon, *J. Electrochem. Soc.* **121**, 416 (1974).
[b]Solutions saturated in As.

and temperature control because of the natural "pulling" of the grown layer toward a lattice-matched composition which minimizes the interfacial dislocation formation.

REFERENCES

1. A. G. Thompson and J. C. Woolley, *Can. J. Phys.* **45**, 255 (1967).
2. D. E. Aspnes, C. G. Olson, and D. W. Lynch, *Phys. Rev. Lett.* **37**, 766 (1976).
3. T. Y. Wu and G. L. Pearson, *J. Phys. Chem. Solids* **33**, 409 (1972).
4. J. C. Woolley, C. M. Gillet, and J. A. Evans, *Proc. Phys. Soc.* **77**, 700 (1961).
5. E. F. Hockings, I. Kudman, T. E. Seidel, C. M. Schmelz, and E. F. Steigmeyer, *J. Appl. Phys.* **37**, 2879 (1966).
6. A. G. Thompson, M. Cardona, K. L. Shaklee, and J. C. Wooley, *Phys. Rev.* **146**, 601 (1966).
7. A. H. Herzog, W. O. Groves, and M. G. Craford, *J. Appl. Phys.* **40**, 1830 (1969).
8. O. Berolo and J. C. Wooley, *Can. J. Phys.* **49**, 1335 (1971).
9. M. R. Lorenz and A. Onton, *Proc. Int. Conf. Phys. of Semicond., 10th* (S. P. Keller, J. C. Hensel, and F. Stern, eds.), p. 574. U. S. Nat. Tech. Informat. Serv., Springfield, Virginia, 1970.
10. J. C. Woolley, S. A. Evans, and C. M. Gillett, *Proc. Phys. Soc.* **74**, 244 (1959).
11. H. Mathieu, D. Auvergne, P. Merle, and K. C. Rustagi, *Phys. Rev. B* **12**, 5846 (1975).
12. B. B. Kosichi, A. Jayaraman, and W. Paul, *Phys. Rev.* **172**, 764 (1968).
13. H. Kressel and I. Ladany, *J. Appl. Phys.* **39**, 5339 (1968).
14. R. J. Chicotka, L. M. Foster, M. R. Lorenz, A. H. Nethercot, and G. D. Pettit, Development of Aluminum Alloy Compounds for Electroluminescent Light Sources, Rep. NASA-CR-111976. Nat. Aeronaut. and Space Administration (1971).
15. C. Alibert, G. Bordure, A. Laugier, and J. Chevallier, *Phys. Rev. B* **6**, 1301 (1972).
16. M. R. Lorenz and A. Onton, *Proc. Int. Conf. Phys. Semicond. 10th, Cambridge, Massachusetts,* p. 444 (1970).
17. G. B. Stringfellow, *J. Appl. Phys.* **43**, 3455 (1972).
18. C. J. Nuese, A. G. Sigai, M. S. Abrahams, and J. J. Gannon, *J. Electrochem. Soc.* **120**, 956 (1973).

19. G. D. Pitt, M. K. R. Vyas, and A. W. Mabbitt, *Solid State Commun.* **14**, 621 (1974).
20. I. Kudman and R. J. Paff, *J. Appl. Phys.* **43**, 3760 (1972).
21. G. B. Stringfellow and P. D. Greene, *J. Phys. Chem. Solids* **30**, 1779 (1969).
22. H. Ilegems, Ph. D. Thesis, Stanford Univ. (1970).
23. L. J. Vieland, *Acta Met.* **11**, 137 (1963).
24. N. N. Sirota, *in* "Semiconductors and Semimetals" (R. K. Willardson and A. C. Beer, eds.), Vol. 4, p. 36. Academic Press, New York, 1968.
25. M. Ilegems and G. L. Pearson, *1968 Proc. Int. Symp. on Gallium Arsenide, 2nd*, p. 18. Inst. Phys., Phys. Soc. Conf., Ser. No. 7.
26. C. D. Thurmond, *J. Phys. Chem. Solids* **26**, 785 (1965).
27. I. Prigogine and R. Defay, "Chemical Thermodynamics." Longmans, London, 1965.
28. G. A. Antypas, *J. Electrochem. Soc.* **117**, 700 (1970).
29. C. S. Darken, *Trans. AIME* **239**, 90 (1967).
30. M. B. Panish and M. Ilegems, *Proc. Int. Symp on Gallium Arsenide, 3rd*, p. 67. Inst. Phys., Phys. Soc. Conf., Ser. No. 9 (1970).
31. E. A. Guggenheim, "Mixtures." Oxford Univ. Press, London and New York, 1952.
32. G. B. Stringfellow, *J. Phys. Chem. Solids* **33**, 665 (1972).
33. L. M. Foster and J. F. Woods, *J. Electrochem. Soc.* **118**, 1175 (1971).
34. H. Rupprecht, J. M. Woodall, and G. D. Pettit, *Appl. Phys. Lett.* **11**, 81 (1967).
35. F. K. Reinhart and R. A. Logan, *J. Appl. Phys.* **44**, 3171 (1973).
36. G. A. Rozgonyi, P. N. Petroff, and M. B. Panish, *J. Crystal Growth* **27**, 106 (1974).
37. R. L. Brown and R. G. Sobers, *J. Appl. Phys.* **45**, 4735 (1974).
38. M. R. Lorenz, R. Chicotka, G. D. Pettit, and P. J. Dean, *Solid State Commun.* **8**, 693 (1970).
39. H. C. Casey, Jr., and M. B. Panish, *J. Appl. Phys.* **40**, 4910 (1969).
40. H. Nelson and H. Kressel, *Appl. Phys. Lett.* **15**, 7 (1969).
41. H. Kressel, H. F. Lockwood, and H. Nelson, *IEEE J. Quantum Electron.* **6**, 278 (1970).
42. J. M. Woodall, H. Rupprecht, and W. Reuter, *J. Electrochem. Soc.* **116**, 899 (1969).
43. L. E. Stone, K. Madden, and R. W. Haisty, *J. Electron. Mater.* **1**, 111 (1972).
44. D. T. Cheung, Thesis, Stanford Univ. Stanford, California, Tech. Rep. 5124–1 (April 1975).
45. H. Kressel, F. Z. Hawrylo, and N. Almeleh, *J. Appl. Phys.* **40**, 2224 (1969).
46. W. G. Rado, W. J. Johnson, and R. L. Crawley, *J. Appl. Phys.* **43**, 2763 (1972).
47. K. K. Shih and G. D. Pettit, *J. Electron. Mater.* **3**, 391 (1974).
48. L. Constantinescu, G. S. Georgescu, A. Goldenblum, and E. Ivan, *Phys. Status Solidi (a)* **24**, 367 (1974).
49. H. Neumann and U. Flohrer, *Phys. Status Solidi (a)* **25**, K145 (1974).
50. Zh. I. Alferov, V. M. Andreev, V. I. Murygin, and V. I. Stremin, *Sov. Phys. Semicond.* **3**, 1234 (1970).
51. H. Kressel, F. H. Nicoll, F. Z. Hawrylo, and H. F. Lockwood, *J. Appl. Phys.* **41**, 4692 (1970).
52. Zh. I. Alferov, D. Z. Garbuzov, O. A. Ninua, and V. J. Trofim, *Sov. Phys. Semicond.* **5**, 987 (1971).
53. Zh. I. Alferov, D. C. Garbuzov, O. A. Ninua, and V. J. Trofim, *Sov. Phys. Semicond.* **5**, 982 (1971).
54. K. Sugiyama and T. Kawakami, *Jpn. J. Appl. Phys.* **10**, 1007 (1971).
55. H. Kressel, H. Nelson, and F. Z. Hawrylo, unpublished; U. S. Patent 3,692,593 (1969).
56. H. Kressel and H. Nelson, Properties and Applications of III–V Compound Films De-

posited by Liquid Phase Epitaxy, *in* "Physics of Thin Films" (G. Hass, M. Francombe, and R. W. Hoffman, eds.), Vol. 7. Academic Press, New York, 1973.

57. G. A. Antypas, *J. Electrochem. Soc.* **117**, 1393 (1970).
58. M. C. Hales, J. R. Knight, and C. W. Wilkins, *Proc. Int. Symp. GaAs, 3rd*, p. 50 (1970).
59. M. B. Panish, *J. Electrochem. Soc.* **117**, 1393 (1970).
60. K. Takahashi, T. Moriizumi, and S. Shirose, *J. Electrochem. Soc.* **118**, 1639 (1971).
61. R. E. Nahory, M. A. Pollack, and J. R. DeWinter, *J. Appl. Phys.* **46**, 775 (1975).
62. G. A. Antypas and T. O. Yep, *J. Appl. Phys.* **42**, 3201 (1971).
63. J. B. Mullin, A. Royle, and B. W. Straughan, *Proc. Int. Symp. GaAs, 3rd*, p. 41 (1970).
64. M. R. Lorenz, W. Reuter, W. P. Dumke, R. J. Chicotka, G. D. Pettit, and J. M. Woodall, *Appl. Phys. Lett.* **13**, 421 (1968).
65. M. B. Panish, *J. Chem. Thermo.* **2**, 319 (1970).
66. Y. Okuno, K. Suto, and J. Nishizawa, *Jpn. J. Appl. Phys.* **10**, 388 (1971).
67. D. R. Scifres, H. M. Macksey, N. Holonyak, Jr., and R. D. Dupuis, *J. Appl. Phys.* **43**, 1019 (1972).
68. B. W. Hakki, *J. Electrochem. Soc.* **118**, 1469 (1971), and references cited therein.
69. A. M. White, E. W. Williams, P. Porteous, and C Hilsum, *Brit. J. Appl. Phys.* **3**, 1322 (1970).
70. C. J. Nuese, D. Richman, and R. B. Clough, *Met. Trans.* **2**, 789 (1971).
71. A. G. Sigai, C. J. Nuese, M. S. Abrahams, and R. E. Enstrom, *J. Electrochem. Soc.* **119**, 98C (1972).
72. A. W. Mabbitt, *J. Mater. Sci.* **5**, 1043 (1970).
73. G. B. Stringfellow, *J. Electrochem. Soc.* **117**, 1301 (1970).
74. A. Onton, M. R. Lorenz, and W. Reuter, *J. Appl. Phys.* **42**, 3420 (1971).
75. H. Rodot, J. Horak, G. Rovy, and J. Bourneix, *C. R. Acad. Sci. Paris* **269**, B381 (1968).
76. E. W. Williams, A. M. White, A. Ashford, C. Hilsum, P. Porteous, and D. R. Wright, *J. Phys. C* **3**, L55 (1970).
77. B. W. Hakki, A. Jayaraman, and C. K. Kim, *J. Appl. Phys.* **41**, 5291 (1970).
78. G. B. Stringfellow, P. R. Lindquist, and R. A. Burmeister, *J. Mater. Sci.* **1**, 437 (1972).
79. R. Z. Bachrach and B. W. Hakki, *J. Appl. Phys.* **42**, 5102 (1971).
80. H. Kressel, C. J. Nuese, and I. Ladany, *J. Appl. Phys.* **44**, 3266 (1973).
81. J. Chevallier and A. Laugier, *Phys. Status Solidi* **8**, 437 (1971).
82. A. Onton and R. J. Chicotka, *Phys. Rev. B* **4**, 1847 (1971).
83. G. A. Antypas and L. W. James, *J. Appl. Phys.* **41**, 2165 (1970).
84. M. B. Panish, *J. Phys. Chem. Solids* **30**, 1083 (1969).
85. K. K. Shih, *J. Electrochem. Soc.* **117**, 387 (1970).
86. G. A. Antypas, *J. Electrochem. Soc.* **117**, 700 (1970).
87. K. Osamura, J. Inoue, and Y. Murakami, *J. Electrochem. Soc.* **119**, 103 (1972).
88. G. B. Stringfellow and P. E. Greene, *J. Electrochem. Soc.* **118**, 805 (1971).
89. K. K. Shih and E. A. Peretti, *Trans. AIME* **48**, 706 (1956).
90. K. K. Shih and E. A. Peretti, *Trans. AIME* **46**, 389 (1954).
91. J. C. Woolley and B. A. Smith, *Proc. Phys. Soc.* **72**, 214 (1958).
92. J. L. Merz and R. T. Lynch, *J. Appl. Phys.* **39**, 1988 (1968).
93. M. B. Panish, R. T. Lynch, and S. Sumski, *Trans. AIME* **245**, 559 (1969).
94. L. M. Foster and J. E. Scardefield, *J. Electrochem. Soc.* **117**, 534 (1970).
95. A. Onton and R. J. Chicotka, *J. Appl. Phys.* **41**, 4205 (1970).
96. Ya. Agaev and N. G. Bekmedova, *Sov. Phys.-Semicond.* **5**, 1330 (1972).
97. O. Madelung, "Physics of III–V Compounds." Wiley, New York, 1964.

98. M. Ilegems and M. B. Panish, *J. Phys. Chem. Solids* **35**, 409 (1974).
99. A. S. Jordan and M. Ilegems, *J. Phys. Chem. Solids* **36**, 329 (1974).
100. A. Antypas and R. L. Moon, *J. Electrochem. Soc.* **120**, 1574 (1973).
101. S. A. Bondar *et al., Sov. J. Quantum Electron.* **6**, 50 (1976).
102. G. A. Antypas and R. L. Moon, *J. Electrochem. Soc.* **121**, 416 (1974).
103. M. Ilegems and G. L. Pearson, *Annu. Rev. Mater. Sci.* **5**, 345 (1975).
104. R. D. Burham, N. Holonyak Jr., and D. R. Scifres, *Appl. Phys. Lett.* **17**, 455 (1970).
105. W. R. Hitchens, N. Holonyak, Jr., P. D. Wright, and J. J. Coleman, *Appl. Phys. Lett.* **27**, 245 (1975)

Chapter 12

Diode Fabrication and Related Topics

The construction of laser diodes includes the following major steps:

1.   Substrate preparation, which typically consists of obtaining a polished surface using combinations of mechanical and chemical treatments (Section 9.5).

2.   Growth of the various epitaxial layers needed including junction formation. Alternatively, diffusion directly into the substrate can be performed for homojunction diodes. In general, however, even for homojunction fabrication it is preferable to grow an epitaxial layer which is likely to be structurally superior to the substrate. Following this step, the wafer thickness is usually reduced by mechanical means to 75–100 μm.

3.   Junction delineation if stripe contacts are used.

4.   Metallization of the wafer on both sides.

5.   Cleaving of bars 200–800 μm wide to form the Fabry–Perot cavity.

6.   Isolation of individual chips by cutting with a wire saw for broad-area lasers, or cleaving of the chips if stripe contacts are used.

7.   The diode is mounted on a header and contacts are attached. Soft solders, such as indium, are used to eliminate possible damage to the diodes.

Figure 12.1.1 summarizes the steps in the fabrication process and shows the type of package commonly used for commercial laser diodes. Also shown is the formation of diode arrays (Section 14.1). In this chapter, we discuss major aspects of the technology with emphasis on the (AlGa)As–GaAs heterojunction and related III–V compound devices. Laser diodes of other materials (e.g, IV–VI compounds) share much of the technology, but with variances in material growth and junction formation (Section 13.2).

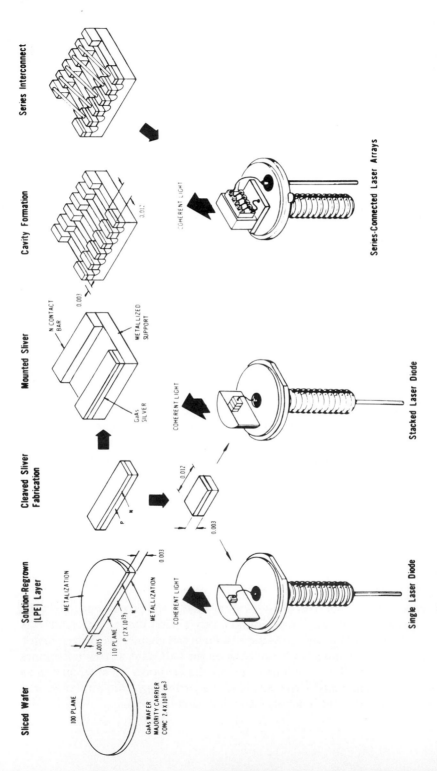

FIG. 12.1.1 Steps in the fabrication of a laser diode, stacked diodes, and linear diode array. All dimensions are in inches. (Courtesy RCA Solid State.)

The fabrication of heterojunction LEDs is similar in most respects, particularly for edge-emitting structures. Of course, cleaving of the facets is not essential (although it does provide a very desirable emitting surface), but stripe contacts are used for devices intended for applications requiring maximum radiance. Surface and edge emission heterojunction LEDs for high radiance applications are discussed in Section 14.4, and other types of heterojunction surface emitters are reviewed in Section 14.6.

12.1 Junction Formation and Layer Characterization

12.1.1 Junction Formation and Related Processes

Multiple-layer growth of heterojunction structures is exacting because it requires layers with widely varying compositions and dopings. In addition, the interfaces between these layers must be flat for laser use; there must be no contamination from one growth solution to the next; the layer thickness must be precisely controlled to submicron tolerance; and the final surface of the processed wafer must be free of any solution, to permit the application of ohmic contacts.

The process of zinc diffusion is widely used in heterojunction laser fabrication for reducing the contact resistance to the p-type region, and to form isolated stripe contacts as described in Section 12.3. Since GaAs will dissociate at the temperatures typically used for the diffusion, it is necessary to use sealed ampules containing As to minimize the surface dissociation. Various aspects of the Zn diffusion process to facilitate ohmic contact are discussed by Shih [1]. The masking of Zn to form isolated diffused regions can be accomplished with SiO_2, Si_3N_4, or Al_2O_3. Standard photolithographic techniques in common use in the silicon device industry are used for this purpose. It is sometimes necessary, however, to add P_2O_5 to SiO_2 to obtain complete masking against Zn during diffusion [1].

Liquid phase epitaxy is the preferred method of making (AlGa)As/GaAs heterojunction devices. The technique used in LPE (Chapter 9) growth consists of sequentially sliding a GaAs substrate into bins containing various solutions. There are many possible designs of the growth apparatus, but variations of the linear multiple-bin graphite boat [2–6] are the most popular for diode fabrication. In a model developed at RCA Laboratories and shown in Fig. 12.1.2a, a GaAs source wafer, usually polycrystalline, precedes the substrate wafer to assure saturation of the solution in each bin before growth on the substrate is initiated [5,6]. Figure 12.1.2b is an improvement over this design in that each solution has its own source wafer, leading to improved layer control. The elimination of oxygen for (AlGa)As growth by careful H_2 gas purification is essential. In a well-fabricated wafer, there are gradual steps on the surface with a height of 0.1 μm or less; thus, the wafer can be processed

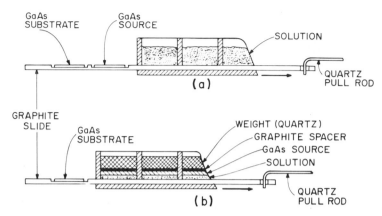

FIG. 12.1.2   Schematic illustration of LPE growth boat. (a) The saturation of the solutions is completed by the source wafer preceding the substrate; (b) each solution is saturated by its own source wafer [5].

for ohmic contact without final polishing. This is especially important for the CW laser where the active layers are within a few microns of the surface. Figure 12.1.3 shows a cross section of such a device.

The determination of the epitaxial layer thickness is conveniently done by first angle lapping and polishing samples at an angle of 1° and then staining or etching the material. Sodium hypochlorite works well on (AlGa)As heterojunction structures. Also, an etch developed by Abrahams and Buiocchi [7] is useful not only for revealing dislocations in the III–V materials, but as a means of delineating junctions as well.*

There is a vast literature concerning ohmic contacts to III–V materials which has been reviewed by Rideout [8]. Preferences vary but a commonly used contact to n-type material consists of sintered Sn or a two-layer Sn–Au

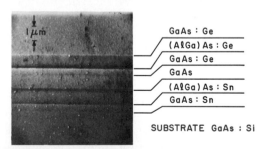

FIG. 12.1.3   Micrograph of the cross section of a six-layer epitaxial film grown using the multiple-bin boat of Fig. 12.1.2b [5].

---

* The A–B etch consists of the following. Solution A: 320 ml AgNO$_3$, 40 ml HF; solution B: 40 g CrO$_3$, 40 ml H$_2$O. The solutions are mixed 1 : 1 just prior to use, and a few seconds of etching time suffice.

contact. For p-type material, particularly where the metal is deposited partly over oxide, a thin Cr layer followed by a Au layer gives good contact, provided the doping level is relatively high (i.e., the GaAs layer is degenerately doped). This is frequently accomplished prior to metallization by a shallow Zn diffusion to provide a surface concentration of $\sim 10^{19}$ cm^{-3}. Tables 12.1.1 and 12.1.2 summarize various contacts used for III–V materials, but the list is far from complete. Ohmic contacts to other semiconductors are reviewed by Sharma and Purohit [9]. The difficulty of making ohmic contacts increases with bandgap energy. To facilitate contacts on (AlGa)As with sufficiently low resistance for CW laser operation, a ~ 1 μm thick GaAs "cap" layer is com-

TABLE 12.1.1

Ohmic Contact Technology for III–V Compound Semiconductors[a]

III–V	E_g (eV)	Type	Contact material	Technique	Alloy temperature (°C)	Application
AlN	5.9	Semi-I[b]	Si	Preform	1500–1800	Bistable resistor
		Semi-I	Al, Al–In	Preform	1000	Bistable resistor
		Semi-I	Mo, W	Sputter	500–1000	Bistable resistor
AlP	2.45	n	Ga–Ag	Preform	150	Hall measurements
AlAs	2.16	n,p	In–Te	Preform	160	Hall measurements
		n,p	Au	Preform	700	Hall measurements
		n,p	Au–Ge	Preform		Hall measurements
		n	Au–Sn	Preform		Hall measurements
GaN	3.5	Semi-I	Al–In	Preform		Bistable resistor
GaP	2.26	p	Au–Zn (99 : 1)	Preform, evap.	700	LED
		p	Au–Ge	Preform	360	LED
		n	Au–Sn (62: 38)	Preform	700	LED
		n	Au–Si (98 : 2)	Evap.	600	LED
GaAs	1.42	p	Au–Zn (99 : 1)	Electroless, evap.		LED
		p	In–Au (80 : 20)	Preform		LED
		n	Au–Ge (88: 12)	Evap.	350–450	Gunn oscillator
		n	In–Au (90 : 10)	Evap.	550	Gunn oscillator
		n	Au–Si (94 : 6)	Evap.	300	Gunn oscillator
		n	Au–Sn (90 : 10)	Evap.	350–700	Gunn oscillator
		n	Au–Te (98 : 2)	Evap.	500	Transistor
GaSb	0.73	p	In	Preform		Hall measurements
		n	In	Preform		Hall measurements
InP	1.34	p	In	Preform	350–600	LED
		n	In, In–Te	Preform	350–600	LED
		n	Ag–Sn	Preform, evap.	600	Gunn oscillator
InAs	0.35	n	In	Preform		Hall measurements
			Sn–Te (99 : 1)	Preform		Hall measurements
InSb	0.17	n	In	Preform		Hall measurements
		n	Sn–Te (99 : 1)	Preform		Hall measurements

[a]From Rideout [8].
[b]Semi-insulating.

TABLE 12.1.2

Ohmic Contact Technology for Mixed III–V Compound Semiconductors[a]

III–V	Type	Contact material	Techniques	Alloy temperature (°C)	Application
$GaAs_{1-x}P_x$	p	Au–Zn	Evap.	500	LED
	p	Al	Evap.	500	LED
	n	Au–Ge–Ni	Evap.	450	LED
	n	Au–Sn	Evap.	450	LED
$Al_xGa_{1-x}As$	p	Au–In	Electroplate	400–450	LED
	p	Au–Zn	Evap.	500	LED
	p	Al	Evap.	500	
	n	Au–Ge–Ni	Evap.	450–485	LED
	n	Au–Sn	Evap., electroless	450	LED
	n	Au–Si	Evap.		LED
$Ga_{1-x}In_xSb$	n	Sn–Te	Evap.		Gunn oscillator
$Al_xGa_{1-x}P$	n	Sn	Preform		LED
$In_xGa_{1-x}As$	n	Sn	Preform		LED
$InAs_xSb_{1-x}$	n	In–Te	Preform		Hall measurements

[a] From Rideout [8].

monly used on such heterojunction devices. The preferred method of attaching leads consists of using a soft solder such as indium because of the possibility of damaging the device with thermocompression bonding.

The performance of laser diodes is very sensitive to the metallurgical perfection of the active region. It is important to have a high internal quantum efficiency (i.e., freedom from nonradiative centers), planar junctions for radiation guiding to minimize scattering, and freedom from clustered defects which produce absorption in the vicinity of the p–n junction. Table 12.1.3 lists the effects of some major metallurgical defects on laser properties. The defects affecting LEDs (Table 12.1.4) are in many cases similar to those affecting laser diodes. However, junction planarity is much less important,

TABLE 12.1.3

Imperfections Affecting Particular Laser Parameters

Laser parameter	Imperfection
Internal quantum efficiency	Small precipitates, nonradiative centers
Absorption coefficient $\bar{\alpha}$	Precipitates, high free carrier density, nonplanar junctions
Nonuniform emission (random "beads" in the near-field pattern)	Nonuniform dopant density, precipitates, nonradiative centers, nonplanar junctions, damaged reflecting facets
Reliability (current density related)	Dislocations, contaminants, strain, precipitates

TABLE 12.1.4

Internal Loss Mechanisms in Electroluminescent Junctions[a]

Loss mechanism	Typical cause
Point imperfections:	
Vacancies	Deviation from stoichiometry during growth
Metal complexes, precipitates	Impurity concentrations approaching solubility in material
Frenkel defects	Generated by external electron bombardment; possibly formed during forward bias operation
Dislocations	Lattice mismatch between substrate and epitaxy; plastic deformation while cooling the material; stressed in assembly
Auger recombination	High carrier concentrations
Deep-level recombination	Contamination (e.g., Cu, O)
Surface or contact recombination	Location of surface or ohmic contact too close to p–n junction
Surface leakage	Work damage; surface contamination during device fabrication

[a]C. J. Nuese, H. Kressel, and I. Ladany, *IEEE Spectrum* **9**, 28 (1972).

the dopant concentrations need not be as precisely controlled, nor are the layer thicknesses as critical. Table 12.1.5 lists the major methods used to increase the external efficiency of LEDs.

TABLE 12.1.5

Methods for Increasing External Diode Efficiency[a]

Objective	Techniques
Minimize absorption coefficient	Keep absorbing layers thin
	Provide optical "window" with higher energy gap material
	Reduce carrier concentrations
	Generate below-bandgap radiation
Maximize surface transmissivity	Shape semiconductor for normal incidence
	Encapsulate diode with transparent material with high refractive index
	Apply antireflection coating

[a]C. J. Nuese, H. Kressel, and I. Ladany, *IEEE Spectrum* **9**, 28 (1972).

It is a common observation in LPE that as-grown surfaces are terraced. If the terracing is small (fraction of a micron in height), lithographic processes are generally unaffected in device preparation. However, there is concern that for active region widths of the same magnitude, the planarity may be inadequate for proper waveguiding. Marcuse [10] analyzed scattering in waveguides containing flaws, and this theory has been extended to heterojunction lasers [11]. Experimental data are as yet inadequate to define the reasonable limits junction planarity However, one expects that the higher the dielectric step and the thinner the guiding region, the more critical junction planarity becomes. Available data concerning J_{th} do suggest that the lack of junction planarity is a cause of scatter in the diode quality [12].

Many defects can be seen in epitaxial layers due to improperly cleaned substrates, nonuniform temperature in the growth apparatus (giving rise to uncontrolled meltback), and the presence of inclusions in the material. These flaws are, of course, not basic to the LPE growth process. The formation of terraces, however, is more closely related to the basic nucleation process as discussed by Lockwood [13], who showed that terracing can be minimized (height of steps $\approx$ 100 Å) in the growth of GaAs on GaAs by avoiding meltback entirely. This may be accomplished by introducing the wafer into the first solution after cool-down of the furnace has been initiated. Since the solution is As-saturated by contact with a GaAs source wafer, there is no possibility of supercooling occurring. The use of a very low cooling rate ensures near-equilibrium growth conditions. Finally, the importance of maintaining essentially oxygen-free growth systems cannot be overemphasized. In practice, this means less than 1 ppm in the gas stream. An infinite list of problems in the growth of alloys [14], particularly those containing Al, can be traced to oxygen contamination. The formation of Al_2O_3 inclusions, for example, is a prime factor in poor growth. Similarly, if the solution contains silicon, detrimental SiO_2 inclusions may form.

Single-Heterojunction "Close Confinement" Lasers. The degree of complexity in fabricating heterojunction lasers varies with the number of layers needed. The simplest heterojunction structure to prepare is the single-heterojunction "close confinement" laser, which requires only the growth of a single* Zn-doped (AlGa)As epitaxial layer on an n-type ($2-4 \times 10^{18}$ cm^{-3}) substrate (Fig. 12.1.4). The Zn diffuses from the epitaxial layer into the substrate a distance of about 2 μm [15]. The diffusion step can accompany the epitaxial growth or be separate. Because the recombination region is actually *within* the substrate, its crystalline perfection as well as the carrier concentration is important. Silicon-doped GaAs substrates grown by the Bridgman technique have been found to yield the best devices because of a moderate dislocation density ($\approx 10^3$ cm^{-2}) and relative freedom from precipitates, a significant difference from GaAs:Te [16]. Note that GaAs:Si grown from

---

* An additional GaAs:Zn "cap" is sometimes used when minimal diode resistance is desired. However, a natural Al concentration reduction in thick layers produces essentially GaAs at the surface, thus facilitating the ohmic contact.

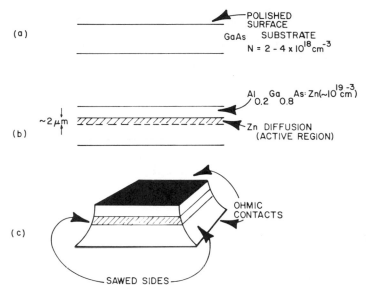

FIG. 12.1.4 Single-heterojunction (close-confinement) laser diode process. The melt-grown substrate in (a), usually Si doped for best results, is overgrown as in (b) with an epitaxial layer of (AlGa)As containing Zn. The diffused recombination region, $\sim 2~\mu$m thick, is formed either during the growth cycle or in a separate heat treatment step.

the melt is always n-type, in contrast to LPE–grown material where the growth temperature determines the majority carrier type (Chapter 10).

The refractive index step between the p-type Zn-diffused recombination region and the n-type region of the single-heterojunction laser strongly affects the device characteristics, particularly at high temperature (Section 7.3.3). The smaller the P–N refractive index step, the lower is the temperature at which mode guiding is lost, and at which the threshold current density increases steeply. Part of the refractive index difference at the p–n junction is due to the high electron concentration in the n-type region. As indicated in Section 12.2.1, the refractive index decreases with increasing free carrier concentration. Substrate carrier concentrations of $\sim 4 \times 10^{18}$ cm^{-3} are desirable for obtaining the best single-heterojunction high temperature diode operation. However, the defect density in such crystals is frequently too high, requiring somewhat lower substrate carrier concentrations to be used for good yields.

Instead of forming the recombination region by diffusion, it is also possible to grow the various regions of the single-hetrojunction laser separately using a multiple-bin boat [17]. However, the added complexity in multiple-layer fabrication is generally justified only for the LOC-type laser because of its improved performance compared to the single-heterojunction device.

Multiple-Layer Lasers. The most widely used acceptor for fabricating multiple-layer lasers is Ge rather than Zn, because of its lower vapor pressure which reduces the cross contamination of the epitaxial layers during growth. Although Ge is amphoteric in GaAs, when prepared by liquid phase epitaxy in the usual growth temperature range below 900°C it introduces predominantly a shallow acceptor. Hole concentrations up to $\sim 3 \times 10^{19}$ cm^{-3} can be obtained (Section 10.1). The ionization energy of Ge increases with Al concentration in (AlGa)As to a much greater extent than Zn, which limits the utility of Ge in Al-rich alloys, as discussed in Section 11.3.1.

The recombination region is commonly doped* with Si (which gives a compensated p-type region), lightly doped with Ge (order 10^{17} cm^{-3}), or left undoped to produce a region that is generally n-type ($\sim 10^{16}$ cm^{-3}) from residual donors. The first LOC lasers [18] had recombination regions formed by Zn outdiffusion from the p$^+$-(AlGa)As layer, but the growth of a Si-doped region is generally preferred and has yielded the best devices [19]. By adjusting the growth conditions, the p-n junction can also be made using only Si [20,21].

The donors used in LPE growth of GaAs and (AlGa)As devices are mostly Sn and Te (Chapters 10 and 11). The low segregation coefficient of Sn compared to Te eases the task of producing moderately doped GaAs layers (i.e., below 10^{18} cm^{-3}). However, the reduced segregation coefficient of Sn with added Al in (AlGa)As (Section 11.3.1) makes it desirable to use Te rather than Sn to obtain the $\sim 10^{18}$ cm^{-3} electron densities desirable in the passive regions of laser diodes to minimize the resistance.

For laser diodes of other III–V ternary compounds, the dopant selection is generally similar. Zinc is a generally useful acceptor dopant because the properties of the group IV impurities must be established for the specific alloy composition and growth conditions. However, Cd may be an alternative acceptor to Zn in some materials.

The extent of the diffusion length limits the maximum width of the recombination region. Table 10.1.3 lists values in GaAs. These are generally in excess of the width of the recombination region of useful laser diodes and do not, therefore, set a limit to their performance. With regard to other materials, it is likely that diffusion lengths of the order of 1 μm are readily achieved, making useful active region widths under that value certainly possible.

Vapor phase epitaxy is not commonly used for the preparation of (AlGa)As alloys, partly because of the reactivity of the gases transporting the Al. Furthermore, the choice of dopants is more restricted than in LPE. In particular, the use of Ge as an acceptor in VPE, desirable because of its low diffusion coefficient, is not possible because it enters GaAs as a donor [22]. The importance of VPE epitaxy is in growing dissimilar alloys combined into

---

* The doping in the active region can affect the diode reliability (Chapter 16).

heterojunction structures, particularly on lattice-mismatched substrates. The advantage of VPE (or molecular beam epitaxy) is in the ability to conveniently grade the composition of the compound in order to minimize the dislocation density of the active region (Chapter 9). Various applications of VPE to heterojunction structures are discussed in Chapter 13. For the moment we note that low J_{th} DH lasers suitable for CW operation have been produced by VPE with lattice-matched $GaAs/InGa_{0.49}P_{0.51}$ heterojunctions as indicated in Section 9.4. With a recombination region width $d_3 = 0.1$–0.2 μm, values of $J_{th} = 1100$ A/cm^2 were obtained at room temperature. These devices are produced by growing 3° from the (100) plane in the [110] direction, a method found to produce the best surfaces [23].

Laser diode fabrication is also possible with *molecular beam epitaxy*, which provides good control of layer thickness. Resonable quality heterojunction (AlGa)As/GaAs lasers have been made capable of 300 K CW operation [24]. Acceptor concentrations in GaAs or (AlGa)As appear relatively low compared to the 10^{19} cm^{-3} from other synthesis techniques. However, a combination of molecular beam and liquid phase epitaxy offers interesting possibilities. The use of MBE for growing over gratings in GaAs, as required for distributed-feedback lasers (Chapter 15), is particularly attractive since no meltback need occur. However, LPE has also been successfully used for this purpose with special precautions to minimize the meltback problem [25].

The growth of epitaxial layers in selected areas of the substrate is possible if a suitable mask is used. In LPE, the solution will not wet an oxide such as SiO_2, thus allowing the growth of layers in desired areas, although edge definition is commonly a problem. Vapor phase epitaxy has been similarly used to produce epitaxial devices in selected areas. The as-grown crystalline facets can furnish the required Fabry–Perot cavity without the conventional cleaving process, and (InGa)As homojunction lasers were thus formed on GaAs substrates [26].

It must be emphasized that the device reliability is intimately related to the fabrication technology and material synthesis method, as discussed in Chapter 16. Therefore, although it is possible to obtain low threshold lasers (and high radiance LEDs) by various epitaxial techniques, the acid test of the technology is the reliability of the devices produced and not simply the convenience of the technique. The greatest success has been achieved with LPE devices, but it is probable that in the future the quality will be matched with other technologies as the factors affecting reliability are better identified.

Facet Coatings. The use of reflecting and antireflecting coatings on laser facets provides increased power emission from one side of the device. In addition, antireflecting coats of appropriate thickness and index increase the device resistance to facet damage (Chapter 16). Gold is the most widely used reflecting film; it has a reflectivity of 97–98% between 7000 and 9000 Å. In principle, it is possible simply to evaporate a thin gold film directly on the diode strip. The thin gold film provides a high resistance which is not sufficient to short the diode at the currents typically used. However, such films do not adhere well enough to survive the diode assembly process and deteriorate further during operation. A more useful coating is provided by first evaporating an insulating layer (e.g., $SiO_2 \approx 300$ Å), followed by the Au layer. It is the practice to mask one diode edge from the Au film to minimize shunt junction leakage.

The deposition of the antireflecting coatings generally involves a single layer adjusted in thickness for the appropriate reflectivity at the laser wavelength. Silicon oxides and Al_2O_3 are used for this purpose. In addition, multiple layers may be used (e.g., involving ZnS).

12.1.2   Material Characterization

In the process of developing device technology, it is desirable to characterize individual layers. The layer characterization of heterojunction structures is difficult by electrical methods because of superimposed n- and p-type layers. In general, Hall measurements are best carried out by growing the desired epitaxial layer individually on a semi-insulating substrate. Alternatively, a p-n junction may be used as the barrier separating one layer from the next. Even with semi-insulating substrates, however, errors in the Hall measurements may be introduced if dopants diffuse during growth from the epitaxial layer into the substrate, because part of the substrate now becomes conducting. Detailed analysis of thin epitaxial layers by electrical measurements is discussed by Wieder [27] and Stillman and Wolfe [28]. Methods for measuring material composition and dopant concentrations are reviewed by Honig [29], and Table 12.1.6 summarizes the major methods and the sensitivities achieved. The electron microprobe is most generally used to determine the Al concentration in (AlGa)As and similar alloys where the lattice parameter changes little with composition. However, for alloys with large lattice parameter variation with composition, x-ray lattice parameter measurements are convenient, although the electron microprobe is increasingly used.

A useful analytical tool consists of photoluminescence (PL) measurements to determine the bandgap energy of the material, and frequently the approximate carrier concentration as well. In the case of GaAs, for example, the hole concentration can be estimated from the position of the peak energy and/or the width of the emitted radiation. Figure 12.1.5 shows this effect in GaAs:Ge and GaAs:Zn at room temperature [30], but for low concentration (under 10^{17} cm^{-3}) PL measurements at 300 or 77 K are not sufficiently sensitive. For n-type GaAs, Fig. 12.1.6a shows the 77 K position of the peak energy in relatively uncompensated material as a function of the 300 K electron concen-

TABLE 12.1.6a

Survey of Major Methods of Materials Characterization[a]

PRIMARY EXCITATION \ DETECTED EMISSION	OPTICAL	X-RAYS	ELECTRONS	IONS (+ AND −)
PHOTONS — OPTICAL	"AA": ATOMIC ABSORPTION "IR": INFRARED VISIBLE } SPEC- "UV": ULTRAVIOLET } TROS- COPY		"ESCA": ELECTRON SPECTR. F. CHEMICAL ANALYSIS — "UPS": VAC. UV PHOTOELECTRON SPECTROSCOPY — OUTER SHELL "XPS": X-RAY PHOTOELECTRON SPECTROSCOPY — INNER SHELL	
PHOTONS — X-RAYS		X-RAY FLUORESCENCE SPECTROMETRY X-RAY DIFFRACTION		
ELECTRONS		"EPM": ELECTRON-PROBE MICRO-ANALYSIS	"AES": AUGER ELECTRON SPECTROSCOPY "SAM": SCANNING AUGER MICROANALYSIS - - - - - - "SEM": SCANNING ELECTRON MICROSCOPY "TEM": TRANSMISSION ELEC-TRON MICROSCOPY	
IONS (+ AND −)	["SCANIIR": Surf. Comp. by Anal. of Neutral and Ion Impact Radiation]	[Ion-Induced X-Rays]		"SIMS": SECONDARY ION MASS SPECTRO-METRY "IPM": ION-PROBE MICRO-ANALYSIS "ISS": ION SCATTERING SPECTROMETRY ["RBS": Rutherford Backscattering Spectrometry]
RADIATION	"ES": EMISSION SPECTROSCOPY			"SSMS": SPARK SOURCE MASS SPECTRO-GRAPHY

[a]From Honig [29].

TABLE 12.1.6b

Survey of Methods for Surface and Thin-Film Analysis[a]

METHOD	PROBE DIAMETER μm	SAMPLING DEPTH μm	SAMPLING DEPTH ATOMIC LAYERS	OPTIMUM DETECTION SENSITIVITY (ppm atomic)	REPRODUCI-BILITY (%)	COVERAGE OF ELEMENTS	SPECIAL FEATURES	APPROX. PRICE (K$)[b]
X-RAY FLUORESCENCE SPECTROMETRY	10^4	3-100	10^4-$3 \cdot 10^5$	1-100	±1	NEARLY COMPLETE ($Z \geqslant 9$)	QUANTITATIVE; NONDESTRUCTIVE; INSULATORS	25
ELECTRON-PROBE MICROANALYSIS	1	0.03-1	10^2-$3 \cdot 10^3$	100-1000	±2	COMPLETE ($Z \geqslant 4$)	QUANTITATIVE; "NONDESTRUCTIVE"	100
SOLIDS MASS SPECTROGRAPHY	10-100	1-10	$3 \cdot 10^3$ -$3 \cdot 10^4$	0.01-10	±20 ±2	NEARLY COMPLETE	SEMI-QUANTITATIVE; ION-SENSITIVE PLATES ELECTRICAL READOUT	100 150
ION SCATTERING SPECTROMETRY	10^3		1	0.1-1%	±20	NEARLY COMPLETE NO H, He	SEMI-QUANTITATIVE; IN-DEPTH CONC. PROF. INSULATORS	40
SECONDARY ION MASS SPECTROMETRY	10^3		3	0.1-100	±2	NEARLY COMPLETE	SEMI-QUANTITATIVE; IN-DEPTH CONCENTRA-TION PROFILE	25-100
ION-PROBE MICROANALYSIS	1-300		10-1000	0.1-100	±2	NEARLY COMPLETE	SEMI-QUANTITATIVE; THREE-DIMENSIONAL CONC. PROFILE	300
AUGER ELECTRON SPECTROMETRY	25-100		2-10	0.01-0.1%	±20	NEARLY COMPLETE NO H, He	SEMI-QUANTITATIVE; THREE-DIMENSIONAL CONC. PROFILE	55
"SAM": SCANNING AUGER MICROANALYSIS	4-15		2-10	0.1-1%	±20	NEARLY COMPLETE NO H, He	SEMI-QUANTITATIVE; THREE-DIMENSIONAL CONC. PROFILE; TWO DIM'L AUGER IMAGES	100
"XPS": X-RAY PHOTOELECTRON SPECTROSCOPY ("ESCA")	10^4		2-10	1%	±20	NEARLY COMPLETE NO H, He	SEMI-QUANTITATIVE; VALENCE STATES	150

[a]From Honig [29].
[b]1975 prices.

TABLE 12.1.6c

Surface and Thin-Film Methods—Capabilities and Limitations[a]

METHOD	DETECTION SENSITIVITY OPTIMUM (ppma)	RANGE FACTOR	EFFECTS MATRIX	GEOMETRICAL	CHARGE-UP & FIELD PROBLEMS	BEAM INDUCED CHEM'L CHANGES	DEPTH RES. RASTER/GATING WITHOUT	WITH	LATERAL RESOL'N	ELEM'L IDENT'N	TYP-ICAL ANAL'L TIME	CAPABILITIES / LIMITATIONS
X-RAY FLUORESCENCE SPECTROMETRY	1-100				NO				NONE	GOOD	15 min	C: NON-DESTRUCTIVE; QUANTITATIVE; FAST; L: Z>9
ELECTRON-PROBE MICROANALYSIS	100-1000	10	SOME	YES	YES	YES			EXC.	GOOD	1 h	C: "NON-DESTRUCTIVE;" QUANTITATIVE; AREA AND LINE SCANS L: Z>4
SOLIDS MASS SPECTROGRAPHY	0.01-10	10			YES				FAIR	EXC.	1 h	C: SENSITIVE SURVEY METHOD
ION SCATTERING SPECTROMETRY	0.1-1%	10		YES	NO	YES	POOR	FAIR	POOR	FAIR	3 h	C: TRUE "SURFACE" ANALYSIS; INSULATORS; DEPTH PROFILE
SECONDARY ION MASS SPECTROMETRY	0.1-100	10^4	SEVERE		YES	YES	POOR	GOOD	FAIR	GOOD	30 min	C: DEPTH PROFILE; L: MATRIX EFFECTS
ION-PROBE MICROANALYSIS	0.1-100	10^4	SEVERE	YES	YES	YES	POOR	GOOD	GOOD	GOOD	30 min	C: AREA AND LINE SCANS; DEPTH PROFILE; L: MATRIX EFFECTS
AUGER ELECTRON SPECTROMETRY	0.01-0.1%	20			YES	YES	GOOD		FAIR	GOOD	30 min	C: DEPTH PROFILE MULTIPLEXING OF SIX ELEMENTS
"SAM": SCANNING AUGER MICROANALYSIS	0.1-1%	20			YES	YES	GOOD		GOOD	GOOD	1 h	C: AREA AND LINE SCANS; DEPTH PROFILES OF SIX ELEMENTS
"XPS": X-RAY PHOTOELECTRON SPECTROSCOPY ("ESCA")	1%				NO				NONE	FAIR	10 h	C: MOLECULAR INFORMATION; VALENCE STATES L: SLOW METHOD

[a]From Honig [29].

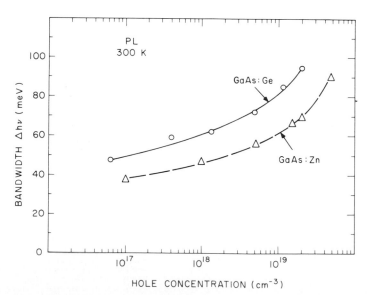

FIG. 12.1.5 Photoluminescence band half-width as a function of hole concentration for GaAs layers doped with Zn and Ge [30].

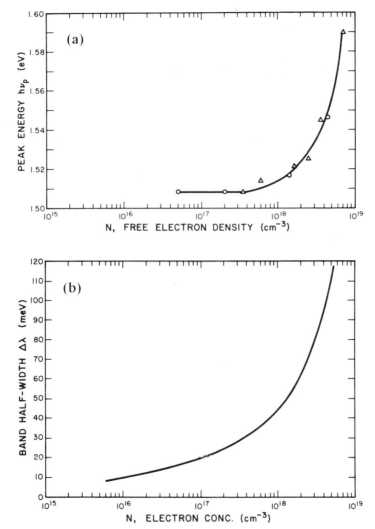

FIG. 12.1.6 Photoluminescence of 77 K from n-type GaAs:Si prepared by vapor phase epitaxy (which produces lightly compensated layers). (a) Peak energy as a function of electron concentration [N determined by Hall measurements ($\triangle$) and from bandgap radiation half-width ($\bigcirc$)]; (b) band half-width.

tration. The band half-width is a particularly useful measurement as shown in Fig. 12.1.6b. However, if the material is rather closely compensated, then PL measurements may be misleading since the peak position and bandwidth depend on the compensation ratio.

The greatest difficulty in characterizing epitaxial layers by PL is encountered with indirect bandgap material where deep centers commonly dominate the radiative processes. In this case, intense excitation using an electron beam (e.g., a demountable 5 keV system) is useful because with sufficient excitation, the deep center recombination saturates, leaving dominant band edge luminescence. Figure 12.1.7 shows a convenient cathodoluminescence apparatus developed by Nicoll [31].

For lightly doped layers, or to study impurity gradients for which photoluminescence measurements are not convenient, evaporated gold Schottky barriers are utilized to determine the carrier concentration, on the basis of capacitance–voltage measurements, using the following equation for an abrupt junction:

$$|N_D - N_A| = \frac{2}{\varepsilon e A^2}\left[\frac{\partial(1/C^2)}{\partial V}\right]^{-1} \tag{12.1.1}$$

where A is the diode area and ε is the dielectric constant.

Following the measurement, the gold dots can be removed in an aqueous KCN solution. Carrier concentrations obtained by this method are typically within 50% of the values obtained from Hall measurements.

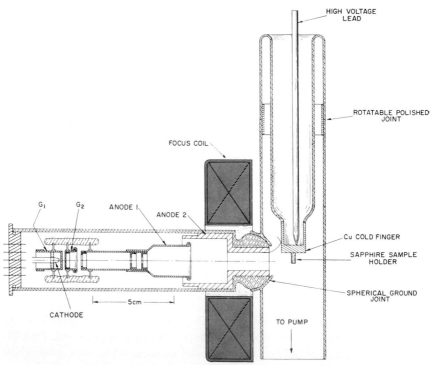

FIG. 12.1.7 Simple cathodoluminescence apparatus suitable for material characterization (F. H. Nicoll, unpublished).

12.2   Some Key Properties of Al$_x$Ga$_{1-x}$As Relevant to Device Design

12.2.1   Refractive Index

The effective refractive index step Δn in GaAs–(AlGa)As heterojunction lasing structures has been determined [32], as a function of the bandgap energy step, from the radiation patterns. These data are shown in the form of the plot (curve A) of Δn vs. x at $\lambda_L \cong 0.9\ \mu$m in Fig. 12.2.1 (where x is the Al concentration in the high bandgap side of the junction), with the relationship $\Delta n \cong 0.6\ \Delta x$.

Figure 12.2.1 (curve B) shows Δn vs. x (at $\lambda_L \cong 0.9\ \mu$m) deduced from direct index measurement of epitaxial layers [33]. Up to $x \cong 0.38$, $\Delta n \cong 0.75\ \Delta x$, with bowing at the high x value end. (The estimated accuracy in determining x is generally ± 0.02.) For comparison we note that the measured refractive index at $\lambda = 0.9\ \mu$m is 3.59 in GaAs and 2.97 in AlAs [34]. Assuming a linear

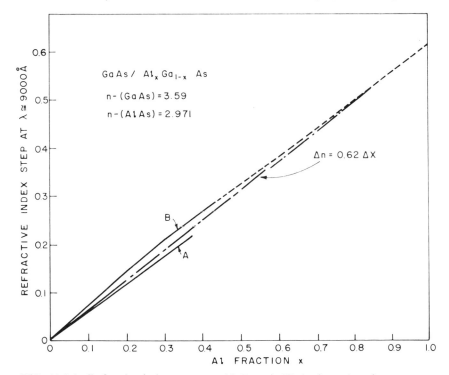

FIG. 12.2.1   Refractive index step at a Al$_x$Ga$_{1-x}$As/GaAs heterojunction at a wavelength of about 9000 Å, as a function of x. Line A is from Kressel *et al.* [32] and line B is from Casey *et al.* [33]. The line $\Delta n = 0.62\ \Delta x$ is a convenient approximation which can be used to determine the refractive index step in the vicinity of the lasing wavelength for heterojunctions with Al in both regions, as long as one side is in the direct bandgap energy composition range.

dependence of n on the Al concentration at $\lambda = 0.9$ μm, we estimate an average value of $\Delta n = 0.62$ Δx. This relationship can also be used to estimate the refractive index step between the active and outer regions of the hetero-junction if the active region contains (AlGa)As instead of GaAs. The reason is that the refractive index *at the lasing wavelength* remains essentially constant at 3.59 [33].

The carrier and dopant concentrations affect the refractive index. The refractive index has been calculated for GaAs at 300 and 77 K from absorption coefficient data [35,36], and measured for photon energies between 1.2 and 1.8 eV at room temperature, using differently doped samples [37]. Figure 12.2.2 shows measured index values for n- and p-type GaAs.

In addition to changes in the density of states distribution with doping (which changes the shape of the absorption curve), a contribution to the refractive index due to intraband absorption of free carriers depresses the index. The approximate expressions given by Stern [35] are useful in estimating the difference in refractive index at p–n junctions, p$^+$–p or n$^+$–n interfaces. For n-type material, the only significant contribution is from *intraband* absorption:

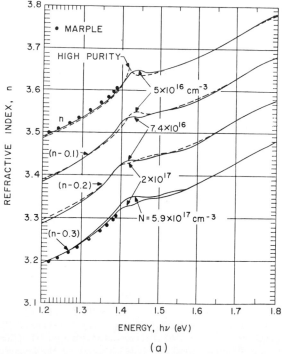

(a)

FIG. 12.2.2 Measured refractive index as a function of wavelength for (a, b) n-type GaAs, and (c, d) p-type GaAs. ●, data of Marple [38], lines from Sell *et al.* [37].

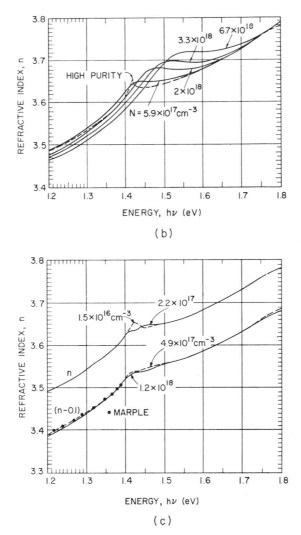

FIG. 12.2.2   Continued

$$\Delta n_{\text{intra}} = -9.6 \times 10^{-21} N/nE^2 \qquad (12.2.1)$$

where N, n, and E are electron concentration, index of refraction, and photon energy, respectively.

For p-type material, *interband* transitions are significant also, and the total free carrier contribution is

$$\Delta n_{\text{inter}} + \Delta n_{\text{intra}} \cong (-1.8 \times 10^{-21} P/nE^2) - (6.3 \times 10^{-22} P/E^2) \qquad (12.2.2)$$

where P is the hole concentration. In GaAs, as an example, for 10^{18} cm^{-3}

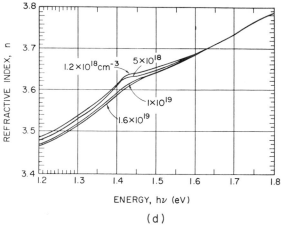

(d)

FIG. 12.2.2 Continued

electrons, $\Delta n = -0.0014$; with 10^{18} cm^{-3} holes, $\Delta n = -0.00026 - 0.00032 = -5.8 \times 10^{-4}$. In the case of injection into a recombination region, the index will be reduced as a result of both the injected electrons and holes. This reduction can significantly lower the index at a p–n junction, an effect important in single-heterojunction lasers as discussed in Section 7.3.3.

12.2.2   Thermal Conductivity

The thermal conductivity of Al$_x$Ga$_{1-x}$As affects the thermal resistance of lasing structures. Figure 12.2.3 shows the data of Afromowitz [39] compared to the theoretical curve of Abeles [40]. It is evident that the (AlGa)As layers between the active region and the heat sink should be thin, requiring a compromise with the need for proper radiation confinement as discussed in Section 7.3.

12.2.3   Internal Quantum Efficiency of Ternary Alloys

The radiative efficiency of the device is ultimately limited by the internal quantum efficiency. In this section, we discuss the limitation set by the distribution of the injected carriers among the direct conduction band valley (Γ) and the indirect valleys, which in the present illustration are the X valleys.

As the energies of the Γ and X conduction band minima approach each other with increasing Al concentration (see Fig. 11.1.5), an increasing fraction of the carriers injected into the recombination region are transferred by thermal activation from the Γ to the X valleys. It is generally assumed that the carriers in the indirect conduction band valleys do not contribute to radiative recombination or stimulated emission. Table 12.2.1 lists the bandgap param-

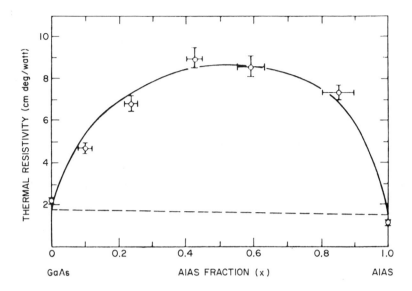

FIG. 12.2.3   The thermal resistivity of the $Al_xGa_{1-x}As$ alloy system [39]. The solid curve is a theoretical fit to the data using the model of Abeles [40].

TABLE 12.2.1

Bandgap Energy and Crossover Composition Values x_c for Four Ternary Alloys[a]

Compound	Bandgap energy range (eV)	E_{gc}	x_c	Lattice constant a_0 range (Å)	Best substrate near E_{gc}	Maximum practical[b] photon energy λ_m for direct bandgap emission (Å)	Color
					GaAs[e]		
$GaAs_xP_{1-x}$	1.42–2.26	1.99	0.452	5.6533–5.4506	($a_0 =$ 5.6533 Å)	1.89 6560	Red
$Al_xGa_{1-x}As$	1.42–2.16	1.92^d	0.37^d	5.6533–5.6607	GaAs	1.82 6800	Red
$In_{1-x}Ga_xP$	1.34–2.26	2.17	0.616	5.8694–5.4506	GaAs[e]	2.07 6000	Yellow
$Al_xIn_{1-x}P$	1.34–2.45	2.23	0.394	5.8694–5.4625	GaAs[e]	2.13 5820	Green

[a]Data collected by R. J. Archer, *J. Electron. Mater.* **1**, 128 (1972) except as noted in (d).
[b]Assuming $h\nu = E_{gc} - 0.1$ eV.
[e]Substantial lattice mismatch between epitaxial layer and the substrate.
[d]Based on electroreflectance data of O. Berolo and J. C. Wooley, *Can. J. Phys.* **49**, 1335 (1971).

eters for ternary alloy systems, in addition to (AlGa)As, of current or potential interest in laser diode fabrication.

The simplest approximation, and one that yields reasonable agreement with experiment, consists of defining the internal quantum efficiency in terms of the fraction of injected carriers ΔN in the Γ valley, $(\Delta N)_\Gamma$, and those in the X (or other indirect) valley $(\Delta N)_X$. We assume that the carriers in the indirect valleys recombine nonradiatively, and that the transfer of carriers between the valleys is rapid compared to the recombination time. Then, in steady state, the internal quantum efficiency is

$$\eta_i = [1 + (\Delta N)_X/(\Delta N)_\Gamma]^{-1} \qquad (12.2.3)$$

When the electron population is degenerate, as appropriate under lasing conditions, then the shift of the quasi-Fermi level E_{Fc} into the conduction band must be considered in determining the distribution of the injected carriers between the Γ and X minima [41]. We recall from Section 1.4 that the carrier population is related to the Fermi level by the integral of the product of the density of states and of the Fermi–Dirac distribution function. Assuming parabolic bands, we obtain for the population in the Γ valley,

$$(\Delta N)_\Gamma = 6.55 \times 10^{21} (m_{c\Gamma}^*)^{3/2} \int_{E_{c\Gamma}}^{\infty} \frac{(E - E_{c1})^{1/2}\, dE}{1 + \exp[(E - E_{Fc})/kT]} \qquad (12.2.4)$$

For the electron population in the X valleys, located at $E_{cX} = E_{c\Gamma} + \Delta E$ above the Γ minimum,

$$(\Delta N)_X = 6 \times 6.55 \times 10^{21} (m_{cX}^*)^{3/2} \int_{E_{cX}}^{\infty} \frac{(E - E_{cX})^{1/2}\, dE}{1 + \exp[(E - E_{Fc})/kT]} \qquad (12.2.5)$$

The following values for effective masses and separation between the direct and indirect valleys have been quoted for $Al_xGa_{1-x}As$ [42]:

$$m_{c\Gamma}^* = 0.0636 + 0.0552x + 0.0092x^2 \qquad (12.2.6)$$

$$m_{cX}^* = 0.39(1 - x) + 0.37x, \qquad m_v^*(AlAs) = 0.85$$

In GaAs, using $\Delta E = 0.38$ [43] for illustration,*

$$E_\Gamma(x) = 1.424 + 1.266x + 0.266x^2, \qquad \Delta E(x) = 0.38 - 0.892x - 0.365x^2$$

To calculate $(\Delta N)_X$, and hence the differential quantum efficiency at lasing threshold, various assumptions can be made concerning the required density of carriers in the Γ conduction band valley. Since the upward shift in the quasi-Fermi level reduces the effective separation from the X minima, the internal quantum efficiency will strongly decrease with the injected carrier density in p-type material. This is seen in Fig. 12.2.4, which shows η_i as a function of x and of $(\Delta N)_\Gamma$. As indicated in Section 3.3, $(\Delta N)_{th} = 1.5$–2×10^{18}

---

* This energy separation between the direct and indirect conduction band minima is approximate and is used here for convenience.

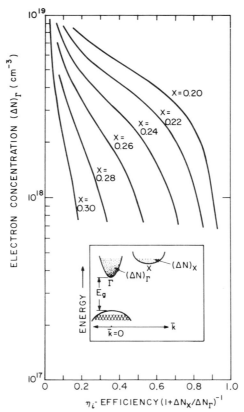

FIG. 12.2.4 Calculated internal quantum efficiency of Al$_x$Ga$_{1-x}$As at 300 K as a function of x for various electron densities in the Γ conduction band valley. The L minima are neglected.

cm^{-3} in GaAs at 300 K. Figure 12.2.5 shows the internal quantum efficiency versus x plotted for $(\Delta N)_\Gamma = 1.5 \times 10^{18}$ cm^{-3}. Other factors being constant, we expect the laser threshold current density to decrease along with the internal quantum efficiency. Experimental data concerning this effect are presented in Section 14.5.

For relatively low carrier injection levels (e.g., as appropriate in typical LED operation), Eqs. (12.2.4) and (12.2.5) can be simplified since a non-degenerate carrier population can be assumed. With this assumption, the carrier distribution among the conduction band valleys follows the effective density of states $N_{c\Gamma}$ and N_{cX} (with the band edges of the Γ and X minima separated by ΔE):

$$\eta_i = [1 + M(m_{eX}^*/m_{e\Gamma}^*)^{3/2} \exp(-\Delta E/kT)]^{-1} \qquad (12.2.7)$$

where M is the number of equivalent indirect valleys.

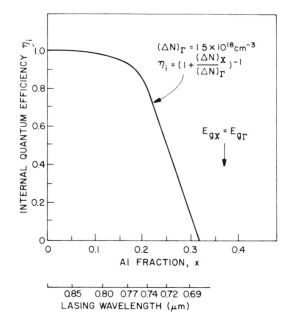

FIG. 12.2.5   Calculated internal quantum efficiency in $Al_xGa_{1-x}As$ at 300 K as a function of x and of the lasing wavelength. It is assumed that the electron density in the Γ conduction band valley is 1.5×10^{18} cm^{-3}. The L minima are neglected.

The reduction in the internal quantum efficiency as a function of alloy composition has been determined experimentally in (AlGa)As, (InGa)P, and Ga(AsP). The data (obtained from spontaneous luminescence measurements) are shown in Fig. 12.2.6 as a function of emission photon energy [44]. The calculated curves (assuming a density of states ratio of 50 [45]) for each of the alloy systems are superimposed on the data with reasonable agreement. [There are no experimental data for (InAl)P.] Note that these data are compared to calculations that neglect the effect of the L conduction band minima on the radiative efficiency in (AlGa)As and Ga(AsP). However, since the direct-to-indirect bandgap crossover is controlled by the X and Γ valleys, this neglect does not significantly change the rapid efficiency reduction predicted from this simple analysis.

12.3   Active Junction Area Definition

The maximum optical power rating of a given construction depends on the thickness of the waveguide region (i.e., the optical flux density) and the extent of the emitting facet region. Originally, CW operation was reported with

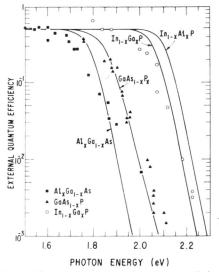

FIG. 12.2.6 Variation of the relative external quantum efficiency (low injection and low doping) in ternary alloys as a function of the emitted photon energy. The internal efficiency may be assumed to follow the external efficiency. The solid curves are calculated assuming a density of states ratio of 50 between the direct and indirect conduction band valleys [44].

broad-area diodes [46], but stripe-contact diodes are now used exclusively for these room temperature lasers for the following reasons:

1. The radiation is emitted from a small area which simplifies coupling of the radiation into low numerical aperture fibers, which have typical diameters of ≤ 100 μm.

2. The operating current is low, usually well under 500 mA.

3. The thermal dissipation of the devices is improved since the heat-generating emission region is partly embedded in a nonactive semiconductor body.

4. The small active area improves the possibility of obtaining a low defect area conducive to long-term reliability.

5. The active region of the device can be isolated from open surfaces on its two major dimensions, which is essential in obtaining reliable operation (see Section 16.2).

Several basic techniques for making stripe-contact diodes are shown schematically in Fig. 12.3.1. The current path is defined as in Fig. 12.3.1a by using oxide masking to limit the ohmic contact area [47]; as in Fig. 12.3.1b by using selective diffusion [48]; as in Fig. 12.3.1c by etching a narrow "deep" mesa and using oxide masking [49] to prevent shorting of the junction during metallization; as in Fig. 12.3.1d by using (AlGa)As to fill in the space between

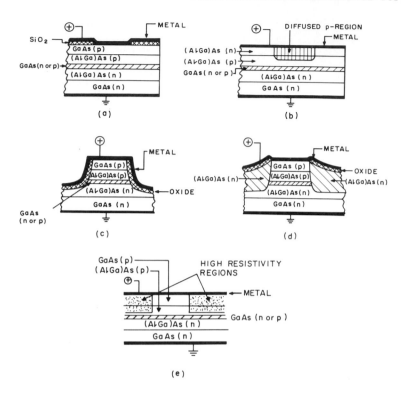

FIG. 12.3.1 Schematic cross section (end view) of various stripe-geometry structures. (a) Oxide isolated; (b) selective Zn diffusion into n-type "cap," thus providing only a selected area for the diode in forward bias; (c) "high" mesa stripe with metal overhang, using oxide coverage on the mesa edges. In another version of this structure (not shown), the "low" mesa is etched only to remove the GaAs surface layer, without exposing the diode edge, thus increasing the effective sheet resistance of the material on top of the active region); (d) buried stripe, in which (AlGa)As is grown into the previously etched out sides of the active region; (e) formation of resistive regions adjoining the active region by proton bombardment or oxygen implantation.

the mesas [50]; or as in Fig. 12.3.1e by using proton bombardment (or oxygen implants) [51] to form high resistivity regions in selective areas [52]. (Instead of using an oxide for isolation, stripe diodes have also been reported using an n-type $Al_{0.5}Ga_{0.5}As$ layer in which a contact area was etched to reach the p-type region [53].)

It is possible to use a shallow ("low") mesa configuration in the mesa-defined stripe-contact devices where the etching removes only the surface layer without exposing the edge of the active region. The removal of the conductive p-type GaAs surface layer does contribute to a reduction of the current spreading, as discussed herein. Although discussed for (AlGa)As devices, the stripe-contact formation techniques are of broad applicability.

Laser diode technology is still evolving and a definitive choice of the best stripe technique is premature, particularly since the laser reliability is affected by the fabrication technique. An important difference between the various stripe structures is in their lateral confinement and resultant effective diode area for a given stripe width. A planar stripe device, lacking lateral blocking regions at the recombination region edges, cannot be made arbitrarily narrow because of current and radiation [54] spread outside the contact area. The current spreading is limited with proton bombardment, a "low" mesa, or selective diffusion by the high resistance of the material surrounding the active area defined by the stripe, but there is some carrier loss by lateral diffusion *within* the recombination region in devices with no potential barrier to laterally confine the carriers [55, 56].

A further limitation of the planar stripe devices results from the lack of a significant refractive index step at the junction sides (Section 7.7). Therefore, as the stripe width is reduced, a greater fraction of the radiation is propagating beyond the stripe edges. Thus, the minimum stripe width of planar structures is limited by current and optical losses, which become increasingly important as the stripe width is reduced to a few light wavelengths. The only way to prevent these losses fully is to provide blocking "walls." This is accomplished by the deep mesa or the use of a high bandgap material deposited in the sides of the junction. However, such strongly laterally confined structures do provide a modal content drawback—high order *lateral* modes are more likely than with the planar devices, unless the stripe width is very narrow (on the order of $\leq 5 \ \mu m$).

The considerations just discussed deal with the problem of obtaining the lowest possible CW operating *current* by limiting the diode area and minimizing the "waste" of injected carriers. In practice, however, two other factors are important: first, the ease of reproducible device construction; and second, the achievement of very reliable operation with the required optical power output. With regard to technology, planar structures tend to be simpler to fabricate. As to reliability, the optical power output scales with emitting region width, and hence the stripe width. As discussed in Section 16.1, laser diodes can fail by a process of facet damage resulting from an excessive optical flux density. A value of approximately 1 mW/μm of stripe width appears a reasonable operating range for typical CW laser diodes. Thus, the device design should reflect the desired power level for sustained operation.

The impact of the stripe fabrication process on the resistance of the device to internal degradation (Section 16.2) is less clearly defined than the facet damage limit. The reason is the complexity of the factors controlling this "gradual" degradation mode in which defects are introduced in the active region of the device in the course of operation. A general rule is that it is essential to minimize the possibility of forming lattice defects (such as dislocations) in the course of fabrication and that the active region of the device must be isolated as much as possible from exposed surfaces or regions containing a high defect density from which migration into the recombination region can occur. In this regard, therefore, the oxide-isolated stripe is a desirable structure since it involves no fabrication process steps which are potentially detrimental (but the surface Zn diffusion requires care). The "deep" mesa device, on the other extreme, is the least desirable since the diode edges are exposed. The shallow mesa device, however, is basically comparable to the oxide-isolated structure. The other techniques all involve process steps in which care is needed to minimize the introduction of damage into the recombination region by careful control of diffusion steps or implantation procedures.

Practical CW laser diode structures typically produce about 10 mW of power (from one facet) and therefore have stripe widths of about 10–15 μm. Planar structures (in which we include the shallow mesa structure) are the most widely used. A convenient figure of merit for the effectiveness of a stripe-contact structure in using the injected carriers is to compare the calculated threshold current density J_{th}, assuming that *all* the current is confined under the stripe, to the threshold current density measured on similar laser material fabricated in the form of broad-area diodes, which we denote here $J_{th}(\infty)$.

A comparison of the ratio $J_{th}/J_{th}(\infty)$ is shown in Fig. 12.3.2 for oxide-isolated stripe diodes and deep mesa stripe lasers. In effect, we are comparing structures with partial and maximum lateral confinement. It is evident from the data that the deep mesa structure provides excellent lateral current confinement down to stripe widths of 10 μm, whereas the $J_{th}/J_{th}(\infty)$ ratio for the oxide-isolated stripes is substantially higher.

Although the planar stripe structures cannot offer the ideal confinement effect, it is still possible to change the vertical structure in order to minimize the current spread beyond the stripe edges. As subsequently discussed in detail, this confinement is accomplished by *maximizing* the sheet resistance of the layers between the recombination region and the *top* diode contact and *minimizing* the resistance between the recombination region and the bottom contact. A theoretical analysis of the subject has been presented by Joyce and Wemple [59]. Here we limit ourselves to a simple analysis of the lateral current spreading problem, neglecting the contribution from lateral diffusion *within* the recombination region.

Figure 12.3.3 shows the structure with a stripe contact width S_t. The distance between the surface of the diode and the recombination region is t_s.

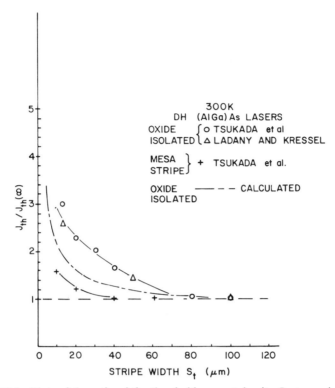

FIG. 12.3.2 Plots of the ratio of the threshold current density J_{th} (assuming that the current is laterally confined under the stripe) to $J_{th}(\infty)$, the threshold value measured on a broad-area device which has *full* lateral confinement. The experimental data are from Tsukada *et al.* [57] and Ladany and Kressel [58]. The calculated curve is from (12.3.5) with the values indicated in the text.

The conductivities of the GaAs surface layer* and of the (AlGa)As p-type layers generally differ, but for the present analysis we will assume an *average* sheet resistance of $r_s =$ resistivity/t_s in ohms/□. Following the analysis of Dumke [60], we consider the origin at the edge of the stripe as shown in Fig. 12.3.3a where $y = 0$. If I is the current conducted along the y direction, $J(y)$ the local current density, and V the potential of the p-type upper layers, then for $y = 0$,

$$dV/dy = r_s I \qquad (12.3.1)$$

and

$$dI/dy = J(y) = -J_{th}(\infty) \exp(eV/akT) \qquad (12.3.2)$$

* This layer can be dispensed with if good ohmic contact can be made to the high bandgap region directly. This provides the most direct means of increasing the sheet resistance.

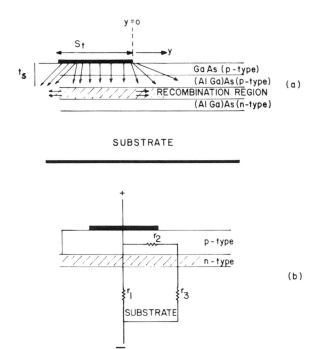

FIG. 12.3.3 Model of stripe using oxide isolation: (a) Current flow pattern; (b) definition of resistance of the various regions used to estimate the effective stripe width due to the current spread.

where $1 \leq a \leq 2$ (Chapter 2), and $J_{\text{th}}(\infty)$ is the current density for a fully laterally confined diode. Combining (12.3.1) and (12.3.2),

$$d^2 V/dy^2 = J_{\text{th}}(\infty) r_s \exp(eV/akT) \qquad (12.3.3)$$

Solving (12.3.3), we can estimate the current spread beyond the stripe edges. The stripe width is increased by ΔS_t to $S_t + \Delta S_t$ and the *effective* laser threshold current density is

$$J_{\text{th}} = J_{\text{th}}(\infty)(1 + \Delta S_t/S_t) \qquad (12.3.4)$$

where

$$\Delta S_t = 2\sqrt{2}[akT/(er_s J_{\text{th}}(\infty))] \qquad (12.3.5)$$

It is evident, therefore, that the lateral current spread in the surface layers can be minimized by increasing the sheet resistance r_s of these layers. This may be accomplished either by making the layers very thin, by etching some of the material away, or by making the layers resistive. However, very thin layers result in high optical losses as discussed in Chapters 7 and 8, whereas very resistive layers can increase the electrical resistance of the device unduly.

To illustrate a practical compromise using oxide-isolated structures, consider the following device values: $a \cong 1$, $r_s = 100$ ohms/$\square$, and $J_{th}(\infty) = 1500$ A/cm². Hence at 300 K,

$$\Delta S_t = 2.8 \left(\frac{0.026}{100 \times 1500}\right)^{1/2} \cong 12 \, \mu m$$

Therefore, a 13 μm-wide stripe would have an effective threshold current density nearly twice the value expected for full confinement, even neglecting other factors which can contribute to the carrier and radiation loss. It is evident that the narrower the stripe, the larger is the relative effect of the lateral carrier loss, which becomes negligible for a 50- or 100-μm-wide stripe.

Figure 12.3.2 shows a calculated plot of $J_{th}/J_{th}(\infty)$ as a function of the stripe width from Eq. (12.3.4) using $\Delta S_t = 12 \, \mu m$, i.e., the values considered for the typical illustration just given. The experimental relative increases in J_{th} with decreasing stripe width are seen to be about 50% higher than the calculated values for stripe widths below about 30 μm. As noted earlier, other factors contribute to the increased J_{th} in addition to the current spreading effect. For very narrow stripes ($\leq 10 \, \mu m$) it is likely that the optical losses due to radiation penetration into the adjoining passive regions of the device and carrier diffusion within the recombination region become increasingly important.

The preceding has assumed that the resistance of the layers *below* the active region is negligible compared to the lateral resistance. In fact, if the Al_xGa_{1-x} As n-type layer has a high series resistance ($x \geq 0.4$, $N \leq 10^{17}$ cm^{-3}), this need no longer be the case. Then, the lateral current spread will be larger than expected from (12.3.5) because the current will be distributed so as to minimize the overall series resistance. The effect can be understood from Fig. 12.3.3b where r_1 is the resistance in series with the stripe below the active region, r_2 denotes the lateral resistance, and r_3 is the resistance below the active region away from the stripe area. If the resistance r_1 is relatively large, then more of the current will tend to flow through the branch containing r_2 and r_3, thus extending the lateral current flow. Consider the following example using our previous values. The lateral resistance limiting the current flow r_2 is approximately

$$r_2 = \rho \, \Delta S_t / 2t_s L = r_s \, \Delta S_t / 2L \tag{12.3.6}$$

where L is the stripe length and ρ is the average resistivity of the two p-type surface layers. With $L = 500 \, \mu m$,

$$r_2 = \frac{(100)(6 \times 10^{-4})}{(2 \times 500 \times 10^{-4})} = 0.6 \text{ ohm}$$

To calculate r_1, assume that the (AlGa)As n-type layer has a resistivity $\rho_l =$

$(eN\mu)^{-1} = 1$ ohm-cm, and is 1 μm thick. The substrate is $D = 75$ μm thick with $\rho_s = 10^{-3}$ ohm-cm. Hence, r_1 consists of the sum of the (AlGa)As and substrate resistances (neglecting a spreading factor),

$$r_1 = \frac{\rho_l t_s}{LS_t} + \frac{\rho_s D}{LS_t} = 1.53 + 0.12 \cong 1.65 \text{ ohm-cm}$$

The effect of r_1 being large with respect to r_2 is to produce a distribution of the current such that the voltage drop across $r_2 + r_3$ equals that across r_1, leading to a reduction in the current flow directly under the stripe.

12.4 Thermal Dissipation of Laser Diodes

Parameters affecting the power emission from a laser diode are the thermal resistance, the temperature dependence of the threshold and differential quantum efficiency, and the electrical resistance. The temperature dependence of J_{th} is analyzed in Section 8.3 and is complex. However, for heterojunction lasers (and many homojunction lasers), the temperature dependence of the threshold current is approximated by the empirical form [61]

$$I_{th} \propto \exp[(T - T_0)/T_0] \tag{12.4.1}$$

where T_0 varies from 50 to 100 K, depending on the dopant concentration in the recombination region, and the magnitude of the bandgap energy steps at the heterojunctions which reduces the temperature dependence of J_{th} (Chapter 8).

The electrical resistance of the diode is reduced* by using highly doped p-type layers ($P > 10^{19}$ cm^{-3}) under the ohmic contact and thinning the various layers in series with the active region. For a typical 13-μm-wide stripe contact, a resistance of 0.5–1 ohm is considered reasonable.

The thermal resistance of the diode can be calculated from the horizontal and vertical geometry [62]. A simple estimate of the *maximum* thermal resistance of the various regions of the laser can be made for a planar stripe-contact double-heterojunction diode on the basis of the schematic shown in Fig. 12.4.1. The resistance of the Al$_{0.3}$Ga$_{0.7}$As, the GaAs contact regions, and the indium solder used to mount the diode p-side down on a copper heat sink is important. Table 12.4.1 shows the calculated thermal resistance of each region (neglecting lateral spreading) and the temperature rise for a power dissipation of 0.5 W. With the 1-μm-thick regions indicated, the resistance of the Al$_{0.3}$Ga$_{0.7}$As is dominant because of its low thermal conductivity.

This estimate for the thermal resistance is too large because of the neglect of the lateral current and heat spread within the semiconductor. As indicated earlier, the current is actually distributed over a width substantially in excess

---

* This requirement must be considered in light of the need to reduce current spread, Section 12.3.

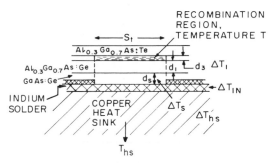

FIG. 12.4.1 Schematic cross section of stripe-contact laser diode, with oxide isolation, used to approximate the thermal resistance. The stripe width is S_t.

TABLE 12.4.1
Thermal Resistance of Laser Structure of Fig. 12.4.1[a]

Layer or region type	Thermal conductivity K_i (W/cm-°C)	Layer thickness d_i (μm)	Thermal resistance R_{th} (°C/W)	ΔT[b] (°C)
$Al_{0.3}Ga_{0.7}As$	0.13	1	14.8[c]	7.4
GaAs	0.5	1	3.9[c]	2
Indium	0.8	1	2.4[c]	1.2
Copper (heat sink)	4	∞	9.6[d]	4.8
Total			30.7	15.4

[a] Fabry–Perot cavity length $L = 400$ μm; stripe width $S_t = 13$ μm.
[b] Power dissipation, $P_i = 0.5$ W.
[c] $R_{th} = d_i/K_i A$, where A is the diode active source area, LS_t.
[d] $R_{th} \cong \ln(4L/S_t)/\pi K_{Cu}L$, where $L \gg S_t$.

of that of the stripe; hence the power is dissipated over a larger volume than assumed in the calculation, although the thickness of the oxide provides a thermal barrier. In fact, the measured [63] thermal resistance of typical stripe lasers of the type described here is in the range of 14–25°C/W, hence substantially below the calculated value of ~31°C/W.

The dissipation within the CW diode is essentially equal to the input power since the power efficiency near threshold is only a few percent. Hence, for a threshold current $I_{th} = 0.3$ A, a bandgap energy $E_g \cong 1.4$ V, and a series resistance of 1 ohm, the power input $P_i = I_{th}E_g/e + (I_{th}^2)R_s \cong 0.51$ W. Assuming a power conversion efficiency of 2%, the dissipated power is 0.5 W. The temperature rise of the active region above the heat sink temperature (far from the device) is therefore 7–12°C.

The maximum output for a pulsed laser occurs at a duty cycle set by the thermal and electrical resistance, the threshold current, and the value of T_0 (in the expression for I_{th}). Since the input power increases the temperature of the active region, lasing will be quenched by too high a duty cycle or diode current. Keyes [64, 65] obtained criteria for CW operation when the power dissipation due to the diode series resistance was small compared to the power dissipation in the junction itself (as was the case in the illustration considered here),

$$I_{th}E_gR_{th}/eT_0 < 0.37 \qquad (12.4.2)$$

where we assume that the junction built-in potential equals E_g/e and I_{th} is the threshold current at the junction temperature.

To illustrate this expression, we calculate the highest possible I_{th} value for which CW operation is possible using our illustrative structure of Fig. 12.4.1. Assuming $T_0 = 70$ K,

$$I_{th}(max) = \frac{0.37T_0e}{E_gR_{th}} = \frac{(0.37)(70)}{(1.4)(30.7)} = 0.6 \text{ A} \qquad (12.4.3)$$

This estimate exceeds the actual limit because of the neglect of ohmic heating, but is within a reasonable range of the actual I_{th} limit for CW operation of such structures, which is 0.5–0.6 A.

Knowing the maximum I_{th} for CW operation, we can estimate the material quality needed for CW operation. For our illustrative 13 μm stripe structure, $I_{th}(max) = 0.5$ A corresponds to an effective J_{th} (as measured on the stripe structure) of $I_{th}/LS_t = 9600$ A/cm^2. From Fig. 12.3.2, $J_{th}(\infty)$ is about one-third the effective J_{th}. Therefore, the material grown must have a threshold current density measured on broad-area structures under 3200 A/cm^2. Of course, if the lateral confinement is more effective in the stripe structure used, it is possible to work with material having somewhat higher broad-area threshold current density values. However, values below 2000 A/cm^2 are readily achieved and are used for producing CW laser diodes. Note the importance of the temperature dependence of the threshold current density in determining I_{th} (max)—the greater the temperature dependence, the lower the threshold current density must initially be.

Turning the laser on is the first objective. The second is to determine the maximum optical power which can be obtained with increasing current above threshold.

Neglecting limitations in the optical power emission due to facet damage (Chapter 16), the maximum laser power output is limited by junction heating. As the current is increased, the junction temperature rises until a point is reached at which the diode current equals the threshold current and lasing ceases. In the ideal case of uniform heating of the emitting area, it is possible to calculate these thermally limited effects on the power output knowing the thermal resistance and the J_{th} and η_{ext} dependence on temperature [65]. Figure 12.4.2 shows a schematic diagram which is helpful in understanding the effect. Initially, the diode current I is below I_{th}, and as the current is increased, the laser turns on at ①. As the current is further increased, the threshold current increases with the junction temperature, but as long as $I > I_{th}$ power is emitted, as shown in the upper sketch. Eventually, a point is reached at ② where again $I = I_{th}$, and beyond I_{th} increases faster than I.

Unfortunately, this calculation for a given device is complicated, even if the thermal resistance and temperature dependence of J_{th} are known, because in CW operation the junction may not be uniformly heated, the region in the center of the stripe being hotter than the edge regions. Therefore, current "pulling" into the hotter region occurs (because of the reduced bandgap energy in the hotter region), and the average temperature may be substantially below the temperature of the hottest portion of the junction. The effect is to produce power saturation at lower currents (and power levels) than anticipated on the basis of the uniform junction temperature model. Some examples of power curves of CW lasers are shown in Section 14.3 for 13- and 100-μm-wide stripe lasers.

In *pulsed operation*, the average power dissipated is simply related to the

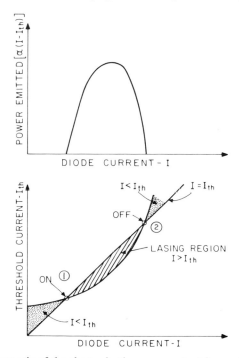

FIG. 12.4.2 Schematic of the change in the power output from a laser diode as a function of increasing current I. Lasing begins at $I = I_{th}$ (point 1) and continues until the junction temperature is such that the threshold current I_{th} reaches I (at point 2). The shaded region is the one in which the output power curve is obtained (it is assumed that the emitted power is proportional to $I - I_{th}$).

duty cycle. For short pulses, the key factor is the thermal diffusion length L_{th}

$$L_{th} = (D_{th}t)^{1/2}$$

where D_{th} is the thermal diffusivity (0.29 cm²/s for GaAs at room temperature) and t is the time. For pulse lengths that are very short, the thermal diffusion length may be less than the distance to the heat sink, and the device heating properties are, therefore, of an essentially adiabatic nature. For longer pulses, thermal diffusion during the pulse limits the temperature rise. For example, with a GaAs device, $L_{th} = 1$ μm for $t = 40$ ns, which sets the approximate conditions for "adiabatic" operation.

The time between pulses is sufficient to return the active region to the heat sink temperature if L_{th} is substantially in excess of the distance between the junction and the heat sink. As an illustration, consider a distance between heat sink and the junction of 10 μm, with the assumed requirement that the thermal diffusion length be twice this value, or 20 μm. Then, the time interval between pulses needed to ensure that the junction returns to the heat sink temperature is 14 μs. Comprehensive calculations of thermal effects in pulsed lasers have been performed by Broom [66].

The simplest method for measuring the diode *thermal resistance* consists of monitoring the emitted spectrum of the diode at a constant peak current (in the spontaneous operating regime) as a function of the duty cycle. As the junction temperature rises, the peak of the emission will shift to lower energy, and from this shift, the junction temperature rise ΔT above the heat sink temperature can be determined. Assuming 100% internal power dissipation, the input power into the diode is determined from the product of the diode current and the voltage applied, $P_i = VI$. The thermal resistance is then

$$R_{th} = \Delta T/P_i \quad (\text{K/W}) \tag{12.4.4}$$

It is commonly found for GaAs that in the vicinity of room temperature the spontaneous spectral peak shifts at a rate of 0.5 meV/°C (see the last paragraph of this chapter). By changing the duty cycle with the current fixed, one obtains a varying input power value from which a plot of ΔT vs. P_i is produced. The slope of the line gives R_{th}. Alternatively, one may change the diode current in dc operation and note the change in the spectral peak energy. However, since the peak position may shift with current density (independent of heating effects), great care must be exercised in using such data to deduce R_{th}.

In the lasing regime itself, it is possible to determine the thermal resistance by using a null measurement of the wavelength shift of a single longitudinal mode with the duty cycle [67].

The shift of the bandgap energy with temperature itself is not a precise reference value for determining the change in the junction temperature with increasing duty cycle, because the spectral peak in spontaneous emission (or lasing) does not necessarily exactly follow the bandgap energy change. With regard to the *lasing peak energy* in undoped GaAs, we discussed in Section 3.5 the fact that the lasing transitions are actually below the bandgap energy and follow a different temperature dependence. In diodes with doped recombination regions, on the other hand, the lasing peak energy depends on the quasi-Fermi level separation. This in turn is related to the bandtail states distribution and their occupancy.

The *spontaneous emission peak* may not precisely follow the bandgap energy either since the spectral shape may be distorted by selective absorption within the diode if the edge emission is measured because the optical path is, on the average, quite long compared to a surface emission diode. Therefore, the safest procedure in thermal resistance measurements consists of first determining the spectral peak as a function of temperature by changing the heat sink temperature (pulsing the diode at low duty cycle), then using these data to determine the junction temperature as a function of power dissipation at a fixed diode current. Figure 12.4.3 shows a typical plot comparing the temperature dependence of the lasing peak at threshold and of the spontaneous emission peak (at a current density of 500 A/cm²). Also shown for comparison is the known GaAs shift of the bandgap energy with temperature (as determined from absorption data) of 0.43 meV/°C. The spontaneous peak energy, on the other hand, shifts by 0.5 meV/°C, and the lasing peak by 0.45 meV/°C in this $Al_{0.5}Ga_{0.5}As$/GaAs DH laser with an undoped recombination region.

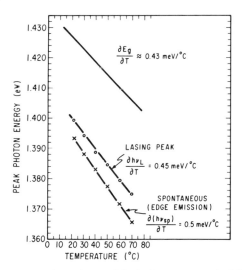

FIG. 12.4.3   Temperature dependence of the lasing energy and of the spontaneous emission peak energy in a double-heterojunction (AlGa)As/GaAs laser containing about $5 \times 10^{17} cm^{-3}$ acceptors in the recombination region.

REFERENCES

1. B. J. Baliga and S. K. Ghandhi, *IEEE Trans. Electron Devices* **19**, 761 (1972). Zinc contact diffusions are discussed by K. K. Shih, *J. Electrochem. Soc.* **123**, 1737 (1977).
2. H. Nelson, U.S. Patent No. 3,565,702 (1971).
3. M. B. Panish, S. Sumski, and I. Hayashi, *Trans. AIME* **2**, 795 (1971).
4. J. M. Blum and K. K. Shih, *J. Appl. Phys.* **43**, 1394 (1972).
5. H. F. Lockwood and M. Ettenberg, *J. Crystal Growth* **15**, 81 (1972).
6. H. F. Lockwood and H. Kressel, *J. Crystal Growth* **27**, 97 (1974).
7. M. S. Abrahams and C. J. Buiocchi, *J. Appl. Phys.* **36**, 2855 (1965).
8. V. D. Rideout, *Solid State Electron.* **18**, 541 (1975).
9. B. L. Sharma and R. K. Purohit, "Semiconductor Heterojunctions." Pergamon, Oxford, 1974.
10. D. Marcuse, "Theory of Dielectric Optical Waveguides," p. 132. Academic Press, New York, 1974.
11. G. H. B. Thompson, P. A. Kirkby, and J. E. A. Whiteaway, *IEEE J. Quantum Electron.* **11**, 481 (1975).
12. F. R. Nash, W. R. Wagner, and R. L. Brown, *J. Appl. Phys.* **47**, 3992 (1976).
13. H. F. Lockwood, *Proc. Biennial Cornell Elec. Eng. Conf.*, **5**th p. 127. (1975).
14. K. K. Shih, G. R. Woolhouse, A. E. Blakesler, and J. M. Blum, *Proc. Int. Symp. GaAs Related Compounds*, **5**th p. 165. Inst. of Phys., London, 1975.
15. H. Kressel, H. Nelson, and F. Z. Hawrylo, *J. Appl. Phys.* **41**, 2019 (1970).
16. H. Kressel, H. Nelson, S. H. McFarlane, M. S. Abrahams, P. LeFur, and C. J. Buiocchi, *J. Appl. Phys.* **40**, 3587 (1969).
17. H. T. Minden and R. Premo, *J. Appl. Phys.* **45**, 4520 (1974).
18. H. F. Lockwood, H. Kressel, H. S. Sommers, Jr., and F. Z. Hawrylo, *Appl. Phys. Lett.* **17**, 499 (1970).
19. H. Kressel, H. F. Lockwood, and F. Z. Hawrylo, *J. Appl. Phys.* **43**, 561 (1972).
20. B. H. Ahn, C. W. Trussel, and R. R. Shurtz, *Appl. Phys. Lett.* **19**, 408 (1971).
21. F. H. Doerbeck, D. M. Blacknall, and R. L. Carroll, *J. Appl. Phys.* **44**, 529 (1973).
22. E. W. Williams, *Solid State Commun.* **4**, 585 (1966).
23. C. J. Nuese, G. H. Olsen, and M. Ettenberg, *Appl. Phys. Lett.* **29**, 54 (1976).
24. H. C. Casey, Jr., A. Y. Cho, and P. A. Barnes, *IEEE J. Quantum Electron.* **11**, 467 (1975).
25. L. Yang and J. M. Ballantyne, *Appl. Phys. Lett.* **25**, 67 (1974).
26. F. A. Blum, K. L. Lawley, and W. C. Holton, *J. Appl. Phys.* **46**, 2605 (1975).
27. H. H. Wieder, *Thin Solid Films* **31**, 123 (1976).
28. G. E. Stillman and C. M. Wolfe, *Thin Solid Films* **31**, 69 (1976).
29. R. E. Honig, *Thin Solid Films* **31**, 89 (1976).
30. H. Kressel and M. Ettenberg, *Appl. Phys. Lett.* **23**, 511 (1973).
31. F. H. Nicoll, Private communication (1970).
32. H. Kressel, H. F. Lockwood, and J. K. Butler, *J. Appl. Phys.* **44**, 4095 (1973).
33. H. C. Casey, Jr., D. D. Sell, and M. B. Panish, *Appl. Phys. Lett.* **24**, 63 (1974).
34. A. Onton, M. R. Lorenz, and J. M. Woodall, *Bull. Am. Phys. Soc.* **16**, 371 (1971).
35. F. Stern, *Phys. Rev.* **133**, A1653 (1964).
36. J. Zoroofchi and J. K. Butler, *J. Appl. Phys.* **44**, 3697 (1973).
37. D. D. Sell, H. C. Casey, Jr., and K. W. Wecht, *J. Appl. Phys.* **45**, 2650 (1974).
38. D. T. F. Marple, *J. Appl. Phys.* **35**, 1241 (1964).
39. M. A. Afromowitz, *J. Appl. Phys.* **44**, 1292 (1973).
40. B. Abeles, *Phys. Rev.* **131**, 1906 (1963).

41. H. P. Maruska and J. I. Pankove, *Solid State Electron.* **10**, 917 (1967).
42. D. L. Rode, *J. Appl. Phys.* **45**, 3887 (1974).
43. G. D. Pitt and J. Lees, *Phys. Rev. B* **2**, 4144 (1970).
44. C. J. Nuese, H. Kressel, and I. Ladany, *IEEE Spectrum* **9**, 28 (1972).
45. R. J. Archer, *J. Electron. Mater.* **1**, 128 (1972).
46. I. Hayashi, M. B. Panish, P. W. Foy, and S. Sumski, *Appl. Phys. Lett.* **17**, 109 (1970).
47. J. C. Dyment, *Appl. Phys. Lett.* **10**, 84 (1967); J. C. Dyment and L. A. D'Asaro, *ibid.* **11**, 292 (1967).
48. H. Yonezu, I. Sakuma, K. Kobayashi, T. Kamejima, M. Unno, and Y. Nannichi, *Jpn. J. Appl. Phys.* **12**, 1585 (1973).
49. T. Tsukada, H. Nakashima, J. Umeda, and D. Nakada, *Appl. Phys. Lett.* **20**, 344 (1972).
50. T. Tsukada, *J. Appl. Phys.* **45**, 4899 (1974).
51. J. M. Blum, J. C. McGroddy, P. G. McMullin, K. K. Shih, A. W. Smith, and J. F. Ziegler, *IEEE J. Quantum Electron.* **11**, 413 (1975).
52. J. C. Dyment, L. A. D'Asaro, J. C. North, B. I. Miller, and J. E. Ripper, *Proc. IEEE* **60**, 726 (1972).
53. K. Itoh, M. Inoue, and I. Teramoto, *IEEE J. Quantum Electron.* **11**, 421 (1975).
54. M. Cross and M. J. Adams, *Solid State Electron.* **15**, 919 (1972).
55. B. W. Hakki, *J. Appl. Phys.* **44**, 5021 (1973).
56. B. W. Hakki, *J. Appl. Phys.* **46**, 2723 (1975).
57. T. Tsukada, R. Itoh, H. Nakashima, and O. Nakada, *IEEE J. Quantum Electron.* **9**, 356 (1973).
58. I. Ladany and H. Kressel, Semiconductor Diode Laser Material and Devices with Emission in Visible Portion of the Spectrum, Contract NAS 1-11421, Final Rep. (1974).
59. W. B. Joyce and L. H. Wemple, *J. Appl. Phys.* **4**, 3818 (1970).
60. W. P. Dumke, *Solid State Electron.* **16**, 1279 (1973).
61. J. I. Pankove, *IEEE J. Quantum Electron.* **4**, 119 (1968).
62. W. B. Joyce and R. W. Dixon, *J. Appl. Phys.* **46**, 855 (1975).
63. H. Kressel and I. Ladany, unpublished.
64. R. W. Keyes, *IBM J. Res. Develop.* **9**, 303 (1965).
65. R. W. Keyes, *IBM J. Res. Develop.* **15**, 401 (1971).
66. R. F. Broom, *IEEE J. Quantum Electron.* **4**, 135 (1968).
67. T. L. Paoli, *IEEE J. Quantum Electron.* **11**, 498 (1975).

BIBLIOGRAPHY

"Gallium Arsenide Lasers," G. H. Gooch (ed.), Wiley (Interscience), London, (1969). Special Issues on Semiconductor Lasers, *IEEE J. Quantum Electron.* **4**, 109–234 (1968); **6**, 275–302 (1970); **9**, 265–392 (1973); **11**, 381–562 (1975).

Special issue on Liquid Phase Epitaxy, *J. Crystal Growth*, **27** (1974). Special issue on Characterization of Epitaxial Semiconductor Films, *Thin Solid Films* **31** (1976).

Chapter 13

Heterojunction Devices of Alloys
Other than GaAs–AlAs

13.1 Introduction

The preparation of various III–V alloys is discussed in Chapters 9–11. The combination of these binary, ternary, and quaternary compounds to produce efficient heterojunction devices emitting at specified wavelengths involves numerous problems of compatible technologies.

The major requirement in the fabrication of useful heterojunction lasers and LEDs is that the lattice parameter be closely matched at the heterojunction *boundaries*. However, the lack of suitable substrates for some alloys means that the epitaxial layers contain dislocations (Chapter 9) due to lattice mismatch with the *substrate*, although the lattice parameters at the active heterojunction boundaries are closely matched. For example, AlGaAsSb/Ga (AsSb) lattice matched structures on GaAs contain inclined dislocations which may impair the device efficiency and reilability, but do not preclude the realization of the optical and carrier confinement benefits of the heterojunctions.

Note that although lattice matching can be realized at one temperature, differences in the thermal coefficient of expansion of the materials comprising the structure lead to a mismatch at other temperatures. As a lesser evil, it appears preferable to *match* the lattice parameters at the *growth temperature* rather than at room temperature. Thus, no (or few) misfit dislocations are incorporated under ordinary conditions, although the structure is strained at room temperature. However, there is little evidence of deleterious effects due to the elastic strain, whereas dislocations may result in reliability problems as discussed in Section 16.2.

Lattice-matched heterojunction configurations can be constructed using combinations of materials, the choice being dependent on the bandgap needed, the technology available, and the lattice parameter. In the following we list three major spectral areas: 1–1.2 μm, far infrared, and the visible emission ranges. (The latter is discussed in greater detail in Section 14.5.)

1. Because of the interest in emitters in the *1–1.2 μm spectral* range for fiber optical communications (Section 14.2), there has been substantial work in producing heterojunctions for this purpose. Three III–V alloy systems are illustrative of possibilities in this range.

a. *(InGa)P/(InGa)As on GaAs.* Here lattice matching at the heterojunctions is possible (see Fig. 14.5.7), but the epitaxial layers are mismatched to the substrate by about 1%. Using VPE, it is possible, however, to grade the composition to minimize the dislocation density in the active region (Section 9.4).

b. *InGaAsP on InP.* This combination is potentially the best since it can produce a lattice-matched heterojunction with no substrate problems (Fig. 11.1.1).

c. *AlGaAsSb/Ga(AsSb) on GaAs substrates.* The lattice mismatch to the substrate is $\sim$ 1%. However, the Al/Ga substitution is convenient by LPE (Section 11.4) and essentially lattice-matched heterojunctions are produced.

2. A second major area in which heterojunction structures are useful is for Pb-salt lasers emitting in the *infrared*, although a significant lattice mismatch at the heterojunctions occurs.

3. A third area of interest is in extending the laser diode operation into the *visible* portion of the spectrum beyond the range of (AlGa)As devices. The subject is reviewed in Section 14.5. The use of (InGa)P/Ga(AsP), InGa AsP/Ga(AsP), and AlGaAsP/Ga(AsP) structures offers the possibility of producing red–yellow light-emitting lasers. However, the lattice mismatch to the GaAs substrate is again quite severe, and the considerations of Chapter 9 with regard to minimizing the dislocation density are relevant to producing good devices.

Although LPE or VPE is more convenient for some III–V alloys, these structures could also be produced by molecular beam epitaxy. The choice of the best technology can only be determined on the basis of the device quality and reliability. In view of the sensitivity of the laser reliability to defect density, extensive testing is needed to establish the comparative merits of various technologies.

13.2   IV–VI Compound Lasers

Injection lasers of $Pb_{1-x}Sn_xTe$ and $PbS_{1-x}Se_x$ can provide emission from 2.5 to $\sim$ 34 μm. In addition to varying the emission wavelength by choice of the appropriate alloy composition, a valuable feature of these alloys is that appreciable spectral tuning is possible by changing external factors such as temperature, magnetic field, or pressure. Practically, however, simple changes in diode current change the emission wavelength by simply changing the junction temperature.

The Pb-salt lasers operate only at cryogenic temperatures, and the smaller the bandgap energy, the lower the operating temperature. They have been used in high resolution spectroscopy [1], including the monitoring of air pollutants, where tunability is highly desirable. Our particular interest here is in the heterojunction devices constructed with these compounds. As a result of the use of heterojunctions the device performance has been significantly increased in recent years compared to earlier homojunctions.

The fabrication of heterojunctions in the Pb salts (rocksalt structure) involves devices with substantial lattice parameter mismatch. As may be seen from the lattice parameter data in Table 13.2.1, the lattice mismatch between PbS and PbSe, for example, is 3%, and therefore changing the bandgap energy involves a substantial lattice parameter change.

TABLE 13.2.1
Lattice Parameter at 300 K

Compound	a_0 (Å)
PbS	5.936
PbSe	6.124
PbTe	6.462
SnTe	6.303

Table 13.2.2 lists the bandgap energy of PbS, PbSe, and PbTe which is seen to increase with temperature (contrary to III–V compounds). Because the valence band maximum and conduction band minimum *both* occur at the L points in the Brillouin zone, these are direct bandgap materials.

The smallest bandgap energy (hence longest lasing wavelength) is achieved with $Pb_{1-x}Sn_xTe$ (and $Pb_{1-x}Sn_xSe$) because of the unusual band structure [2], shown in Fig. 13.2.1. The conduction and valence bands are believed to *invert*, producing a zero bandgap energy material with $x = 0.4$ at 77 K. However, on both sides of the inversion point, where $E_g = 0$, the direct bandgap transitions permit stimulated emission at low temperatures. $Pb_{1-x}Sn_xSe$ has similar properties and has produced homojunction lasers to 34 μm, while $Pb_{1-x}Sn_xTe$ lasers have operated to 28 μm. The best threshold current densities are low. For example, Bi-doped PbSnTe lasers emitting at 24.6 μm lased

TABLE 13.2.2

Minimum Direct Bandgap Energy $E_g{}^a$

T (K)	PbS	PbSe	PbTe	Ref.
4.2	0.286 ± 0.003	0.165 ± 0.005	0.190 ± 0.002	b
77	0.307 ± 0.003	0.176 ± 0.005	0.217 ± 0.002	b
300	0.41	0.27	0.31	c
373	0.44	0.31	0.34	c

[a] In electronvolts.

[b] D. L. Mitchell, E. D. Palik, and J. N. Zemel, *Phys. Semicond.: Proc. Int. Congr.*, *7th, Paris* (M. Hulin, ed.), p. 325. Academic Press, New York, 1964.

[c] J.N. Zemel, J.D. Jensen, and R.B. Schoolar, *Phys. Rev.* **140**, A330 (1965).

at 71 A/cm² at 12 K, and at 1400 A/cm² at 77 K, where the lasing wavelength decreases to 15.5 μm [3, 4].

Figure 13.2.1b shows the range of possibilities with regard to bandgap energy and lattice parameter, and Fig. 13.2.1c summarizes the potential range of heterojunction devices with the spectral range achievable and the maximum lattice parameter mismatch with various combinations. It is evident that the PbSnSe system is preferable over the PbSnTe system from the point of view of

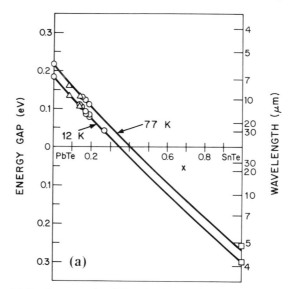

FIG. 13.2.1 (a) Bandgap energy of $Pb_{1-x}Sn_xTe$ as a function of x, the mole fraction of SnTe as determined from various measurements. $\bigcirc$ = laser emission, $\triangle$ = photovoltaic effect, $\square$ = tunneling [3]. (b) Range of heterojunction device possibilities with maximum lattice parameter mismatch between the recombination region of the heterojunction structure and the higher bandgap bounding layers (A. Groves, unpublished). (c) ($\bullet$) Lattice parameter and 77 K bandgap energy of various IV–VI materials.

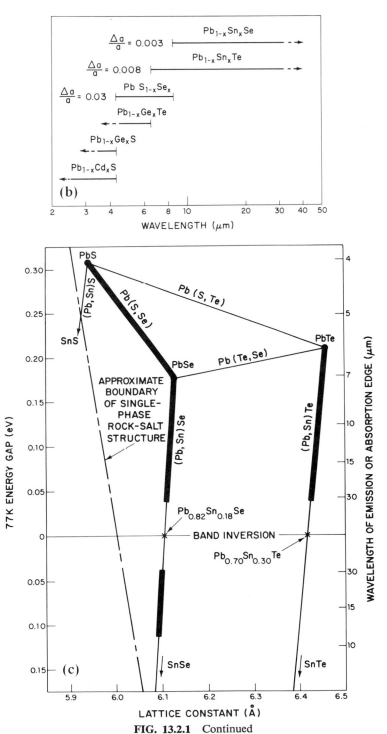

FIG. 13.2.1 Continued

producing lattice-matched heterojunctions (other factors remaining constant).

The technology of the Pb-salt devices is intimately connected with the control of crystal stoichiometry because metal atoms in excess of the stoichiometric density are donors, whereas excess chalcogenide atoms are acceptors. The required carrier concentration and type are sometimes achieved by controlling deviations from stoichiometry, rather than by the addition of dopants. In fact, p–n junctions can be formed by stoichiometric control only (achieved by heating the material in a suitable ambient). However, even with the addition of dopants, the control of stoichiometry remains a key problem.

The fabrication of lasing structures is similar to that used for III–V compound devices, with cleaved facets forming the Fabry–Perot cavity mirrors. Ohmic contact to the p-type material is commonly made using Pt or Au followed by In, whereas In or Au is used for the n-type material. Despite the low bandgap energy, the choice of suitable ohmic contacts is essential to minimize the device resistance. In fact, metal Schottky barriers have been used by Nill et al. [5] to produce rectifying junctions in PbTe and $Pb_{0.8}Sn_{0.2}Te$ suitable for laser diode operation without p–n junctions. Cold compression bonding with In is used to attach the laser to the header—with great care since the materials are very soft.

Stripe-geometry lasers [1] using oxide isolation are coming into increasing use, replacing earlier broad-area devices. Stripe structures are particularly interesting because of the requirement that the devices operate CW for most convenient use in spectroscopy. Furthermore, it is desirable that CW operation be extended to as high a heat sink temperature as possible because operation at 77 K and above greatly simplifies the cooling requirements compared to operation below 77 K.

Several methods may be used to obtain material suitable for laser diode fabrication. Homojunction devices are made by forming a simple p–n junction by diffusion or heat-treating of bulk-grown material. The heterojunction devices, however, require epitaxial layers. The various technological aspects of thin-film preparation have been reviewed by Zemel [6]. Evaporation and vapor transport are the most widely used techniques for heterojunction laser fabrication, with LPE a more recent addition.

The evaporation process basically consists of the method quite similar to that now denoted as molecular beam epitaxy in that the constituents of the alloy are provided by heated ovens under vacuum.* Control of the rate of arrival of the constituents on the heated substrate provides the desired alloy composition. In the method of Holloway et al. [7] heated cells with apertures

---

* Note, however, that in MBE of III–V compounds the source materials are frequently the elemental constituents. Here, on the other hand, the alloys in powdered form are commonly used as a source in the evaporator.

of different size are used to compensate for the different evaporation rates of the source materials. Here, the walls of the apparatus are cold, but the heated substrate is in direct line with the sources.

Another vacuum method, a hot-wall technique, uses a baffle between the heated source (or sources) and the substrate [8]. The sources and baffle are enclosed inside a heated furnace, with the substrate being independently heated and placed either inside or outside the furnace. The baffle may be maintained at a temperature above that of the source and substrate to prevent deposition on the baffle, which thus acts as an effective diffuser because only indirect or reflected molecules strike the substrate.

Vapor phase epitaxy has been successfully used by Rolls et al. [9] to prepare epitaxial layers of PbSnTe on PbTe substrates using H_2 transport in an open tube, at a growth rate of about 0.3 μm/hr. A single-heterojunction laser [10] of $Pb_{0.83}Sn_{0.17}Te/PbTe$ ($\Delta a_0/a_0 = 0.31\%$) emitting at 12.2 μm (77 K) was produced by VPE.

Liquid phase epitaxy has been used to prepare Pb salts by Longo et al. [11], and applied to PbSnTe homojunction and heterojunction laser diodes by Tomasetta and Fonstad [12] using PbTe substrates. The solutions consist of Pb and Sn with polycrystalline PbTe to saturate the solution. The carrier type and concentration are determined by the growth temperature and solution composition, in a manner consistent with the data of Harmon [13], shown in Fig. 13.2.2. The growth temperature was between 550 and 600°C and a multiple-bin boat of the type conventionally used for multiple-layer LPE was used. The layer thicknesses obtained were in the 10–20 μm range.

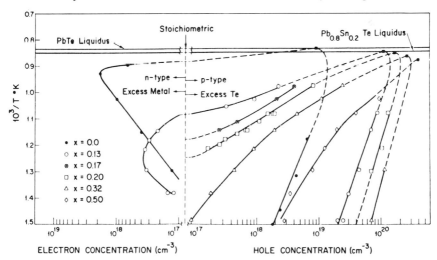

FIG. 13.2.2 Carrier concentration of $Pb_{1-x}Sn_xTe$ as a function of growth temperature [13]. (■) Estimated hole concentration of solid at composition corresponding to maximum melting point.

A troublesome feature of LPE at these temperatures for the growth of thin heterojunction structures is interdiffusion of Pb, Sn, and Te during growth. As a result, the p–n junction can shift several microns away from the desired heterojunction boundary. Although not disastrous for single-heterojunction devices, this interdiffusion makes the growth of double-heterojunction lasers difficult. Groves et al. [14] avoided this difficulty in growing DH PbSnTe/PbTe lasers by doping the PbTe substrate with Tl, a dopant which appears to make Pb-rich PbTe p-type and which diffuses slowly enough during the growth period to prevent the conversion of the grown layers from p- to n-type. Another interesting feature of their LPE devices was the use of MgF_2 as a selective mask during growth, thus providing stripe-geometry lasers in the as-grown form with stripe widths of 50 μm. These lasers operated CW at temperatures as high as 77 K ($\lambda = 8.2$ μm).

An evaporation process similar to that of Holloway et al. [7] was used by Walpole et al. [15] to produce the first single-heterojunction lasers of $Pb_{0.88}Sn_{0.12}Te$/PbTe ($\lambda = 8.9$ μm at 77 K) with markedly improved performance compared to homojunction devices, as shown in Fig. 13.2.3. The substrate temperature was only 300°C, which minimizes interdiffusion.

The same growth technique, in which the individual layers are grown by evaporation of different polycrystalline sources with the desired composition of the layer, was used to grow double-heterojunction stripe-geometry lasers with MgF_2 windows [16]. The active region contained $Pb_{0.782}Sn_{0.218}Te$ and the laser operated CW up to a heat sink temperature of 114 K. It could be temperature-tuned between 15.9 and 8.54 μm, with emission at 77 K at about 11.5 μm. Because of the favorable thermal properties, CW operation of this device was possible despite the rather high J_{th} values, which ranged from 5000 A/cm² at 10 K to $\sim$ 18,000 A/cm² at $\sim$ 110 K. The CW power emitted was in the hundreds of microwatts range.

Double-heterojunction PbS/PbSe lasers were also grown by a hot-wall evaporation process by Preier et al. [17] using a method described by Duh and Preier [18]. The active layer of $PbS_{0.6}Se_{0.4}$ (about 1 μm thick) provided devices emitting in the range of 6.4–4.6 μm between 20 and 180 K. CW operation was possible up to 96 K with a threshold current density of 1000 A/cm². Note that the J_{th} value is about four times lower than that achieved with a homojunction laser at the same temperature, despite the large lattice mismatch of $\sim$ 1.2%. It appears, therefore, that the heterojunction lasers produced with the Pb-salts are less sensitive to the interfacial lattice parameter mismatch than those made using III–V compounds, where $\Delta a_0/a_0 < 0.3\%$ appears necessary (Section 13.3). This difference is probably connected to a puite different defect structure associated with dislocations.

A vacuum deposition method in which the substrate was rotated from one source to another was used to grow DH $PbS_{1-x}Se_x$/$PbS_{1-y}Se_y$ lasers by Mc-

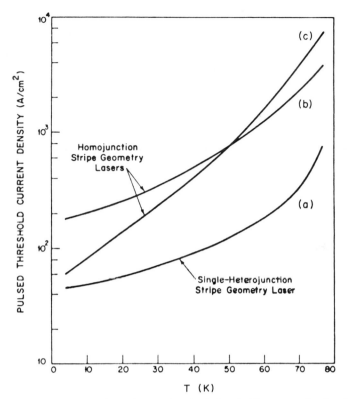

FIG. 13.2.3 Temperature dependence of pulsed threshold current density for $Pb_{0.88}$ $Sn_{0.12}Te$ diode lasers: (a) A single-heterojunction stripe-geometry laser, (b) a homojunction stripe-geometry laser with unusually low 4.2 K threshold, and (c) a typical homojunction stripe-geometry laser [15].

Lane and Sleger [19]. A feature of their system was the use of an independently heated Se source (to 130°C) to provide the required Se concentration for p-type layers. When this source was left unheated, n-type material was grown. The substrate temperature was 290–320°C, and the source temperature was 450–500°C. Typical growth rates were 0.20–2 μm/hr. Threshold current densities as low as 60 A/cm² were obtained at 12 K with $\lambda = 6.1$ μm.

The internal quantum efficiencies of the Pb-salt lasers reported to date appear low (3–10%) compared to state of the art devices of GaAs and related compounds. The reason for the low efficiency, despite very low threshold current densities, remains unexplained in the literature. The nonradiative processes may be involved with defects in the material. The power emitted is commonly limited to a few milliwatts.

The lasers far-field patterns depend, of course, on the width of the mode guiding region. In the homojunction devices of $Pb_{0.88}Sn_{0.12}Te$ reported by

Ralston *et al.* [20], the beam width perpendicular to the junction plane was about 8–10° because of the long diffusion length of the minority carriers, which can reach $\sim 60 \, \mu m$ owing to the high carrier mobility. In the plane of the junction the beam width is also 8–10° (comparable to III–V lasers). Wider beams in the direction perpendicular to the junction plane will be observed in heterojunction structures.

The spectral purity of the lasers varies with the fabrication technology. Single longitudinal mode operation is encountered in some cases near threshold and line widths as narrow as 54 kHz were reported by Hinkley and Freed [21] for a single mode laser emitting 240 μw.

In spectroscopy [1], the diode is mounted in a Dewar flasc on a cold finger for multimode lasers. A spectrometer is used as a filter. Wavelength tuning can be conveniently obtained by changing the diode temperature by either increasing the current or changing the heat sink temperature. Alternatively, but more complicated, is the use of hydrostatic pressure or magnetic fields to change the emission wavelength. In fact, by applying hydrostatic pressure to 15 kbar, a diode laser was tuned between 8.5 and 22 μm [22].

An idea of the useful operating range of a Pb-salt laser as relevant to spectroscopy is obtained from Fig. 13.2.4a. The laser shown (made of PbSnSe) can be temperature-tuned over a range of frequencies which corresponds to the absorption lines of the gases shown. Figure 13.2.4b shows the full range covered by IV–VI laser diodes with the gases which can be detected.

13.3   III–V Compound Lasers

Heterojunction lasers have been fabricated from various combinations of materials, the more successful ones having a close lattice match ($\Delta a_0/a_0 <$ 0.3%). The degree of success is defined by the reduction in J_{th} achieved compared to homojunction lasers operating at the same temperature and emission wavelength. Some representative laser results are shown in Table 13.3.1.

Some structures were constructed as alternatives to (AlGa)As/GaAs lasers. The GaAs$_{0.9}$P$_{0.1}$/GaAs single-heterojunction laser has been studied in detail [25] using both an abrupt and a slightly graded heterojunction. The lattice mismatch here is about 0.36%. The heterojunction lasers are at best only comparable to homojunctions, indicating serious defect-related problems in the addition of the heterojunction.

The In$_{0.5}$Ga$_{0.5}$P/GaAs/In$_{0.5}$Ga$_{0.5}$P LOC heterojunction diodes have a close lattice match; their characteristics are similar to those of an (AlGa)As/GaAs LOC with equally spaced heterojunctions. These diodes were prepared by VPE, as were DH lasers with $J_{th} \approx 1000$–2000 A/cm^2 [26].

In the 1–1.2 μm spectral range, lasers have been fabricated using ternary, binary–quaternary, and ternary–quaternary combinations. The first devices

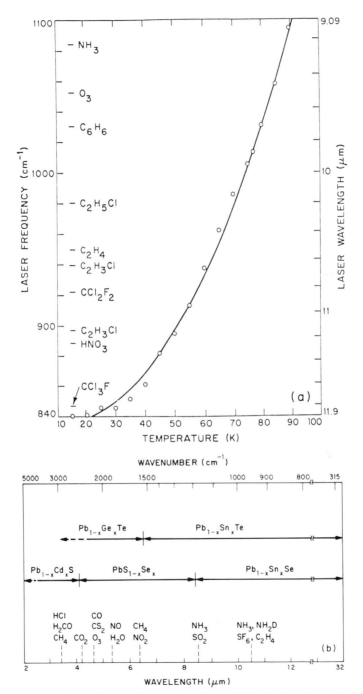

FIG. 13.2.4 (a) Change in emission wavelength of a PbSnSe single-heterojunction laser with temperature. The absorption lines of various gases which can be detected with such a laser are shown. A spectrometer is used to filter out a single longitudinal mode emission line with power output of tens of microwatts [23]. (b) Spectral range covered by IV–VI lasers and relevant absorption lines of various gases [24].

TABLE 13.3.1

Illustrative Heterojunction Laser Diodes Using Alloys Other Than AlAs–GaAs

Materials	Laser type	J_{th} (A/cm^2)	d_3 (μm)	λ_L (Å)	Operating temperature (K)	Growth technique	References[a]
GaAsP–GaAs	SH	$1.4 \times 10^5-$ 8×10^4	1 to ~10	~9,000 Å	300	VPE	a
GaAsSb–AlGaAsSb	DH	9×10^3	0.8	9,800	300	LPE	b
GaAs$_{0.88}$Sb$_{0.12}$/Al$_{0.4}$–Ga$_{0.6}$As$_{0.88}$Sb$_{0.12}$	DH	2×10^3	0.45	~10,000	300	LPE	c
InGa$_{0.5}$P$_{0.5}$–GaAs	LOC	8×10^3	2.5^d	~8,900	300	VPE	e
InGaP–InGaAs	LOC	1.49×10^4	1.6^d	10,750	300	VPE	f
InGaAsP–GaAsP	SH	6.2×10^4	1	6,300	77	LPE + VPE	g
AlGaAsP–GaAsP	SH	6.6×10^4	1.24	~8,100	300	LPE	h
AlGaAsP–GaAsP	DH	1.6×10^4	1.25	8,450	300	LPE + VPE	i
PbSnTe–PbTe	SH	780	—	~89,000	77	Evaporation	j
PbSnTe–PbTe	DH	4.2×10^3	9	~83,500	77	LPE	k
PbSnTe–PbTe	DH	1.3×10^3	5	~84,000	77	LPE	l
InGa$_{0.5}$P$_{0.5}$–Al$_{0.69}$Ga$_{0.31}$As	SH	2.5×10^3	1	6,380	77	LPE	m
PbS$_{0.72}$Se$_{0.28}$–PbS$_{0.78}$Se$_{0.22}$	SH	~200	~3	47,800	12	Evaporation	n
In$_{0.88}$Ga$_{0.12}$As$_{0.23}$P$_{0.77}$–InP	DH	2.8×10^3	0.6	11,000	300	LPE	o
GaAsP–InGaP	LOC	5.5×10^4	4^d	6,750	273	VPE	p
	DH	3.4×10^3	0.2	7,010	300	VPE	q

[a] M. G. Craford, W. O. Groves, and M. J. Fox, *J. Electrochem. Soc.* **118**, 355 (1971). The abrupt heterojunction barrier was formed using $GaAs_{0.9}P_{0.1}$–GaAs ($\Delta E_g \approx 0.1$ eV). Graded heterojunctions with 4% P per micron were also studied with similar device results.

[b] K. Sugiyama and H. Saito, *Jpn. J. Appl. Phys.* **11**, 1057 (1972).

[c] R. E. Nahory et al., *Appl. Phys. Lett.* **28**, 19 (1976).

[d] Distance between the two heterojunctions, d^0.

[e] C. J. Nuese, M. Ettenberg, and G. H. Olsen, *Appl. Phys. Lett.* **25**, 612 (1974).

[f] C. J. Nuese and G. Oslen, *Appl. Phys. Lett.* **26**, 528 (1975). The heterojunction barrier consisted of the near-lattice-matching compositions $In_{0.68}Ga_{0.32}P$–$In_{0.16}Ga_{0.84}As$. The highest $\Delta a_0/a_0$ value used was 0.2%. The threshold values obtained were about five times lower than obtained with homojunction lasers emitting at the same wavelength.

[g] J. J. Coleman, W. R. Hitchens, N. Holonyak, Jr., M. J. Ludowise, W. O. Groves, and D. L. Keune, *Appl. Phys. Lett.* **25**, 725 (1974); J. J. Coleman et al., *IEEE J. Quantum Electron.* **11**, 471 (1975).

[h] R. D. Burnham, N. Holonyak, Jr., and D. R. Scifres, *Appl. Phys. Lett.* **17**, 455 (1970).

[i] R. D. Burnham, N. Holonyak, Jr., H. W. Korb, H. M. Macksey, D. R. Scifres, J. B. Woodhouse, and Zh. I. Alferov, *Appl. Phys. Lett.* **19**, 25 (1971).

[j] N. Walpole, A. R. Calawa, R. W. Ralston, T. C. Harman, and J. P. McVittie, *Appl. Phys. Lett.* **23**, 620 (1973). The structure used consisted of $Pb_{0.88}Sn_{0.12}Te$–$PbTe$ ($\Delta a_0/a_0 \cong 0.24\%$). The J_{th} values obtained were reported to be about one-third those measured for homojunction lasers.

[k] S. H. Groves, K. W. Nill, and A. J. Strauss, *Appl. Phys. Lett.* **25**, 331 (1974).

[l] R. Tomasetta and C. Fonstad, *Appl. Phys. Lett.* **25**, 440 (1974); see also *Appl. Phys. Lett.* **24**, 567 (1974). A high dislocation density (10^8–10^9 cm^{-2}) in the substrate was noted.

[m] G. Schul and P. Mischel, *Appl. Phys. Lett.* **26**, 394 (1975).

[n] K. G. Sleger, G. F. McLane, U. Strom, S. G. Bishop, and D. Mitchell, *J. Appl. Phys.* **45**, 5069 (1974). $\Delta a_0/a_0 \cong 0.2\%$ at the n–n heterojunction.

[o] J. J. Hsieh, *Appl. Phys. Lett.* **28**, 283 (1976).

[p] I. Ladany, H. Kressel, and C. J. Nuese, NASA Rep. Contract NASI-13739B4 (March 1976).

[q] H. Kressel, G. Olsen, and C. J. Nuese, *Appl. Phys. Lett.* **30**, 249 (1977).

in this range were LOC laser diodes, $In_{0.68}Ga_{0.32}P/In_{0.16}Ga_{0.84}As$ on GaAs, and showed a factor of about 5 reduction in J_{th} at room temperature compared to homojunctions emitting at $\lambda \approx 1$ μm [27]. Figure 13.3.1 shows the cross section of this LOC laser (made by VPE) with the p–n junction between the two lattice-matched heterojunctions. Figure 13.2.2 shows the temperature dependence of J_{th} for the (InGa)P/(InGa)As lasers (with the lattice mismatch indicated). Note that reasonable performance was observed with a $\Delta a_0/a_0 \approx 0.2\%$, although J_{th} is still two to three times higher than that for a comparable (AlGa)As/GaAs or $In_{0.5}Ga_{0.5}P/GaAs$ LOC laser.

Reducing the interfacial lattice mismatch improved control of the interfacial defects thereby enabling production of (InGa)As/In(GaP) double-heterojunction laser diodes with $J_{th} \cong 1000$ A/cm^2, and capable of room temperature CW operation in the 1–1.1 μm range [27a]. The use of very thin (fraction of a micrometer) active region width plays an important role in reducing the misfit dislocation formation process in double heterojunction lasers despite a significant lattice mismatch (Chapter 9).

Although insufficient data exist to compare accurately the experimental results to the analysis of Section 8.1 concerning the role of interfacial defects, it is nevertheless interesting to analyze the (InGa)As/(InGa)P LOC lasers with parameter mismatch $\Delta a_0/a_0 = 0.2\%$, having the threshold characteristics shown in Fig. 13.3.2. As just noted, the J_{th} at room temperature is two to three times higher than that of comparable dimension GaAs LOC lasers, and factors other than nonradiative interfacial recombination could well be responsible. In the following we estimate the interfacial surface recombination velocity S needed to *fully* account for their high threshold by assuming $\gamma^* = 0.4$ (see Section 8.1). The p-type recombination region is 0.7 μm thick, and we assume $L_e = 3$ μm, $D_e = 50$ cm^2/s, and $d_3/L_e = 0.23$. From Fig. 8.1.2, we estimate $SL_e/D_e = 0.5$, from which we conclude that $S \leq 8 \times 10^4$ cm/s. This value compares surprisingly well to $S = 5 \times 10^4$ cm/s calculated from Eq. (8.1.22), assuming that *all* the atomic sites associated with misfit interfacial dislocations contribute to the formation of nonradiative recombination centers and that the capture cross section $\sigma_t = 10^{-15}$ cm^2 for the states associated with the dislocations.

Other devices for the ~ 1 μm spectral range were produced by LPE. The first AlGaAsSb/Ga(AsSb) DH lasers emitted at 0.98 μm, and had a J_{th} value about four to five times lower than those of homojunction lasers emitting at the same wavelength [28]. Subsequently, J_{th} values of 2000 A/cm^2 at $\lambda_L \approx 1$ μm were achieved, making room temperature CW operation possible [29]. These lasers had active region widths $d_3 = 0.45$ μm with a composition $Al_{0.4}Ga_{0.6}As_{0.88}Sb_{0.12}/GaAs_{0.88}Sb_{0.12}$. To minimize the dislocation density in the recombination region, three layers of Ga(AsSb), with increasing Sb content,

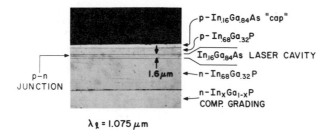

$\lambda_{\ell} = 1.075 \, \mu m$

FIG. 13.3.1 (InGa)As–(InGa)P LOC laser structure designed for room temperature lasing at 1.075 μm [27].

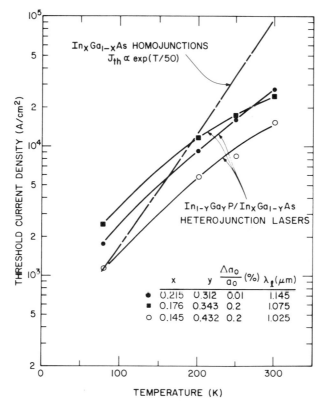

FIG. 13.3.2 Temperature dependence of the threshold current density of LOC In_xGa_{1-x} As–In_yGa_{1-y}P structures with the lattice mismatch ($\Delta a_0/a_0$) indicated as well as the room temperature lasing wavelength. A curve for a (InGa)As homojunction laser is shown for comparison. The low temperature J_{th} is not impaired by the lack of heterojunctions. The diodes were prepared by vapor phase epitaxy [27].

were grown on the GaAs substrate prior to the deposition of the AlGaAsSb n-type layer.

Devices capable of CW lasing at ~ 1.1 μm at room temperature were also obtained with DH structures of $In_{0.88}Ga_{0.12}As_{0.23}P_{0.77}/InP$ prepared by LPE [30]. These lasers, with $J_{th} = 2800$ A/cm^2 ($d_3 = 0.6$ μm), were grown on p-type InP substrates with (111) B orientation. (The first such devices did not lase at room temperature [31].)

Of course, LED structures can be produced by similar technologies. Particularly for emission in the 1–1.2 μm spectral range, there is considerable interest for optical communications. These are discussed in Section 14.4.

The other early quaternary alloy heterojunctions [32–34] listed in Table 13.3.1 first demonstrated the concept of using alloys for lattice matching, but their performance at room temperature did not match that achieved at the same wavelength with (AlGa)As diodes. They most likely contained rather gross metallurgical defects, including nonplanar junctions, which further technological improvements would eliminate. This also applies to the first Ga(AsP)/(InGa)P LOC laser structures, which are of interest for visible emission. These visible lasers are discussed in Section 14.5.

13.4 Summary

From the work reported in this chapter, we can draw certain conclusions regarding the expanded spectral range of semiconductor laser diodes using materials other than GaAs–AlAs alloys.

1. The IV–VI compound heterojunction lasers have greatly improved performance compared to their homojunction counterparts. In particular, the increased CW operating temperature (to ~ 100 K) made possible by the heterojunctions is extremely useful. These improvements have occurred despite rather significant lattice parameter mismatch values at the heterojunctions, perhaps indicative of a reduced sensitivity to lattice defects compared to III–V laser diodes. Three epitaxial technologies have been used: vapor phase epitaxy, liquid phase epitaxy, and evaporation. The latter method appears to have yielded the most flexible approach toward producing heterojunction lasers. The improved molecular beam epitaxy equipment now becoming generally available promises to expand the use of vacuum technology for preparing these devices.

2. Great strides have been made with III–V compounds in producing lattice-matched structures. Devices produced in the 1–1.2 μm spectral range have threshold current densities adequate for CW operation; such lasers have been made using at least three approaches: AlGaAsSb/GaAsSb, InGaAsP/InP, and (InGa)As/In(GaP). The first two systems were grown by LPE, the third

by VPE. Progress has also been made in extending laser operation into the visible (Chapter 14).

The lattice mismatch does not exceed a fraction of 1% in the successful structures, although the limits remain to be established. The ability to produce good quality double-heterojunction lasers is aided by two effects: first, the growth of very thin recombination regions (well under 1 μm) which can remain misfit-dislocation free for small misfit values (Section 9.4); second, the "pulling" effect in LPE where the material composition tends to adjust to minimize the lattice mismatch. This is particularly important in the quaternary alloy growth. Of these, the InGaAsP alloys promise to be of the greatest continuing interest since they provide a broad spectral range and lattice-matching potential extending also into the visible (Section 14.5).

Note that although low threshold lasers have been produced, early devices had shorter operating lifetimes in CW operation than (AlGa)As lasers, probably because of a defect density that was excessive. Technological improvements can be expected, however, with a maturing process.

REFERENCES

1. For a review of small bandgap lasers and their use in spectroscopy, see A. R. Calawa, *J. Luminescence* **7**, 477 (1973).
2. For a review of the band structure of small bandgap semiconductors, see M. Balkanski, *J. Luminescence* **7**, 451 (1973).
3. I. Melngailis, *J. de Phys. Colloque Suppl.* **C4**, 11–12 (1968).
4. I. Melngailis, *Proc. Conf. Short Pulses Coherent Interactions*, Chania, Greece (1969).
5. K. W. Nill, A. R. Calawa, T. C. Harman, and J. N. Walpole, *Appl. Phys. Lett.* **16**, 375 (1970).
6. J. N. Zemel, *J. Luminescence* **7**, 524 (1973).
7. H. Holloway, D. K. Honke, R. L. Crawley, and E. Silkes, *J. Vac. Sci. Technol.* **7**, 586 (1970).
8. R. F. Bis, J. R. Dixon, and G. Lowney, *J. Vac. Sci. Technol.* **9**, 226 (1972).
9. W. Rolls, R. Lee, and R. J. Eddington, *Solid State Electron.* **13**, 75 (1970).
10. L. N. Kurbatov *et al.*, *Sov. J. Quantum Electron.* **5**, 1137 (1976).
11. J. T. Longo, J. Harris, E. Gertner, and J. Chu, *J. Crystal Growth* **15**, 107 (1972).
12. L. R. Tomasetta and C. G. Fonstad, *Appl. Phys. Lett.* **24**, 567 (1974).
13. T. C. Harmon, *J. Nonmetals* **1**, 183 (1973).
14. S. H. Groves, K. W. Nill, and A. J. Strauss, *Appl. Phys. Lett.* **25**, 331 (1974).
15. J. N. Walpole, A. R. Calawa, R. W. Ralston, T. C. Harman, and J. P. McVittie, *Appl. Phys. Lett.* **23**, 620 (1973).
16. J. N. Walpole, A. R. Calawa, T. C. Harman, and S. H. Groves, *Appl. Phys. Lett.* **28**, 552 (1976).
17. H. Preier, M. Bleicher, W. Riedel, and H. Maier, *Appl. Phys. Lett.* **28**, 669 (1976).
18. K. Duh and H. Preier, *J. Mater. Sci.* **10**, 1360 (1975).
19. G. F. McLane and K. J. Sleger, *J. Electron. Mater.* **4**, 465 (1975).
20. R. W. Ralston, I. Melngailis, A. R. Calawa, and W. T. Lindley, *IEEE J. Quantum Electron.* **9**, 350 (1973).

21. E. D. Hinkley and C. Freed, *Phys. Rev. Lett.* **23**, 277 (1969).
22. J. M. Besson, W. Paul, and A. R. Calawa, *Phys. Rev.* **173**, 699 (1968).
23. K. J. Linden, J. F. Butler, and K. W. Nill, unpublished. Commercial lasers are produced by Laser Analytics, Inc. 38 Hartwell Avenue, Lexington, Massachusetts 02173.
24. E. D. Hinkley, K. W. Nill, and F. A. Blum, *Laser Focus*, p. 47 (April 1976).
25. M. G. Craford, W. O. Groves, and M. J. Fox, *J. Electrochem. Soc.* **118**, 355 (1971).
26. C. J. Nuese, M. Ettenberg, and G. H. Olsen, *Appl. Phys. Lett.* **25**, 612 (1974); **29**, 54 (1976).
27. C. J. Nuese and G. H. Olsen, *Appl. Phys. Lett.* **26**, 528 (1975).
27a. C. J. Nuese *et al. Appl. Phys. Lett.* **29**, 807 (1976).
28. K. Sugiyama and H. Saito, *Jpn. J. Appl. Phys.* **11**, 1057 (1972).
29. R. E. Nahory, M. A. Pollack, E. D. Beebe, J. C. DeWinter, and R. W. Dixon, *Appl. Phys. Lett.* **28**, 19 (1976).
30. J. J. Hsieh, *Appl. Phys. Lett.* **28**, 283 (1976); J. J. Hsieh, J. A. Rossi, and J. P. Donnelly, *ibid.* **28**, 709 (1976).
31. A. P. Bogatov *et al.*, *Sov. J. Quantum Electron.* **4**, 1281 (1975).
32. R. D. Burnham *et al.*, *Appl. Phys. Lett.* **19**, 25 (1971).
33. J. J. Coleman, W. R. Hitchens, N. Holonyak, Jr., M. J. Ludowise, W. O. Groves, and D. L. Keune, *Appl. Phys. Lett.* **25**, 725 (1974).
34. R. D. Burnham, N. Holonyak, Jr., and D. R. Scifres, *Appl. Phys. Lett.* **17**, 455 (1970).

Chapter 14

Devices for Special Applications

Various aspects of diode design and construction have been reviewed in the preceding chapters. Although specific characteristics can be obtained by suitable structural design, no single device can perform all the desirable functions required in various optoelectronic systems. In this chapter, we consider lasers designed for high peak power operation, CW operation, emission in the visible or near-visible spectral range, as well as various types of infrared light emitting diodes.

14.1 High Peak Power, Pulsed Operation Laser Diodes

Heterojunction laser diodes designed for high peak power pulsed operation have been commercially available since 1969 and are used in systems such as ranging (optical radar), infrared illumination, and intrusion alarms. The pulse width is typically between 50 and 200 ns and the pulse rate is in the kilohertz range. The operating current density (at the rated emitted power level; see below) is typically as high as 40,000 A/cm², with $J_{th} \approx 10,000$–14,000 A/cm². The maximum diode operating range is limited by facet damage rather than gradual degradation, because of the low duty cycle (order 0.1 %). The devices are designed with emitting widths which scale with the required peak power. It has been experimentally established that the single-heterojunction laser is capable of many thousands of hours of reliable operation at the ~ 1 W/mil (400 W/cm) level (see Section 16.1), and the diode size is adjusted accordingly. Commercial lasers have emitting widths from 75 to 600 μm with corresponding peak power from 4 to 36 W. Very wide lasers are not desirable because of

455

the possibility of "cross lasing" in the structure, which grossly reduces the external differential quantum efficiency. However, with special precautions to reduce the reflectivity of the diode sidewalls, lasers as wide as 1500 μm have been made, emitting 100 W of peak power. In general, the use of stripe lasers (with stripe widths appropriate to the peak power needed) ensures the highest possible reliability because of the reduced probability of facet damage induced by defects at the edges of the older type of sawed-side laser diodes (Chapter 16).

To increase the power emitted from a small source size, diodes can be stacked by soldering one on top of the other (Fig. 12.1.1), thus in effect providing a series-connected module, or the diodes can be laid out in series as shown in Fig. 14.1.1a using a metallized BeO substrate. To fabricate such an array, a strip of diode material is soldered on the BeO substrate, and each diode is isolated from its neighbor by sawing through the strip into the BeO to remove the metallization between the diodes. Then the diodes are individually wired in series, the top of one diode being connected to the metallized strip extending behind the neighboring diode. Figure 14.1.1b shows a photograph of a completed series-connected array following assembly on a header. The width of the series-connected strips can be adjusted; in some cases as many as 60 diodes are so assembled in series. In general, the advantage of this construction is the low thermal resistance of the devices since each diode is individually heat sunk.

In the stacked diodes (as many as six diodes can be stacked commercially) the thermal resistance is higher, limiting the duty cycle to 0.01% compared to 0.1% for a single diode. A commercial six-stack device can emit as much as 180 W, which provides a convenient 500 × 500 μm source.

Series-connected linear arrays are used also in cooled systems where the duty cycle of operation (at 77 K) can be several percent, thus providing the potential of assembly infrared sources for illumination with several watts of *average power*.

The high peak power laser diodes are not designed for minimal threshold current density, but rather for maximum reliability under the rated power operating conditions, as well as minimal beam width to ease the problem of designing collimating optical systems. Furthermore, because of the need for diode arrays, it is important to construct devices as uniform in their characteristics as possible. An additional constraint is added in some cases by the need for efficient operation at ambient temperatures as high as 100°C. Here the LOC devices become particularly useful because they do not suffer the loss of radiation confinement above 60–70°C common with the single-heterojunction diodes as discussed in Section 7.3.3. As shown in Fig. 14.1.2, the best LOC lasers have threshold current densities (with heterojunction spacing of

IMPORTANT!

Your blanket control works like a thermostat
your home heating system.

Do not expect the blanket to heat if the bedr
temperature is warmer than the control dial
ting.

For example, if the bedroom temperatu
70° Fahrenheit, the blanket will not begin h
until the control is adjusted approxima
Position 5.

If more warmth is desired, adjust dial to
setting. Please refer to instruction book
plete details of the automatic blanket

P.N. 16

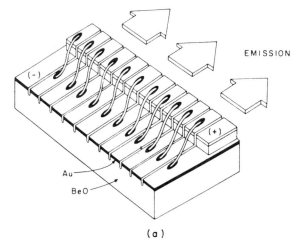

(a)

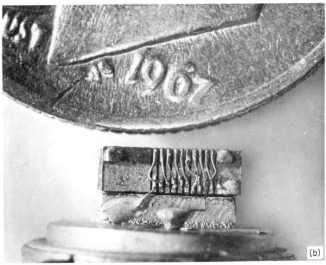

FIG. 14.1.1   (a) Series-connected laser diode array on BeO substrate. (b) Photograph of actual array mounted on package for room temperature operation. (Courtesy RCA Solid State, Lancaster, Pennsylvania.)

2 μm) below 10,000 A/cm^2, hence substantially below single-heterojunction values [1].

However, it is important to ensure fundamental transverse mode operation in such structures because of the disadvantage of "rabbit ear" far-field patterns observed with higher order modes [2] (Chapter 7). To ensure fundamental

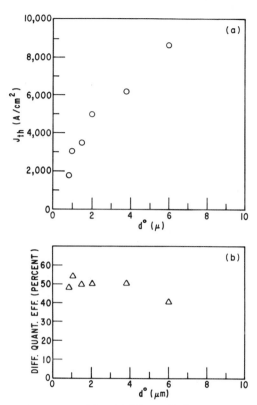

FIG. 14.1.2 Best values reported for LOC laser diodes at room temperature operated at low duty cycle. The width of the mode guiding region between the heterojunctions, $d°$, is indicated; $T = 300$ K; $L = 400$–500 μm [1].

mode operation, the structure of Fig. 14.1.3 is used. This structure incorporates some Al in region 4 for mode control, as discussed in Chapter 8, thus forming a three-heterojunction LOC. Typical data for such a structure are listed in Table 14.1.1. Note the high differential quantum efficiency of 50% combined with a moderate beam width $\theta_\perp = 30°$C, as well as moderate increase in the threshold current density at 75°C compared to room temperature. The advantage of this structure for production is that none of the dimensions are too critical to obtain the desired performance. The safe operating range is ~ 400 W/cm. Four-heterojunction devices (Chapters 7 and 8) can produce comparable electrical performance, but with additional fabrication complexity since an additional region is needed.

The single-heterojunction laser needs but a single basic epitaxial layer. Such devices reproducibly have $\theta_\perp$ values of about 20°. Because the junction is formed directly in melt-grown substrates, excellent uniformity can be ob-

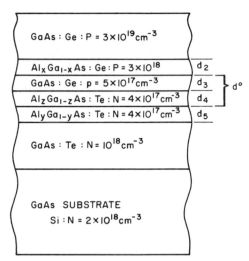

FIG. 14.1.3 Cross section of three-heterojunction structures designed for high power operation in the fundamental mode. The mode guiding region width $d° = 2 \mu m$ [2].

TABLE 14.1.1
Typical LOC Laser Characteristics[a]

$J_{th}(A/cm^2)$ at			$\eta_{ext}(\%)$ at				λ_L at	
23°C	75°C	100°C	23°C	75°C	$\theta_\perp$	$\theta_\parallel$	23°C	75°C
9000	15,000	30,000	50	35	28°	13°	8900 ± 50 Å	9050 ± 50 Å

[a]Structure of Fig. 14.1.3 [2].

tained under manufacturing conditions, the junction depth being controlled by the Zn diffusion step (Section 12.1). Figure 14.1.4 shows typical curves of power output versus current up to 60°C of a commercial stripe-contact single-heterojunction laser, (the RCA SG 2007).

The relative radiant flux collected versus collection angle for a typical single-heterojunction laser diode is shown in Fig. 14.1.5. The data were obtained by placing an iris of fixed aperture between the laser and the photodetector. The collection angle θ_c is then defined as

$$\theta_c = \tan^{-1}(r/l) \tag{14.1.1}$$

where r is the radius of the detector aperture and l is the distance from the source to the detector aperture. With drive conditions fixed, the power output was measured for various aperture-to-diode spacings [3].

The power conversion efficiency depends on the basic diode parameters and the operating current relative to the threshold current. It is given by

$$\eta_p \cong \frac{P_\theta}{I^2 R_s + (E_g/e)I} \tag{14.1.2}$$

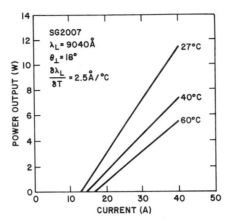

FIG. 14.1.4 Typical power output curves as a function of current and heat sink temperature for a commercial stripe-contact single-heterojunction laser diode, SG 2007. The stripe width is 225 μm. (Courtesy RCA Solid State, Lancaster, Pennsylvania.)

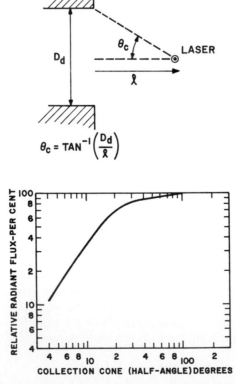

FIG. 14.1.5 Relative radiant flux as a function of collection angle for typical single-heterojunction laser diode. The adjoining schematic shows the method for determining these values. (Courtesy RCA Solid State, Lancaster, Pennsylvania.)

where R_s is the diode resistance, I the diode current, and P_θ the output power. Sommers [4] has calculated the relationship between the device properties and η_p, which peaks at $\sim 3-4I_{th}$ for high power lasers. The highest reported [1] power efficiency (two-sided emission) at room temperature is $\sim 22\%$, as shown in Fig. 14.1.6 for an LOC laser operating at a duty cycle of 1% and a current $I \approx 4I_{th}$.

High power operation can be obtained at other emission wavelengths with (AlGa)As lasers in the range of composition where the threshold current density is reasonable (Section 14.5). In practice, this means emission wavelengths at room temperature above 7800 Å for convenient reproducibility. Array assembly techniques comparable to those used for GaAs devices can be utilized to obtain high peak power operation.

In the vicinity of 1 μm, (InGa)As homojunction laser diodes have been operated at 77 K with peak emission values, from 12-diode linear arrays, of about 20 W [5].

The operation of laser diodes in the pulsed mode generally requires pulsers with provisions for eliminating the possibility of damaging reverse-bias operation during portions of the cycle. The pulse may be obtained by either a capacitive discharge circuit, in which a silicon controlled rectifier (SCR) is used to discharge a capacitor through the laser, or alternatively, a transistor-switched source may be used as the driving element. Each circuit has its partic-

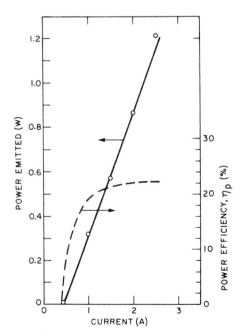

FIG. 14.1.6 Power output versus current and power efficiency (emission from both facets) of LOC laser diode at room temperature [1].

ular advantages and disadvantages, and the overall system performance will determine the optimum drive circuit design. Figures 14.1.7–14.1.9 show three different circuit designs, each with uniquely different features.

The circuit in Fig. 14.1.7 is an adjustable drive, general purpose SCR driver circuit in which the transistors Q_1 and Q_2 regulate the level to which the storage element C is charged by the supply voltage. The SCR acts as the discharge switch and, when triggered, drives the laser diode. This circuit may be used for pulse repetition rates in the range of 5–10 kHz. The value of C is determined by the combination of current and pulse width desired. For best results, a high quality Mylar-type capacitor, or equivalent, is recommended.

When higher repetition rates and shorter pulse widths are required, the circuit shown in Fig. 14.1.8 may be used. In general, most commercially available SCRs are not fast enough to deliver short, high current pulses at repetition rates in excess of 10 kHz. The GA-201 (Unitrode, Inc.), when used in

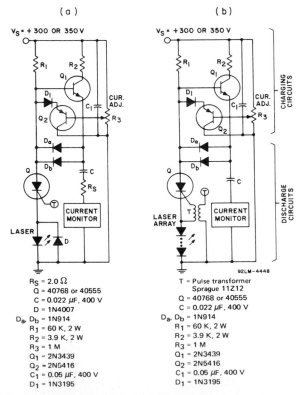

(a)

$R_S = 2.0\ \Omega$
Q = 40768 or 40555
C = 0.022 μF, 400 V
D = 1N4007
D_a, D_b = 1N914
R_1 = 60 K, 2 W
R_2 = 3.9 K, 2 W
R_3 = 1 M
Q_1 = 2N3439
Q_2 = 2N5416
C_1 = 0.05 μF, 400 V
D_1 = 1N3195

(b)

92LM-4448

T = Pulse transformer
   Sprague 11Z12
Q = 40768 or 40555
C = 0.022 μF, 400 V
D_a, D_b = 1N914
R_1 = 60 K, 2 W
R_2 = 3.9 K, 2 W
R_3 = 1 M
Q_1 = 2N3439
Q_2 = 2N5416
C_1 = 0.05 μF, 400 V
D_1 = 1N3195

FIG. 14.1.7   Laser driver using SCR: (a) for single diode; (b) for array. (Courtesy RCA Solid State, Lancaster, Pennsylvania.)

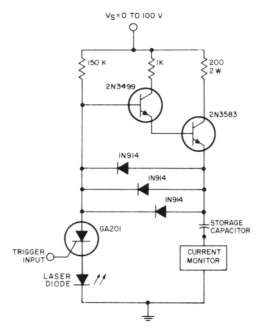

FIG. 14.1.8 Laser drive circuits, utilizing high speed SCR. (Courtesy RCA Solid State, Lancaster, Pennsylvania.)

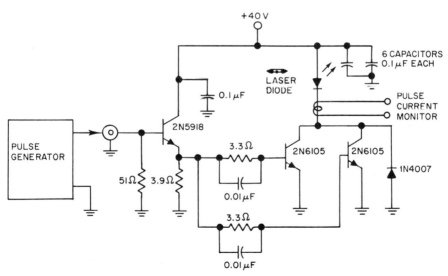

FIG. 14.1.9 Laser drive circuit utilizing high speed transistor. (Courtesy RCA Solid State, Lancaster, Pennsylvania.)

the circuit of Fig. 14.1.8, can deliver pulses as short as 25 ns at pulse repetition rates up to 25 kHz.

The transistor circuit of Fig. 14.1.9 is useful when repetition rates in excess of 25 kHz are needed. This circuit delivers pulses as short as 10 ns at pulse repetition rates beyond 100 kHz, but its maximum peak current is limited to about 20 A.

The packages for the laser diodes conventionally used are shown in Fig. 14.1.10. These consist of Kovar cases with central leads and screw bases for convenient heat sinking.

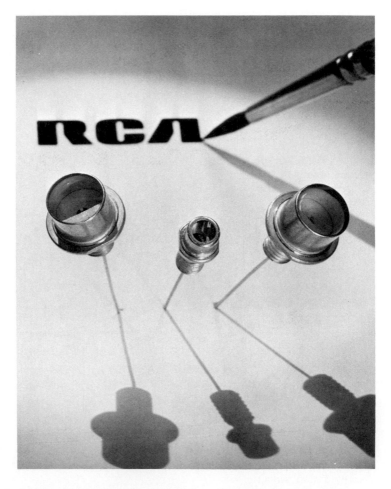

FIG. 14.1.10 Laser packages with hermetic enclosure. (Courtesy RCA Solid State, Lancaster, Pennsylvania.)

14.2 Fiber Concepts Relevant to Optical Communications

In this section we briefly review the major relevant concepts which affect the use of laser diodes and LEDs in optical communications using fibers. For a comprehensive treatment of the optical communications field (particularly systems and fibers) we refer to several extensive reviews [6–10].

Three major features of the fiber are of prime importance with respect to the choice of light source: (a) the attenuation versus wavelength, (b) pulse broadening which limits the transmitted data rate, and (c) coupling efficiency of the radiation into the fiber.

14.2.1 Fiber Properties

Absorption due to impurities in the fiber is the most important cause of light attenuation in the fiber, with absorption due to metallic contaminants and the OH ions in silica fibers being the most troublesome. The OH ions result in absorption peaks at 0.95, 0.72, and 2.7 μm, and their elimination is more difficult than that of most other contaminants. However, the concentration is low enough to permit low loss fiber fabrication. Figure 14.2.1 shows the attenuation (in dB/km) of a commercial step index multimode fiber [11]. The attenuation is low (about $\sim$4–6 dB/km) in the vicinity of 0.85 and 1.1 μm. These spectral "windows," which skirt the OH absorption peaks, are most fortunate for the use of the devices described here because it is not essential to eliminate all water traces from the silica manufacturing process. Note that the losses can be increased by several decibels in the course of cabling these fibers, although these losses are expected to decrease with improving technology.

In addition to this other significant optical losses result from Rayleigh scattering, which decreases with wavelength as λ^{-4} and contributes about 1 dB/km attenuation at $\lambda = 1$ μm. For very high optical power levels propagating in the fiber (order of a watt in a typical fiber) other loss mechanisms involving stimulated Brillouin scattering can become important. However, the typical operating level is much below this range. Additional losses of a few decibels per kilometer in long fibers may occur due to slight variations in the width of the fiber, radiation losses at bends in the fiber, and cross talk in parallel fibers within the same jacket.

The most widely used fibers, shown in Fig. 14.2.2, differ in the refractive index profile and core dimensions. The simplest, shown in Fig. 14.2.2a, is the "step index" fiber. Because of interference effects between rays propagating inside the fiber, the number of modes which propagate is limited by the dimension of the core, the wavelength, and the refractive index difference $\Delta n = n_1 - n_2$. The maximum number N_m of modes which can propagate is [10]

$$N_m \cong (2\pi a/\lambda)^2(n_1{}^2 - n_2{}^2) \approx (2\pi a/\lambda)^2(n_2 \, \Delta n) \qquad (14.2.1)$$

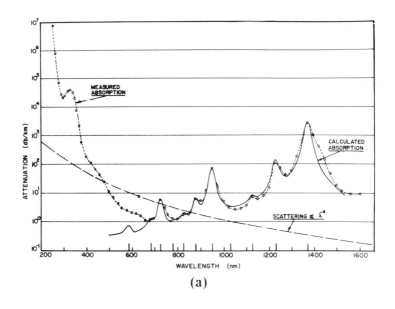

(a)

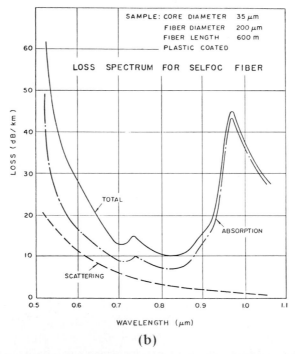

(b)

FIG. 14.2.1 (a) Attenuation of step index fiber produced by the Corning Glass Works. The various components contributing to the total attenuation are indicated. The important low loss regions are in the vicinity of 800 and 1100 nm (0.8 and 1.1 μm) [11]. (b) Attenuation of graded index Selfoc fiber produced by the Nippon Electric Company.

It is evident from (14.2.1) that by reducing the core radius a and minimizing Δn, it is possible to produce a fiber capable of propagating only a single mode. In fact, for ~ 1 μm radiation, a core diameter $2a \approx 5$ μm produces the desired effect, with $\Delta n \approx 0.01$ when $n_2 = 1.5$. Commercial Corning step index, multimode fibers have typical core diameters $2a = 80$–100 μm, a loss of ~ 6 dB/km at 0.85 and ~ 1.1 μm, and $\Delta n = 0.0068$. Hence, for $\lambda = 1$ μm and $a = 50$ μm, the maximum mode number $N_m \approx 1000$.

Figure 14.2.2b shows the second important type of fiber in which the refractive index is graded. The first of these, a graded index fiber (denoted Selfoc by the Nippon Electric Co. [12]), can be approximated by a parabolic profile of the form

$$n = n_1[1 - (x^2/a^2)(\Delta n/n_1)] \qquad (14.2.2)$$

An advantage of this type of fiber is that it supports fewer modes than the step index fiber with equal diameter and Δn value since [13]

$$N_m \cong \tfrac{1}{2}(2\pi a/\lambda)^2(n_1 \Delta n) \qquad (14.2.3)$$

Note that (14.2.3) is half of (14.2.1). (Single-mode graded index fibers are also possible by restricting the core diameter sufficiently.) As shown in Fig. 14.2.1 the Selfoc fiber loss is ~ 10 dB/km at $\lambda \cong 0.8$ μm, and the core diameter $2a \approx 35$ μm, with $\Delta n = n_1 - n_2 = 0.02$.

Pulse broadening is a basic limitation to the data rate. Assuming a "delta function" pulse imput, if the pulse is lengthened to Δt in a distance traversed L, then the maximum data rate in bits per second is approximately $(2 \Delta t)^{-1}$. The two major factors contributing to pulse broadening are as follows:

1. *Material dispersion.* The refractive index changes with wavelength which in turn changes the velocity of the components of a pulse having different

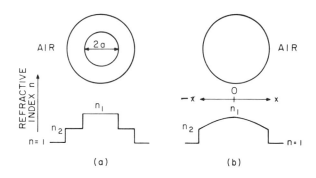

FIG. 14.2.2   Refractive index profile of commonly used fibers: (a) Step index fiber with core radius $2a$; (b) graded index fiber.

wavelengths. This effect is particularly important for LEDs since the emitted spectral width is several hundred angstroms.

2. *Modal dispersion.* Various modes in the fiber have different path lengths, hence their effective velocity changes. The larger the mode density, the greater this effect becomes, which explains the interest in single-mode fibers, or fibers with graded index profiles.

In addition, a third minor dispersive property exists which is related to the fact that even for a *single mode* the group velocity varies with wavelength. Similar to modal dispersion, this is a basic "waveguide property" rather than a material property; the calculated $\Delta t/L < 1$ ns/km.

Material dispersion is fundamentally related to the change in refractive index with wavelength, a parameter characterized for the present purpose by its second derivative. For a pulse containing a spectral width (half-intensity) $\Delta\lambda$, the broadening in a fiber length L is [14]

$$\frac{\Delta t}{L} = \frac{1}{c}\left(\frac{\Delta\lambda}{\lambda}\right)\lambda^2\left(\frac{d^2n}{d\lambda^2}\right) \tag{14.2.4}$$

An important aspect of the material dispersion is its wavelength dependence. The fact that $(d^2n/d\lambda^2)$ decreases with wavelength, as shown in Fig. 14.2.3, suggests that devices with an emission wavelength at about 1.1 μm, for example, are superior in this respect to devices emitting at 0.8 μm [15]. At 0.8 μm the material dispersion is about three times greater than that at 1.1 μm. The pulse broadening for typical LEDs can be estimated as follows. Consider a typical device:

$$\Delta\lambda = 300 \text{ Å}, \quad \lambda = 8000 \text{ Å}, \quad \lambda^2\left(\frac{d^2n}{d\lambda^2}\right) \cong 3 \times 10^{-2}, \quad c = 3 \times 10^5 \text{ km/s}$$

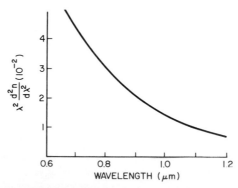

FIG. 14.2.3   Estimated variation of the key term contributing to pulse broadening by the process of "material dispersion" [Eq. (14.2.4)], as a function of wavelength in a Corning fiber with a silica-rich core material [15].

Then $\Delta t/L \cong 3.75$ ns/km. However, for a source emitting at 1.1 μm, with the same $\Delta\lambda/\lambda = 3.75\%$, $\Delta t/L \cong 1.3$ ns/km.

The modal dispersion contribution can be estimated, from a simple ray analysis, to produce a traversal time difference Δt between the fastest and slowest mode in a fiber of length L with a step index Δn:

$$\Delta t/L \cong c^{-1} \Delta n \qquad (14.2.5)$$

The predicted pulse broadening is very large. For example, with $\Delta n = 0.0068$, $\Delta t/L = 20$ ns/km. Fortunately, it is found experimentally [16,17] that the pulse width increase with fiber length (in a step index fiber) is closer to a $L^{1/2}$ dependence, as shown in Fig. 14.2.4 for $L > 0.5$ km. This occurs because the various modes in the guide exchange energy, the slowest modes feeding the faster moving ones as a result of mode mixing due to inhomogeneities in the fiber and in the cladding. In addition, the highest order modes, which are also the slowest, tend to have higher losses than the lower order modes. Thus, the actual number of modes present in the fiber over very long distances is smaller than the calculated value [Eq. 14.2.1].

The benefits of using graded index fibers in increasing the information bandwidth can be large because of the reduced modal dispersion. As shown by Marcuse [19],

$$\Delta t/L = (\Delta n)^2/2cn_2 \qquad (14.2.6)$$

With $\Delta n = 0.0068$, $n_2 = 1.5$, we calculate $\Delta t/L = 0.5$ ns/km—a value much lower than that just calculated for a step index fiber with the same index difference Δn.

The experimental values for Selfoc fibers do indeed show very low modal dispersion. Values of ≤ 1 ns/km have been reported, consistent with (14.2.6), which predicts 0.4 ns/km [20]. In other graded index fibers $\Delta t/L$ values of 2–3 ns/km are common [21], the difference being related to the detailed nature of the gradient, which is not optimum.

Measurements of fibers as long as 2.5 km show that the modal dispersion in graded index fibers is a linear function of the fiber length, as shown in Fig. 14.2.5. Note that the actual values observed for the pulse broadening differ slightly depending on the axis of the laser with respect to the fiber, because the density of excited modes changes. The calculated pulse broadening in Fig. 14.2.5 is for a fiber with the index profile shown in Fig. 14.2.5a, assuming no mode mixing. The measured values are seen to be in reasonable agreement, and the fact that the pulse broadening is linear with distance suggests that the mode mixing effects present in step index fibers are minimal in the graded index ones.

In Section 14.4 we discuss experimental values of the bandwidth transmitted over fibers using various LEDs. The reference point for the fiber quality

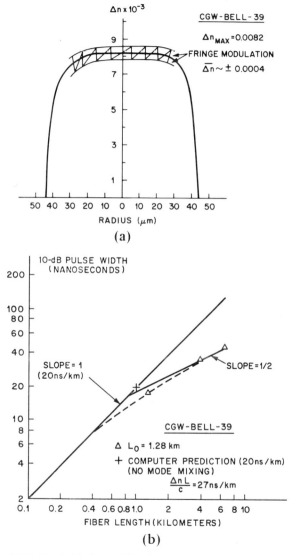

FIG. 14.2.4 (a) Refractive index profile of a Corning *step index fiber,* as deduced from interference microscopy. (b) Pulse width between 10-dB points plotted versus fiber length for a fiber with the index profile shown in (a). The numerical aperture of the fiber is 0.16 and the loss at 9000 Å is about 6 dB/km [17]. For relatively short fiber lengths, a large number of modes are excited and the pulse width increases with length L, as classically expected. For longer lengths (about 800 m in this case) mode mixing effects reduce the mode density to a steady state value, and the pulse width then increases as $L^{1/2}$. Also, the angle of incidence of the radiation entering the fiber affects the excited mode density and thus the length of fiber needed to reach a steady state condition, as discussed by Schicketanz [18].

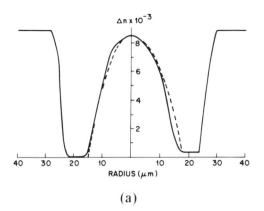

(a)

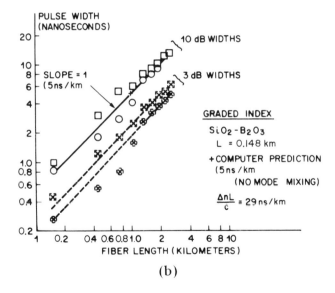

(b)

FIG. 14.2.5   (a) Graded refractive index profiles across the core of a SiO_2-B_2O_3 fiber. The dashed curve describes parabolic profile. (b) Pulse widths between 3 and 10-dB power points are plotted versus fiber length for coaxial ($\bigcirc$) and off-axis ($\square$) alignment between the fiber input and the injected laser beam. Computed 10-dB pulse widths predict 5-ns/km pulse spreading [21].

in this regard is the pulse broadening due to modal dispersion, which is measured using a laser.

14.2.2 Coupling Considerations

The fiber is characterized by a numerical aperture which is used in estimating the fraction of the radiation emitted from a diode which can enter the fiber. In practice, however, such coupling efficiency measurements can be misleading if clad short fiber lengths are used because much of the power can enter the fiber cladding rather than the core, and hence will be quickly attenuated.

The simplest approximation consists in characterizing the fiber with a numerical aperture which takes into account the incidence of rays on the fiber end. The rays enter the fiber if the angle is less than the critical angle θ_c,

$$\theta_c = \sin^{-1}(n_1^2 - n_2^2)^{1/2} \tag{14.2.7}$$

where $\sin \theta_c = (n_1 - n_2)^{1/2}$ is the numerical aperture (NA). For example, for a step index fiber, $\Delta n = n_1 - n_2 = 0.0068$, $NA \cong (2n_2 \Delta n)^{1/2} \approx 0.14$, since $n_2 \cong 1.5$.

For a source smaller than the core of the fiber (which is placed in proximity to the fiber) the coupling efficiency η_c is simply found by integrating the angular distribution $I(\theta)$ of the radiation between θ and θ_c, and dividing by the total output of the diode:

$$\eta_c = \frac{\int_0^{\theta_c} I(\theta) \sin \theta \, d\theta}{\int_0^{\pi/2} I(\theta) \sin \theta \, d\theta} \tag{14.2.8}$$

If the source is Lambertian, as is the case for a surface-emitting LED, then $I(\theta) = I_0 \cos \theta$. Neglecting a small factor accounting for Fresnel reflection at the fiber tip,

$$\eta_c \cong \sin^2 \theta_c \cong (NA)^2 \tag{14.2.9}$$

Hence, for an $NA = 0.14$ fiber, $\eta_c \cong 2\%$.

For other diode emission patterns, such as lasers or LED edge emitters described in Section 14.4, Eq. (14.2.8) must be used to calculate the coupling efficiency. It is evident, however, that the coupling efficiency can decrease to rather low numbers if the index steps (and hence NA) are small. As will be described in Sections 14.3 and 14.4, the coupling efficiency of laser diodes into step index fibers with $NA \cong 0.14$ is about -3 dB, whereas it is between -10 and -17 dB for LEDs, depending on their construction.

Improved coupling efficiency from LEDs can be obtained by using a lens to focus the radiation. The simplest technique consists of forming a spherical lens at the end of the fiber by melting the tip [22, 23]. This can easily provide a factor of ~ 2 improvement in the LED coupling efficiency.

The emission of the diode is sometimes characterized in terms of its radiance. If the diode emission fills the fiber core, and the emission is uniform, then the power coupled into a fiber

$$P_{\theta i} = (\text{radiance})(\text{diode area})(\text{solid acceptance angle of the fiber})$$

For small Δn values,

$$P_{\theta i} \cong \pi(\text{radiance})(\text{diode area})(\text{NA})^2 \qquad (14.2.10)$$

14.3 Near-Infrared CW Laser Diodes of (AlGa)As

The CW laser diodes emitting in the 0.8–0.85 μm spectral range are used in optical communications using fibers because of their high radiance, relatively narrow spectral width, and modulation capability extending to the gigahertz range. In addition, other applications exist for which a laser diode source may be competitive with low power gas lasers, including optical scanning systems [24], holographic readout, optical range finders, and the readout of information stored on disks. However, wavelengths shorter than 0.8 μm are desirable for improved depth of field in scanning systems, making it desirable to shift the emission further toward the visible (Section 14.5). In general, these applications require CW power emission levels of a few milliwatts, with long-term reliability being a very important consideration. In this section we review some representative lasers designed for room temperature CW operation which have demonstrated lifetimes well in excess of 20,000 hr.

14.3.1 Laser Construction and Packaging

Figure 14.3.1a shows a typical cross section of an oxide-isolated stripe-contact CW-type (AlGa)As laser diode* [25]. The active region ($d_3 = 0.2$–0.3 μm) contains about 10% Al, and the surrounding regions contain 30–35% Al. Although these lasers do not have the very lowest threshold current densities in broad-area form (values of 1200–2000 A/cm^2 are typical), the use of direct bandgap (AlGa)As in the "walls" of the structure minimizes the diode resistance. The diode shown is produced using the oxide stripe isolation process. Proton bombardment is another commonly used method for the production of planar stripe-geometry diodes (Chapter 12). It appears desirable to prevent the proton-bombarded region from reaching to the junction in order to minimize the possibility of point defects getting into the active region. Other stripe fabrication techniques described in Chapter 12, such as "buried

*Lasers of this type are produced in commercial quantities.

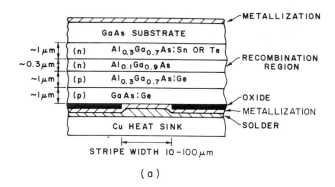

(a)

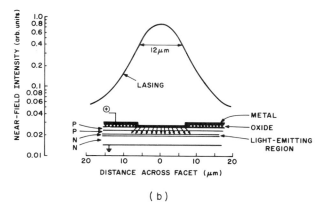

(b)

FIG. 14.3.1 (a) Typical cross section of double-heterojunction CW laser diode designed for room temperature operation with oxide stripe isolation. (b) Near-field emission pattern in the lasing condition. The half-intensity point in this particular structure occurs at the stripe edges [26].

stripes" or selective diffusion, are of a more experimental nature because of the greater control difficulty under manufacturing conditions.

The distance between the recombination region and the heat sink is typically about 2 μm to minimize the device thermal resistance. A stripe width of 10–15 μm offers a reasonable compromise between adequate and reliable power emission (about 10 mW) and moderate operating currents.

A diode package is evidently not suitable for all applications, particularly because of the need to attach fibers for optical communications. Commercial CW lasers designed for general purpose use are mounted on hermetically scaled coaxial cases of the type shown in Fig. 14.3.2. These are similar to those used for pulsed operation power lasers, with the difference that a copper base is mounted inside the package to reduce the thermal impedance of the structure. The thermal resistance of such lasers is 14–20 K/W which means a

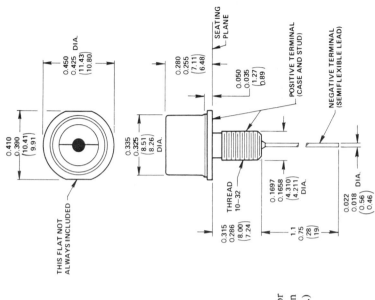

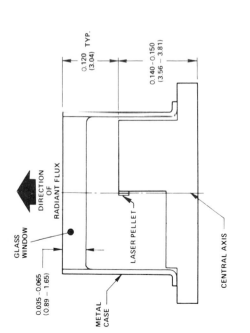

FIG. 14.3.2 Cross section of general purpose package used for commercial CW laser diodes. Dimensions (in parentheses) are in millimeters. (Courtesy RCA Solid State, Lancaster, Pennsylvania.)

modest 7–10°C junction temperature rise with a typical power dissipation of ≤ 0.5 W.

14.3.2   Power Emission

Figure 14.3.3a shows a typical curve of power output as a function of current of a 13-μm stripe laser operated pulsed and CW at room temperature [26]. The CW threshold is slightly higher than the pulsed one because of somewhat higher junction temperature, which also decreases the differential quantum efficiency. Higher power emission is obtained by widening the stripe, with 100 μm a practical limit because of the nonuniform thermal distribution in wider stripes due to the center of the stripe becoming substantially warmer than the edges. As a result, current crowding occurs, which leads to a saturation of the emitted CW power. Figure 14.3.3b shows the power emission from a 100-μm-wide stripe laser, with a maximum of 100 mW from one facet being obtained prior to saturation.

Some lasers show "kinks" in the light output versus current curve, i.e., a nonlinear behavior that is unrelated to obvious junction heating. Kinks can be caused by several factors. A possible cause is a nonuniform lasing region in which several "thresholds" are seen with increasing current. However, lateral mode change with current provides a more fundamental reason for nonlinear behavior. We now illustrate some of the more common observations.

Kinks can be classified into two broad categories. The first type involves "spikes," as seen in diode A of Fig. 14.3.3c. This effect is frequently observed in filamentary lasers (as shown in the spotty near-field photograph), the filaments being due to defects in the laser's active region. A second type of kink is due to the changes in the dominant lateral mode of the laser as the current is changed. Figure 14.3.3c shows the power curve of laser B where the far field in the plane of the junction indicates a change from lasing in the dominant fundamental lateral mode (s = 1) to the second mode (s = 2) in a current region corresponding to the change of slope. (The near-field photograph shows a typically nonfilamentary behavior.) The cause for the slope change is the gradual saturation in the emission of the fundamental mode in a current range still below the threshold for stimulated emission into the higher order mode [27]. As the higher order mode "turns on" and becomes dominant, the power emitted versus current curve slope increases once again. Accompanying the mode change, one observes increased noise in the optical output, as expected when threshold is reached by a mode (Chapter 17). Since this noise may be troublesome in modulation of the laser, it is generally desirable to limit the modulation range to current ranges outside the kink region.

The increase in the lateral modes with current was already noted in Section

7.7, an effect particularly prevalent in wide stripe lasers. Concurrent with these mode changes small kinks can sometimes be seen.

Figure 14.3.3d shows an example of changing lateral mode content in a laser diode with a stripe width of 25 μm (oxide isolated). As the current is increased, the kinks in the CW output curve are clearly seen. Various regions are shown in the curve correlated with increasing complexity in the lateral beam profile, reflecting the change from fundamental lateral mode operation very near threshold, to a very complex pattern reflecting many modes at 500 mA.

The typical series resistance of a 13-μm-wide stripe laser is 0.4–1 ohm. Hence with a *junction* voltage drop of 1.5 V, the total voltage drop across the diode at a current of 300 mA is 1.7–1.8 V (Fig. 2.1.3). With 10 mW emitted from *one facet*, the power efficiency is therefore about 2%. Of course, this efficiency can be improved by operating further above threshold, but the utmost in reliability is generally preferred to high power efficiency in such devices, and reliability considerations make it desirable to minimize the operating current, and thus limit the power output (Chapter 16).

The temperature dependence of the CW threshold current generally follows that of the pulsed operation value, with a factor of about 1.5 between 20 and 60°C being a reasonable J_{th} increase for the structure of Fig. 14.3.1a. (As noted in Section 8.3, however, a lower J_{th} temperature dependence is obtained by using higher Al concentration differences between the recombination region and the two bounding regions.) To maintain the power level constant with increasing heat sink temperature it is, therefore, necessary to increase the current level.

The simplest solution to the problem of maintaining constant output under ambient conditions where the temperature changes is to use a temperature-stabilized heat sink which incorporates thermoelectric devices. A thermistor placed on the heat sink provides the temperature-sensitive element for control when used in conjunction with the circuit shown in Fig. 14.3.4.

Optical feedback is another commonly used method for maintaining constant power output. Here, a small detector senses the emitted power level and appropriate circuitry is used to adjust the diode current to maintain the power level constant. It is important to limit the current range to minimize the possibility of laser damage.

14.3.3 Near- and Far-Field Patterns

The near-field intensity distribution is a function of the stripe width. With a relatively narrow (≤ 10 μm) stripe device, formed by a planar process in which the lateral optical confinement (i.e., in the plane of the junction) is relatively poor, the fundamental lateral mode is usually dominant at low power levels, giving rise to a single intensity maximum in the center of the 13-μm

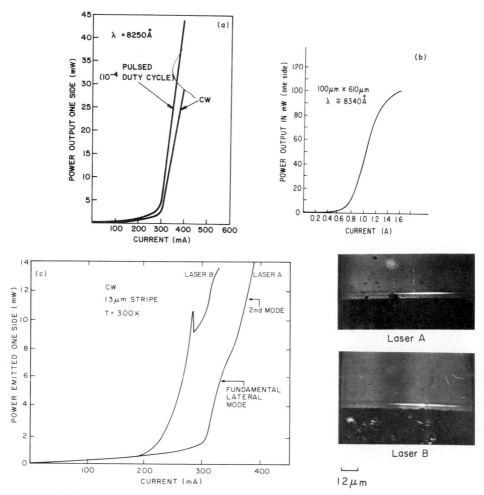

FIG. 14.3.3 Power output at room temperature as a function of dc current from an
(AlGa)As double-heterojunction laser diode with a stripe width of (a) 13 μm and (b) 100 μm.
The saturation effect is thermal in origin as discussed in Section 12.4 [26].   (c) Two types of
"kinks" in the light versus current curves of CW lasers. Laser A has a behavior related to
filamentary emission due to defects as shown in the near-field photograph. Laser B is representative of behavior related to change in the dominant lateral mode from the fundamental to the first higher-order one. The near-field shows no evidence of "beady" emission
due to defects.   (d) Power output (CW) as a function a current of a stripe-contact laser
diode (25 μm wide stripe) at room temperature showing evidence of slight "kinking," and
the corresponding far-field patterns in the plane of the junction. At low current, very near
threshold, the device operates in the fundamental lateral mode. The mode content changes
with increasing current, as deduced from the increasing complexity of the radiation patterns
shown. (H. Kressel and I. Ladany, unpublished.)

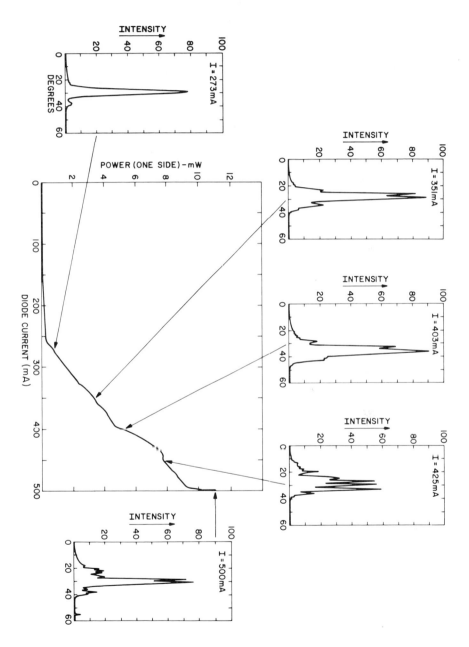

FIG. 14.3.3d

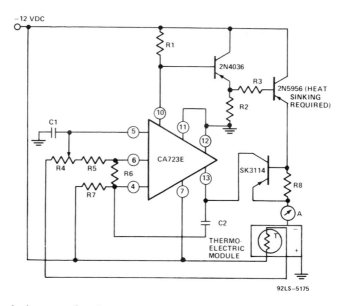

92LS–5175

A: Ammeter, 0 to 5 amperes
C_1: 0.001 μF, 100 V
C_2: 0.01 μF, 100 V
R_1: 1 kΩ, 1/2 W
R_2: 1 kΩ, 1/2 W
R_3: 100 Ω, 1/2 W
R_4: 5 kΩ potentiometer (Temperature adjustment)
R_5: 10 kΩ, 1/2 W
R_6: 3 kΩ, 1/2 W
R_7: 3.6 kΩ, 1/2 W
R_8: 0.287 Ω, 3 W

T: Thermistor Fenwall Part GB41P2
    (10 kΩ at 25° C), or equivalent
Thermo-Electric Module: Melcor Part
    CP1.4-17-10, or equivalent

FIG. 14.3.4 Temperature stabilization circuit used for laser diodes. (Courtesy RCA Solid State, Lancaster, Pennsylvania.)

stripe as shown in Fig. 14.3.1b and in the microphotograph of Fig. 7.7.1. The far-field pattern in the plane of the junction consists in this case of only a single dominant lobe about 6–9° wide at the half-intensity point (defined as $\theta_\parallel$; Fig. 14.3.5). With wide stripes, however, higher order lateral modes are generally dominant as seen in the near-field micrograph of Fig. 7.7.1. The resultant far-field pattern in the *plane* of the junction then consists of several

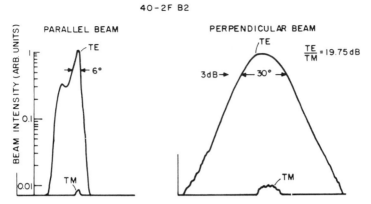

FIG. 14.3.5 Typical far-field pattern of a 13-μm-wide stripe laser showing the dominant TE polarization. These patterns remain essentially constant as the device temperature is increased to its maximum practical operating limit (I. Ladany and H. Kressel, unpublished).

lobes as shown in Fig. 7.7.2a. Note that the lateral mode content can increase with current as indicated in Section 7.7, and therefore unless the active region width in the plane of the junction is very narrow, a complex modal pattern is likely.

Note that with strong lateral confinement, such as obtained with buried stripe lasers, high order lateral mode operation is unavoidable unless the stripe width is made sufficiently narrow (Section 7.7). In practice, this may mean stripe widths of 1–2 μm for high Al concentration steps at the edges of the stripe. Since fundamental lateral mode operation is generally desirable, these dimensional considerations must be carefully considered in diode design.

In the plane *perpendicular* to the junction, only the fundamental mode exists in typical CW lasers, as expected on the basis of the theory of Chapters 5 and 6. Figure 14.3.6 shows scans of the near-field emission pattern, with a half-width of about 0.5 μm, independent of the drive current. The resultant far-field pattern in the direction perpendicular to the junction plane consists of a single lobe, as analyzed in Chapters 5 and 6 and shown in Fig. 14.3.5. Typical CW laser diodes have $\theta_\perp$ values of 30–45°, which are independent of temperature, indicative of no change in the radiation confinement. The radiation is strongly polarized TE (consistent with the theory of Chapter 5), as shown in Fig. 14.3.5.

14.3.4 Spectral Emission

Even though they commonly operate in the fundamental lateral and transverse mode, narrow stripe lasers generally exhibit multimode emission due to

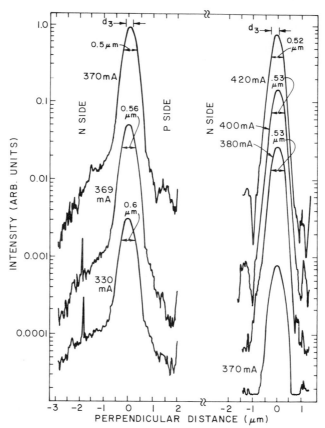

FIG. 14.3.6 Near-field distribution in the direction *perpendicular* to the junction plane of a typical CW laser diode (pulsed) (H. S. Sommers, Jr., unpublished).

the contribution of several longitudinal modes, as shown in Fig. 14.3.7. However, some lasers with stripe widths of 13 μm (or less) operate in a single longitudinal mode over significant current ranges above threshold, and thus emit a few milliwatts in basically single mode operation. Figure 14.3.7 shows the evolution of the spectra from such a laser with increasing current. Figure 14.3.8 shows a high resolution resolution scan with the line half-width at a maximum of 0.16 Å (order gigahertz) [28]. (Note the absence of the satellite lines associated with higher order lateral modes, which were present in the spectrum from the stripe laser of Fig. 5.7.2.) It is probable that the 0.16 Å half-width is experimentally limited because of temperature inhomogeneities in the laser. Narrower line widths have in fact been observed at ≈ 77 K in measurements of CW homojunction GaAs lasers, with $\Delta\nu$ values as low as $\sim 10^5$ Hz reported [29]. The theoretical values are probably still lower (Appendix E).

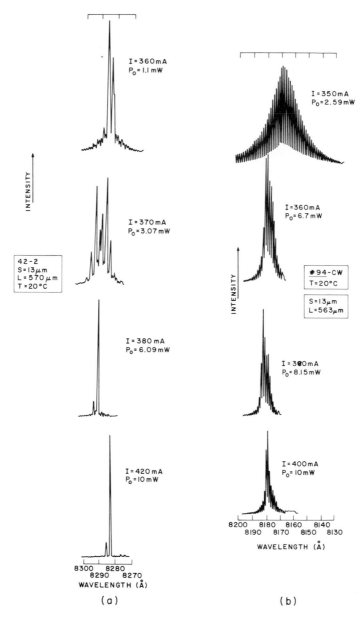

FIG. 14.3.7 Emission spectra of room temperature CW laser as a function of current showing the diversity of spectral purity seen. (a) "Pure" spectrum at relatively high drive with one dominant longitudinal mode. (b) More typical multimode spectrum. The power values indicated are emission from one facet only (H. Kressel and I. Ladany, unpublished).

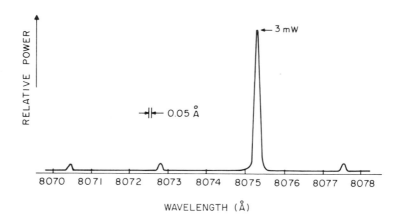

FIG. 14.3.8 Lasing spectrum of a CW laser diode operating at 300 K in the fundamental transverse and lateral mode and in mostly a single longitudinal mode. The stripe width is 5 μm formed by oxide isolation [28].

The reason for the differences in the spectral purity with regard to longitudinal mode content of the lasers is still not clear. The uniformity of the material in the recombination region may be a factor in the spectral purity. In fact, lasers exhibiting obvious inhomogeneities do show much more pronounced multimode behavior than good quality devices. Furthermore, lasers which have degraded by the process of internal defect generation (Section 16.2) exhibit much more pronounced multimode behavior than present initially. However, experience has shown that the control of the longitudinal mode content in Fabry–Perot structures is chancy. The distributed-feedback lasers (Chapter 15) were specifically designed for longitudinal mode control.

14.3.5 Modulation

As indicated in Section 8.1, the delay caused by the spontaneous carrier lifetime limits the modulation rate of lasers if they are completely turned off after each pulse. However, biasing the laser to threshold ensures that it is always operating in the stimulated mode, and high modulation rates are thereby possible. This is because the stimulated carrier lifetime is shortened with increasing injection (Section 3.4) which in turn changes the intensity of the electromagnetic field above lasing threshold. Using homojunctions of GaAs, modulation of laser emission as high as 11 GHz was obtained by Goldstein and Weigand [30], and Nishizawa [31] extended the modulation to 46 GHz, all indicative of carrier lifetimes below 10^{-10}s, sufficiently above threshold. Thus, it appears that laser diodes provide modulation capabilities extending into the gigahertz range. In practice, there are limitations associated with optical fluctuations in CW lasers which must be considered in practical systems. These effects are discussed in Chapter 17.

Double-heterojunction laser diodes have been modulated at 1 GHz by using the transistor circuit shown in Fig. 14.3.9 in which the laser is dc biased to threshold [32]. However, the resonance effects due to intrinsic high frequency fluctuation in the optical output do represent a limiting factor in obtaining 100% modulation and "clean" short pulses at arbitrary current levels above threshold. Chown *et al.* [32] found that distortion-free optical modulation at about 1 GHz was best achieved in a current range just above threshold where multimode (longitudinal) spectral emission was observed. In general, the resonance frequency increases with current above threshold, but complications and additional noise appear to be introduced in lasers containing significant kinks in the light versus current curves.

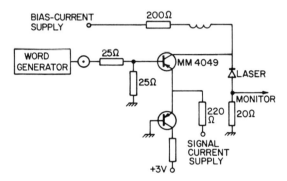

FIG. 14.3.9 Circuit used to modulate a CW laser diode (dc biased to threshold) up to about 1 GHz. The MM 4049 (Motorola) transistor is a p–n–p 4 GHz device designed for 200 mW dissipation and capable of 30 mA dc operation [32].

14.4 High Radiance Light-Emitting Diodes

The spectral bandwidth of the LED is typically 300–400 Å at room temperature, hence at least one order of magnitude broader than the typical laser diode emission. Because of the increased material dispersion discussed in Section 14.2, this can represent a drawback with regard to bandwidth for long-distance communication through fibers. However, the LED has the advantage of smaller temperature dependence of the emitted power and simpler construction. For example, there is typically only a factor of 1.5–2 reduction in power output between room temperature and 100°C at constant current. This reduced temperature dependence permits a simplified drive circuit and reduces the need for temperature stabilization.

Assuming that the emission wavelength is suitable and the reliability sufficient, the major factors of interest in the application of an LED to fiber systems is the modulation capability and the power that can be coupled into a desired fiber. The latter is related to the radiance of the source.

Heterojunction structures are advantageous for high radiance LEDs because they allow the combination of an appropriately doped recombination region with surrounding material having a higher bandgap energy, hence low absorption of the emitted radiation. Furthermore, waveguiding leads to improved edge emission efficiency and a more directional beam than achieved from a surface-emitting LED.

14.4.1   Diode Construction

The basic high radiance heterojunction LED technology is similar to that used for the fabrication of heterojunction laser diodes. The major differences between the LED and the laser are in the device geometry. Two basic structures for obtaining maximum radiance have evolved—surface and edge emitters.

For the *uncoated surface emitter*, the efficiency is limited by the refractive index difference between the semiconductor and air:

$$\eta_{sp} = [n(n + 1)^2]^{-1} \qquad (14.4.1)$$

With $n = 3.6$ in GaAs, the external efficiency is limited to about 1.3%, even with unity internal quantum efficiency. (The radiation which is not emitted is absorbed in the diode substrate or contact areas.) In order to increase the

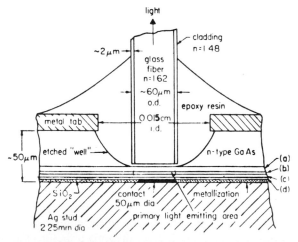

FIG. 14.4.1   Cross-sectional drawing (not to scale) of small-area double–heterojunction electroluminescent diode coupled to optical fiber. Layer (a), n-type $Al_xGa_{1-x}As$, 10 μm thick; emitting layer (b), p-$Al_yGa_{1-y}As$, ≈ 1 μm thick; layer (c), p-type $Al_xGa_{1-x}As$, 1 μm thick; layer (d), p-GaAs, ≈ 0.5 μm thick (for contact purposes) [33].

diode external efficiency, it is common practice to encapsulate it in materials having a refractive index higher than 1, or to use spherical shapes to produce an angle of incidence at the emitting face as close to perpendicular as possible. However, the divergence of the rays so produced is not very helpful in coupling radiation into low numerical aperture fibers.

The first surface-emitting LED specifically designed for single-fiber coupling is shown in Fig. 14.4.1 [33]. It consists of a standard (AlGa)As double-heterojunction diode in which the active area is defined by an oxide-isolated metal contact. Since the radiation emitted from the diode is absorbed in the substrate, a well is etched into the substrate which terminates at the (AlGa)As layer. A fiber can then be inserted into the well and glued into place. (The attachment of the fiber requires great care to minimize damage to the diode.) The diode emission is Lambertian and the coupling efficiency can be computed from (14.2.9).

In the second basic approach, the *edge-emitting* heterojunction structure, the diode is mounted upside down (similarly to a laser diode), and a stripe geometry is used with the striped width adjusted for the diameter of the fiber being used [23, 34, 35]. As shown in Fig. 14.4.2a, a restricted contact at the edge of the chip provides a convenient means of restricting the emitting area to maximize the diode efficiency. Such restricted edge-emitting (REED) structures provide substantially improved output efficiency compared to the long stripe contact similar to that used for the laser diodes. With edge emitters, the fiber is attached to the package as shown in Fig. 14.4.2c and no stress is placed on the diode material itself [23]. In all edge-emitting structures, it is desirable to add an antireflecting film on the diode facet in order to improve the efficiency. The edge emission is directional, as described in Section 14.4.2, dependent on the heterojunction configuration.

Note that both of these structures are capable of operation at very high current densities (order 1000 A/cm^2) without excessive junction heating because the diode is mounted with the active region close to the heat sink. However, for low power emission levels, where current densities of only a few hundred amperes per square centimeter are needed, other surface emission structures may be used, closer to the conventional surface-emitting diode used for general purpose applications (see Section 14.6) with the diode substrate side on the heat sink. Such structures have substantially higher thermal resistance values than the diodes mounted p-side down.

Some applications require fiber bundles. In this case, a parabolic package of the type shown in Fig. 14.4.3 is useful. The emission from the diode surface and edges can be collected and a relatively uniform source is provided for the fibers in the bundle. However, since such bundles are costly, single fibers are expected to be preferred whenever practical.

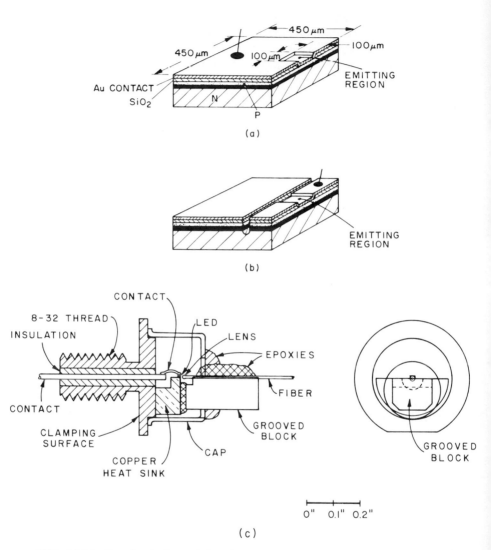

FIG. 14.4.2   Restricted edge-emitting diodes (REED) with (a) a continuous surface and (b) a slotted back to improve the external efficiency [35]. (c) Cross section of package used for edge-emitting diodes (or lasers) with fiber "pigtail" [23].

14.4.2   Modulation Capability

As shown in Section 2.5, the inherent modulation speed of an LED is a function of the minority carrier lifetime. Assuming a constant lifetime independent of the injected carrier density, the power output of a diode falls off with frequency ω for a constant modulation current amplitude:

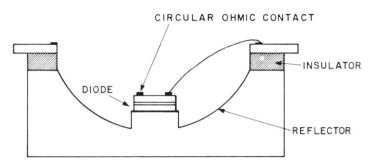

FIG. 14.4.3   Reflector package for LED useful for coupling into fiber bundles.

$$P(\omega) = \frac{P_\theta}{[1 + (\omega\tau)^2]^{1/2}} \tag{14.4.2}$$

where P_θ is the dc power output for the same diode current, $P(\omega)/P_\theta$ is the response R in Fig. 14.4.4b.

It is evident, therefore, that the fabrication of a high speed diode requires the lowest possible minority carrier lifetime. We first consider results obtained using diodes with highly doped recombination regions. It is important to reduce the *radiative* lifetime τ_r and not the nonradiative lifetime τ_{nr} because of the decrease in the internal quantum efficiency η_i with τ_{nr} (see Section 1.5),

$$\eta_i = [1 + \tau_r/\tau_{nr}]^{-1} \tag{14.4.3}$$

Unfortunately, it is a common observation in GaAs and related compounds that nonradiative centers are formed when the dopant concentration approaches the solubility limit at the growth temperatures. As mentioned in Section 10.1.2, Ge is a particularly useful acceptor in GaAs prepared by liquid phase epitaxy. Its concentration can reach values in the low 10^{19} cm^{-3} range without introducing an excessive density of nonradiative centers, and $\tau \cong 1 - 2$ ns can be achieved. The experimental data shown in Fig. 14.4.4 for edge-emitting diodes [36] follow (14.4.2) quite well, with τ ranging from 27 to ~ 1.1 ns. A similar dependence of modulation capability on minority carrier lifetime was found to hold for both stripe-contact and broad-area diodes [37].

While useful devices can be produced with high doping in the recombination region, their efficiency is reduced compared to lightly doped (i.e., slower) devices. An alternative to the use of high doping levels to reduce the carrier lifetime is to operate lightly doped devices at a current density such as to produce a *high injected carrier density*. As discussed in Section 1.5, in the bimolecular recombination regime the carrier lifetime decreases with carrier density. Thus, even if the lifetime is initially long because of a low background carrier population, it is possible to envision a very narrow recombination region device where the lifetime can be short at moderate current densities. Experimental results [23, 38] have indeed shown that important benefits ac-

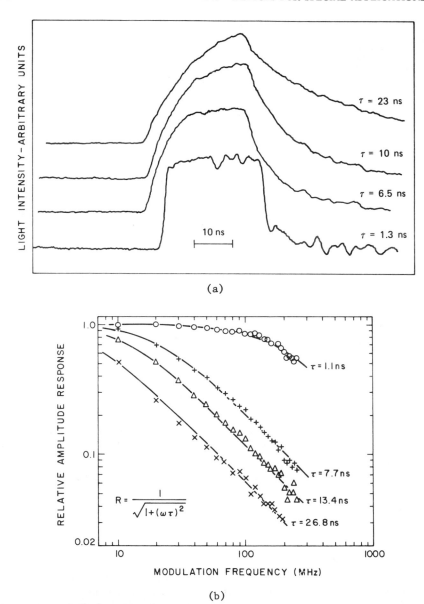

FIG. 14.4.4   (a) Light output response to a 25-ns square-wave current pulse and (b) response of LEDs with various carrier lifetimes (indicated) as a function of frequency. The response R follows (14.4.2) [36].

crue from using narrow (~0.05–0.1 μm) DH LEDs with undoped recombination regions: (1) the efficiency is high and the lifetime short; and (2) the emitted radiation is directional, increasing the coupling efficiency into fibers.

Figure 14.4.5 shows the stripe-geometry structure described by Ettenberg *et al.* [38]. In Fig. 14.4.6 is shown the spectral line shape which is narrow (225 Å) at 100 mA, increasing to 300 Å at 400 mA because of heating in the structure (which also increases the peak wavelength somewhat). Figure 14.4.7 shows that the relative diode response increases with current as the carrier lifetime decreases (as $J^{-1/2}$) to 1–2 ns at ~ 4000 A/cm² ($I = 400$ mA). However, the modulation depth so achieved must be analyzed for specific system needs.

Of course, the frequency response of the diode itself is only one aspect of the problem of obtaining high data rates with LEDs since the material dispersion in the fiber can easily represent the limiting factor for significant fiber lengths. As expected from (14.2.4), the bandwidth should decrease with increasing diode line width $\Delta\lambda$, other factors remaining constant. Figure 14.4.8 shows the measured relative response of various LEDs through a 1-km length of graded index multimode fiber produced by Corning. Taking the 50% response frequency as a comparative number, we see from Table 14.4.1 that the material dispersion, as estimated from (14.2.4), scales very well with the falloff in frequency response with increasing $\Delta\lambda/\lambda$. The manufacturer's modulation

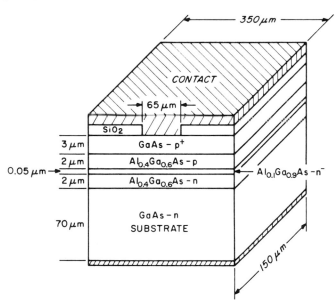

FIG. 14.4.5 Schematic of edge-emitting double-heterojunction LED with highly directional beam perpendicular to the junction [38].

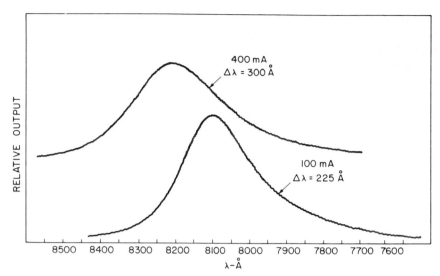

FIG. 14.4.6   Spectral emission of diode of Fig. 14.4.5 at 100 and 400 mA drive current showing the spectral broadening and shift to longer peak wavelength because of junction heating. This effect is related to the thermal resistance of the diode, and is not fundamental [38].

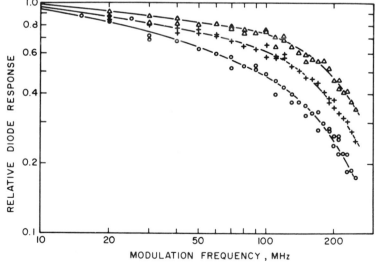

FIG. 14.4.7   Modulation response of stripe-contact diode of Fig. 14.4.5 as a function of frequency for various fixed bias current values. The carrier lifetime τ decreases with current I following approximately $\tau \propto I^{-1/2}$, which is reflected in an increasing high frequency response; ($\triangle$) $I = 400$ mA, ($+$) $I = 200$ mA, ($\bigcirc$) $I = 100$ mA [38].

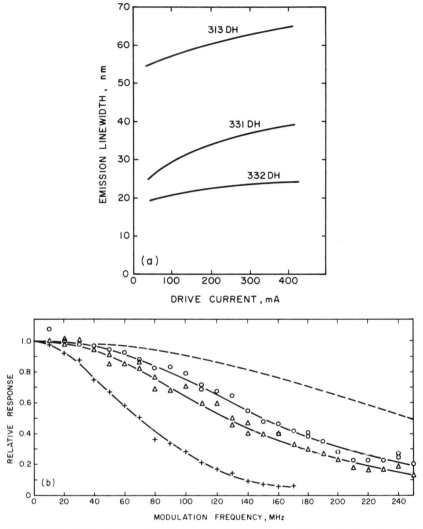

FIG. 14.4.8   Data showing the effect of the LED spectral width on the fiber dispersion. (a) Broadening of the emitted diode spectral bandwidth with increasing current (a result of junction heating). (b) Frequency response (50% optical power point) through graded index Corning fiber for the three diodes of (a) [313 DH (+), 331 DH (△), 332 DH (○)]. The dashed curve is the fiber response curve as limited by modal dispersion. (The pulse broadening is about 2 ns/km due to modal dispersion.) See Table 14.4.1 for a comparison between calculated and observed values [23].

TABLE 14.4.1

Material Dispersion Contribution in LED–Corning Graded Index Fiber System[a]

λ (Å)	$\Delta\lambda/\lambda$	Measured frequency response[b] (MHz)	Calculated[c] Δt ($L = 1$ km) (ns)	Calculated bandwidth $(2\Delta t)^{-1}$ (MHz)	Calculated[d] overall bandwidth (MHz)
8120	0.075	70	7	71	69
8000	0.043	127	4	125	112
8030	0.025	151	2.3	217	164

[a]See Fig. 14.4.8.

[b]-6 dB signal power point (50% optical power level). From Wittke *et al.* [23].

[c]Assuming $\lambda^2 d^2 n/d\lambda^2 = 2.8 \times 10^{-2}$; hence $\Delta t/L \cong 9 \times 10^{-8} \Delta\lambda/\lambda$ s/km (-6 dB signal power level).

[d]Using $(\Delta t)^2 = (\Delta t)^2_{mat\ dis} + (\Delta t)^2_{mod\ dis}$ (Gaussian pulse shape), with $(\Delta t)_{mod\ dis} = 2$ ns. (Here, mat. dis. denotes material dispersion and mod. dis. denotes modal dispersion.)

limit shown in Fig. 14.4.8b is measured using a laser under conditions in which the material dispersion is negligible. This provides an upper limit to the data transmission rate with a monochromatic source. Therefore, in addition to the material dispersion, modal dispersion contributes to the falloff in frequency response.

The additive pulse broadening effects can be estimated (for Gaussian pulses) by the square of the individual pulse broadening contributions. Thus, the total pulse width is [39] $(\Delta t)^2 = \Sigma(\Delta t)_i^2$, where $(\Delta t)_i$ is the contribution of the *i*th factor.

Finally, we note measurements of noise from GaAs homojunction [40] and heterojunction LEDs. Poor ohmic contacts provided the dominant noise source; with good contacts, the measured frequency-dependent noise would be well below the shot noise in a practical system [41].

14.4.3 Emission Pattern and Power into Fibers

The emission from a surface emitter is, as indicated earlier, Lambertian, and appropriate estimates of the coupling efficiency [42] into fibers can be made using Eq. (14.2.9). The emission pattern of the edge emitters in the direction perpendicular to the junction is more complicated, being dependent on the width of the active region and the refractive index step at the heterojunctions. However, the beam is very broad in the plane of the junction.

To understand the emission pattern of the edge-emitting LED, we must consider that the incoherent radiation is being partially guided as described in Chapter 5 for lasing structures. Because of the spontaneous nature of the emission, however, the overall external quantum efficiency for emission from one edge is about 1%—at least a factor of 10 lower than in stimulated emission. The difference arises from the fact that the stimulated emission is into the Fabry–Perot modes of the cavity which are incident at normal or nearly normal angles to the facet. Of course, radiation guiding in the LED occurs only because of the heterojunctions, but, parallel to the junction plane no such effect occurs and the emission is therefore broad. Figure 14.4.9 shows the asymmetry of the edge emission from the LED of Fig. 14.4.5: The beam width perpendicular to the junction is $\theta_\perp = 35°$, whereas in the plane of the junction, $\theta_\parallel = 120°$.

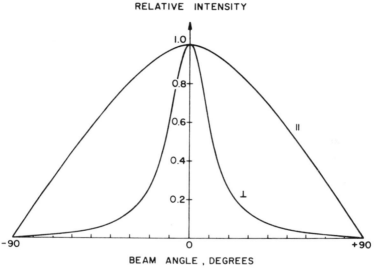

FIG. 14.4.9 Emission pattern from diode (LED 297) shown in Fig. 14.4.5 in the direction perpendicular ($\perp$) and parallel ($\parallel$) to the junction plane. Other data of similar devices are shown in Table 14.4.2. For the present diode $\theta_\perp \approx 25°$ and $\theta_\parallel \approx 120°$ [38].

In fact, the value of $\theta_\perp$ correlates for narrow DH LEDs with the refractive index step and the heterojunction spacing d_3. Table 14.4.2 shows results obtained for a series of such devices. The calculated value of $\theta_\perp$ is obtained from the approximation [43] valid only for very small heterojunction spacings (Chapter 7),

$$\theta_\perp \cong 20d_3(\Delta x)/\lambda \quad \text{(radians)} \qquad (14.4.4)$$

where Δx is the fractional Al concentration difference between the recombination region and the outer confining regions of the symmetric DH structure.

The radiance of such narrow beam devices can be as high as $\sim 1000 \text{ W/cm}^2$ sr, as determined from scanning the beam intensity [38]. The important parameter for fiber applications is coupling into low numerical aperture fibers. The measured coupling loss into $\text{NA} = 0.14$ (step index) fibers from a diode with $\theta_\perp \cong 25°$ and $\theta_\parallel \sim 120°$ is 10 dB compared to 17 dB for a surface emitter, and substantial amounts of power can be coupled into fibers. Figure 14.4.10 shows the toal power output from the diode as well as the amount of power transmitted through 350 m of fiber having an 8 dB/km loss at the diode

TABLE 14.4.2

Summary of Properties of Double-Heterojunction (AlGa)As LEDs[a]

Sample no.	$d_s(\mu m)$	Δx^b	$\theta_\perp$ (exp. degrees)	λ (μm)	$\theta_\perp{}^c$ (calc. degrees)
295	0.08	0.25	35	0.88	26
297	0.05	0.48	25	0.88	31
298	0.08	0.45	65	0.82	50
305	0.04	0.32	30	0.81	18
309	0.06	0.35	25	0.81	17
313	0.06	0.35	28	0.83	29
314	0.10	0.50	67	0.81	70
321	0.10	0.25	30	0.81	35
327	0.07	0.35	31	0.80	35
344	0.03	0.65	29	0.87	25

[a]From Ettenberg *et al.* [38].
[b]Al concentration difference at heterojunctions.
[c]Using Eq. (14.4.4).

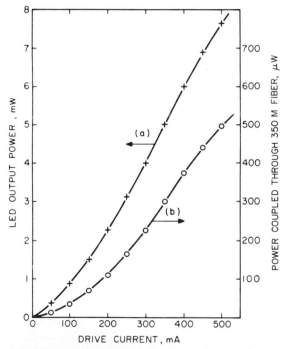

FIG. 14.4.10 Total power output from one edge of a stripe-contact diode and power coupled through 350 m of 8-dB/km attenuation, NA = 0.14, 90-μm-diameter fiber. All measurements made with a 1-cm-diameter calibrated silicon photodiode [38].

wavelength of ~8000 Å. Note that 500 μW is transmitted down the length of that fiber with a diode output power of 7.7 mW. A surface-emitting structure of the same power output would couple 2% or 150 μW into the fiber, of which about half, ~ 80 μW, would be transmitted through the fiber length of 350 m.

A comparison of the measured and calculated fractional power coupled into fibers with varying acceptance angles is shown in Fig. 14.4.11. The device studied is diode No. 297 from Table 14.4.2 with $\theta_\perp = 25°$, and the calculated fractional power coupled is from Eq. (14.2.8) using the measured radiation pattern. The agreement between theory and experiment is seen to be good.

The power emission from an LED and its linearity with current is limited by (1) heating, which reduces the diode efficiency and hence produces a sublinear increase in power with current eventually leading to a saturation in the output; and (2) reliability, because of the undesirability of operating the diode at excessive current densities over long periods of time. As discussed in Chapter 16, current densities of a few thousand amperes per square centimeter are considered acceptable for the best (AlGa)As devices with stripe-geometry edge emitters or isolated contacts of the type used for the surface emitter of Fig. 14.4.1. For illustrative purposes, we note that all the better LED structures provide a few milliwatts of output power in the kiloampere per square centimeter range. At 2000 A/cm², the REED [36] emits at one edge ~ 3 mW at ~ 8000 A. The "lensed" surface emitter has emitted a total of 6 mW at a current density of 3.4×10^3 A/cm² [44], and the emitter of Fig. 14.4.1 has emitted a total of 2 mW at 7.5×10^3 A/cm².

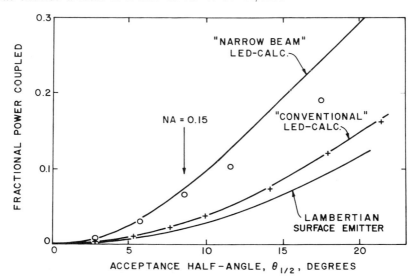

FIG. 14.4.11 Calculated and measured coupling efficiencies from three diode types into cones of various numerical apertures. Experiments: $\bigcirc$ = LED 297, + = LED 294 ($\theta_\perp \approx 70°$) [23].

With regard to the diode power required for various fiber systems, the requirement depends on the desired signal-to-noise ratio at the detector, the band width, and the detector. With Si avalanche photodiodes, the received detector power requirement may be as low as a few nanowatts. With a PiN silicon diode detector several tens of microwatts will commonly prove adequate. Therefore, the power levels available from the devices described here, used in conjunction with low loss fibers, are potentially capable of satisfying systems with multikilometer-long fiber links. With LEDs, the bandwidth achievable rather than the power loss may provide a limiting factor in the interrepeater spacing. Figure 14.4.12a shows the calculated fiber length related to the power emission from the source, the power coupled into the fiber $P_{\theta i}$, and the typical required power level at the detector for three bandwidths. Figure 14.4.12b shows generalized plots which allow the power needed at the detector to be calculated for a desired signal to noise ratio, bandwidth, and load resistor on the detector. A simple detector with no gain, and an avalanche detector with a gain $G = 100$ are considered.

From a systems point of view, the relative independence of the LED output on ambient temperature is an important advantage. Figure 14.4.13 shows that the relative change in output between 22 and 100°C is less than a factor of 2 for an edge-emitting structure [36]. Surface emitters have similar properties.

14.4.4   LEDs for 1–1.2 μm Emission

Diodes emitting in the 1–1.2 μm spectral range have been made with homojunction and heterojunction structures. The fact that (InGa)As (or other low bandgap material) is grown on GaAs or InP (materials with a higher bandgap energy) is advantageous because the diode emission is not absorbed, thus making it possible to produce surface emission structures in which the radiation is taken out through the substrate. Early homojunction (InGa)As LEDs reported in the literature [45] have been conventional surface emission structures capable of emission of about 1 mW at ~1 μm.

Double-heterojunction LEDs have been constructed [46] using $In_{0.83}Ga_{0.17}$ $As_{0.34}P_{0.66}$/InP structures emitting at about 1.1 μm, and power levels of at least 1 mW should be achievable in a Lambertian emission pattern. However, one of the negative aspects in these early devices is that the spectral width of the emitted radiation it much broader than that of (AlGa)As diodes—1000 vs. 300 Å. Thus, the benefits of the reduced material dispersion (Section 14.2) due to the longer wavelength is not fully realized since the factor of about 3 reduction in $d^2n/d\lambda^2$ between 0.8 and 1.1 μm (Fig. 14.2.3) is compensated by the wider emission half-width. The excessive line width could be the result of an inhomogeneous composition in the recombination region, which may be expected to be improved with a maturing technology.

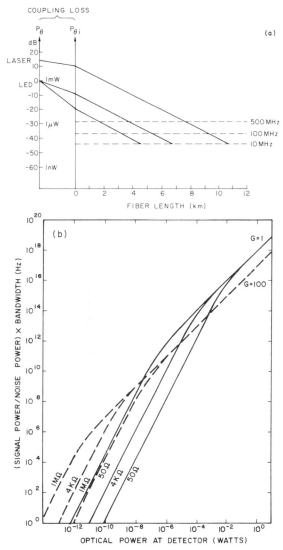

FIG. 14.4.12 (a) Calculated fiber link length using typical LED and laser diode power emission values P_θ and coupled power into fiber $P_{\theta i}$. An avalanche detector is assumed with the following system parameters: response, 0.57 A/W; gain, 100; load, 50 Ω. The bit error rate is 10^{-10} (S/N $\approx$ 23 dB); the amplifier noise is 6 dB; and the fiber loss is 5 dB/km. The dashed lines denote the fiber length where the minimum power level at the detector is reached at frequencies of 10, 100, and 500 MHz, neglecting limitations set by the LED modulation or dispersion in the fiber. (b) Typical (signal-to-noise ratio) × (bandwidth) product available for different silicon detector gains G and load resistors, as a function of the optical power reaching the detector. Hundred percent power modulation depth of the signal source is assumed, the amplifier noise is 6 dB and the detector responsivity is 0.57 A/W. A signal/noise ratio of 23 dB is a commonly used value. The allowable load resistor value decreases as the required bandwidth is increased (J. P. Wittke, unpublished).

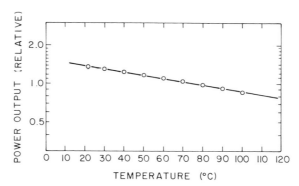

FIG. 14.4.13   Power emission as a function of temperature from a double-heterojunction LED, measured through one edge. Spontaneous emission is $100 \times 300 \ \mu m$.

The DH LEDs using $GaAs_{0.88}Sb_{0.12}/Al_{0.17}Ga_{0.83}As_{0.88}Sb_{0.12}$ emitting at 1 μm had spectral half-widths of about 500 Å [47]. However, in contrast to these devices grown on InP, the diodes contained a higher dislocation density because of the substantial lattice parameter mismatch with the GaAs substrate. These dislocations could limit the ultimate operating lifetime of these devices (Chapter 16).

In principle, the modulation speed of these longer wavelength LEDs should be as high as those achieved with (AlGa)As by appropriate dopant control in the recombination region. Furthermore, the edge-emission beam narrowing effects should be similarly realizable by control of the index profile. Of course, the technological difficulties are greater than in (AlGa)As because of the precise alloy composition control needed to minimize the lattice parameter mismatch at the heterojunctions.

14.5   Visible Emission Laser Diodes

Ternary alloys of InP and AlP provide the highest III–V compound direct bandgap ($E_{gc} = 2.3$ eV) materials capable of being doped p- and n-type (Table 12.2.1). However, as pointed out in Section 11.3.9, these materials are difficult to prepare, which leaves (InGa)P and InGaAsP alloys with the most practical potential for visible emission at room temperature.

At room temperature (InAl)P lasers should operate to 2.13 eV (5820 Å), (InGa)P lasers to 2.07 eV (6000 Å), Ga(AsP) lasers to 1.89 eV (6560 Å), and (AlGa)As lasers to 1.82 eV (6800 Å). However, these limits are without consideration of the threshold current density which in each case would be too high for CW operation (i.e., well in excess of 10,000 A/cm²) because of the low internal quantum efficiency due to carrier loss to the indirect conduction band valleys discussed in Section 12.2.3. This would occur even if appropriate carrier and radiation confinement could be achieved within the active region with heterojunctions. For CW operation $J_{th} < 5000\,A/cm^2$ is desirable. Then, the alloy composition must be further removed from the cross-over composition to provide a separation of about 0.2 eV between the direct and indirect conduction band minima.

In this section, we review state of the art devices emitting in the visible portion of the spectrum. Of these, the (AlGa)As devices have operated near their theoretical limits at room temperature as dictated by the internal quantum efficiency. Difficulties in producing heterojunction configurations of sufficient metallurgical quality have limited the performance of the other devices at room temperature. However, the role of heterojunctions is not as essential at 77 K as at more elevated temperatures, and the internal quantum efficiency is higher. Thus, yellow lasing emission has been achieved, close to the limit set by the available materials.

14.5.1 Homojunction Lasers

The first visible homojunction lasers were fabricated using $GaAs_{1-x}P_x$ alloys [48, 49]. The lowest threshold lasers of this alloy were prepared by vapor phase epitaxy on GaAs substrates. Both the p- and n-type regions were grown rather than diffused. These devices have lased at 6750 Å (300 K, $J_{th} = 10^6\,A/cm^2$) and 6350 Å (77 K). Figure 14.5.1 summarizes the best experimental results obtained with Ga(AsP) homojunction lasers. Note that all these lasers with emission in the visible portion of the spectrum are produced in material containing a significant dislocation density, because of the lattice mismatch of the epitaxial layer with the GaAs substrate (Table 12.2.1).

Homojunction laser diodes of (InGa)P have been prepared by VPE and LPE. Using VPE, lasing at 77 K was obtained to 5980 Å, but with J_{th} values in excess of 10,000 A/cm² [52]. With LPE devices, formed by the sequential growth of an n-type layer followed by a p-type layer and interdiffusion to form the p–n junction within the n-type region of $In_{0.37}Go_{0.63}P$, lasing was obtained to 5900 Å. A further reduction to about 5700 Å is believed possible with (InGa)P. Indeed, using electron beam excitation, lasing was achieved at 5800 Å (77 K) [53]. Difficulties in constructing quality p–n junctions are a major problem in this material. This may be partly related to the fact that the achievement of high p-type doping levels needed for homojunctions is difficult in this alloy without the formation of an excessive density of nonradiative centers. For example, the radiative efficiency of $In_{0.5}Ga_{0.5}P$:Zn drops sharply [54] with increasing hole concentration above $10^{18}\,cm^{-3}$. The use of Cd may be an alternative to Zn doping, but its incorporation by LPE is rather difficult, its solubility is uncertain, and it cannot be used as a convenient diffusant because of its low diffusion coefficient.

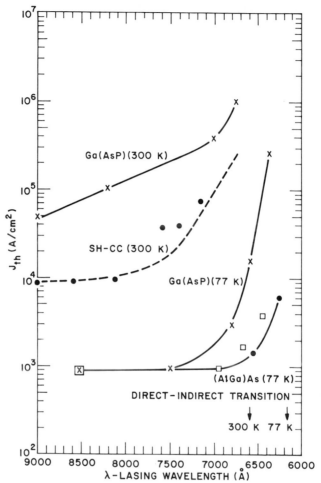

FIG. 14.5.1 Threshold current density as a function of emission wavelength for Ga(AsP) homojunction laser diodes produced by vapor phase epitaxy [49] ($\times$), and single-heterojunction (AlGa)As lasers produced by liquid phase epitaxy [50] ($\square$) and [51] ($\bullet$).

14.5.2   *Heterojunction Lasers*

It is evident that heterojunction structures are essential for visible lasers capable of useful room temperature operation. It is noteworthy that small shifts of the emission wavelength toward the red substantially increase the brightness of the laser emission. This is illustrated in Fig. 14.5.2 which shows the relative visibility of the emission from a laser as a function of wavelength. For example, an order of magnitude increase in visibility is obtained by

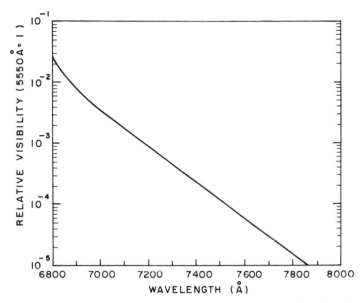

FIG. 14.5.2 Relative visibility of devices emitting at various wavelengths with constant beam width, source size, and power emission.

shifting the emission from 7850 to 7500 Å. Laser emission at 7400 Å is clearly visible in ordinary room illumination, particularly in CW operation.

In the (AlGa)As alloy system, single-heterojunction [50, 51], double-heterojunction [55–59], and LOC lasers [53] have been constructed in the direct bandgap alloy composition region ($x \leq 0.37$). Figure 14.5.3 shows the dependence of the emission wavelength ($h\nu_L = E_g - 0.03$ eV) on the alloy composition; J_{th} as a function of lasing wavelength at 300 and 77 K is shown in Fig. 14.5.1 for broad-area single-heterojunction ($d_3 \approx 2 \mu$m) lasers. The lowest threshold current density values achieved at 300 K with broad-area DH lasers are shown in Fig. 14.5.4. Lasing has been achieved at 6900 Å with $J_{th} = 30,000$ A/cm². Table 14.5.1 shows the differential quantum efficiency as well as the J_{th} values of lasers spanning the emission wavelength range in (AlGa)As. At 77 K (Fig. 14.5.5), pulsed laser operation is conveniently obtained to about 6300 Å [61], with the lowest $\lambda_L = 6190$ Å [62]. Assuming that the direct-to-indirect bandgap energy crossover occurs at ~2 eV at 77 K, this wavelength represents the normally achievable limit within the direct bandgap material composition range. (However, the use of isoelectronic dopants could extend the lasing range to shorter wavelengths).

Stripe-geometry lasers of (AlGa)As have operated CW at room temperature to 7400 Å [59], although operation nearer 7000 Å is believed achievable with

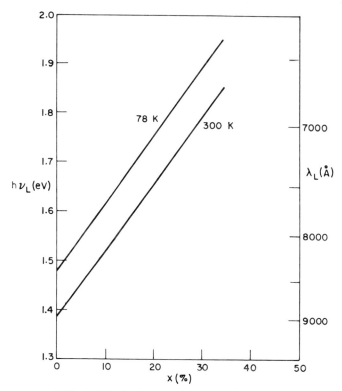

FIG. 14.5.3   Lasing wavelength in $Al_xGa_{1-x}As$.

appropriate heat sinking and reduction of the thermal resistance of the devices. Figure 14.5.6 illustrates the performance of a CW laser at 7400 Å, constructed using an oxide-isolated stripe 13 μm wide. The rather broad beam width ($\theta_\perp = 52°$) in the direction perpendicular to the junction plane is indicative of the strong radiation confinement ($\Gamma = 0.47$) achieved with this structure of $Al_{0.6}Ga_{0.4}As/Al_{0.2}Ga_{0.8}As$ with an undoped recombination region $d_3 = 0.08$ μm.

Note that these (AlGa)As lasers use Zn as the acceptor dopant, since Ge provides too low a carrier concentration in the Al-rich bounding region (Section 11.3.1). Unfortunately, carrier freeze-out in the Ge-doped material greatly increases the resistance of such lasers at cryogenic temperatures, but zinc doped lasers can readily operate to 77 K. Since CW operation is more easily achieved at low temperatures than at room temperature, because of the low thresholds at 77 K, CW power values in excess of 50 mW have been obtained in the 6500–6600 Å range [61].

It is of interest to compare the J_{th} laser data to the calculated decrease of the internal quantum efficiency η_i with increasing Al content discussed in

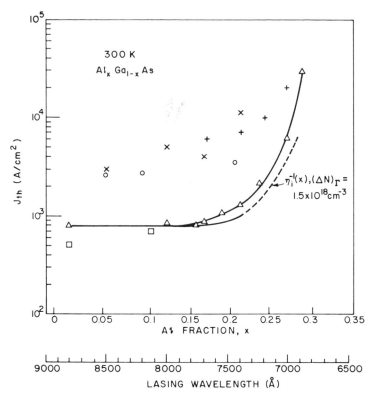

FIG. 14.5.4 Lowest values of threshold current density reported by various investigators. All devices are double-heterojunction structures, and the J_{th} differences for the same x value are due to different active region widths, junction quality, and degree of radiation and carrier confinement. The calculated curve of internal quantum efficiency η_i^{-1} is normalized to unity in GaAs and is presented to show the inherent limitation for a given active region width, degree of confinement, and junction quality. This curve assumes that the electron population in the Γ valley is 1.5×10^{18} cm^{-3}. Data from ($\triangle$) [59], ($\square$) [60], ($+$) [58], ($\bigcirc$) [56], $\times$ [57].

TABLE 14.5.1
(AlGa)As DH Laser Data (300 K)[a]

λ_L wavelength (Å)	J_{th} (A/cm^2)	η_{ext} (%)
8800	800	35
7760	800	35
7690	900	24
7530	1,140	14
7400	1,300	24
7240	2,230	14
6900	30,000	3

[a]Broad-area diodes, 100 μm × 500 μm; pulsed operation: 100 ns pulse length, 1 kHz rate; two-sided emission. From Kressel and Hawrylo [59].

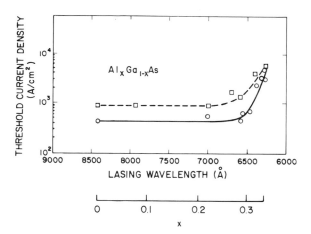

FIG. 14.5.5   Threshold current density as a function of lasing wavelength of (□) single- and (○) double-heterojunction broad-area lasers at 77 K (pulsed operation). The single-heterojunction data ($d_3 \approx 2\ \mu m$) are from Kressel *et al.* [51]. The double-heterojunction data ($d_3 \cong 1\ \mu m$) are from [61].

Section 12.2.3. Other factors remaining constant, we expect $J_{th} \propto \eta_i^{-1}$. Figure 14.5.4 shows η_i^{-1} (normalized to unity in GaAs) as a function of the Al concentration and emission wavelength. It is assumed that the population of the direct conduction band valley is $(\Delta N)_\Gamma = 1.5 \times 10^{18}\ cm^{-3}$ and that six equivalent X valleys are relevant to the internal quantum efficiency calculation. The experimental J_{th} values follow quite well the reduction in η_i except for high Al values where there is some loss of confinement, and the junction quality may be inadequate.

Turning our attention to other heterojunction structures, consider devices with Ga(AsP) in the recombination region as a means of obtaining moderately low threshold lasers with $\lambda_L \lesssim 7000$ Å at room temperature. The lattice constant of $In_yGa_{1-y}P$ alloys spans a range from 5.451 Å (for GaP) to 5.869 Å (for InP), and therefore can be used to lattice-match any desired alloy of $GaAs_{1-x}P_x$, whose lattice constant ranges from 5.451 Å (for GaP) to 5.653 Å (for GaAs). For a particular alloy of $GaAs_{1-x}P_x$ the unique lattice-matching alloy of $In_yGa_{1-y}P$ can be determined from the expression [63]

$$y = 0.483(1 - x) \qquad (14.5.1)$$

For emission near 7000 Å, the $GaAs_{1-x}P_x$ alloy composition should have $x = 0.3$; from (14.5.1), the appropriate $In_yGa_{1-y}P$ composition for lattice-matching $GaAs_{0.7}P_{0.3}$ should therefore have $y = 0.34$.

The energy bandgap for alloys of $In_yGa_{1-y}P$ and $GaAs_{1-x}P_x$ at their lattice-matching compositions is illustrated in Fig. 14.5.7. The energy difference of about 0.5 eV over the wavelength range of interest provides carrier and

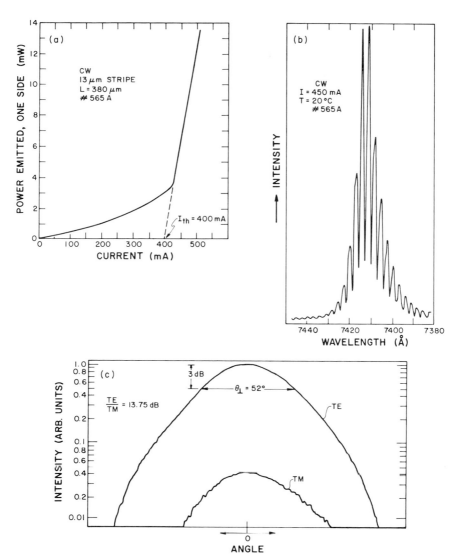

FIG. 14.5.6 Performance characteristics of oxide-isolated $Al_{0.6}Ga_{0.4}As/Al_{0.2}Ga_{0.8}As$ DH laser at room temperature. (a) Power output, one side, as a function of current. (b) Spectral emission at 450 mA (6 mW of power emitted). (c) Far-field pattern in the direction perpendicular to the junction plane. The actual emitting region width is 40 μm; thus $J_{th} \cong$ 2600 A/cm^2 [59].

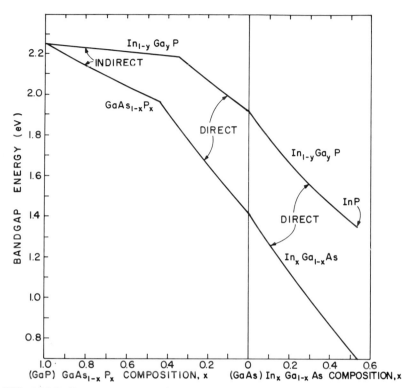

FIG. 14.5.7   Room temperature bandgap energy values of $In_yGa_{1-y}P$, $GaAs_{1-x}P_x$, and $In_xGa_{1-x}As$ alloys for lattice-matched structures of $In_{1-y}Ga_yP/GaAs_{1-x}P_x$ (left of zero composition) and $In_{1-y}Ga_yP/In_xGa_{1-x}As$ (right of zero composition) [63].

radiation confinement within the active $GaAs_{1-x}P_x$ region. Hence, $GaAs_{1-x}$ $P_x/In_yGa_{1-y}P$ structures are a reasonable choice for room temperature hetero-junction lasers, although a lattice mismatch to the GaAs substrate is unavoidable.

As an illustration, consider the structure shown [63] in Fig. 14.5.8. The substrate consists of an n-type commercial $GaAs_{0.7}P_{0.3}$ epitaxial wafer grown on GaAs (100), doped with Te to 1–2×10^{17} cm^{-3}. Two $In_yGa_{1-y}P$ ($y \sim$ 0.34) confining layers, each 2–3 μm thick, and a $GaAs_{1-x}P_x$ ($x \sim 0.3$) laser cavity, 3–4 μm thick, containing a p–n junction approximately in its center, were grown by VPE. A zinc-doped $GaAs_{1-x}P_x$ "cap" was employed as the final layer to facilitate making ohmic contact to the higher bandgap p-type $In_yGa_{1-y}P$ uppermost confining layer. The n-type layers of $GaAs_{1-x}P_x$ and $In_yGa_{1-y}P$ were doped with sulfur (from H_2S) to a carrier concentration of about 5×10^{17} cm^{-3}, while the p-type $GaAs_{1-x}P_x$ and $In_yGa_{1-y}P$ layers were zinc doped to a carrier concentration between 3×10^{18} and 1×10^{19} cm^{-3}.

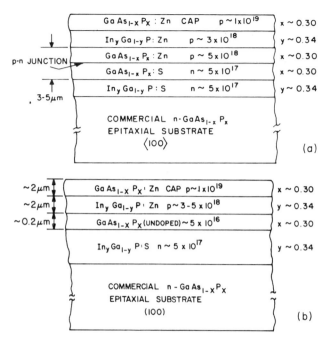

FIG. 14.5.8   Schematic presentation of vapor-grown GaAs$_{1-x}$P$_y$/In$_y$Ga$_{1-y}$P heterojunction structure prepared for visible-light-emitting laser diodes [63]. (a) Large optical cavity (LOC) structure; (b) double-heterojunction structure.

Devices made with the LOC configuration of Fig. 14.5.8 have lased to 273 K ($\lambda_L = 6790$ Å) with J_{th} values of 55,000 A/cm^2 (or $J_{th}/d° = 14,000$ A/cm^2 μm); at 77 K, $J_{th} = 5000$ A/cm^2 ($\lambda_L = 6470$ Å) [63]. Improved fabrication and material synthesis, together with narrower heterojunction spacings, substantially reduce J_{th}. In fact, similar devices in the double-heterojunction configuration with $d_3 = 0.2$ μm have J_{th} as low as 3400 A/cm^2 and have operated CW at 10°C at $\lambda_L = 7030$ Å [63a].

Alternative to these (InGa)P layers for confinement is the use of AlGaAsP or InGaAsP alloy layers prepared by LPE. At 77 K, InGaAsP/Ga(AsP) (on GaAs) lasers have operated with $J_{th} = 62,000$ A/cm^2 ($\lambda_L = 6300$ Å) [64]. Using AlGaAsP/Ga(AsP) DH configurations, lasing at 300 K was obtained at 8450 Å with $J_{th} = 16,000$ A/cm^2 (Table 13.3.1). The performance of such lasers is clearly limited by metallurgical difficulties, and improved performance can be expected, including room temperature operation.

As noted earlier, the highest practical III-V direct bandgap alloy is currently (InGa)P with $\sim$30% P, which has a bandgap energy of about 2.2 eV at room temperature. The partial substitution of As (10%) for P, thus forming a quaternary alloy In$_{0.3}$Ga$_{0.7}$P$_{0.9}$As$_{0.1}$ in the recombination region, permits the construction of a lattice-matched double heterojunction to $In_{0.34}Ga_{0.66}$ P (see Fig. 11.1.1). The bandgap energy of the recombination region is about 2.15 eV at 77 K, while that of the outer regions is about 2.3 eV, thus providing for carrier and radiation confinement. Lasers of this construction operated to 5850 Å at 77 K, the shortest wavelength laser diode obtained. Similarly constructed devices (with variations in composition) have operated at room temperature to 6470 Å ($J_{th} \approx 40,000$ A/cm^2) [65], with slightly altered material composition.

In considering the extension of semiconductor laser diode operation toward the visible, it is important to keep in mind potential limitations set by the low mobilities of the carriers in the bounding layers of the heterojunctions as the bandgap energy is increased. Because of the low mobilities, and the difficulty encountered in producing very highly doped materials, the series resistance of the devices is apt to be high relative to values encountered in lower bandgap lasers. As a result, the duty cycle in pulsed operation is limited by excessive thermal dissipation in the device, and CW operation could become difficult to sustain, even if the threshold current densities are reduced to the low values ordinarily needed.

In this discussion we have not delineated the lasing mechanism in the various alloys. With regard to the (AlGa)As visible emission lasers, the lowest threshold DH lasers were obtained with recombination regions which were not deliberately doped, but probably contained some Zn contamination. Similar uncertainty exists concerning the doping level of other visible emission lasers. However, interesting effects in Ga(AsP) and (InGa)P alloys are associated with the role of deliberately introduced nitrogen (Section 1.7). In a Ga(AsP):N lasing region there are indications that the nitrogen center is active in the stimulated emission process [66] extending operation into the indirect bandgap region. Evidence for bound states of ion-implanted N in (AlGa)As has also been found [67] and these could be important in stimulated emission.

14.6 General Purpose Heterojunction LEDs

The most widely used homojunction GaAs LEDs are made either by diffusion of Zn into bulk-grown substrates, or by liquid phase epitaxy with Si doping to produce compensated p- and n-type regions. The latter diodes have typical external quantum efficiencies of about 10%, considerably in excess of the diffused diodes, and are widely used for applications requiring several milliwatts of power. These commercial devices are basically surface emission structures.

Heterojunction diodes of (AlGa)As with provision for surface emission have been reported in the literature. Although some of the earlier work was motivated by the interest in producing visible emission diodes, no commercial devices of this type have ever been realized because of the economically more favorable Ga(AsP) technology. In this section we review some of the major approaches toward the fabrication of LEDs of GaAs and related compounds with emphasis on the heterojunction structures.

14.6.1 GaAs:Si LEDs

A unique application of the LPE process has come from the use of amphoteric Si doping to produce GaAs diodes that are much more efficient than Zn-diffused ones [68]. The layers are grown from a solution of Ga, GaAs, and Si with compositions and growth conditions chosen to provide for the generation of n-type material during the first (high temperature) part and p-type material during the last part of the growth cycle (Chapter 10). External quantum efficiency values as high as 32% have been reported [69] at room temperature after diode shaping and coating with a high refractive index glass dome, but reproducible values are about one-third lower. Although the *internal* quantum efficiency is comparable in both Zn-diffused and Si-compensated diodes, the external quantum efficiency in the Si-doped diodes is higher because

1. the junctions are graded with the material being closely compensated, which reduces free carrier absorption; and

2. the energy of the emitted radiation is below the bandgap energy because the acceptor terminal states are mainly connected with an ~ 0.1 eV Si complex level [70]. This eliminates the normal "band-to-band" absorption processes which accompany recombination via shallow impurity states.

The diode properties depend on the growth plane as well as on the Si concentration in the material [71]. Thus, Ladany [69] has shown that emission peaking at long wavelengths (due to a high Si concentration) is more efficient for diodes grown on the (111) As than on the (100) plane. Diodes can be made in which the emission peak wavelength ranges from 9300 to 10,000 Å without significant change in the external quantum efficiency. (It is not possible to obtain such a broad spectral range by Zn diffusion.) However, the GaAs:Si diodes have long carrier lifetimes, limiting their application in high data rate optical communication.

Owing to the involvement of the shallow acceptor only (as in the case of Zn), high external diode efficiencies are not obtained using Ge as noted by Morizumi and Takahashi [72], who studied diodes in which the p-type Si or Ge-doped layer was grown on n-type melt-grown substrates. The efficiency of their GaAs:Si diodes reached 2%, whereas the GaAs:Ge diodes of similar mechanical configuration had an efficiency of only 0.2% (see Section 14.6.3).

Although the GaAs:Si LEDs are the most efficient diodes at this time (particularly if a GaAs dome is used) [73], the (AlGa)As–GaAs single-hetero-junction LED (see below) may be competitive for some applications, especial-ly if rapid switching is needed. Note that the combined rise and fall time of a typical GaAs:Si diode is several hundred nanoseconds, whereas for a Zn-doped diode it is 30–80 ns, typically.

14.6.2   (AlGa)As Diodes

Since GaAs diodes emit only in the infrared, (AlGa)As is employed to ex-tend the emission range of LEDs into the visible. Efficient emitters of this material can be made by several different techniques.

It is possible to generate p–n junctions in the course of LPE growth in a vertical furnace by the addition of Zn to a Te-doped solution [74]. A vertical growth system of the type discussed in Section 9.1.1 can be used. The gradient in the Al content of the material was used to good advantage by Woodall et al. [75] who exposed the initially grown n-region by removing the GaAs substrate following growth. Thus, from diodes of the type shown in Fig. 14.6.1a,

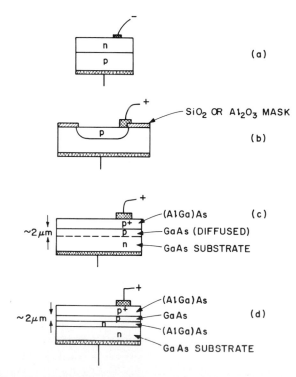

FIG. 14.6.1 $Al_xGa_{1-x}As$ LED structures: (a) Simple diode chip with small-area contact to high bandgap n-type $Al_xGa_{1-x}As$ light-emitting surface; (b) planar LED structures with small-area contact to Zn-diffused region in n-type $Al_xGa_{1-x}As$ material; (c) single-hetero-junction surface emission diode; and (d) double-heterojunction surface emission diode.

the light is emitted through the higher bandgap n-region, and is therefore not strongly absorbed. Room temperature efficiency values of 1.2 and 6% have been obtained (with encapsulation) at $hv_p = 1.8$ and 1.6 eV, respectively. Kressel *et al.* [76] employed a modified version of this technique to achieve high efficiencies. Tellurium and Zn were replaced by Si as the sole dopant to obtain the advantage of a Si-compensated p–n junction region. Results for diodes of different Al content, covering a 1.4–1.8 eV emission energy range, are shown in Fig. 14.6.2. The falloff in the efficiency with increasing photon energy shown in Fig. 14.6.2 is consistent with the predicted behavior based on the thermal depopulation of the Γ conduction band minimum. (AlGa)As:Si junction luminescence also has been studied by Mischel and Schul [77].

(AlGa)As LEDs have also been prepared by LPE growth of an n-type layer on a GaAs substrate followed by the formation of a p–n junction by Zn diffusion [78]. This technique is particularly useful for the fabrication of planar diodes and monolithic numeric displays (see Fig. 14.6.1b). Blum and Shih [79, 80] have described an LPE growth procedure resulting in a smooth film surface suitable for the fabrication of planar Zn-diffused junctions. The efficiency of these planar diodes, however, is lower than those obtained by the first technique described in this section ($\eta_{ext} \cong 0.25\%$ at 6750 Å). Also of in-

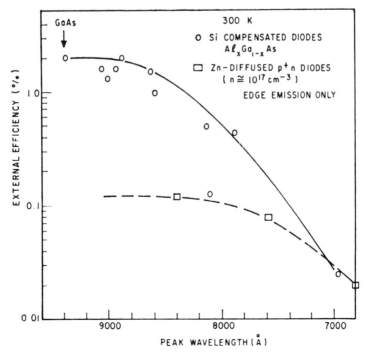

FIG. 14.6.2 External quantum efficiency of $Al_xGa_{1-x}As$: Si LEDs versus emission wavelength ($\bigcirc$). The efficiency of Zn-diffused diodes is shown for comparison ($\square$).

terest with regard to reducing the absorption in the diode is the growth of (AlGa)As on transparent GaP substrates instead of GaAs substrates [81]; however, for this structure, one must contend with the added problem of lattice mismatch between the GaP substrate ($a_0 \sim 5.45$ Å) and the (AlGa)As epitaxial layer ($a_0 \sim 5.65$ Å).

A heterojunction can be incorporated into the diode to obtain higher external efficiencies. A single-heterojunction diode, similar to that used for the room temperature lasers, also has a higher external *spontaneous* efficiency than a homojunction p^+–p–n diode [82]. LEDs of this type have been studied in detail by Ulmer [83], who used surface emission devices with small ohmic contacts, as shown in Fig. 14.6.2c. These diodes have improved external efficiencies, not only because the radiation is not significantly absorbed in the (AlGa)As p-type surface layer, but also because the nonradiative recombination which occurs at the free surface of conventional diodes is eliminated by the presence of a p^+–p (AlGa)As–GaAs barrier. Diodes embedded in epoxy have been made with external efficiencies as high as 10% at 9100 Å, which is 8–10 times higher than those obtained with diffused diodes or similarly made LEDs with a GaAs p^+-region instead of an (AlGa)As p^+-region. The same structure can, of course, be used with different Al concentrations in the active region or with other materials, so long as the lattice parameter mismatch is small.

Double-heterojunction structures of (AlGa)As in which the active p-region is sandwiched between higher bandgap p^+- and n-regions have also been employed for the fabrication of LEDs. As described in Section 14.4 the DH structure is convenient for the study of the effect on radiative diode properties of various dopants and Al concentrations in the active regions. In their study, Dolginov *et al.* [84] used Ge as a dopant in the active region in a spectral range extending from $h\nu_p \cong 1.4$ (~ 9000 Å) to $h\nu_p = 1.85$ eV (6700 Å) at 300 K. At this lower wavelength, an efficiency of 0.03% was obtained. It appears probable that this result will be improved by optimizing the geometry and by changing the dopant or its concentration.

The structures shown in Fig. 14.6.1 can be used for coupling power into fibers as long as the current density is moderate (less than < 1000 A/cm^2) because of the mounting of the structure with the p-side upward and consequent long thermal path. The use of a selectively diffused area is attractive since it allows a definition of an emitting area comparable to that of the fiber. Figure 14.6.3 shows a surface emission single-heterojunction LED designed for optical communications. The heterojunction is first grown in the form of an n–n isotype junction [85]. Then selective diffusion is performed, forming the p–n homojunction in the substrate a preselected distance below what has now become the p–p heterojunction (which provides carrier confinement). The low absorption in the (AlGa)As surface layer is advantageous for reasonable

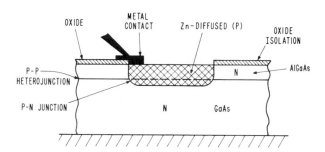

FIG. 14.6.3   Single-heterojunction LED designed for optical fiber coupling. The n–n heterojunction is first grown by LPE, then a selective Zn diffusion is performed to move the p–n junction below the original (as-grown) p–p heterojunction. The metal contact is at the edge of the active area and overlaps the oxide isolation [85].

efficiency. Diodes of this type have fall times of about 10 ns, from which the modulation characteristics can be computed using Eq. (14.4.2).

14.6.3   GaAs:Ge LEDs

In this section we summarize some of the results obtained with homojunction LEDs containing varying concentrations of Ge in the recombination region. As noted earlier (Chapter 9), the use of Ge instead of Zn is advantageous for GaAs doping for devices fabricated by liquid phase epitaxy because of the ease of controlling the hole concentration, the low diffusion coefficient, and the vapor pressure which minimizes cross contamination of the solutions by Ge vapor transport. These are edge-emitting devices, and the spectral properties are thereby affected because of selective absorption. The magnitude of these effects can be judged by comparing the diode electroluminescence spectrum to the photoluminescence spectrum of material comparable to that in the recombination region. In fact, as we will show, the spectral structure seen in photoluminescence is sometimes not seen in electroluminescence where the injected carrier density is generally much higher.

Figure 14.6.4 shows the peak energy of the GaAs:Ge photoluminescence (PL) and diode electroluminescence (EL) at room temperature as a function of hole concentration [86]. Since the n-side of the junction is heavily doped in all the diodes, electron injection into the p-side with consequent radiative recombination is dominant. In the most lightly doped samples, the photoluminescence results from band-to-band recombination; due to increasing bandtailing with doping, the peak shifts downward in energy as the hole concentration increases. Note that the EL peak (which is independent of current density in the 50–5000 A/cm^2 range tested) is lower in energy than the PL peak for a given hole concentration. The lower EL peak energy is due to selective absorption in the material, an effect well known in all GaAs diodes

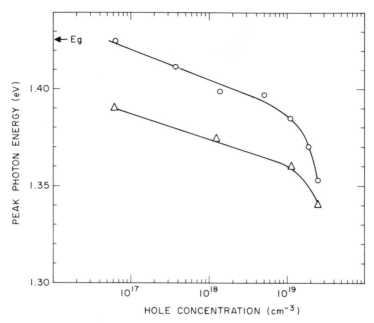

FIG. 14.6.4 Peak photon energy versus hole concentration as observed at 300 K by photoluminescence (○) of GaAs: Ge at room temperature and in electroluminescence (△) of p–n junctions in which the p-side of the junction was GaAs: Ge and the n-side of fixed composition ($N = 2 \times 10^{18}$ cm^{-3}, melt grown) [86].

in which the radiation is observed through the edge. [However, in diodes in which the radiation is observed through the surface via an (AlGa)As heterojunction, the EL and PL peak positions agree closely at room temperature.]

Figure 14.6.5 shows the peak photon energy for photoluminescence and electroluminescence at 77 K as a function of the room temperature hole concentration. The three major bands observed are denoted A, B, and C. Band A, seen in the lightly doped material, is due to the usual near-band edge recombination seen in lightly doped GaAs. Band B involves the shallow Ge acceptors as terminal states; its importance relative to A increases with Ge concentration. The fact that band A is not seen in the diode emission is probably the result of more severe internal absorption of the higher energy radiation. Note, however, that the energy of the PL and that of the EL are identical at 77 K due to the small absorption loss for the slightly deeper "B" transition. Band C, prominent only in the photoluminescence of samples with $P \gtrsim 10^{19}$ cm^{-3}, shifts downward in energy with increasing hole concentration. This band is not seen in the diode emission in the current density range studied.

Figure 10.1.10b shows the 300 K dependence of the relative radiative efficiency on the hole concentration as determined from photoluminescence

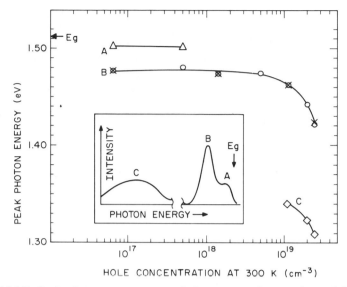

FIG. 14.6.5 Peak photon energy versus hole concentration as observed by photoluminescence ($\triangle$, $\bigcirc$, $\square$) of GaAs: Ge at 77 K and in electroluminescence ($\times$) of p–n junctions in which the p-side of the junction was GaAs: Ge and the n-side of fixed composition ($N = 2 \times 10^{18}$ cm^{-3}, melt grown). The insert shows the relative positions of the three dominant bands—A, B, and C. Band B is the only significant band seen in electroluminescence [86].

measurements and from the electroluminescent diode efficiency. The edge emitting diode efficiency was measured in an integrating sphere with a calibrated silicon solar cell. Pulsed measurements were also made in the 300–5000 A/cm^2 current density range to check that the light output was linear with current. This was found to be the case for all the diodes tested. An efficiency peak at $P \sim 10^{19}$ cm^{-3} is observed in both types of measurements, with a rather sharp efficiency falloff at higher hole concentrations. The absolute *edge* emission diode efficiency at $P \sim 10^{19}$ cm^{-3} was 0.4% at 300 K. The PL efficiency decrease for $P \gtrsim 10^{19}$ cm^{-3} is in agreement with previous photoluminescence measurements made at very low temperatures (12 K) [87]. It is evident from the available data that the achievement of efficient *very* highly doped diodes is improbable.

Theoretically, it is anticipated that nonradiative band-to-band Auger recombination becomes important in p-type GaAs only when $P \gtrsim 6 \times 10^{19}$ cm^{-3} [88]. Thus, the radiative efficiency falloff at high doping levels in the present material is most likely due to other factors. Of these, the formation of deep complex centers involving Ge and point defects and the formation of small precipitates are the most likely possibilities. Note that the PL efficiency decrease at high doping levels coincides with the increase in the relative intensity at 77 K of the broad low energy emission band C. It is possible that band C is related to the nonradiative centers responsible for the efficiency decrease. Despite the fact that some radiative emission due to this complex center is seen at low temperatures, much of the recombination through these centers may be nonradiative, possibly via an Auger process (Section 1.8). Whether this complex center is a compensating donor or neutral level cannot be determined from the available data, but it is known that the hole concentration above 10^{19} cm^{-3} is much lower than the total Ge concentration in the crystal [91] (Fig. 10.1.5).

One application for LEDs emitting in the vicinity of 8000 Å is in replacing lamps used for pumping solid state laser rods. For Nd:YAG lasers, several absorption bands exist, but the one in the vicinity of 8000 Å is most attractive for (AlGa)As diodes. For this purpose, the highest possible diode efficiency (and power) is desirable and the line width should be as narrow as possible. Diodes designed for this purpose were described by Dierschke et al. [89] and Ono et al. [90], who used devices in which a thick (AlGa)As substrate served as the transmitting window with a homojunction on the opposite side. Power outputs of 50 mW (at currents up to ~0.5 A) were reported at 8100 ± 15 Å (for Nd:YAG pumping). Operating lifetimes in excess of 10,000 hr were obtained.

Room temperature CW operation has been obtained using a single LED pumping the end of a small Nd:YAG crystal. The current of the LED needed to reach threshold was 45 mA (7 mW emitted power) and the emitting diode diameter was 85 μm [92]. The interest in such Nd:YAG devices arises from potential utility as light sources for fiber communications. However, external modulation of the laser emission is needed, which is a disadvantage compared to semiconductor lasers that are directly modulated.

REFERENCES

1. H. Kressel, H. F. Lockwood, and F. Z. Hawrylo, *J. Appl. Phys.* **43**, 561 (1972).
2. H. F. Lockwood and H. Kressel, Techn. Rep. AFAL-TR-75-13, Wright-Patterson Air Force Base, Dayton, Ohio (March 1975).
3. J. O'Brien, *Electronics*, August 5, 94 (1976).
4. H. S. Sommers, Jr., *Solid State Electron.* **11**, 909 (1968).
5. C. J. Nuese, M. Ettenberg, R. E. Enstrom, and H. Kressel, *Appl. Phys. Lett.* **24**, 224 (1974).
6. M. K. Barnoski (ed.), "Fundamentals of Fiber Optic Communications." Academic Press, New York, 1976.
7. J. A. Arnaud, "Beam and Fiber Optics." Academic Press, New York, 1976.
8. M. Balkanski and P. Lallemand (eds.), "Photonics." Gauthier-Villars, Paris, 1975.
9. S. E. Miller, E. A. J. Marcatili, and T. Li, *Proc. IEEE* **61**, 1703 (1973).

10. D. Marcuse, "Light Transmission Optics." Van Nostrand-Reinhold, Princeton, New Jensey, 1972.
11. D. B. Keck, R. D. Mauer, and P. C. Schultz, *Appl. Phys. Lett.* **22**, 307 (1973).
12. T. Ushida, M. Furukawa, I. Kitano, K. Koizumi, and H. Matsumuru, *IEEE J. Quantum Electron.* **6**, 606 (1970).
13. D. Gloge, *Appl. Opt.* **10**, 2252 (1971).
14. R. D. Dyott and J. R. Stern, *Electron. Lett.* **7**, 82 (1971).
15. K. P. Kapron and D. B. Keck, *Appl. Opt.* **10**, 1519 (1971).
16. E. L. Chinnock, L. G. Cohen, W. S. Holden, R. D. Standley, and D. B. Keck, *Proc. IEEE* **61**, 1499 (1973).
17. L. G. Cohen and S. D. Personick, *Appl. Opt.* **14**, 1357 (1975).
18. D. Schicketanz, *Electron. Lett.* **9**, 5 (1973).
19. D. Marcuse, *Bell Syst. Tech. J.* **52**, 1169 (1973).
20. D. Gloge, E. L. Chinnock, and K. Koizumi, *Electron. Lett.* **8**, 526 (1972).
21. L. G. Cohen and H. M. Presby, *Appl. Opt.* **14**, 1361 (1975).
22. D. Kato, *J. Appl. Phys.* **44**, 2756 (1973).
23. J. P. Wittke, M. Ettenberg, and H. Kressel, *RCA Rev.* **37**, 159 (1976).
24. I. Gorog, P. V. Goedertier, J. D. Knox, I. Ladany, J. P. Wittke, and A. H. Firester, *Appl. Opt.* **15**, 1425 (1976).
25. H. Kressel and I. Ladany, *RCA Rev.* **36**, 230 (1975).
26. I. Ladany and H. Kressel, *Appl. Phys. Lett.* **25**, 708 (1974).
27. H. Kressel, J. P. Wittke, and H. F. Lockwood, unpublished.
28. H. Kressel, I. Ladany, M. Ettenberg, and H. F. Lockwood, *Phys. Today* **29**, 38 (1976).
29. W. E. Ahearn and J. W. Crowe, *IEEE J. Quantum Electron.* **2**, 597 (1966).
30. B. S. Goldstein and R. M. Weigand, *Proc. IEEE* (*Lett.*) **53**, 195 (1965).
31. J. Nishizawa, *IEEE J. Quantum Electron.* **4**, 143 (1968).
32. M. Chown, A. R. Goodwin, D. F. Lovelace, G. B. H. Thompson, and P. R. Selway, *Electron. Lett.* **9**, 34 (1973).
33. C. A. Burrus and R. W. Dawson, *Appl. Phys. Lett.* **17**, 97 (1970).
34. M. Ettenberg, H. F. Lockwood, J. P. Wittke, and H. Kressel, Digest, International Electron Devices Meeting, Washington, D.C., IEEE Catalog No. 73CH0781-SED (1974).
35. H. Kressel and M. Ettenberg, *Proc. IEEE* **63**, 1360 (1975).
36. M. Ettenberg, J. P. Wittke, and H. Kressel, Final Report, Office of Naval Res , Contract N00014–73–C–0335 (1975).
37. H. F. Lockwood, J. P. Wittke, and M. Ettenberg, *Opt. Commun.* **16**, 193 (1976).
38. M. Ettenberg, H. Kressel, and J. P. Wittke, *IEEE J. Quantum Electron.* **12**, 360 (1976).
39. D. N. Payne and W. A. Gambling, *Electron. Lett.* **11**, 176 (1975).
40. J. Conti and M. J. O. Strutt, *IEEE J. Quantum Electron.* **8**, 815 (1972).
41. T. P. Lee and C. A. Burrus, *IEEE J. Quantum Electron.* **8**, 370 (1972).
42. J. Colvin, *Opto-Electronics* **6**, 387 (1974).
43. W. P. Dumke, *IEEE J. Quantum Electron.* **11**, 400 (1975).
44. F. D. King and A. J. Springthorpe, *J. Electron. Mater.* **4**, 243 (1975).
45. C. J. Nuese and R. E. Enstrom, *IEEE Trans. Electron. Devices* **17**, 1067 (1972).
46. T. P. Pearsall, B. I. Miller, R. J. Capik, and K. J. Bachmann, *Appl. Phys. Lett.* **28**, 499 (1976).
47. R. E. Nahory, M. A. Pollack, E. D. Beebe, and J. C. DeWinter, *Appl. Phys. Lett.* **27**, 356 (1975).
48. N. Holonyak, Jr., and S. F. Bevacqua, *Appl. Phys. Lett.* **1**, 82 (1962).

49. J. J. Tietjen, J. I. Pankove, I. J. Hegyi, and H. Nelson, *Trans. AIME* **239**, 285 (1967).
50. H. Nelson and H. Kressel, *Appl. Phys. Lett.* **15**, 7 (1969).
51. H. Kressel, H. F. Lockwood, and H. Nelson, *IEEE J. Quantum Electron.* **6**, 278 (1970).
52. W. R. Hitchens, N. Holonyak, Jr., M. H. Lee, and J. C. Campbell, *Sov. Phys. Semicond.* **8**, 1575 (1975).
53. I. Ladany and H. Kressel, Final Report, NASA Contract NAS1-11421 (December 1974).
54. H. Kressel, C. J. Nuese, and I. Ladany, *J. Appl. Phys.* **44**, 3266 (1973).
55. H. Kressel and F. Z. Hawrylo, *Appl. Phys. Lett.* **17**, 169 (1970).
56. B. I. Miller *et al.*, *Appl. Phys. Lett.* **18**, 403 (1971).
57. Zh. I. Alferov *et al.*, *Sov. Phys. Semicond.* **6**, 495 (1972).
58. K. Itoh, M. Inone, and I. Teramoto, *IEEE J. Quantum Electron.* **11**, 421 (1975).
59. H. Kressel and F. Z. Hawrylo, *Appl. Phys. Lett.* **28**, 598 (1976).
60. M. Ettenberg, *Appl. Phys. Lett.* **27**, 652 (1975).
61. H. Kressel and F. Z. Hawrylo, *J. Appl. Phys.* **44**, 4222 (1973).
62. K. Itoh, *Appl. Phys. Lett.* **24**, 127 (1974).
63. I. Ladany, H. Kressel, and C. J. Nuese, Final Report, NASA Contract NSAl-13739B4 (March 1976).
63a. H. Kressel, G. H. Olsen, and C. J. Nuese, *Appl. Phys. Lett.* **30**, 249 (1977).
64. J. J. Coleman, N. Holonyak, Jr., M. J. Ludowise, P. D. Wright, W. O. Groves, and D. L. Keure, *IEEE J. Quantum Electron.* **11**, 471 (1975).
65. W. R. Hitchens, N. Holonyak, Jr., P. D. Wright, and J. J. Coleman, *Appl. Phys. Lett.* **27**, 245 (1975). Room temperature operation was reported by J. J. Coleman, N. Holonyak, Jr., M. J. Ludowise, and P. D. Wright, *ibid.* **29**, 167 (1976). See also Zh. I. Alferov, I. N. Arsentyev, D. Z. Garbuzov, S. G. Konnikov, and V. D. Rumyantsev, *Pisma Zh. Tekh. Fiz.* **1**, 305 (1975).
66. J. J. Coleman *et al.*, *Phys. Rev. Lett.* **33**, 1566 (1974).
67. Y. Makita, H. Ijuin, and S. Gonda, *Appl. Phys. Lett.* **28**, 287 (1976).
68. H. Rupprecht, J. M. Woodall, K. Konnerth, and D. G. Pettit, *Appl. Phys. Lett.* **9**, 221 (1966).
69. I. Ladany, *J. Appl. Phys.* **42**, 654 (1971).
70. H. Kressel, J. U. Dunse, H. Nelson, and F. Z. Hawrylo, *J. Appl. Phys.* **39**, 2006 (1968).
71. B. H. Ahn, R. R. Shurtz, and C. W. Trussell, *J. Electrochem. Soc.* **118**, 1015 (1971).
72. T. Morizumi and K. Takahashi, *Jpn. J. Appl. Phys.* **8**, 348 (1969).
73. W. N. Carr, *IEEE Trans. Electron. Devices* **12**, 531 (1965).
74. H. Rupprecht, J. M. Woodall, and G. D. Pettit, *Appl. Phys. Lett.* **11**, 81 (1967).
75. J. M. Woodall, H. Rupprecht, and W. Reuter, *J. Electrochem. Soc.* **116**, 899 (1969).
76. H. Kressel, F. Z. Hawrylo, and N. Almeleh, *J. Appl. Phys.* **40**, 2224 (1969).
77. P. Mischel and G. Schul, *Proc. Int. Symp. Gallium Arsenide, 3rd,* Inst. Phys. Phys. Soc. Conf., Ser. No. 9, p. 188 (1970).
78. K. J. Linden, *J. Appl. Phys.* **40**, 2325 (1969).
79. J. M. Blum and K. K. Shih, *Proc. IEEE* **59**, 1488 (1971).
80. J. M. Blum and K. K. Shih, *J. Appl. Phys.* **43**, 1394 (1972).
81. J. M. Woodall, R. M. Potenski, S. E. Blum, and R. Lynch, *Appl. Phys. Lett.* **20**, 375 (1972).
82. H. Kressel, H. Nelson, and F. Z. Hawrylo, *J. Appl. Phys.* **41**, 2019 (1970).
83. E. A. Ulmer, *Solid State Electron.* **14**, 1265 (1971).
84. L. M. Dolginov, L. D. Libov, V. Yu. Rogulin, and A. A. Shlenskii, *Sov. Phys. Semicond.* **5**, 569 (1971).

85. J. Lebailly, *in* "Photonics" (M. Balkanski and P. Lallemand, eds.). Gauthier-Villars, Paris, 1975.
86. H. Kressel and M. Ettenberg, *Appl. Phys. Lett.* **23**, 511 (1973).
87. F. E. Rosztoczy, F. Ermanis, I. Hayashi, and B. Schwartz, *J. Appl. Phys.* **41**, 264 (1970).
88. K. H. Zschauer, *Solid State Commun.* **7**, 1709 (1969).
89. E. G. Dierschke, L. E. Stone, and R. W. Haisty, *Appl. Phys. Lett.* **19**, 98 (1971).
90. Y. Ono, M. Morioka, K. Ito, A. Tachibana, and K. Kurata, *Hitachi Rev.* **25**, 129 (1976).
91. F. E. Rosztoczy and K. B. Wolfstirn, *J. Appl. Phys.* **42**, 426 (1971).
92. J. Stone, C. A. Burrus, A. G. Dentai, and B. I. Miller, *Appl. Phys. Lett.* **29**, 37 (1976).

Chapter 15

Distributed-Feedback Lasers

15.1 Introduction

The interest in integrated optical circuits [1, 2] in which modulators, switches, waveguides, and radiation sources are formed monolithically has led to interest in laser diodes in which cleaved facets are not required for optical feedback. In addition to the elimination of facets, such a structure offers a "purer" spectral emission by limiting the longitudinal modes which can propagate.

A distributed-feedback (DFB) laser is fabricated similarly to the Fabry–Perot type of structures, but the lasing action is generally obtained by the addition of periodic variations of the refractive index along the direction of wave propagation. The feedback in the cavity occurs because the energy of a wave propagating in one direction is continuously fed back in the opposite direction by Bragg scattering. Kogelnik and Shank [3, 4] first investigated characteristics of DFB using thin-film dye lasers.

15.2 Coupled Mode Analysis

Various techniques can be used for the analysis of DFB lasers, but the application of the concepts of coupled wave theory to grated structures appears to be the most fruitful [5–9]. The use of this theory allows one to determine the threshold gain and frequency characteristics in terms of the grating and waveguide geometry. The coupled mode analysis uses perturbation methods.

For simplicity, we consider only the TE modes in a three-layer waveguide.

523

Assume regions 1 and 5 bracket a center slab region 3 with index $n_3 > n_1, n_5$. The trapped waveguide modes are of the form

$$E_y = \psi_m(x) \exp[i(\omega t \pm \beta_m z)] \tag{15.2.1}$$

which are solutions to Maxwell's equations for an unperturbed reactive structure. The transverse behavior of the mth mode is $\psi_m(x)$, and β_m is the longitudinal propagation constant. We now introduce corrugations in the structure as indicated in Fig. 15.2.1. The set of trapped modes and the leaky modes form a complete set of eigenfunctions so that the fields in the perturbed structure can be expanded in terms of the unperturbed modes. Limiting our discussion to the coupling between a forward and a backward trapped mode of identical order, the waveguide field is

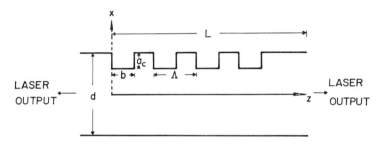

FIG. 15.2.1 Waveguide geometry of the idealized distributed-feedback laser. The periodic variations (period Λ) of the refractive index produce a frequency-sensitive feedback of the optical fields.

$$E_y = (A_m^+(z) \exp(-i\beta_m z) + A_m^-(z) \exp(i\beta_m z)) \psi_m(x) \tag{15.2.2}$$

where A_m^+ and A_m^- satisfy the differential equations

$$dA_m^+/dz = -\alpha A_m^+ + \kappa_{fb} \exp(i\Delta z)A_m^- \tag{15.2.3a}$$

$$dA_m^-/dz = \kappa_{bf} \exp(-i\Delta z)A^+ + \alpha A_m^- \tag{15.2.3b}$$

Here κ_{fb} and κ_{bf} are the coupling coefficients, Δ is a phase factor depending on β_m and the grating geometry, and α represents the attenuation due to losses in all regions, which we treat here as part of the perturbed dielectric constant.

From Fig. 15.2.1, the real part of the perturbed dielectric constant can be written

$$\Delta\kappa' = (n_3^2 - n_1^2)[u(x - d_3/2 + a) - u(x - d_3/2)]f(z) \tag{15.2.4}$$

where $u(x - x_0)$ is the unit step turning on at x_0 and $f(z)$ is a periodic function whose Fourier expansion is

$$f(z) = \sum_{l=-\infty}^{\infty} C_l \exp\left(i\frac{2l\pi}{\Lambda} z\right) \tag{15.2.5}$$

with

$$C_l = (\pi l)^{-1} \sin[\pi l b/\Lambda] \exp(-i\, l\pi b/\Lambda) \tag{15.2.6}$$

Equation (15.2.4) assumes the form

$$\Delta\kappa'(x, z) = \sum_l \Delta\kappa_l'(x) \exp(i\, 2l\pi/\Lambda\, z) \tag{15.2.7}$$

The imaginary part of the perturbed dielectric constant is

$$\Delta\kappa''(x) = k_0^{-1} n(x)\alpha(x) \tag{15.2.8}$$

where $n(x)$ is the unperturbed index distribution and $\alpha(x)$ the absorption constant. Note that in region 3, $-d_3/2 < x < d_3/2$, $\alpha(x) = \alpha_3 = (\alpha_{fc} - g)$. The total dielectric perturbation $\Delta\kappa = \Delta\kappa' + i\,\Delta\kappa''$. Using standard analytical techniques, we substitute Eq. (15.2.2) into Maxwell's equations, which yields

$$\frac{dA_m^+}{dz} = \frac{k_0^2}{2i\beta_m} [A_m^+ + A_m^- \exp(i2\beta_m z)] \int_{-\infty}^{\infty} \Delta\kappa\psi_m^2(x)\, dx \tag{15.2.9a}$$

$$\frac{dA_m^-}{dz} = -\frac{k_0^2}{2i\beta_m} (A_m^+ \exp(-i2\beta_m z) + A_m^-) \int_{-\infty}^{\infty} \Delta\kappa\psi_m^2(x)\, dx \tag{15.2.9b}$$

where we have normalized the wave functions according to

$$\int_{-\infty}^{\infty} \psi_m^2(x)\, dx = 1$$

Note that the term $\Delta\kappa$ in the integrand of Eq. (15.2.9) contains spatial harmonics along z. The product of these spatial harmonics with the term in parentheses gives phase terms varying with z. The terms of primary importance are those which give small phase terms, or produce the so-called *matched-phase* condition. This condition can be understood if we assume that A_m^+ and A_m^- are slowly varying functions of z. If a phase term is large, then the product of A_m^+ or A_m^- and a rapidly oscillating function produces a highly oscillating function. On the other hand, some terms will be slowly varying with z. If we multiply both sides of Eq. (15.2.9) by dz and integrate, those terms with small phase form the major part of the integration, whereas the terms with rapid oscillation contribute very little.

The perturbed dielectric constant has both a real and an imaginary part. Only the real part contains spatial harmonics. The "dc component," $\int_{-\infty}^{\infty} \Delta\kappa_0'(x) \psi_m^2(x)\, dx$, of the expansion in Eq. (15.2.9a) has a zero phase term which we will not consider here. Physically, this term relates to the fact that the effective width of the waveguide is modified by the corrugation which in turn modifies the propagation constant of both forward and backward waves.

Substituting the perturbed dielectric constant into Eq. (15.2.9) and comparing with Eq. (15.2.3), we obtain

$$\kappa_{fb}^{-l} = \frac{k_0^2}{2i\beta_m} \int_{-\infty}^{\infty} \Delta\kappa'_{-l}(x)\psi_m^2(x)\, dx \tag{15.2.10a}$$

$$\alpha = \frac{k_0}{2\beta_m} (n_1\alpha_1 a_1 + n_3\alpha_3 a_3 + n_5\alpha_5 a_5) \qquad (15.2.10b)$$

$$\Delta = 2\beta_m - \frac{2l\pi}{\Lambda} \equiv 2\delta \simeq 0 \qquad (15.2.10c)$$

where a_i is the portion of the unperturbed mode intensity in the ith region (Section 5.6). The quantity δ represents the deviation of the wave number of the unperturbed mode and $l\pi/\Lambda$; l is the spatial harmonic responsible for the scattering.

Consider now the case where $m = 1$, i.e., fundamental transverse mode operation. For a symmetric structure, $n_1 = n_5$, the fundamental mode wave function $\psi_1 \equiv \psi$ is

$$\psi(x) = \frac{1}{N_n} \begin{cases} \cos(h_3 d_3/2) \exp[h_1(d_3/2 - x)], & d_3/2 < x \\ \cos h_3 x, & -d_3/2 < x < d_3/2 \\ \cos(h_3 d_3/2) \exp[h_1(d_3/2 + x)], & -d_3/2 > x \end{cases} \qquad (15.2.11)$$

where the normalization factor N_n is

$$N_n^2 = \frac{1}{2}\left[\frac{d_3}{2} + \frac{\sin h_3 d_3}{2h_3} + \frac{\cos^2(h_3 d_3/2)}{h_1}\right] \qquad (15.2.12)$$

The coupling coefficient is

$$\kappa_{fb}^{-l} = \frac{k_0^2}{4i\beta N_n^2} C_l(n_3^2 - n_1^2)\left[a + \frac{\sin h_3 a \cos h_3(d_3 - a)}{h_3}\right] \qquad (15.2.13)$$

The backward–forward coupling coefficient κ_{bf}^l satisfies

$$\kappa_{bf}^l = (\kappa_{fb}^{-l})^* \qquad (15.2.14)$$

It is important to note here that in Eq. (15.2.10) the integral is equal to the product of the dielectric step and the fraction of the unperturbed field in the corrugation region, which we define as Ω. The distributed feedback coefficient $\kappa^l = |\kappa_{fb}^{-l}|$ is

$$\kappa^l = (k_0^2/2\beta) C_{-l}(n_3^2 - n_1^2) \Omega \simeq k_0 C_{-l}(n_3 - n_1)\Omega \qquad (15.2.15)$$

15.3 Solution of Coupled Modes

Consider now a structure with corrugations extending from $z = 0$ to $z = L$. The lasing modes are determined by solving Eq. (15.2.3) with appropriate boundary conditions. At $z = 0$, the forward wave is launched with zero amplitude, whereas the backward one starts at $z = L$ with no energy. The waves in the DFB region upon reaching the boundaries at $z = 0, L$, transfer all their energies into the uncorrugated waveguide regions. Consequently, the appropriate boundary conditions are

$$A^+_{z=0} = A^-_{z=L} = 0 \qquad (15.3.1a)$$

$$|A^+_{z=L}| = |A^-_{z=0}| \qquad (15.3.1b)$$

The wave solutions, found by elementary techniques, are

$$A^+(z) = a_0 \sinh(\gamma z) \exp(i\delta z) \qquad (15.3.2)$$

$$A^-(z) = \pm a_0 \sinh \gamma(L - z) \exp(-i\delta z) \qquad (15.3.3)$$

where

$$\gamma = [(\kappa')^2 + (\alpha + i\delta)^2]^{1/2} \qquad (15.3.4)$$

The secular equation defining the different longitudinal modes is

$$\gamma \coth \gamma L = -(\alpha + i\delta) \qquad (15.3.5)$$

Equation (15.3.5) contains complex quantities, and thus the roots γ_m will be complex. There are several regimes in which (15.3.5) can be simplified; for example, the high gain region where $-\alpha \gg \kappa'$ corresponds to weak feedback compared to the active region gain. Equation (15.3.5) can thus be separated into its real and imaginary parts, leading to

$$2 \tan^{-1} \frac{\delta_q}{\alpha_q} + 2\delta_q L - \frac{\delta_q L(\kappa')^2}{\alpha_q^2 + \delta_q^2} = (2q - 1)\pi \qquad (15.3.6a)$$

$$\frac{\exp(2\alpha_q L)}{\alpha_q^2 + \delta_q^2} = \frac{4}{(\kappa')^2}, \qquad q = 0, \pm 1, \pm 2 \quad (15.3.6b)$$

Near the Bragg frequency, the longitudinal modes are given by

$$\delta_q L = (q - \tfrac{1}{2})\pi \qquad (15.3.7)$$

which corresponds to the longitudinal modes in a Fabry–Perot cavity. The condition defining the optical cavity gain g_{th} at threshold for a specific longitudinal mode number q is

$$\frac{\exp[\Gamma(g_{th} - G_{th} - \alpha_{fc})L]}{\Gamma^2(g_{th} - G_{th} - \alpha_{fc})^2 + 4\delta_q^2} = \frac{1}{(\kappa')^2} \qquad (15.3.8)$$

where Γ is the optical wave confinement factor and G_{th} is the active region gain required to offset losses in the regions exterior to the active region. The key result deduced from Eq. (15.3.8) is the strong discrimination between longitudinal modes because the value of G_{th} depends on δ_q. This produces spectral purity of the output. Note that the threshold gain g_{th} just derived has not taken into consideration the possible coupling between different transverse cavity modes.

15.4   GaAs–(AlGa)As DFB Lasers

Nakamura and co-workers [10–12] and Shank and Schmidt [13] observed lasing in corrugated structures of GaAs–(AlGa)As by optical pumping at low

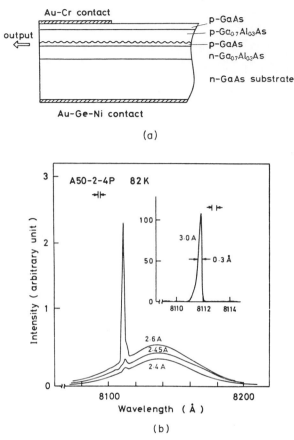

FIG. 15.4.1   (a) Schematic cross section of the double-heterojunction DFB laser, and (b) emission spectra of the double-heterojunction DFB laser. The active region $d_3 = 1.3$ μm, $L = 630$ μm, $a = 0.09$ μm, and $\Lambda = 0.3416$ μm [12].

temperatures ($\sim$77 K). Injection DFB lasers fabricated with GaAs–(AlGa)As have operated at low temperatures [14], and a four-heterojunction configuration has first lased pulsed at room temperature, [15, 16] and then Nakamura *et al.* [17] obtained CW operation at room temperature.

In (AlGa)As–GaAs heterojunction DFB structures corrugations are commonly introduced by ion milling (although etching can also be used), and then material is grown into the grooves so formed. The periodicity used is $\sim$0.3 $-$0.4 μm. The most successful devices to date (operating at 300 K with $J_{th} < 5000$ A/cm²) have used the large optical cavity concept in which the recombination region is smaller than the waveguide region, thus allowing part of the optical energy to couple to the periodic structures in the waveguide. The introduction of corrugations within the double-heterojunction configuration itself has not been as successful because of possible excessive non-radiative recombination due to defects introduced in the process of ion milling, although such structures have exhibited DFB behavior. Figure 15.4.1a shows a schematic cross section of a simple double-heterojunction DFB laser in which corrugations separate the p-type GaAs active region from the p-type (AlGa)As [12]. Figure 15.4.1b shows the optical output as a function of wavelength from the device operating in a single longitudinal mode.

The DFB structure used to obtain CW operation at room temperature is shown in Fig. 15.4.2. This laser, a mesa stripe-geometry diode, used a separate confinement region to avoid nonradiative recombination of the injected carriers in the corrugation region. As shown in Fig. 15.4.2, the p-GaAs forms both the optical waveguide and the active layer. The n-$Al_{0.3}Ga_{0.7}$As and the p-$Al_{0.17}Ga_{0.83}$As layers confine the optical field to the p-GaAs layer, which has a width of 0.2 μm; the p-layer also acts as a barrier for the injected electrons, confining them to the active layer. A weak distributed-feedback coefficient is obtained because only part of the optical field leaks across the thin p-$Al_{0.17}Ga_{0.83}$As layer ($\sim$0.1 μm) into the corrugated layer of p-$Al_{0.07}Ga_{0.93}$As. Figure 15.4.3 shows its threshold current density and lasing wavelength as a function of junction temperature; the corrugation length $L = 730$ μm and $\Lambda = 3814$ Å. For comparison, the threshold characteristics of a Fabry–Perot (FP) laser made from the same wafer are also shown in Fig. 15.4.3. The length of the cleaved laser was 570 μm. The DFB laser was capable of operation in two transverse modes, denoted $m = 1$ and $m = 2$, but between 300 and 350 K, only the fundamental mode was observed with a threshold current

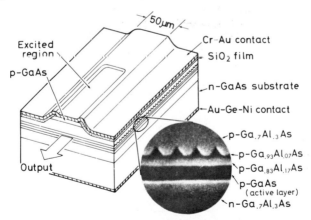

FIG. 15.4.2 A mesa stripe-geometry DFB laser. The corrugations are separated from the active region to minimize nonradiative recombination of injected carriers. Distributed feedback is produced because the optical field leaks across the thin p-wall of $Al_{0.17}Ga_{0.83}$As (~ 0.1 μm) which confines most of the field to the active p-GaAs layer [17].

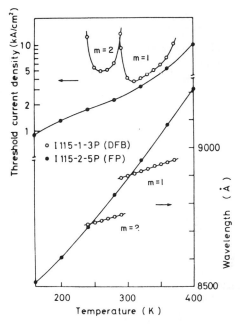

FIG. 15.4.3 Threshold characteristics of a DFB laser compared with that of a standard Fabry–Perot cavity laser. The corrugation period $\Lambda = 0.3814\ \mu$m. These data were obtained by varying the heat sink temperature under pulsed conditions. The DFB laser operated in either the fundamental transverse mode $m = 1$, or the second mode $m = 2$ depending on the temperature [17].

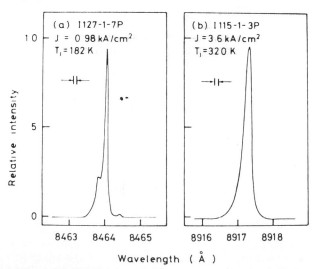

FIG. 15.4.4 The lasing spectra for CW operation. In (a) $\Lambda = 0.3648\ \mu$m and in (b) $\Lambda \sim 0.3814\ \mu$m. The diodes lased in a single longitudinal mode but with numerous lateral modes often found in mesa stripe lasers. The broadening of the spectra and the substructure are attributed to the multiple lateral modes [17].

about 1.2 times that of the Fabry–Perot device. Figure 15.4.4 shows the lasing spectra obtained under CW conditions for two different temperatures. The fine structure at 182 K is attributed to operation in several lateral modes. These could also contribute to the broadening of the longitudinal mode line at 320 K. Thus, a narrower line width could be achieved if the laser operation is restricted to a single longitudinal and fundamental lateral mode. (See Appendix E for a discussion of the theoretical line width of a laser). Insufficient data exist at this time to establish the current range (or power emission level) over which single longitudinal mode operation can be maintained in DFB devices.

REFERENCES

1. S. E. Miller, *Bell Syst. Tech. J.* **48**, 2059 (1969).
2. P. K. Tien, R. Ubrich, and R. J. Martin, *Appl. Phys. Lett.* **14**, 291 (1969).
3. H. Kogelnik and C. V. Shank, *Appl. Phys. Lett.* **18**, 152 (1971).
4. H. Kogelnik and C. V. Shank, *J. Appl. Phys.* **43**, 2327 (1972).
5. D. Marcuse, "Light Transmission Optics." Van Nostrand-Reinhold, Princeton, New Jersey, 1972.
6. A. Yariv, *IEEE J. Quantum Electron.* **9**, 919 (1973).
7. H. F. Taylor and A. Yariv, *Proc. IEEE* **62**, 1044 (1974).
8. H. Kogelnik, *Bell Syst. Tech. J.* **48**, 2909 (1969).
9. S. Wang, *J. Appl. Phys.* **44**, 767 (1973).
10. M. Nakamura, A. Yariv, H. W. Yen, S. Somekh, and H. L. Garvin, *Appl. Phys. Lett.* **22**, 315 (1973).
11. M. Nakamura, H. W. Yen, A. Yariv, E. Garmire, S. Somekh, and H. L. Garvin, *Appl. Phys. Lett.* **23**, 224 (1973).
12. M. Nakamura, K. Aiki, J. Umeda, A. Yariv, H. W. Yen, and T. Morikawa, *Appl. Phys. Lett.* **25**, 487 (1974).
13. C. V. Shank and R. V. Schmidt, *Appl. Phys. Lett.* **25**, 200 (1974).
14. D. R. Scifres, R. D. Burnham, and W. Streifer, *Appl. Phys. Lett.* **25**, 203 (1974).
15. K. Aiki, M. Nakamura, J. Umeda, A. Yariv, A. Katzir, and H. W. Yen, *Appl. Phys. Lett.* **27**, 145 (1975).
16. H. C. Casey, Jr., S. Somekh, and M. Ilegems, *Appl. Phys. Lett.* **27**, 142 (1975).
17. M. Nakamura, K. Aiki, J. Umeda, and A. Yariv, *Appl. Phys. Lett.* **27**, 403 (1975).

Chapter 16

Device Reliability

Factors controlling laser diode and LED reliability have been extensively studied because of the poor life of the early devices. Although the problem is complicated and all aspects are not yet fully understood, enormous progress has been made since 1968 in solving the reliability problems. In this chapter we review the major failure modes and mechanisms so far identified, as well as the solutions which have evolved to produce devices with years of operating lifetimes.

Our discussion is concerned with the two major subdivisions of the problem, which are denoted *catastrophic* and *gradual* degradation. The first depends on the optical flux density in the emitting region and on the pulse length, and results in *facet damage*; the second (an internal process) is related to the electron–hole recombination process and is strongly affected by the laser technology. This degradation mode is similar in LEDs and laser diodes.

16.1 Facet (Catastrophic) Degradation

Complete or partial laser failure may occur as a result of mechanical damage of the facet in the region of intense optical emission [1,2]. The nature of the damage suggests local dissociation of the material [3] (see Fig. 16.1.1), and the damage sometimes extends a significant distance into the crystal [5].

It is well established that facet damage is caused by the optical flux density at the laser facet and that it is *not* a function of the operating current [1]. The width of the emitting region and the pulse length are important factors deter-

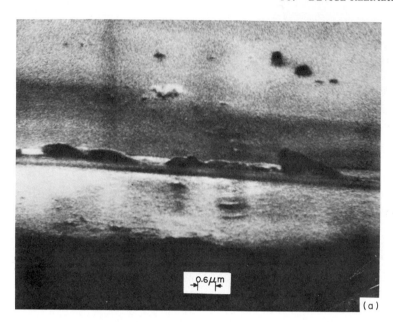

0.6 μm

(a)

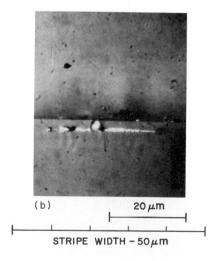

(b)   20 μm

STRIPE WIDTH – 50 μm

FIG. 16.1.1 (a) Appearance of laser diode facet following catastrophic damage in pulsed operation, as viewed by scanning electron microscopy. (b) Appearance of laser facet following catastrophic damage as a result of CW operation at room temperature at excessive optical power level. The damaged region is smaller than the stripe-contact width of 50 μm, and is centered in the region of initially highest optical power density [4].

mining the failure level defined in terms of a figure of merit, P_c, the critical damage level in watts per centimeter of emitting facet. For example, for a given operating condition, P_c decreases with the recombination region width of *wide* double-heterojunction lasers (or near-field distribution for thin DH lasers). With a pulse length of 100 ns, $P_c \approx 200$ W/cm for a broad-area DH laser with $d_3 = 1$ μm, whereas $P_c = 400$ W/cm with $d_3 = 2$ μm.

It is important to note that the damage threshold can be reduced if mechanical flaws exist at the laser facet because the optically induced facet damage initiated at these faults will spread into the other regions of the facet [6]. In particular, facet damage can be initiated at the edges of the diode in broad-area sawed-side lasers and thus reduce the laser's reliability. Therefore, planar stripe-contact devices are highly desirable for the minimization of facet damage [6].

The determination of the *optical power density* is not easily made at the failure point because of the nonuniform optical energy distribution in the direction perpendicular to the junction plane. Furthermore, in stripe-contact lasers, the optical intensity is also not uniform in the plane of the junction. Therefore, the power density estimates are at best within a factor of 2. The experimental results obtained for double-heterojunction *broad-area* devices operated with 100-ns-long pulses indicate that failure occurs at about 2–4 × 10^6 W/cm^2 [7]. Studies of planar *stripe-contact* lasers gave an estimate of 4–8 × 10^6 W/cm^2 [5], consistent with the reduced susceptibility to facet damage.

For a given device, P_c decreases with increasing pulse length t as $t^{-1/2}$ [8], as illustrated in Fig. 16.1.2 for various devices, including LOC, FH, and

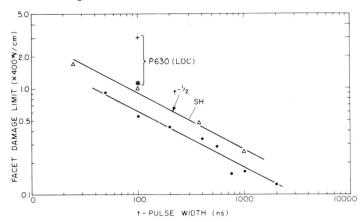

FIG. 16.1.2 Dependence of facet damage on pulse width for uncoated lasers. The data points for P-630 LOC-type lasers are given for dielectric-coated (+) and uncoated (*) facet structures and correspond closely to data for single-heterojunction lasers (△). The lower curve (●) is data taken on four-heterojunction lasers.

single-heterojunction devices. (Data reported by Eliseev [9] for DH lasers follow a similar behavior.)

The safe operating level is increased by antireflecting films on the laser facet (e.g., SiO), which lower the ratio between the optical flux density inside and outside the crystal. This is illustrated in Fig. 16.1.3 for single-heterojunction lasers on which the facet reflectivity R was changed [10]. Despite the significant scatter in the data, the trend of increased P_c with reduced R is evident. It has been suggested [5] that facet failure occurs at a constant electric field intensity of 120 kV/cm (for a 100-ns pulse length) and that the ratio P_c'/P_c for a facet reflectivity R can be expressed as

$$\frac{P_c'}{P_c} = n \frac{(1 - R)}{(1 + R^{1/2})^2} \tag{16.1.1}$$

where n is the GaAs refractive index (~ 3.6) and P_c is the measured value for the GaAs–air interface (i.e., uncoated laser). The "best fit" curve to the data of Fig. 16.1.3 shows agreement with (16.1.1).

Lasers operating CW can also fail by facet damage if the optical flux density is excessive [4]. For stripe-contact lasers with oxide isolation and stripe widths of 13 and 50 μm, the values found were on the order of 20–40 W/cm or 2–4×10^5 W/cm^2. (These laser diodes were thin DH lasers, $d_3 \simeq 0.2$–0.3 μm, with Al$_{0.1}$Ga$_{0.9}$As in the recombination region and Al$_{0.3}$Ga$_{0.7}$As in the

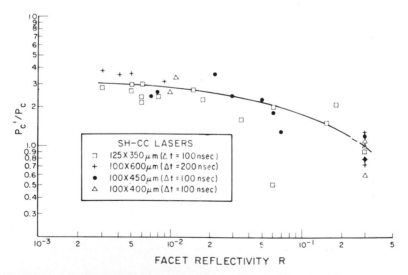

FIG. 16.1.3 Ratio of the linear power density at catastrophic laser failure P_c', to the power density for failure for GaAs–air interface, P_c ($R = 0.32$), with decreasing facet reflectivity R of single-heterojunction lasers. The curve represents the best empirical fit [10].

adjoining n- and p-type regions.) The facet failure is generally initiated under the central portion of the stripe contact where the optical flux density is generally highest, as seen in Fig. 16.1.1b.

It is sometimes desirable to operate narrow stripe lasers in the pulsed mode of operation instead of CW. In this case, the allowable peak power is increased with decreasing pulse width. Table 16.1.1 shows values obtained with (AlGa)As DH lasers, emitting at about 8200 Å, operated with pulse lengths of 100 and 400 ns, and CW. Note that the damage limit decreases from 240 mw (power emitted from one facet) at 100 ns to 30 mW in CW operation. These lasers had uncoated facets; higher levels are expected with dielectric coatings.

TABLE 16.1.1
Catastrophic Damage Limit of Uncoated AlGaAs CW Laser Diodes[a]

Pulse Length (ns)	Catastrophic damage limit (mW)[b]
100 (1kHz)	240
400 (0.25 kHz)	90
CW	30

[a]Stripe width 13 μm. From Kressel and Ladany [4].
[b]Average of four diodes. All diodes selected from the same wafer.

This discussion concerns a failure mode which occurs in a short period of time (order of hours). Facet damage ("erosion") can also appear gradually over a long operating time (many thousands of hours) for diodes operated below P_c, an effect accelerated by moisture on the facet [11]. The damage can be seen in Fig. 16.1.4 to consist of a delineation of the junction. The effect of this damage is typically to decrease the differential quantum efficiency, and to increase the threshold current density because of the change in facet reflectivity. Thus the laser continues to operate but with reduced efficiency. To minimize such damage, significant (factor of $\sim$ 3) derating below P_c is recommended for systems use of CW laser diodes requiring operating lifetimes of years. The use of dielectric facet coatings also minimizes the formation of such facet damage [4]. Good success has been achieved with coatings, including Al_2O_3 facet coatings, which are impervious to moisture; lasers so protected have operated stably for many thousands of hours (Section 16.3). The thickness of the dielectric coatings (half-wave) used for the CW lasers is such that the facet reflectivity is essentially unchanged. Their function, therefore, is mainly in protecting the device from its surroundings and preventing facet erosion via loss of constituents such as As.

Although it is clear that catastrophic damage is basically an optically induced effect, the basic physical mechanism whereby the optical field interacts with the crystal is uncertain. It is noteworthy that below-bandgap energy ra-

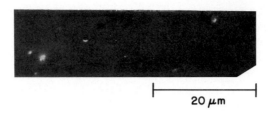

FIG. 16.1.4   Facet damage ("erosion") observed after long-term CW operation of a
laser diode, stripe width 13 μm, at room temperature in a dry air ambient, but with no facet
coating. The laser was operated for 10,721 hr with 5–10 mW of power emitted. The active
region of this laser consisted of $Al_{0.1}Ga_{0.9}As$.

diation can induce damage in GaAs comparable to that seen in catastrophic
degradation at power densities of the same order of magnitude [9]. Two
major mechanisms have been proposed: (1) an effect whereby the optical
flux generates acoustic waves [1], thus leading to either massive damage at the
facets (which sometimes occurs) or strong local heating where the acoustic
waves are damped; (2) absorption of the radiation at inhomogeneities in the
crystal, leading to local overheating and hence to the dissociation of the
crystal [3]. A discussion of the various mechanisms has been published by
Eliseev [9]. However, insufficient data exist to completely rule out either of the
two effects.

The fact that facet damage is initiated preferentially at mechanical flaws at
the facet may be explained by the weakness of the crystal in those regions.
Once damage is initiated, adjoining regions become susceptible, giving rise
to a "zipper" effect which continues until the whole of the strongly emitting
region is eventually damaged. In view of this effect, the average P_c values
observed should be interpreted as statistical values which may be limited due
to technology rather than fundamental.

16.2   Internal Damage Mechanisms

16.2.1   General Observations [12]

The gradual degradation observed in laser diodes (without evidence of
facet damage) consists of a reduction in the differential quantum efficiency
and an increase in J_{th}. Erratic variations in reliability and fabrication-depen-
dent effects were characteristic of early laser diodes, which suggested imperfect
control of the device metallurgy and led to detailed investigations of the
relevant factors [13]. In LEDs, the diode efficiency decreases with time, usually
with no significant spectral changes.

Major changes in the *bulk* of a laser diode occurring during high current
density operation ($J > 1000$ A/cm^2) were first observed in GaAs homojunc-

tion lasers by Kressel and Byer [13]; these lasers showed a drop in internal efficiency and an increase in internal absorption. Similar observations were later made on double-heterojunction diodes [14], which confirmed that permanent changes *within* the recombination region, rather than a simple increase in the excess current, are mainly responsible for degradation.

A characteristic feature of gradual degradation is the increasing "spottiness" of the lasing emission, as shown in Fig. 16.2.1. At the start of the test, the laser's CW near-field pattern is seen to be relatively uniform, with the maximum optical intensity at the center of the stripe. After degradation, the emission is greatly reduced at the originally most intense region (where the current density was also the highest). Simultaneously, the carrier lifetime is decreased from 6 to 3.5 ns, suggestive of a decrease in the average nonradiative lifetime, and hence of the internal quantum efficiency. No evidence of facet damage is noted. It is evident, therefore, that the laser is *internally* damaged and that these changes can affect the incoherent emission as well as the lasing properties. A drop in internal quantum efficiency lowers the output of both the spontaneous and coherent emission, as will an increase in internal absorption. The effects may differ quantitatively, however, since the spectral patterns and internal dynamics change when lasing occurs. Moreover, a low density of nonradiative centers may be important in reducing the efficiency at the low current densities of some LEDs but not at the laser threshold where the injected carrier density is relatively high.

Results obtained by various investigators often differ, but the following

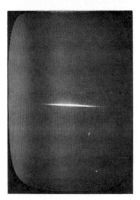
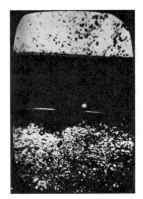

START: END: 700 hr at 800 mA ($3 \times I_{th}$)
τ = 6 ns τ = 3.5 ns

FIG. 16.2.1 Evidence of gradual degradation (internal defect formation) in a CW coated laser diode (13 μm stripe width). At the start of the test, the near-field emission is continuous under the stripe contact and the spontaneous carrier lifetime is 6 ns. After long-term operation at a very high current of 800 mA, the emission is nonuniform, with the middle portion (under the stripe) no longer contributing. The average carrier lifetime is reduced to 3.5 ns.

observations of device changes with time appear to be generally valid for degradation effects.

1.   The threshold current density increases while the differential quantum efficiency usually (but not always) decreases.

2.   Heterojunction diodes operated at high current densities degrade similarly whether or not lasing [14] (as long as facet damage does not occur), the degradation rate being a superlinear function of the operating current density. The degradation rate may increase by as much as the square of the average diode current density [14,15].

3.   The carrier lifetime decreases with the spontaneous efficiency [16]. The change of τ with η_i suggests a reduction in the nonradiative lifetime by the formation of nonradiative recombination centers. Although the changes in τ and J_{th} are often found to be related [17], good correlation between the reduction in τ and the increase in J_{th} is not always possible because any large area defects created will increase the absorption coefficient [18–20].

4.   Degradation does not require the presence of a p–n junction. It has been observed both above and below lasing threshold [21] in n-type GaAs *optically* pumped. No evidence of damage was observed in the transparent (AlGa)As window region of the heterojunction structure, indicating that the *presence of excess electron–hole pairs was necessary* for degradation to occur.

5.   There are successive gradual degradation stages. In the early stages, when the density of newly formed nonradiative recombination centers is low, the *spontaneous* efficiency decreases with only minor effects on the *lasing* properties. As degradation proceeds, "dark lines" may appear when the emission is viewed through the surface of the diode [20,22]. The dark lines constitute regions of concentrated nonradiative centers and are believed responsible for the spotty near-field emission pattern of degraded lasers, and the *rapid* fall off in the output of CW lasers at room temperature.

Figure 16.2.2 shows the formation of nonradiative centers in the vicinity of the ohmic contact to the LED surface [12]. Although the power is initially reduced without evidence of such concentrated "dark" regions, they do appear when the degradation in power emission is substantial. Hence, *dispersed* nonradiative centers exist in addition to the concentrated nonradiative areas. The dark regions can have several origins, including impurity precipitation at existing dislocations. In some structures examined by transmission electron microscopy, evidence was found that the dark regions were *dislocation networks* formed by climb starting at initially present dislocation sources [23, 24]. Dislocation climb (i.e., motion out of its plane) requires the addition or removal of atoms by diffusion to or from existing dislocations. Therefore, the growth of networks of dislocations is direct evidence for a diffusion process being a cause of gradual degradation (see later).

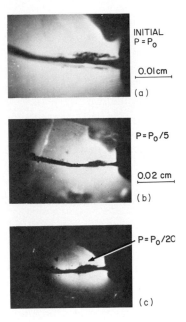

INITIAL
P = P₀

0.01cm

(a)

P = P₀/5

0.02 cm

(b)

P = P₀/2C

(c)

FIG. 16.2.2 Effect of continuing operation on the surface emission from a double-heterojunction diode. (a) Microphotograph of the infrared emission in the vicinity of the ohmic contact showing a clear emission pattern. (b) The diode output is reduced to one-fifth of the initial value P_0, but no evidence of visible damage is seen. (The spots are on the surface of the diode.) (c) The diode output is reduced to one-twentieth its initial value and dark lines are seen in the region of initial highest emission density (AlGa)As–GaAs: Si DH diode [12].

In one case the dark lines were found to originate in regions of the crystal which had originally low radiative efficiency as measured by photoluminescence [25]. By using intense external laser photoexcitation, it has been possible to promote the rapid growth of these dark regions. As an alternate process to dislocation climb, it was suggested that the dislocation increase can occur via a process of glide (on {111} planes, ⟨110⟩ directions) in the device. The process of glide may be eased by electron–hole recombination which reduces the energy needed for dislocation motion at room temperature. Such motion is sometimes very rapid, resulting in degradation in periods of hours.

6. There is evidence that the degradation rate increases with temperature from a comparison of diodes operating at 77 K and at room temperature. Additional evidence [26] found under conditions of CW laser operation shows a strong temperature dependence above room temperature for the specific DH devices studied (GaAs in the recombination region, proton-bombardment stripe-contact diodes).

7. A frequent accompaniment of laser degradation is the appearance of

high frequency oscillation in the optical emission [27,28]. Such oscillations often occur in laser diodes in which some regions are lasing and others are absorbing. Yang *et al.* [28] have suggested that the microwave oscillations after degradation result from the internal Q-switching from saturable absorption in the degraded region [29] similar to the effect described in Chapter 17 in diodes with nonuniform population inversion.

8. It is a common observation that the current–voltage characteristics change as degradation proceeds. The reverse I–V characteristic "softens" while the excess current increases in forward bias. These I–V changes are consistent with the formation of localized defects in the junction region and a reduction in the minority carrier lifetime. However, the current–voltage measurements usually show no measurable change indicative of gross junction gradient changes.

16.2.2 Material-Related Factors Affecting Gradual Degradation

The first direct evidence of strong metallurgical effects on the degradation rate was obtained by a study of the effect of dislocations on GaAs homojunction lasers made by LPE [30]. It was shown that a high dislocation density (order 10^5 cm^{-2} introduced by plastic deformation of a wafer containing the junction at elevated temperatures) led to erratic degradation rates, as shown in Fig. 16.2.3a. Such behavior is consistent with a nonuniform dislocation distribution among the diodes introduced by the plastic deformation. In light of the observation of dislocation network growth, these results are, of course, easily understood, because existing dislocations provide the nuclei for expanding networks.

In similar experiments, it was shown that GaAs diodes made using different dopants degrade at different rates [30]. For example, Be-doped diodes degrade much more rapidly than Zn-doped diodes. The effect was attributed to the smaller ionic radius of Be with its consequent higher probability of displacement by the energy released in nonradiative electron–hole recombination.

Contaminants such as Cu in GaAs are definitely detrimental; experiments with Cu in GaAs:Zn-diffused homojunctions [31] yielded an activation energy of 0.45 ± 0.1 eV for the spontaneous emission quantum efficiency degradation process, suggestive of Cu diffusion. However, since Cu can be effectively removed by various leaching techniques, it is unlikely that Cu is significant for the degradation of diodes made by liquid phase epitaxy, where the Ga melt is an excellent "getter" for Cu. However, it could be a factor in diodes made using other technologies.

Care is needed in the assembly of diodes to prevent stresses, in particular when "hard" solders should not be used to bond the diodes to the heat sink [32]. The effect of stress on accelerating degradation has been well known in the commercial LED and laser diode field, but the more demanding CW operating conditions of laser diodes make it even more imperative to avoid diode strains. The use of indium solders appears sufficient in this regard. The effect of the strain due to hard solders is probably connected with the formation of dislocation networks, even in the process of diode assembly itself, since GaAs and related alloys are relatively plastic (compared to Si) at a few hundred degrees centigrade.

There are great differences in the degradation rates of diodes using different compounds, an effect of important technological impact. Most noteworthy is that diodes in which the recombination region consists of $Al_xGa_{1-x}As$ are less susceptible to gradual degradation than comparable diodes with GaAs in the recombination region [33]. This is illustrated in Fig. 16.2.3b which shows the half-life of diodes operated at 1000 A/cm^2 (spontaneous emission) as a function of the decreasing emission wavelength [i.e., increasing Al content in the (AlGa)As recombination region]. In a variety of homojunction and heterojunction devices, the general trend of improved life with increasing Al content is evident. These experiments were limited to $x \leq 0.1$ and *sawed-side* diodes. Therefore, the GaAs diode data shown are *not* indicative of state of the art values with stripe-contact devices, which have much longer operating lifetimes. On the low bandgap energy side of GaAs, it has been found that (InGa)As LEDs showed a reduced degradation rate with increase in In [34]. (These experiments were limited to a spectral range of 1.1 μm at room temperature, and have not been carried out with lasers or under high current density conditions.)

Other factors being constant, an effect controlling long-term laser or LED reliability arises from work-damaged diode sidewalls. It is firmly established that exposed diode edges can lead to accelerated degradation as demonstrated by the performance of similar dimension oxide stripe and broad-area CW laser diodes cut from the same wafer [11, 27]. The broad-area lasers that had sides formed by sawing degraded in a few hours, whereas the stripe-contact diodes (with the sides embedded in the GaAs) operated quite stably for thousands of hours. These experiments also showed that a possible source of defects is a highly doped Zn-diffused region in close proximity to (or extending into) the recombination region. Figure 16.2.4 illustrates the dramatic difference observed with deep Zn diffusion on a laser diode's reliability, compared to a diode in which Zn was eliminated from the active region.

The growth rate used to prepare the GaAs:Ge recombination region by liquid phase epitaxy can strongly affect the degradation rate [35]. This effect on the degradation rate was attributed to the influence of the vacancy density in the material grown at the various rates. The best material was obtained at a very high growth rate where the As vacancy concentration is believed to be lower than in the slowly grown material.

In view of the strong evidence for the motion of point defects, the effect of crystal stoichiometry can be expected to play a key role in the reliability of the

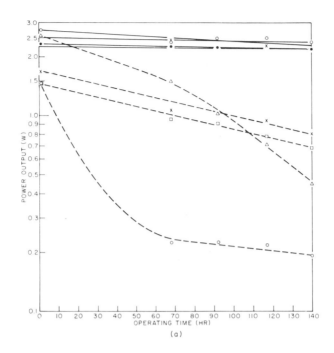

(a)

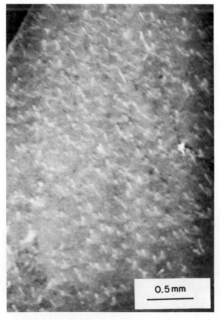

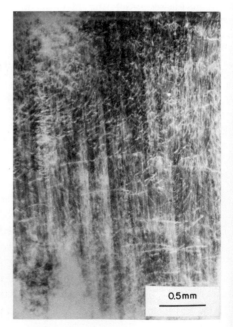

(b)

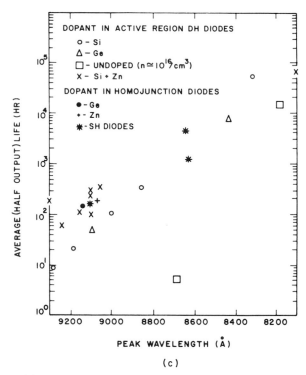

(c)

FIG. 16.2.3 (a) Power output as a function of operating time (pulse length 100 ns, repetition rate 4 kHz) of LPE lasers made from as-grown (solid curve) and plastically deformed (dashed curve) substrates to introduce a high dislocation density. Note the random degradation rate of the lasers containing a high dislocation density [30]. (b) X-ray topographs of undeformed (left) and plastically deformed GaAs (right) used for a reliability experiment with the results shown in (a). (c) Average half-life of LEDs operating at 1000 A/cm² as a function of their emission wavelength. For each dopant type in the recombination region the shift to shorter wavelength represents additions of Al to the recombination region. Both single and double-heterojunction and homojunction diodes were tested as indicated, all with sawed sides [33].

devices (Section 16.3). In fact, initial differences in native point defects and aggregates are known to be present due to differences in the material synthesis technique (Chapter 9). Molecular beam epitaxy, vapor phase epitaxy, and liquid phase epitaxy produce GaAs with different concentrations of vacancies, interstitials, and defect clusters, which may partly explain (in addition to different contaminants) the different gradual degradation rates observed under similar operating conditions. For example, early GaAs/(AlGa)As DH lasers grown by MBE were reported to have lifetimes of only hours [36] in CW operation, despite otherwise reasonable performance. A similar problem was encountered with GaAs/(InGa)P CW DH diodes prepared by vapor phase epitaxy [37].

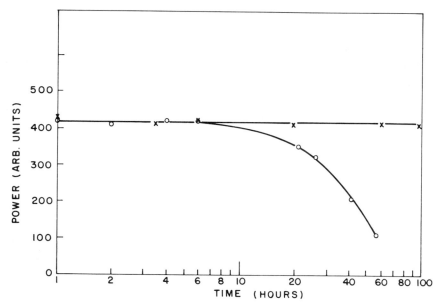

FIG. 16.2.4 Experiment illustrating the possible negative impact of Zn diffusion into CW laser diode recombination regions. Shown is the power output as a function of time for two (AlGa)As DH laser diodes with oxide-isolated stripe contacts fabricated from the same wafer but processed differently. One diode (○) has a deep Zn diffusion (extending to the active region) from an excess Zn source (providing a very high surface concentration) prior to ohmic contact application. The other diode (×) was not diffused. Both were operated at 0.5 A [11].

Most of the CW laser diode development with systems impact has been concentrated on the use of Al in the recombination region because of the improved degradation resistance and because the emission at $\lambda \approx 8200$ Å is desirable for fiber transmission. However, work has also been reported on diodes with GaAs in the recombination region but with phosphorus added to the outer (AlGa)As regions in order to match their thermal coefficient of expansion and hence reduce the elastic strain. There are insufficient published reliability data at this time to determine whether, in fact, this process improves laser reliability [26]. In these experiments, the lattice mismatch at the growth temperature was about 10^{-4}. However, by keeping the active region width below about 1 μm misfit dislocation formation was prevented, as discussed in Section 9.4.

16.2.3   Basic Causes of Gradual Degradation

It is clear from Section 16.2.2 that nonradiative recombination centers can be introduced into the recombination region during forward bias operation and that the internal degradation process is typically spatially nonuniform, although distributed defects are also present. That vacancies or interstitials are formed and diffuse into the recombination region is established by the observed growth of dislocation networks by climb, but the origin of these point defects is uncertain. Gold and Weisberg [38], in their tunnel diode degradation studies, suggested that nonradiative electron–hole recombination at an impurity center (Zn in their case) could result in its displacement into an interstitial position, leaving a vacancy behind. A similar process of enhanced diffusion of point defects is also conceivable. This is the basic "phonon kick" model in which multiphonon emission gives an intense vibration of the recombination center, thus reducing its activation energy for displacement. Applying this mechanism to electroluminescence, the assumption is that the vacancy and interstitial formed would have a large cross section for nonradiative recombination. Repeated nonradiative transitions would gradually move it to internal sinks.

The probability of obtaining a lattice atom displacement via the phonon kick process is evidently small. However, it was estimated [13] that the probability of vacancy formation need only be as small as one displacement in 10^{15} recombinations within the diode active region to produce a measurable change in the laser or LED efficiency, In fact, a density of nonradiative centers $N_t = 10^{17}$ cm^{-3} with a capture cross section $\sigma_t = 10^{-15}$ cm^2 would produce a nonradiative lifetime $\tau_{nr} = (N_t \sigma_t v_{th})^{-1} = 10^{-9}$ s which is much lower than $\tau_r \cong 3$–5 ns in a typical laser diode.

Although there is no *definitive* evidence for the phonon kick model in degradation, experimental results do indicate that the energy released in (presumably nonradiative) electron–hole recombination is a factor in the degradation process. The (InGa)As LED experiments showed [34] that the degradation rate decreased with increasing In. This could be related to the decreasing (bandgap) energy available for atomic displacement processes. The experiments of Lang and Kimerling [39] provided more direct support for this hypothesis by showing that the lattice defects introduced into GaAs diodes by irradiation with 1 MeV electrons anneal more readily under forward bias (i.e., in the presence of carrier recombination). The activation energy for motion of the unidentified point defects (probably vacancies and/or interstitials) was reduced to ~ 0.34 eV, by forward bias, from ~ 1.4 eV in the unbiased diode similarly heat-treated.

Although these experiments showed that a reduction in the activation energy for some point defects can occur in a region containing excess carriers, they do not directly explain the degradation results. A driving force for the point defects has to be postulated to explain their accumulation with time, rather than annihilation as observed by Lang and Kimerling. The simplest hypothesis is that the growth of existing dislocation networks, which constitute ideal sinks for the point defects, produces a reduction in the free energy of the crystal. Kimerling *et al.* [40] have indeed directly observed, in the transmission electron microscope, the growth of dislocation networks following annealing of point defects introduced with 1 MeV electron irradiation. This suggests an energetically favorable situation since the energy of the crystal is reduced when the point defect becomes part of the dislocation network compared to its being in a "free" state, i.e., isolated.

So far we have concentrated on the motion of *native* point defects. Dark lines can also form by a precipitation process. If some particularly mobile species are present in the device, such as O, Cu, or interstitial Be or Zn atoms, then their diffusion rate can also be accelerated and they may eventually cluster within the strain field of existing dislocations, or newly expanded networks. Thus, dislocations can become "decorated" by an atmosphere of impurities which can increase the local absorption coefficient. This effect could well occur in diodes containing high Zn concentrations [22]. Finally, the process of dislocation glide into the active region from the surrounding passive regions is another possibility, as mentioned in Section 16.2.1, for diodes under stress.

In summary, knowledge of the detailed kinetics of the degradation process is still too limited for a comprehensive model. However, major degradation effects are explained on the theory that the energy released in nonradiative recombination enhances the diffusion of vacancies and/or interstitials. (Whether any point defects are actually *formed* within the recombination region remains unclear.) Hence, if nonradiative electron–hole recombination occurs, for example, at the damaged surface of a diode (as in the case of the sawed-edge diode experiment already described), it accelerates the motion of point defects into the active region of the device. Another source of native point defects could be excess vacancies or interstitials in, or close to, the active region (i.e., a region of intense electron–hole recombination). Although contamination level differences could also be relevant (see later), differences in initial vacancy density compared to GaAs could contribute to the improved degradation resistance of (AlGa)As diodes, as well as differences between VPE, MBE, or LPE devices. Finally, regions in which nonradiative recombination occurs will tend to grow in size, leading to the strongly nonuniform degradation process commonly observed.

The role of dopants and contaminants in degradation cannot be ignored. Active regions containing high concentrations of species such as Zn, Be, or Cu, which diffuse rapidly by an interstitial process, are likely to be prone to rapid degradation. Oxygen is another possible troublesome contaminant, the nature of which has not been established. In fact, it is possible that the introduction of Al in the LPE solutions is an effective "gettering" mechanism for oxygen, thus preventing its incorporation into the active region and increasing the diode life.

16.3 Technology of Reliable Devices

From the discussion of Section 16.1, it is clear that facet damage is avoidable by controlling the operating conditions, by the use of dielectric facet coatings, by planar stripes, and by minimizing mechanical defects on the laser facet. Therefore, catastrophic degradation or facet "erosion" does not represent a practical limit to laser life.

The control of gradual degradation, however, is more difficult. The discussion in Section 16.2 has emphasized the role of defects on gradual degradation—a phenomenon which can occur in both laser diodes and LEDs. Although all the factors needed to eliminate gradual degradation completely are not fully known, it is believed that the major ones have been identified, making it possible to produce devices with operating lifetimes expected to be comparable to those of conventional silicon devices. Of course, the reliability requirements depend on the application, with optical communications being the most demanding. In telephone systems, for example, a value of 100,000 hr operating mean time to failure is considered essential. For instruments, on the other hand, where the on-time is generally limited, a few thousand hours of life is adequate, and 1000 hr is a common benchmark number.

The question of what constitutes reliable operation must be further defined for the specific application. Since few devices exhibit *no* measurable change during long-term operation, some overdesign is accepted procedure with respect to system needs. This overdesign is easily made in an LED because of its linear current–power output characteristics. A reduction in the power output of 20%, for example, is not important in a well-designed optical communications system. However, in a laser diode, because of the nonlinearity introduced by the threshold current, an increase of 20% in J_{th} can result in a cessation of lasing if the device is operated CW. Thus, in order to prevent actual system failure, increases in the current may be necessary to compensate for either increases in the ambient temperature or degradation. An optical feedback loop provides this process automatically, and this feature is likely to be introduced in systems designed for very long term, unattended operating life.

In high power pulsed laser operation, on the other hand, the problem of shifts in the threshold current with time (or temperature) is not as severe as in CW operation, since high power lasers are operated at currents several times their threshold current.

The most reliable CW laser diodes and high radiance LEDs are the $Al_{0.3}Ga_{0.7}As/Al_{0.1}Ga_{0.9}As$ devices. We limit ourselves here to a few examples. Liquid phase epitaxy has produced the most reproducible devices from the reliability point of view, but it has also received the most attention. The use of oxide stripe-geometry configurations (which provides a defect-free, edge-isolated device) in LEDs, with careful construction to minimize defect introduction during material growth and device assembly, produces diodes operating at 1000 A/cm² (1 mW output) havng a constant output for times in excess of 10,000 hr, as shown in Fig. 16.3.1. In fact, it is difficult to predict the ultimate lifetime of such diodes since their output either increases or remains constant. Surface emission diodes of the type shown in Fig. 14.4.1 should also have long lifetimes, if no damage is introduced in the course of attaching the fiber [41] and the assembly is otherwise stress-free.

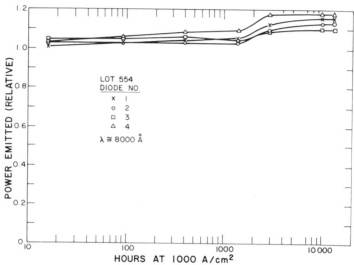

FIG. 16.3.1   Power output as a function of time of LEDs in stripe-contact configuration operating at 1000 A/cm². The active region of the double-heterojunction diodes contains $Al_{0.1}Ga_{0.9}As$ [8].

Pulsed operation high power GaAs single-heterojunction laser diodes have also proven to be very reliable. Figure 16.3.2 shows data obtained on commercial wide stripe-contact RCA lasers operating at the rated power value of ∼ 1 W/mil of facet (400W/cm) at a duty cycle of 0.1%. The average power reduction in 10 lasers is less than 20% in 5000 hr. Since in these lasers the life is linearly related to the duty cycle (at constant pulse width and current), at a lower duty cycle, 0.01% for example, the data of Fig. 16.3.2 are equivalent to 50,000 hr of operation.

Historically, most difficulties were encountered initially with CW laser diodes at room temperature because small shifts in threshold cause significant changes in power output, and because of the high current densies of a few thousand amperes per square centimeter. However, as the technology matured and key defects were better identified, the yield of long-lived CW lasers continued to improve, making commercial devices feasible in 1975.

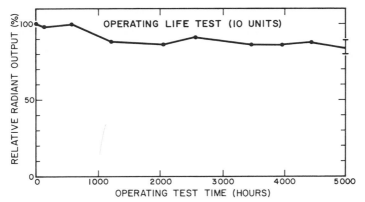

FIG. 16.3.2 Average power output as a function of time of 10 commercial RCA (AlGa) As/GaAs single-heterojunction laser diodes (with stripe contacts) operating (300 K) pulsed at a duty cycle of 0.1 % (200 ns, 5 kHz) with an emitted power level of about 1 W/mil of facet (400 W/cm); diode width is 9 mils. (Courtesy RCA Solid State, Lancaster, Pennsylvania.)

The use of (AlGa)As in the recombination region, careful LPE growth methods on good quality substrates to minimize the dislocation density in the active region, and finally the use of Al_2O_3 dielectric coatings on the facets, all contributed to CW laser diodes with excellent stability for periods of time exceeding 10,000 hr, as shown in Fig. 16.3.3. It is noteworthy that lasers, even without

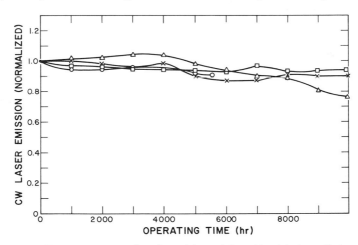

FIG. 16.3.3 Power output as a function of time of CW (AlGa)As laser diodes operating at a heat sink temperature of 22°C at *constant current*. The power emitted is from 5 to 15 mW from one facet. The diode facets are coated, but operation is in an unprotected laboratory ambient. Lot A ($\times$), 3 diodes; lot B ($\bigcirc$), 2 diodes; lot C ($\square$), 3 diodes; lot D ($\triangle$), 1 diode [8, 44].

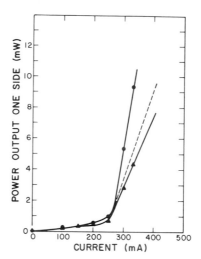

FIG. 16.3.4 Power output versus diode current of CW (AlGa)As laser diode operated in a dry air ambient without facet coatings. The efficiency reduction is attributed for the most part to facet "erosion" of the type shown in Fig. 16.1.4. (●) indicate before life test, (▲) indicate after 15,000 hr at 330 mA dc, (– – –) indicate after 5000 hr [8].

a facet coating, have operated for over 20,000 hr, although some reduction in the diode efficiency occurred, as shown in Fig. 16.3.4.

Accelerated life tests to predict "mean time to failure" are an accepted part of the semiconductor device world. It is evidently desirable to establish such tests for lasers and LEDs. With LEDs, it is possible to operate the devices at higher current densities than in the actual application because the degradation rate increases superlinearly with current density, i.e., $\propto J^{3/2}$ [42]. With lasers this test is more difficult since operation at high current densities can lead to failure by facet damage. However, one possible accelerated laser life test consists of increasing the ambient temperature. If, in fact, the diffusion of point defects is a dominant degradation cause, then the lifetime of the diodes could decrease with temperature following a well-defined law representative of a thermally activated process. In practice, it is difficult to define the specific device property which would be measured as representative of this thermally activated degradation process. A study [43] of CW (AlGa)As/GaAs DH lasers (made using proton-bombarded stripes) was conducted in which the operating temperature was varied and the time for total laser failure, even with increasing current was noted. It was found that the laser life so defined decreased with temperature proportional to $\exp(E_0/kT)$, where $E_0 = 0.7\text{–}0.8$ eV. Assuming the general validity of such an expression, the lifetime of a laser operating at 330 K is $\sim$ 20 times shorter than one operating at 300 K. Such a relationship clearly suggests the need to maintain the temperature of such lasers as close to room temperature as possible for long life, until the cause for the degradation is eliminated. However, available data suggests, on the basis of high-temperature testing, that room temperature CW laser lifetimes could exceed 100,000 hrs.

REFERENCES

1. H. Kressel and H. P. Mierop, *J. Appl. Phys.* **38**, 5419 (1967).
2. C. D. Dobson and F. S. Keeble, *Proc. Int. Symp. on GaAs, Reading, England.* Inst. Phys. and Phys. Soc. London (1967).
3. D. A. Shaw and P. R. Thornton, *Solid State Electron.* **13**, 919 (1970).
4. H. Kressel and I. Ladany, *RCA Rev.* **36**, 230 (1975).
5. B. W. Hakki and F. R. Nash, *J. Appl. Phys.* **45**, 3907 (1974).
6. H. F. Lockwood and H. Kressel, Tech. Rep. AFAL–TR–75–13. Wright-Patterson Air Force Base, Ohio (March 1975).
7. V. I. Borodulin, G. M. Malyavkina, G. T. Pak, A. I. Petrov, N. P. Chernousov, V. I. Shveikin, and I. V. Yashumov, *Sov. J. Quantum. Electron.* **2**, 294 (1972).
8. H. Kressel, I. Ladany, M. Ettenberg, and H. F. Lockwood, Technical Digest, Int. Electron Devices Meeting, p. 477. Washington, D. C. (1975).
9. P. G. Eliseev, *in* "Semiconductor Light Emitters and Detectors" (A. Frova, ed.). North-Holland Publ., Amsterdam, 1973; *J. Luminescence* **7**, 338 (1973).
10. M. Ettenberg, H. S. Sommers, Jr., H. Kressel, and H. F. Lockwood, *Appl. Phys. Lett.* **18**, 571 (1971).
11. I. Ladany and H. Kressel, *Appl. Phys. Lett.* **25**, 708 (1974).
12. A comprehensive discussion of the literature until 1973 was presented by H. Kressel and H. F. Lockwood, *J. Phys.* Suppl. **35**, **C3**, 223 (1974).
13. H. Kressel and N. E. Byer, *Proc. IEEE* **38**, 25 (1969).
14. D. H. Newman, S. Ritchie, and S. O'Hara, *IEEE J. Quantum Electron.* **8**, 379 (1972).
15. N. E. Byer, *IEEE J. Quantum Electron.* **5**, 242 (1969).
16. E. S. Yang, *J. Appl. Phys.* **42**, 5635 (1971).
17. N. Chinone, R. Ito, and O. Nakada, *IEEE J. Quantum Electron.* **10**, 81 (1974).
18. B. W. Hakki and T. L. Paoli, *J. Appl. Phys.* **44**, 4113 (1973).
19. H. Yonezu, M. Urno, T. Kamejima, and I. Sakuma, *Jpn. J. Appl. Phys.* **13**, 835 (1974).
20. B. C. DeLoach, B. W. Hakki, R. L. Hartman, and L. A. D'Asaro, *Proc. IEEE* **61**, 1042 (1973).
21. W. D. Johnston and B. I. Miller, *Appl. Phys. Lett.* **23**, 192 (1973).
22. J. R. Biard, G. E. Pittman, and J. F. Leezer, *Proc. Int. Symp. GaAs, Reading, England.* Inst. Phys. and Phys. Soc. London (1967).
23. P. Petroff and R. L. Hartman, *Appl. Phys. Lett.* **23**, 469 (1973); *J. Appl. Phys.* **45**, 3899 (1974).
24. P. W. Hutchinson, P. S. Dobson, S. O. O'Hara, and D. H. Newman, *Appl. Phys. Lett.* **26**, 250 (1975).
25. R. Ito, H. Nakashima, and O. Nakada, *Jpn. J. Appl. Phys.* **13**, 1321 (1974). The glide phenomena are discussed by J. Matsui *et al., ibid.* **14**, 1561 (1975) and by R. Itoh *et al., IEEE J. Quantum Electron.* **11**, 551 (1975).
26. R. L. Hartman and R. W. Dixon, *Appl. Phys. Lett.* **26**, 239 (1975).
27. I. Ladany and H. Kressel, "Gallium Arsenide and Related Compounds, 1974," p. 192. Inst. Phys. and Phys. Soc., Conf. Ser. No. 24, London, 1975.

28. E. S. Yang, P. G. McMullin, A. W. Smith, J. Blum, and K. K. Shih, *Appl. Phys. Lett.* **24**, 324 (1974).
29. N. V. Basov and V. N. Morozov, *Sov. Phys.-JEPT* **30**, 338 (1970).
30. H. Kressel *et al., Met. Trans.* **1**, 635 (1970).
31. A. Bahraman and W. G. Oldham, *J. Appl. Phys.* **43**, 2383 (1972).
32. R. L. Hartman and A. R. Hartman, *Appl. Phys. Lett.* **23**, 147 (1973).
33. M. Ettenberg, H. Kressel, and H. F. Lockwood, *Appl. Phys. Lett.* **25**, 82 (1974).
34. M. Ettenberg and C. J. Nuese, *J. Appl. Phys.* **46**, 2137 (1975).
35. M. Ettenberg and H. Kressel, *Appl. Phys. Lett.* **26**, 478 (1975).
36. A. Y. Cho, R. W. Dixon, H. C. Casey, Jr., and R. L. Hartman, *Appl. Phys. Lett.* **28**, 501 (1976).
37. C. J. Nuese, G. H. Olsen, and M. Ettenberg, *Appl. Phys. Lett.* **29**, 54 (1976).
38. R. D. Gold and L. R. Weisberg, *Solid State Electron.* **7**, 811 (1964).
39. D. V. Lang and L. C. Kimerling, *Phys. Rev. Lett.* **33**, 489 (1974).
40. L. C. Kimerling, P. Petroff, and H. J. Leamy, *Appl. Phys. Lett.* **28**, 297 (1976).
41. F. D. King, A. J. Springthorpe, and O. I. Szentesi, Technical Digest, Int. Electron Devices Meeting, p. 480. Washington, D. C., (1975).
42. H. Kressel, M. Ettenberg, and H. F. Lockwood, J. Electron. Mat. **6**, 467 (1977).
43. R. L. Hartman and R. W. Dixon, *Appl. Phys. Lett.* **26**, 239 (1975).
44. I. Ladany, M. Ettenberg, H. F. Lockwood, and H. Kressel, *Appl. Phys. Lett.* **30**, 87 (1977).

Chapter 17

Transient Effects in Laser Diodes

17.1 Introduction

Fluctuations in the output of laser diodes have been studied experimentally and theoretically. Our purpose is to review the major effects seen and to highlight dominant features. We are particularly interested in phenomena which affect the modulation of laser diodes at high frequencies.

1. Transient oscillatory effects can be seen when the laser is turned on. These oscillations can be approximated by a damped high frequency sine wave over a significant portion of their duration. Such effects are related to the interdependence of the electron and photon populations which require a finite time to reach a steady state value.

2. Even in CW operation oscillations are observed in both the light output and the current, and are believed related to quantum shot noise effects.

3. Oscillatory effects occur in devices with uneven population inversion, i.e., containing regions of net gain and loss within the cavity where saturable absorption phenomena are possible. Lasers containing two lasers in tandem, each of which can be individually pumped, exhibit such controlled effects by changes in the current in the two diode parts.

4. Transient effects, oscillatory effects, and "noise" of ill-defined origin occur in laser diodes containing defects, filaments, or weak mode guiding subject to change with small changes in temperature and current. Section 8.4 described such anomalies in some asymmetrical laser diodes.

In addition to the discussion of transient effects, we also take the opportunity to review the steady state solution of the rate equations. This leads us into a discussion of the "ideal" laser above threshold, and deviations from ideality further discussed in Appendix B.

17.2   Turn-On Effects

17.2.1   The Rate Equations

The starting point for the analysis of the laser kinetics involves the coupled rate equations formulated by Statz and deMars [1, 2]. These are appropriate for laser diodes under the following simplifying assumptions: (a) The laser is operating in a *single mode* above threshold. (b) We consider an ideal cavity with homogeneous population inversion. The spontaneous carrier lifetime is assumed constant at τ_s while the photon lifetime is τ_{ph}. (c) The gain coefficient is a linear function of the injected carrier density N_e above a minimal value N_{0m}. (d) Noise sources are excluded.

We describe the rate of change of the injected electron density N_e (in p-type material) and of the photon density N_{ph} (in the single mode),

$$\frac{dN_e}{dt} = \frac{J}{ed_3} - A(N_e - N_{0m})N_{ph} - \frac{N_e}{\tau_s} \tag{17.2.1}$$

$$\frac{dN_{ph}}{dt} = A(N_e - N_{0m})N_{ph} - \frac{N_{ph}}{\tau_{ph}} + \gamma\frac{N_e}{\tau_s} \tag{17.2.2}$$

Here A (in cm^3/s) is a proportionality constant, d_3 is the width of the recombination region, and γ is the probability that a photon is emitted spontaneously into the mode. Nonradiative processes are neglected (i.e., unity internal quantum efficiency).

The terms on the right-hand sides of (17.2.1) and (17.2.2) are (1) rate of carrier injection; (2) carrier decrease rate due to stimulated emission (R_{st}); (3) decrease rate due to spontaneous recombination (R_{sp}); (4) rate of increase due to stimulated photon emission; (5) rate of loss of photons by radiation and absorption; and (6) spontaneous emission rate into the mode.

An approximate estimate of N_{0m} can be obtained from Fig. 3.3.2 for un-doped GaAs where we see that a nominal current density of 4000 A/cm^2 μm is needed to obtain $g > 0$ at 300 K. Hence, assuming a spontaneous lifetime at threshold of $\tau_s = 2 \times 10^{-9}$ s,

$$N_{0m} \cong \frac{J\tau_s}{ed_3} \approx \frac{(4000)(2 \times 10^{-9})}{(1.6 \times 10^{-19})(10^{-4})} \cong 5 \times 10^{17} \text{ cm}^{-3}$$

17.2.2   Steady State Solution of the Rate Equations

It is instructive to analyze the steady state solution of the coupled rate equations since it provides useful insights into some basic "ideal" laser principles. After some possible turn-on transient effects, the laser may be expected to reach a condition under which fluctuations of the carrier pair density and photon density are eliminated. Then $dN_e/dt = 0$, $dN_{ph}/dt = 0$, and steady state populations $\bar{N}_e$ and $\bar{N}_{ph}$ are reached.* If the laser is just turned on to threshold, from (17.2.1) we obtain at threshold (where $N_{ph} \approx 0$)

$$J_{th} \cong e\bar{N}_e d_3/\tau_s \qquad (17.2.3)$$

However, even for $J > J_{th}$, we see from (17.2.2) that the steady state injected carrier, population $\bar{N}_e$ remains constant when stimulated emission occurs, *being independent of the photon population in the mode,*

$$\bar{N}_e \cong 1/A\tau_{ph} + N_{0m} \qquad (17.2.4)$$

where we have neglected the spontaneous emission rate term $\gamma N_e/\tau_s$ which is much smaller than the stimulated emission term above threshold. The fact that the carrier population is constant above threshold means that the quasi-Fermi level separation remains ideally fixed in the highly simplified model.

A further result from the steady state solution of (17.2.1) and (17.2.2) is the linear dependence of the photon density on current above threshold. Neglecting the small spontaneous emission terms for $J > J_{th}$,

$$J = \{ed_3 A(\bar{N}_e - N_{0m})\} \bar{N}_{ph} \qquad (17.2.5)$$
$$J = (ed_3/\tau_{ph}) \bar{N}_{ph}$$

Hence, above J_{th} the change in the photon density with respect to the current is

$$\partial\bar{N}_{ph}/\partial J = \tau_{ph}/ed_3 \qquad (17.2.6)$$

This linear relationship results from the fact that each injected carrier produces a photon by stimulated emission; as a consequence the photon emission rate ($\propto \bar{N}_{ph}/\tau_{ph}$) and hence the power emitted is a linear function of the current above threshold.

It also follows from this that the *total* spontaneous emission rate is constant above threshold because the carrier concentration $\bar{N}_e$ is constant. This is evident from the fact that the spontaneous recombination rate is $\bar{N}_e/\tau_s$. Similarly, the gain coefficient is predicted to saturate at threshold, because it is also a function of the injected carrier concentration (Chapter 3).

Experimentally, one finds significant deviations from the "ideal" laser analysis based on the "one mode" rate equations, although some predictions of the analysis are valid:

1. The photon density, as determined from the emitted power increase with current above threshold, is indeed substantially linear (barring "kinks") as discussed in Chapter 3. This occurs despite the fact that the internal quan-

---

*As discussed in Section 17.2.4, the carrier pair density does not quite reach $\bar{N}_e$ but only approaches that value very closely in this simple model.

tum efficiency is *not* unity above threshold. In fact, one would expect that the nonradiative recombination rate, characterized by a lifetime τ_{nr} on the order of 10^{-9} s, would remain constant above threshold in the face of the competition of the simulated recombination, and that the internal quantum efficiency would therefore reach unity. If this occurred, then the linear increase of the power emission with the diode current would be consistent with expectation. The fact that available measurements indicate that the internal quantum efficiency is not unity above threshold, and yet the linearity is maintained, suggests that the "branching ratio" between radiative and nonradiative processes remains constant above threshold as a result of a process so far unexplained.

2. Equation (17.2.3) does provide a reasonable basis for estimating the carrier concentration at threshold, and numbers so estimated are in good agreement with theory (Chapters 3 and 8).

3. A limitation of the simple theory is in the neglect of the impact of a strong optical field on the gain coefficient. The conclusion that the power in a mode increases linearly with current can only be valid within some bounds. We know that the stimulated recombination rate into a mode is inversely proportional to the photon population in the mode. However, as the stimulation rate increases to a level where the effective carrier lifetime is comparable to the equilibration time of carriers in the bands (order 10^{-12} s), we begin to deplete the population of the relevent states involved in the stimulated emission process. Thus, the inversion is decreased and with it the gain coefficient. In this simple picture, a few thousand photons in a mode are capable of reducing the inversion significantly. This represents only power levels in the few milliwatt range in the mode.

4. The present simple analysis predicting saturation of the inverted population assumes an homogeneously broadened atomic system under conditions where the modal field and the region of inverted population coincide. Both of these assumptions are dubious in practical devices. Inhomogeneities will clearly produce a nonuniform device, as will small spatial variations of the bandgap energy in lasers produced from alloys, and we are then surely not dealing with a system which behaves as a homogeneously broadened one. Furthermore, if we consider a stripe-contact device, the current spread beyond the edges of the region of inversion may increase with drive above threshold. Hence, the carrier population in those external regions is surely not "clamped" within the assumptions of the model. Therefore, the observation of increasing spontaneous emission above threshold in many laser diodes may or may not reflect fundamental parameters, and interpretations are to be approached with caution. Appendix B discusses a model proposed to explain the increase of spontaneous emission above threshold in terms of a fundamental limitation of the performance of the lasing system in a strong field.

With these limitations, the analysis of the rate equations does provide a very useful insight into the laser operation and justifies the further analysis in this chapter.

17.2.3 Transient Solution of the Rate Equations

When the laser switch is opened in Fig. 17.2.1a, transient phenomena occur because of the time required for the electron and photon populations to come into equilibrium (Fig. 17.2.1). As we show in the following, theory predicts a damped oscillatory optical output, the characteristics of which depend on the diode current relative to the threshold current and on the spontaneous carrier lifetime and photon lifetime. These *relaxation oscillations* are important when it is desired to modulate the laser output at frequencies near the oscillation frequency. Basically, the functional dependence of the high output behavior is analogous to the current and voltages in a tuned circuit. Consequently, a resonant condition will appear in the system transfer function which is the ratio of light output and current density at some driving frequency. Depending on the system application some modulation schemes may be optimized; however, for straight AM modulation, distortions can occur at frequencies near resonance. Modulation is further discussed in Section 17.5.

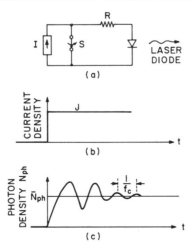

FIG. 17.2.1 (a) Simple circuit with laser diode in series with a resistor. At $t = 0$ the switch is opened and current from the current generator is supplied to the diode. (b) The current density applied to the diode is a step function beginning at $t = 0$. (c) The photon density transient solution. At $t = 0$ the photon density grows according to a solution of the rate equations. For larger values of t, the solution is represented by a decaying exponential modulating a sinusoidal function; $N_{ph} \to \bar{N}_{ph}$ as $t \to \infty$. (The initial delay in the build up of the photon density resulting from stimulated emission is not shown. See Fig. 17.2.4 which shows numerical solutions.)

The present analysis is based on the rate equations [3–6] introduced in the preceding section. We assume a current step function to turn the diode on to what will eventually become steady state values $\bar{N}_e$ and $\bar{N}_{ph}$. However, during the transience the electron and photon populations deviate slightly from their equilibrium values by ΔN_e and ΔN_{ph}, respectively. This assumption will allow us to obtain a solution to the equations by linearization. Thus,

$$\Delta N_e = N_e - \bar{N}_e \tag{17.2.7a}$$

$$\Delta N_{ph} = N_{ph} - \bar{N}_{ph} \tag{17.2.7b}$$

It is assumed that the deviations from equilibrium of the electron and photon populations are sufficiently small to permit the following Taylor expansion around the median values (neglecting higher order terms), for the stimulated and spontaneous recombination rates,

$$R_{st} = \bar{R}_{st} + \frac{\partial \bar{R}_{st}}{\partial N_e} \Delta N_e + \frac{\partial \bar{R}_{st}}{\partial N_{ph}} \Delta N_{ph} \tag{17.2.8a}$$

$$R_{sp} = \bar{R}_{sp} + \frac{\partial \bar{R}_{sp}}{\partial N_e} \Delta N_e \tag{17.2.8b}$$

The second term of (17.2.8a) does not appear in (17.2.8b) since the spontaneous recombination rate is independent of the photon density.

The current density is assumed constant following the step increase, and we ignore noise sources (these are discussed in Section 17.3). Hence, using (17.2.8) the rate equations (17.2.1) and (17.2.2) are

$$\frac{d}{dt} \Delta N_e = \left\{ \frac{J}{ed_3} - A(\bar{N}_e - N_{0m})\bar{N}_{ph} - \frac{\bar{N}_e}{\tau_s} \right\}$$
$$- \left\{ A\bar{N}_{ph}\Delta N_e + A(\bar{N}_e - N_{0m}) \Delta N_{ph} + \frac{\Delta N_e}{\tau_s} \right\} \tag{17.2.9}$$

and neglecting the spontaneous emission term into a single mode,

$$\frac{d}{dt} \Delta N_{ph} = \{A(\bar{N}_e - N_{0m}) - 1/\tau_{ph}\} \Delta N_{ph} + A\bar{N}_{ph} \Delta N_e$$
$$+ \{A(\bar{N}_e - N_{0m}) - 1/\tau_{ph}\} \bar{N}_{ph} \tag{17.2.10}$$

From the steady state solution of the rate equations we know that the three terms in the first brace of (17.2.9) and the two terms in the braces of (17.2.10) add up to zero, respectively. Hence,

$$\frac{d}{dt} \Delta N_e = -(A\bar{N}_{ph} + 1/\tau_s) \Delta N_e - A(\bar{N}_e - N_{0m}) \Delta N_{ph},$$
$$\frac{d}{dt} \Delta N_{ph} = A\bar{N}_{ph} \Delta N_e \tag{17.2.11}$$

Equations (17.2.11) can be combined into identical differential equations for ΔN_e and ΔN_{ph}

$$\frac{d^2}{dt^2}(\Delta N_e) + \left(A\bar{N}_{ph} + \frac{1}{\tau_s}\right)\frac{d}{dt}(\Delta N_e) + \frac{A\bar{N}_{ph}}{\tau_{ph}}\Delta N_e = 0$$

$$\frac{d^2}{dt^2}(\Delta N_{ph}) + \left(A\bar{N}_{ph} + \frac{1}{\tau_s}\right)\frac{d}{dt}(\Delta N_{ph}) + \frac{A\bar{N}_{ph}}{\tau_{ph}}\Delta N_{ph} = 0$$

(17.2.12)

A solution to (17.2.12) is of the form

$$\Delta N_e = (\Delta N_e)_0 \exp[-(a - i\omega_c)t],$$

$$\Delta N_{ph} = (\Delta N_{ph})_0 \exp[-(a - i\omega_c)t]$$

(17.2.13)

with the values

$$a = \tfrac{1}{2}\left(A\bar{N}_{ph} + \frac{1}{\tau_s}\right)$$

(17.2.14)

$$\omega_c = \left(\frac{A\bar{N}_{ph}}{\tau_{ph}} - \frac{A^2\bar{N}^2_{ph}}{4} - \frac{A\bar{N}_{ph}}{2\tau_s} - \frac{1}{4\tau_s^2}\right)^{1/2}$$

(17.2.15)

The values of a and ω_c are determined most easily if they are expressed in terms of the diode current density J as follows. We recall from (17.2.5),

$$A\bar{N}_{ph} = J/[ed_3(\bar{N}_e - N_{0m})]$$

and from (17.2.3),

$$1/\tau_s = J_{th}/ed_3\bar{N}_e$$

Hence, since $N_e \gg \bar{N}_{0m}$,

$$a \cong \frac{1}{2\tau_s}\left(\frac{J}{J_{th}} + 1\right)$$

(17.2.16)

$$\omega_c \cong \left[\frac{1}{\tau_s\tau_{ph}}\left(\frac{J}{J_{th}} - 1\right) - a^2\right]^{1/2}$$

(17.2.17)

the photon lifetime is of the order of 10^{-12} s (Section 3.4) in a typical laser structure, and τ_s is in the low 10^{-9} s range. Equation (17.2.17) becomes (in the present case of a linear dependence of gain coefficient on carrier density)

$$\omega_c = 2\pi f_c \cong \left[\frac{1}{\tau_s\tau_{ph}}\left(\frac{J}{J_{th}} - 1\right)\right]^{1/2}$$

(17.2.18)

Having arrived at the result desired, it is appropriate to review the practical implications of these oscillations. From (17.2.16) we see that the envelope of the oscillations is such that the oscillations disappear in a period of time on the order of the spontaneous carrier lifetime, or a few nanoseconds. Also, the higher the current is relative to J_{th}, the shorter the decay time $\sim 1/a$.

The resonance frequency f_c is seen to increase with decreasing spontaneous carrier lifetime and photon lifetime. Also, f_c is dependent on the ratio J/J_{th}, and thus it increases with current density above J_{th}. For example, with $J = 2J_{th}$, $\tau_s = 2 \times 10^{-9}$ s, and $\tau_{ph} = 10^{-12}$ s, $f_c = 4$ GHz. The existence of this resonance frequency means that if attempts are made to apply a modulating current density $J = J_0 e^{i\omega t}$ to the diode, distortion effects are expected as ω approaches ω_c, but the modulation efficiency will be observed to peak at $\omega = \omega_c$. However, if attempts are made to modulate the diode at frequencies *above* the resonant frequency ω_c, the modulation efficiency will be found to decrease rather steeply with frequency.

The resonant effect in modulation has been seen by Ikegami and Suematsu [6] in homojunction GaAs lasers, and moderate agreement with theory has been obtained using values of $\tau_s = 2$ ns and $\tau_{ph} \cong 10^{-12}$ s. Moderate agreement with regard to the predicted f_c values appears to exist experimentally in (AlGa)As DH laser diodes operating at room temperature, although the damping time of about 1 ns was shorter than predicted from (17.2.1) [6a].

Means have been proposed for reducing the resonant effect by the use of optical pumping of the laser being modulated by a similar diode operating CW [7]. The effect of injecting photons at the stimulated emission energy from an external source is similar to the effect of increasing the diode current density J noted above, and is helpful in decreasing the initial amplitude of the oscillations. The required radiation entering the active region of the modulated laser is estimated to be only a few percent of the emitted power level for substantial improvements in the diode performance to be noted.

17.2.4 Numerical Solution of Rate Equations

In this section we discuss some numerical solutions to the rate equations, neglecting gain perturbations due to the optical field. We will find it convenient to normalize the various quantities in the rate equations (17.2.1) and (17.2.2) as follows:

$$\mathcal{t} = t/\tau_s \tag{17.2.19a}$$

$$n_e = A\tau_{ph}N_e \tag{17.2.19b}$$

$$n_{om} = A\tau_{ph}N_{0m} \tag{17.2.19c}$$

$$n_{ph} = A\tau_s N_{ph} \tag{17.2.19d}$$

$$j = A\tau_s\tau_{ph}(J/ed_3) \tag{17.2.19e}$$

$$w = \tau_s/\tau_{ph} \tag{17.2.19f}$$

Accordingly, (17.2.1) and (17.2.2) become, respectively,

$$dn_e/d\mathcal{t} = j - n_{ph}(n_e - n_{om}) - n_e \tag{17.2.20}$$

$$dn_{ph}/d\mathcal{t} = w[n_{ph}(n_e - n_{om} - 1) + \gamma n_e] \tag{17.2.21}$$

From (17.2.21), the steady-state solution is given by

$$\bar{n}_{ph} = \gamma \bar{n}_e / (1 + n_{om} - \bar{n}_e) \qquad (17.2.22)$$

It is important to note that $\bar{n}_e$ cannot equal or be greater than $1 + n_{om}$, because the photon density would be infinite negative.

It is well known that to start oscillation, every electronic oscillator, including of course the laser, must have a gain *slightly* in excess of the losses. However, the steady state is established by a damping mechanism which prevents a "runaway" situation from developing as the signal level is increased. In the laser this damping mechanism can be visualized as follows. Suppose that the current is increased, tending to inject more carriers than needed to produce the gain value which just matches the losses. The photon density builds up to a higher steady state value (higher stimulated recombination rate), which "uses up" the extra carriers at a rate which *just* matches the supply of these extra carriers less the carrier loss via other relaxation processes. As a result, the carrier population (and hence gain value) reached at threshold is maintained, which is the value just needed to match the losses. In other words, the carrier lifetime for stimulated emission into the mode of our single mode laser adjusts itself with changing carrier injection to produce a constant *steady state* inversion level value above threshold. This is the essence of the lasing process within the limits of the rate equation model presented here. Fluctuations in the carrier and photon population about the steady value will occur, with the tendency to equilibrium being reestablished in a time dependent on the spontaneous carrier lifetime, the photon lifetime, and the injection level. These interactions and perturbations give rise to fluctuations in the laser output, which we analyze later in this chapter.

From the numerical solutions of the steady-state rate equations we show that $\bar{n}_e$ becomes infinitesimally close to the value of $1 + n_{om}$ under lasing conditions. As a result, we define the normalized inversion at threshold as

$$n_{eth} = 1 + n_{om} \qquad (17.2.23)$$

The steady-state solution of (17.2.20) is

$$j = \bar{n}_{ph}(\bar{n}_e - n_{om}) + \bar{n}_e \qquad (17.2.24)$$

If j is sufficiently small, $\bar{n}_{ph}(\bar{n}_e - n_{om}) \ll \bar{n}_e$, and the device behaves as an LED. When $\bar{n}_{ph}(\bar{n}_e - n_{om}) \gg \bar{n}_e$, the diode acts as a laser. The important point to note here is that when $\bar{n}_{ph}(\bar{n}_e - n_{om})$ becomes the dominant term, the device is a laser; however, when j obtains its largest value under the condition when $\bar{n}_e$ is dominant, we define that value of j as j_{th}, the normalized threshold current density. Since $\bar{n}_e \simeq n_{eth}$,

$$j_{th} \equiv n_{eth} = 1 + n_{om} \qquad (17.2.25)$$

We now consider the numerical solution to the steady-state rate equations.

Eliminating $\bar{n}_{\rm ph}$ in (17.2.22) and (17.2.24) and using the definitions given in (17.2.23) and (17.2.25),

$$(1 - \gamma)\left[\frac{\bar{n}_{\rm e}}{n_{\rm eth}}\right]^2 - \left[\frac{j}{j_{\rm th}} + (1 - \gamma) + \frac{\gamma}{j_{\rm th}}\right]\left[\frac{\bar{n}_{\rm e}}{n_{\rm eth}}\right] + \frac{j}{j_{\rm th}} = 0 \quad (17.2.26)$$

The value $\bar{n}_{\rm e}/n_{\rm eth}$ can be determined as a function of $j/j_{\rm th}$ by solving the simple quadratic equation. Numerical results give two solutions with only one being physically meaningful. (One solution gives $\bar{n}_{\rm e}/n_{\rm eth}$ values greater than unity, which makes $\bar{n}_{\rm ph} < 0$.) Figure 17.2.2 shows the value of $\bar{n}_{\rm e}/n_{\rm eth}$ as a function of $j/j_{\rm th}$. It is clear that when $j = j_{\rm th}$, the normalized pair density $\bar{n}_{\rm e}$ is close to its asymptotic value. The curve was derived with $\gamma = 10^{-3}$, $n_{\rm om} = 10^{-1}$; the value of $n_{\rm om}$ was obtained by assuming that $n_{\rm eth}/n_{\rm om} = N_{\rm e}/N_{\rm 0m} \simeq 10$. Actually, similar curves for $n_{\rm om}$ values lying between 1 and 10^{-6} are almost identical to that shown in Fig. 17.2.2.

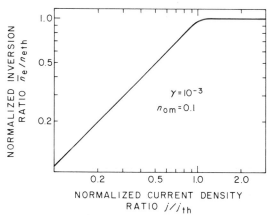

FIG. 17.2.2 The normalized steady-state inversion level as a function of current density. The inversion essentially saturates at currents above threshold, although $n_{\rm e}/n_{\rm eth}$ always remains slightly under unity.

The steady-state values of $\bar{n}_{\rm ph}$ can now be determined from (17.2.22) as shown in Fig. 17.2.3. Near threshold, there is a rapid increase in $\bar{n}_{\rm ph}$ and for $j/j_{\rm th} > 1$, $\bar{n}_{\rm ph}$ increases linearly with j. Note that the shape of the curve in Fig. 17.2.3, derived from the theoretical model, is similar to the experimental curve shown in Fig. 2.4.1.

Next we show the time dependence of the normalized inversion level $n_{\rm e}$ and the photon density $n_{\rm ph}$ for a step current j, which turns on at $t = 0$. Solutions of the differential equations (17.2.20) and (17.2.21) were obtained using an analog computer. In Fig. 17.2.4a, we show $n_{\rm e}$ and $n_{\rm ph}$ for $j = 7.5$, while in Fig. 17.2.4b, $j = 18$. Note that the values of normalized current in both cases are well above threshold. The peak values of $n_{\rm ph}$ are slightly inaccurate be-

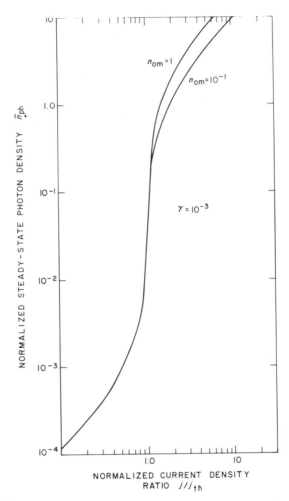

FIG. 17.2.3 The normalized steady-state photon density as a function of normalized current density. At current values well above threshold, n_{ph} is a linear function of j. Near threshold, n_{ph} rises extremely fast then reaches a linear dependence on current density.

cause of the inability of the printer pin to follow the rapid oscillations; this is particularly true for the conditions illustrated in Fig. 17.2.4b, where we show the values of n_{ph} rising above 40. It is interesting to note that there is a delay time prior the rapid rise of the photon density (already mentioned in Section 8.1). This delay is due to the fact that the inversion density must rise to a certain level before stimulated recombination occurs. In the transient state, the inversion level can rise above the threshold value; however, stimulated recombination rapidly pulls the inversion level to lower values.

17.3 Continuous Oscillations

17.3.1 Theory

In Section 17.2 we discussed transient effects during a short period following laser turn-on by a step functional current. These oscillations are predicted to last only for a period of time about twice the spontaneous carrier lifetime. In this section we turn our attention to *continuous, self-sustaining oscillations* of CW lasers in which both the light output and the current can exhibit high frequency oscillations. These effects arise from quantum shot noise effects,

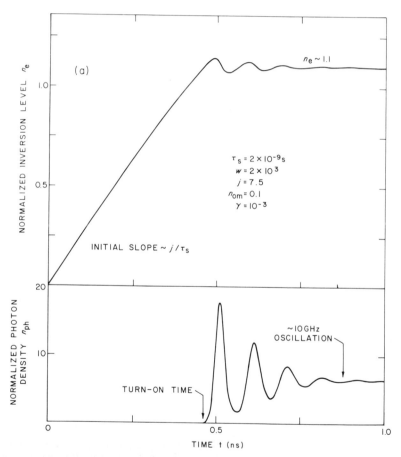

FIG. 17.2.4 The time-dependent solutions of $n_e(t)$ and $n_{ph}(t)$ for different dc injection levels. In (a) $j = 7.5$, while in (b) $j = 18$. In both cases $j_{th} = 1.1$. Note that the delay time for n_{ph} and the frequency of the oscillations are current dependent. (R. Brockie and M. Schell, unpublished.)

i.e., intrinsic fluctuations in the photon generation rate and hence of the carrier concentration.

The starting point for the theoretical analysis again involves the simple coupled rate equations (17.2.1) and (17.2.2). However, we now add a shot noise term $F(t)$ which can be calculated from the photon density and other basic

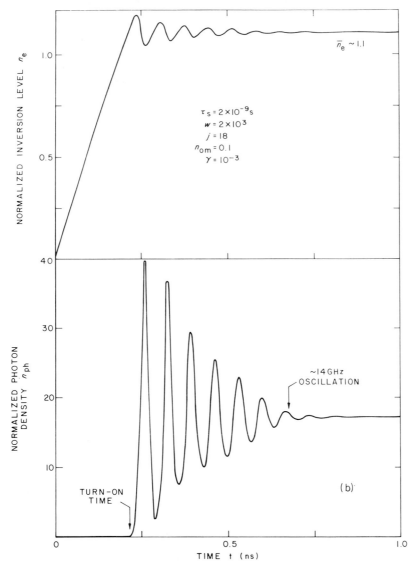

FIG. 17.2.4 Continued

parameters [8–11]. The interesting result is that the high frequency oscillations peak at a frequency f_n given by [11]

$$\omega_n = 2\pi f_n = \left(\bar{R}_{sp}^t \frac{\partial \bar{R}_{st}}{\partial N_e}\right)^{1/2} \left(\frac{J}{J_{th}} - 1\right)^{1/2} \tag{17.3.1}$$

where R_{sp}^t is the total mean spontaneous emission rate into all modes, and the other terms have the meaning assigned to them in Section 17.2.

The functional form of (17.3.1) resembles (17.2.18), but the detailed calculations of the electron and noise spectrum involve assumptions concerning the relationship between the gain coefficient and the carrier concentration, as well as a determination of the spontaneous emission rates at various temperatures and for various material parameters. Haug [10] calculated the GaAs laser noise spectrum assuming parabolic bands with **k** selection for the electron–hole recombination process. Figure 17.3.1 shows his calculated noise spectrum at 80 K as a function of the normalized pump rate J/J_{th}, and Fig. 17.3.2 shows the variation of the peak intensity oscillation frequency with temperature and pump rate.

The following observations are relevant concerning the preceding calculations: (1) The frequency of the oscillations where the spectrum peaks can vary from the megahertz region well into the gigahertz region depending on the pump rate and the temperature. (2) The relative *magnitude* of the noise spectrum decreases with increasing pump rate, i.e., a maximum is expected near threshold which should rapidly decrease above threshold (Fig. 17.3.1b). Hence, by biasing the laser diode slightly above threshold, it is theoretically possible to obtain a reduction in the noise compared to operation very near threshold.

17.3.2 Experiment

A major difficulty in comparing theory to experiment on a quantitative basis lies in the fact that the theory is basically a "single mode" small signal one, whereas practical laser diodes are generally multimode devices operating at high optical fields. In addition, the condition of uniform inversion of the active region is rarely encountered in practice, nor is it generally certain that filamentary behavior is not observed, i.e., sections of the laser are operating nearly independently of each other as the diode current is increased. This would have the effect of producing multiple laser operation, with each small area having a noise spectrum characteristic of its local carrier and photon population. Furthermore, as we noted in Section 14.3.2 the modal content of laser diodes is commonly a function of the diode current, with changes in both the longitudinal and lateral mode density. Therefore, any description of the laser in terms of a simple model based on one mode, or even several modes which remain invariant with current, must be treated with caution.

Among the earliest observations of microwave oscillations which could

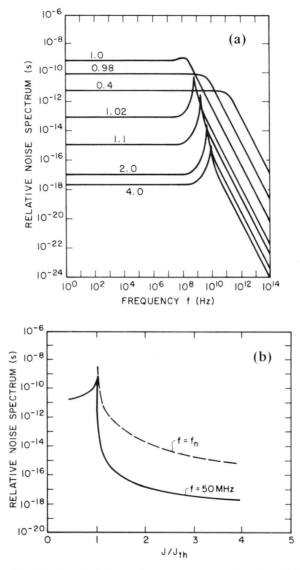

FIG. 17.3.1 (a) Calculated relative noise spectrum as a function of the frequency f for pure GaAs at 80 K (assuming parabolic bands and k selection) with the normalized pump rate J/J_{th} as a variable. (From Haug [10].) (b) Relative noise spectrum from above at 50 MHz and at the resonance frequency f_n as a function of J_{th}. The noise spectrum is seen to peak sharply at the threshold current density.

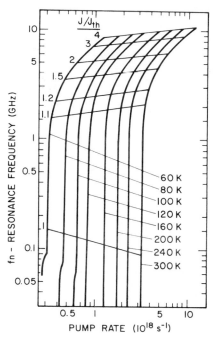

FIG. 17.3.2   Calculated resonance frequency f_n of the noise spectrum as a function of the pump rate J/J_{th} for pure GaAs. The temperatures for the various curves are indicated. (From Haug [10].)

be qualitatively related to the theory of Section 17.3.1 were those of D'Asaro *et al.* [12], who studied CW GaAs homojunction lasers at low temperatures. Oscillations in the 0.5–3 GHz range were observed in the optical output and the diode current, depending on the temperature and diode current. In fact, the peak resonant frequency of the noise spectrum was found to increase with an increase in J above J_{th}, qualitatively consistent with Fig. 17.3.1a.

Room temperature studies of DH (AlGa)As laser diodes [13] have produced a complex picture not easily related to theory beyond the fact that high frequency (measured at 4 GHz) oscillations are seen. But these are not necessarily reduced in intensity as the current is increased above threshold (Fig. 17.3.3), as theoretically expected. However, the low frequency noise (measured at 50 MHz) does exhibit a maximum in the vicinity of J_{th}, decreasing in intensity as the current is increased above J_{th}. This is consistent with Fig. 17.3.1b.

The complicated behavior of various diode samples of CW laser diodes is partly related to their structural perfection, uniformity, and mode content stability. For example, Fig. 17.3.4 shows the curve of the power emission ver-

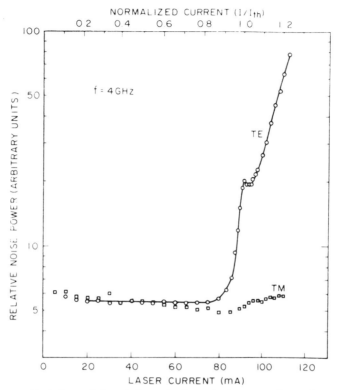

FIG. 17.3.3 Variations of the relative noise intensity in 1-MHz intervals centered 200 MHz above and below 4 GHz as a function of the current in a CW (AlGa)As/GaAs laser at room temperature. Note the continuing increase of the noise spectrum with current, an effect inconsistent with simple theory. (From Paoli [13].)

sus diode current and the obvious kink in the curve (Section 14.3.2) at $I = 200$ mA. Note that the low frequency noise spectrum peaks near threshold, then increases again beyond the kink, suggesting the onset of another small lasing region going through its threshold behavior, or perhaps the threshold of a lateral mode.

It is evident from this that the noise characterization of CW laser diodes is experimentally complex and that detailed comparisons between theory and experiment require devices with a carefully selected degree of perfection and modal content. From the practical point of view, it appears that noise properties are affected by lateral mode shifts and by structural parameters, of which kinks in the light output versus current curves are indicative. For example, the modulation of diodes in a current range which traverses a kink could well result in the emission of random pulses in a frequency range cor-

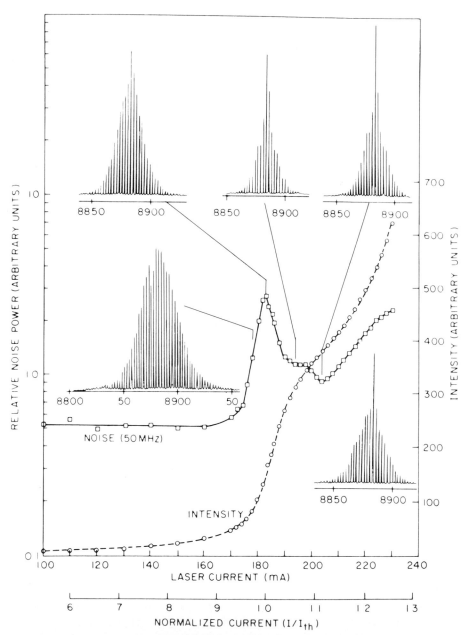

FIG. 17.3.4 Variations of the relative noise intensity at 50 MHz and the total intensity of the laser emission of a device exhibiting a kink in its characteristics. The longitudinal mode spectra are obtained for selected currents shown. Note the peak in the noise intensity at threshold, and the additional increase just beyond the kink. (From Paoli [13].)

responding to the modulation frequency of the device and hence bothersome from the systems point of view in optical communications. However, since devices free of kinks (over a useful power emission level) are fabricated, this evidently does not represent an inherent limitation to the use of laser diodes.

In all experiments concerning modulation of laser diodes at high frequencies it is important to keep in mind the need to maintain the "proper" dc bias condition for minimum optical pulse distortion. Figure 17.3.5 shows a comparison of the optical pulse output relative to the current pulse for a CW laser being modulated at 250 Mbits/s. In Fig. 17.3.5a the dc bias was set at a level too close to threshold, which resulted in optical pulse distortion. A change in the current level resulted in the much improved modulation characteristics shown in Fig. 17.3.5b.

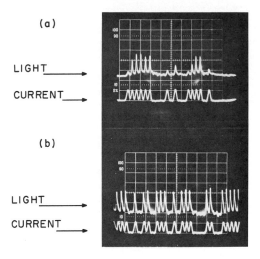

250 Mbit/s MODULATION

FIG. 17.3.5 Comparison of current pulses with optical pulses emitted by (AlGa)As DH laser at room temperature (250 Mbits/s modulation). (a) The dc bias is too close to threshold, resulting in pulse distortion; (b) proper dc bias improves the modulation characteristics. (Courtesy S. Maslowski, AEG–Telefunken.)

17.4 Oscillations Related to Nonuniform Population Inversion

Lasher [14] proposed that self-sustaining pulse generation from a laser diode can be produced by placing an emitting region in tandem with an absorbing region, each region being separately driven by a current as shown in Fig. 17.4.1. Both regions are encompassed within the same optical cavity because the two facets of the Fabry–Perot cavity enclose both regions. The dimensions of the two regions and the material parameters are relevant to the

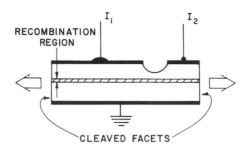

FIG. 17.4.1 Two-section laser diode (tandem structure) with an individual terminal for each section. Both regions are enclosed within the same Fabry–Perot cavity.

operation of the device, which is based on the principle that the absorbing region constitutes a *saturable* absorber, i.e., its absorption coefficient is a function of the photon density. A detailed analysis of such structures can be found in the original paper by Lasher [14] and in the articles by Lee and Roldan [15] and Basov *et al.* [16].

Briefly summarized, the principle of repetitive pulse generation is as follows. Suppose that the emitting region 1 is strongly pumped with current I_1 to a level which produces stimulated emission, while region 2 is less strongly pumped with current I_2 to a level just below that needed for stimulated emission. (Of course, if *both* regions are equally pumped to a level above threshold, then we are dealing with a conventional laser diode operating stably.) Consider what happens when a photon emitted from the emitting region 1 enters the absorbing region 2. Here it produces a new electron–hole pair by absorption, in effect increasing the quasi-Fermi level separation in region 2. If we now suppose that this is just sufficient to yield the required condition for stimulated emission—that the quasi-Fermi level separation must be greater than the photon energy (Chapter 3)—then a following photon entering region 2 from region 1 will produce stimulated emission. However, this latter process again reduces the carrier population within region 2 to the absorbing state for the subsequent photon. Therefore, the net effect of our experiment is the observation of a single stimulated photon being emitted from region 2 (i.e., the whole structure), followed by a pause, and so on. In other words, we have a means of producing short pulses of light on a repetitive basis.

This effect occurs evidently only under rather restrictive conditions dependent on the spontaneous carrier lifetime, the photon lifetime, the dimensions of the structure, basic band parameters (which affect the gain coefficient dependence on carrier density), and the current ratio in the two sections. Lee and Roldan [15] measured repetition rates in the 450–1000 MHz range with pulse lengths of a small fraction of a nanosecond.

Although the specific tandem structure described here has found no practical application to date, the basic concept of oscillations due to inhomogeneous population inversion is a general one. It is possible that optical anomalies in devices containing defects within the active region are related to this process, although characterization of such devices via reasonable models is evidently not possible unless the detailed internal configuration is known. In fact, self-sustaining oscillations increasing in frequency with current in some room temperature DH (AlGa)As laser diodes have been attributed to this effect [17], although other factors cannot be easily dismissed.

It is noteworthy that saturable absorption effects involving traps have been suggested as responsible for Q-switching seen in certain diffused GaAs diodes at cryogenic temperatures. It was postulated [18] that lasing will not occur during the application of the current pulse because the optical losses due to absorption by the traps are too large. At the end of the current pulse, however, the traps (having a special property) transfer from the absorbing to the nonabsorbing state. Thus, the internal loss decreases rapidly as the trap state changes, and the remaining electrons in the conduction band recombine with holes in the valence band giving rise to a narrow burst of emitted light. Although the mathematical model postulated does produce the required effect, no evidence has been found for the existence of such very special traps in GaAs or other materials.

17.5 Diode Modulation

In Section 17.2 we developed the steady-state solution of the rate equations and the transient oscillations near steady state. In this section the rate equations will be developed using a perturbation technique. In particular, the input current to the diode will be split into a "dc" term and a time varying one. The results give a pair of differential equations defining the perturbed (modulated) inversion level and cavity photon density in terms of the steady-state values. Of course, it should be understood that the resulting analysis is only applicable to situations when the perturbing current is small compared to the steady-state dc value. In addition, both the perturbed inversion density and photon density levels must be small compared to their respective dc levels.

Before proceeding with the mathematical development, we consider the various types of modulation applicable to laser diodes. Basically, two types of modulation schemes are useful for optical communication systems: (1) analog modulation and (2) digital or pulse modulation. Here we separate pulse modulation from analog; however, in a strict sense, some pulse modulation schemes are analog in nature.

Analog modulation is obtained by making the perturbing current proportional to the base-band information signal. In this case it is necessary to make the laser light intensity proportional to the modulation signal. Consequently, a linear relation between the light output and current input must be achieved.

A pulsed signal is obtained by appropriately sampling the base-band signal at a rate larger than the Nyquist rate. The total information content of the signal is contained in the amplitudes of the samples. Pulse amplitude modulation (PAM) is a waveform consisting of a series of flat-topped pulses with the height of each pulse corresponding to the value of the message signal.

A pulse-width modulated (PWM) waveform is one consisting of a series of pulses, the width of each pulse being proportional to the value of the message signal at the sampling instants.

Pulse-position modulation (PPM) consists of pulses in which the pulse displacement from a specified time reference is proportional to the sampled values of the signal.

Pulse-code modulation (PCM) is produced by: (1) sampling the base-band signal, (2) quantizing the amplitudes of the samples, and (3) generally encoding the quantized samples into a binary sequence. The binary sequence is then transmitted as a series of "ones" and "zeros" obtained by sending two types of pulses. For example, a binary "one" can be represented by a light pulse, while a binary "zero" can be represented by the absence of a pulse.

Due to the inherent nature of the laser diode (its highly nonlinear characteristics) PCM schemes are desirable. For analog modulation of the laser diode, the device must be stable with respect to power output versus current; diode stability is far less critical for a transmitter designed for PCM.

17.5.1 *Perturbational Solution to the Rate Equations*

The normalized rate equations (17.2.20) and (17.2.21) serve as a starting point for our development. The relevant quantities are

$$j = j^0 + j^1 \tag{17.5.1}$$

$$n_e = n_e{}^0 + n_e{}^1 + n_e{}^2 + \cdots \tag{17.5.2}$$

$$n_{\text{ph}} = n_{\text{ph}}^0 + n_{\text{ph}}^1 + n_{\text{ph}}^2 + \cdots \tag{17.5.3}$$

The dc or steady-state solutions are $n_e{}^0$ and n_{ph}^0 and are due to the dc current j^0. Note that, for the sake of standard nomenclature, we assume in this analysis that $n_e{}^0$ and n_{ph}^0 are the steady-state solutions instead of $\bar{n}_e$ and $\bar{n}_{\text{ph}}$ as used earlier in this chapter The superscriptes here refer to the perturbation order. The *zero* order is assumed to be time independent.

Substituting (17.5.1), (17.5.2) and (17.5.3) into (17.2.20) and (17.2.21) gives for zero order

$$\dot{j}^0 - n_{ph}^0(n_e^{\ 0} - n_{0m}) - n_e^{\ 0} = 0 \tag{17.5.4a}$$

$$n_{ph}^0(n_e^{\ 0} - n_{0m} - 1) + \gamma n_e^{\ 0} = 0 \tag{17.5.4b}$$

The first-order equations are

$$dn_e^{\ 1}/dt = \dot{j}^1 - (n_{ph}^0 + 1) n_e^{\ 1} - (n_e^{\ 0} - n_{0m}) n_{ph}^1 \tag{17.5.5a}$$

$$dn_{ph}^1/dt = w(n_{ph}^0 + \gamma)n_e^{\ 1} + w(n_e^{\ 0} - n_{0m} - 1)n_{ph}^1 \tag{17.5.5b}$$

and the second-order equations are

$$dn_e^{\ 2}/dt = -(n_{ph}^0 + 1)n_e^{\ 2} - (n_e^{\ 0} - n_{0m})n_{ph}^2 - n_e^{\ 1}n_{ph}^1 \tag{17.5.6a}$$

$$dn_{ph}^2/dt = w(n_{ph}^0 + \gamma)n_e^{\ 2} + w(n_e^{\ 0} - n_{0m} - 1)n_{ph}^2 + wn_e^{\ 1}n_{ph}^1 \tag{17.5.6b}$$

The equations defining the zero-order perturbation simply govern the static solution. Equations (17.5.5) can be used to evaluate the time dependence of the inversion level and the photon density to first order and (17.5.6) give second-order dependence. Note that the driving function for the first-order equations is the perturbed current density $\dot{j}^1$, while the driving force of the second order equations is $n_e^{\ 1}n_{ph}^1$, first-order quantities. Consequently, the rate of convergence of this approximate method is dependent upon how the value of $\dot{j}^1$ affects $n_e^{\ 1}$ and n_{ph}^1 relative to $n_e^{\ 0}$ and n_{ph}^0. Accordingly, one has to be particularly careful using only the first-order results when $\dot{j}^0 < \dot{j}_{th}$, while $\dot{j}^0 + \dot{j}^1 > \dot{j}_{th}$ for any t value.

17.5.2   Diode Transfer Function

Using the first-order perturbation equation, we now estimate the frequency characteristics of a laser diode. Frequency information can be conveniently described by a diode transfer function which we define as the ratio of the photon density n_{ph}^1 and the perturbed current $\dot{j}^1$ at a driving frequency f. The harmonic time dependence of the drive current is

$$\dot{j}^1(t) = \dot{j}^1 \exp(i\omega t)$$

and we assume that $n_e^{\ 1}(t)$ and $n_{ph}^1(t)$ also vary harmonically. Equations (17.5.5) become

$$i\omega\tau_s n_e^{\ 1} - \dot{j}^1 - (n_{ph}^0 + 1)n_e^{\ 1} - (n_e^{\ 0} - n_{0m})n_{ph}^1 \tag{17.5.7a}$$

$$i\omega\tau_s n_{ph}^1 = w(n_{ph}^0 + \gamma)n_e^{\ 1} + w(n_e^{\ 0} - n_{0m} - 1)n_{ph}^1 \tag{17.5.7b}$$

Eliminating $n_e^{\ 1}$ in the above equations and solving for the ratio $n_{ph}^1/\dot{j}^1$ we get the transfer function

$$H(\omega) = \frac{w(n_{ph}^0 + \gamma)}{(i\omega\tau_s + n_{ph}^0 + 1)\{i\omega\tau_s - w(n_e^{\ 0} - n_{0m} - 1)\} + w(n_{ph}^0 + \gamma)(n_e^{\ 0} - n_{0m})} \tag{17.5.8}$$

For the case when $\gamma = 0$, the above simplifies to

$$H(\omega) = \frac{w n_{ph}^0}{w n_{ph}^0 - (\omega \tau_s)^2 + i\omega \tau_s (n_{ph}^0 + 1)} \qquad (17.5.9)$$

Figure 17.5.1 shows the transfer function when $\gamma = 0$, $w = 2000$, and $\tau_s = 2$ ns. When $n_{ph}^0 = 1$, the transfer function shows a resonance at $f \cong 3.5$ GHz, while for $n_{ph}^0 = 10$, resonance occurs at $f \cong 11.25$ GHz. These plots can be used to qualitatively analyze the pulsed response of laser diodes. When current pulses are applied to the diodes, high-frequency ringing will occur because the high-frequency components of the pulse spectra are highly amplified compared to the low-frequency ones.

17.6 Summary

Theory exists for predicting (1) transient oscillatory effects during laser turn-on; (2) continuous self-sustaining oscillations in both the photon emis-

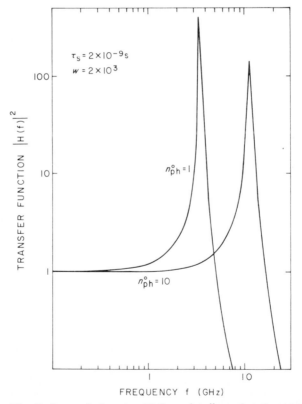

FIG. 17.5.1 The diode transfer function $H(f) = n_{ph}^1/f^1$ as a function of frequency. The resonance frequency is dependent upon the dc injection level as discussed in Section 17.2.

sion and the current density; and (3) repetitive Q-switching effects involving lasers containing emitting and absorbing regions in tandem.

Experimentally, these phenomena are indeed observed, although the specific comparison between theory and experiment is sketchy except for the tandem laser structure. Among the reasons complicating the experimental work are the difficulty of defining the required degree of structural perfection of lasers and, in particular, the filamentary behavior of many laser diodes which can result in noisy characteristics [19,20] in the megahertz range, In addition, multimode behavior is common in laser diodes, with the mode content changing very frequently with the junction current. This makes modeling in terms of a single mode theory difficult. (See Appendix B for other observations concerning deviations from simple theory.)

Other effects which give rise to anomalies in the light output, including instabilities, are related to *weak* mode guiding (Section 8.4), the presence of defects, and isolated absorbing regions within the diode active region. For example, laser diodes that have been seriously degraded by the internal formation of nonradiative centers (Chapter 16) in the course of operation sometimes exhibit oscillatory outputs not seen prior to degradation.

REFERENCES

1. H. Statz and G. DeMars, *in* "Quantum Electronics" (C. H. Townes, ed.). Columbia Univ. Press, New York, 1960.
2. A comprehensive analysis of the maser rate equations is given by D. A. Kleinman, *Bell Syst. Tech. J.* **43**, 1505 (1964).
3. W. Kaiser, C. G. B. Garrett, and D. L. Wood, *Phys. Rev.* **123**, 766 (1961).
4. P. P. Sorokin, M. J. Stevenson, J. R. Lankard, and G. D. Pettit, *Phys. Rev.* **127**, 503 (1962).
5. An introductory discussion of transient behavior in lasers is given by W. V. Smith and P. P. Sorokin, "The Laser," p. 86. McGraw-Hill, New York, 1966.
6. T. Ikegami and Y. Suematsu, *IEEE J. Quantum Electron.* **4**, 148 (1968).
6a. H. Yanai, M. Yano, and T. Kimiya, *IEEE J. Quantum Electron.* **11**, 519 (1975).
7. R. Lang and K. Kobayashi, *IEEE J. Quantum Electron.* **12**, 194 (1976).
8. D. E. McCumber, *Phys. Rev.* **141**, 306 (1966).
9. H. Haug and H. Haken, *Z. Phys.* **204**, 262 (1967).
10. H. Haug, *Phys. Rev.* **184**, 338 (1969).
11. D. J. Morgan and M. J. Adams, *Phys. Status Solidi. (a)* **11**, 243 (1972).
12. L. A. D'Asaro, J. M. Cherlow, and T. L. Paoli, *IEEE J. Quantum Electron.* **4**, 164 (1968).
13. T. L. Paoli, *IEEE J. Quantum Electron.* **11**, 276 (1975).
14. G. J. Lasher, *Solid-State Electron.* **7**, 707 (1964).
15. T. Lee and R. H. R. Roldan, *IEEE J. Quantum Electron.* **6**, 338 (1970).
16. N. G. Basov, V. N. Morozov, V. V. Nikitin, and A. S. Semenov, *Sov. Phys.-Semicond.* **1**, 1305 (1968).
17. T. Ohmi, T. Suzuki, and J. Nishimaki, *Oyo Buturi (Suppl.)* **41**, 102 (1971).

18.   J. E. Ripper and J. C. Dyment, *IEEE J. Quantum Electron.* **5**, 396 (1969).
19.   M. Cross, *Phys. Status Solidi (a)* **16**, 167 (1973) (theory).
20.   G. Guekos and M. J. O. Strutt, *IEEE J, Quantum Electron.* **6**, 423 (1970).

Appendix A

Physical Constants

Name	Symbol	Value	Dimension
Avogadro's number	N_0	6.0249×10^{23}	molecules/g-mole
Boltzmann's constant	k	1.3804×10^{-23}	joule/deg K
		1.3804×10^{-16}	erg/deg K
Electron charge	e	-1.6018×10^{-19}	coulomb
		-4.8029×10^{-10}	esu
		-1.6018×10^{-20}	emu
Electron rest mass	m_0	9.1083×10^{-31}	kg
		9.1083×10^{-28}	g
Electron volt	eV	1.6018×10^{-19}	joule
		1.6018×10^{-12}	erg
Permittivity of free space	ε_0	8.8541×10^{-12}	farad/m
		1	esu
		1.1126×10^{-21}	emu
Permeability of free space	μ_0	$4\pi \times 10^{-7}$	henry/m
		1.1126×10^{-21}	esu
		1	emu
Planck's constant	h	6.6252×10^{-34}	joule-s
		6.6252×10^{-27}	erg-s
Product of photon wave-length and energy	λE	1.2398	μm-eV
Velocity of light under vacuum	c	2.9979×10^8	m/s
		2.9979×10^{10}	cm/s

Major Symbols

The symbols used are defined in the context of each chapter. The following symbols are used throughout and occur frequently.

a_0	Lattice parameter		measure of distance in Section 14.2
CW	Continuous wave		
DFB	Distributed feedback	LOC	Large optical cavity laser
DH	Double-heterojunction laser	LPE	Liquid phase epitaxy
d°	Total width of optical wave-guide perpendicular to the junction. $d^\circ = d_2 + d_3 + d_4$	L_e, L_h	Minority carrier length for electrons and holes, respectively
d_i	Slab width with d_3 the recombination region width	m	Transverse mode number ($m = 1, 2 \ldots$)
e	Electron charge	MBE	Molecular beam epitaxy
E_F	Fermi level	n	Refractive index, with n_i refractive index in region i
E_g	Bandgap energy; ΔE_g bandgap energy step at heterojunction	n_e	effective refractive index
$E_i(E_A, E_D)$	Ionization energy of a recombination center (acceptor, donor)	N (N_A, N_D)	Electron concentration (acceptors, donors)
E_x, E_y, E_z	Electric field components	N_0	Initial electron concentration in recombination region (prior to injection)
FH	Four-heterojunction laser	N_{ss}	Surface state density
f	Frequency	P	Hole concentration
g	Gain coefficient of the recombination region	P_c	Linear power density (in W/cm) for catastrophic damage with semiconductor–air interface
g_{th}	Gain coefficient of the recombination region at threshold		
G_{th}	Gain coefficient of the recombination region at threshold with no free carrier absorption in the recombination region and no cavity end losses	P_θ	Total power radiated from device
		q	Longitudinal mode number
		R, R_a, R_b	Facet reflectivity, of facets a and b; ideal gas constant
h	Planck's constant	R_m	Facet reflectivity of mth transverse mode
h_1, h_2, h_3	Transverse propagation constants	R_s	Diode series resistance
H_x, H_y, H_z	Magnetic field components	R_{th}	Diode thermal resistance
I	Diode current	s	Lateral mode number ($s = 1, 2 \ldots$)
I_{th}	Diode threshold current	S	Surface recombination velocity
J	Current density; J_{th} threshold current density		
k	Boltzmann constant	S_t	Contact stripe width
k_0	Free space wave number ($2\pi/\lambda$)	t_d	Time delay
K_i	Thermal conductivity of ith layer	t	Pulse length; time
		T	Temperature
L	Fabry–Perot cavity length;	T_0	Constant appearing in equation for temperature dependence of threshold

	current	η_{ext}	Differential quantum efficiency
v_{th}	Thermal velocity of carriers	η_p	Power conversion efficiency
VPE	Vapor phase epitaxy	η_0	Free-space wave impedance
W	Fabry–Perot cavity width	$\theta_\perp, \theta_\parallel$	Full angular beam width at
x_i	Al fraction in region (Al_{x_i}-		half-power (direction per-
	$Ga_{1-x_i}As$)		pendicular and parallel to
Δx	Difference in Al fraction be-		the junction plane).
	tween two layers	κ	Relative dielectric constant
α	Absorption coefficient		$(\varepsilon/\varepsilon_0)$
α_{end}	Equivalent absorption asso-	κ'	Real part of dielectric constant
	ciated with cavity end radi-	κ''	Imaginary part of dielectric
	ation loss		constant
α_{fc}	Free carrier absorption of the	κ_{fb}, κ_{bf}	Forward and backward dis-
	recombination region		tributed reflection constants
$\bar{\alpha}$	Weighted modal absorption	κ^l	Distributed-feedback coeffi-
	coefficient due to passive		cient of l_{th} Fourier com-
	regions		ponent
α_i	Bulk absorption coefficient of	$\lambda_L(\lambda_0)$	Lasing wavelength (or relevant
	the ith layer		wavelength)
β_m	Longitudinal mode propaga-	Λ	Grating spacing in DFB laser
	tion constant	ρ_l	Linear dislocation density
γ^*	Minority carrier utilization	σ_t	Capture cross section of states
	(radiative recombination)	$\sigma(x)$	Material conductivity seen by
Γ	Fraction of wave energy con-		the optical field
	fined to the recombination	τ	Minority carrier lifetime
	region	$\tau_r(\tau_s)$	Minority carrier lifetime for
Δn_{ij}	Index discontinuity between		radiative (spontaneous) re-
	regions i and j. For sym-		combination
	metrical double-heterojunc-	τ_{nr}	Minority carrier lifetime for
	tion structures Δn denotes		nonradiative recombination
	the index step between the	τ_{ph}	Photon lifetime
	recombination region and	ϕ	Minority carrier potential barri-
	the outer regions		er at isotype heterojunction
ε	Dielectric constant	ψ_m	Modal wave function
η	Dielectric asymmetry factor	ω_p	Plasma frequency
η_i	Internal quantum efficiency	ω	Angular frequency

Appendix B

Gain in Strong Fields and Lateral Multimoding

B.1 Introduction

There is extensive theory relating the gain coefficient to the population inversion for various models of the energy bands (Chapter 3). They lead to rate equations (Chapter 17) useful for discussing the operation of the idealized laser. However, the effect of the optical field leads to perturbation of the lasing medium, and two interactions have been examined: (1) a dependence of the carrier inversion on optical power at fixed carrier injection rate, and (2) a dependence of optical gain at fixed inversion on optical power. The importance of these two effects on laser-diode operation is still being examined by comparison of model calculations to observable parameters, in particular to the dependence on junction voltage (or spontaneous intensity) of the total power, the mode thresholds and modal power distribution, and the polarization. Our discussion touches on the causes for lateral multimoding (Chapter 7).

B.2 Spatial Modulation of the Gain and Multimoding

It has long been recognized that high optical fields in laser media may depress the local inversion level and hence the gain coefficient [1]. The depression may be spatially uniform or may reflect the pattern of the optical modes. Phenomena associated with this effect are commonly denoted "spatial hole burning." The effect depends in detail on the lasing media.

Consider a semiconductor laser where the standing wave pattern associated

585

with a lateral mode produces variation in optical field intensity. As the current is increased above threshold, the inversion in the regions of peak intensity will be gradually reduced. The spatial inhomogeneity produced is a balance between injection, recombination, and diffusion currents. Hakki [2] used the idea of local gain depletion and carrier redistribution to explain the shift from the dominant fundamental to the next mode in narrow stripe-contact lasers. His analysis includes consideration of the relationship of the diffusion length to the stripe width and the ability of the structure to distribute the injected current. Index changes or other factors that perturb the field distribution are neglected in the simple model.

The proposed sequence of events as the laser is turned on is as follows. Assume a planar stripe laser (say 10 μm stripe width). The fundamental mode reaches threshold first, since it couples most effectively to the injected carrier distribution, which peaks under the stripe contact. As we increase the current, the prorated gain of the fundamental mode remains at its threshold value; however, there is gain depletion near the stripe center, where the standing wave peaks, and an enhancement away from the center sufficient to keep the overall gain constant. Eventually, a current level is reached where the perturbed gain distribution begins to couple effectively to the second mode (with its two optical field peaks symmetrically placed under the stripe contact). Thus, we reach threshold for the second mode, which now shares power with the fundamental mode.

No direct experimental support for the model has been presented. Hakki's calculations are consistent with the observation that fundamental mode operation is more easily sustained in 10 μm-wide planar stripe lasers than in lasers with 20 μm stripes (Chapter 17). Note that in this model the *average* inversion level may be constant and thus the *average* spontaneous emission is constant with drive, although local variations (difficult to measure) are occurring. As discussed in Section B.4, a nearly constant spontaneous emission level has been seen in some stripe lasers, but its importance is still controversial. No correlations of this effect with lateral mode changes have been made.

B.3   Optically Induced Saturation of Transition Probabilities

North [3] described the time evolution of the stimulated emission by a rate equation with an inherent nonlinearity,

$$dQ/dt = [g/(1 + Q/Q^*) - \alpha]Q + \text{spontaneous term} \qquad (B.3.1)$$

Here, Q is the Poynting vector of a traveling wave and g and α are the customary gain and loss coefficients prorated over a round trip of the cavity. Q^* is an optical constant characteristic of the optical nonlinearity that controls the amplitude of the lasing oscillations. For calculation, it is assumed to be independent of the lasing mode. In contrast to the classical treatment [1], it concentrates on the effect of the running waves and ignores any interaction with standing waves.

It can be shown [3] that (B.3.1) leads to the power in mode k above threshold

$$P_k = P_k^*[(g_k/\alpha_k - 1)], \qquad g_k \geq \alpha_k \qquad (B.3.2)$$

g_k and α_k are the prorated gain and loss coefficients (including end loss); and p_k^* is the critical power in mode k describing the nonlinearity. The total radiated coherent power P_θ is

$$P_\theta = (1 - R) \sum P_k^*[(g_k/\alpha_k - 1)] \qquad (B.3.3)$$

R is the facet reflectivity (averaged over the excited modes) and Σ means summation over all positive values of the summand.

In this model, to increase the power, the inversion must be increased, and new modes become excited as their thresholds are crossed. The simple experimental prediction is a monotonic increase of gain (or junction voltage or spontaneous emission) with lasing power throughout the lasing region.

Quantitative test of North's model requires modeling of the gain and loss coefficients of all the lasing modes. With narrow stripe lasers, no appropriate modeling has been performed, and so the experimental tests have been restricted to wide lasers. In these, many lateral modes are excited, and average modal properties can be used to test the theory. Most of the tests are on diodes with sawed sides, in which the modal loss coefficient was dominated by Rayleigh scattering from the granular walls, an effect that can be calculated.

The basis for determining the loss of various lateral box modes of the wide laser is that the roughness of the side walls introduces a scattering loss proportional to the square of the glancing angle of the propagating plane wave. The dependence of the loss coefficient on lateral mode number s is [3]

$$\alpha \doteq \alpha_0 + b(s - 1)^2 \doteq \alpha_0 + B\theta^2, \qquad s = 1, 2, \ldots \qquad (B.3.4)$$

with b and B being geometric constants depending on the sawing, and $\pm \theta$ the lateral deviation from the normal to the facet of the pair of principal lobes radiated by a mode with lateral index s; α is independent of longitudinal mode number. All propagating modes have the same transverse index. (For single-heterojunction lasers, this is generally the lowest, $m = 1$).

The predicted dependence of the full beam width at half power in the junction plane on power emitted by the laser is

$$\theta_\parallel \sim P_\theta^{1/4} \qquad (B.3.5)$$

Equation (B.3.5) was satisfied at all high powers in a variety of broad-area lasers [4]. In a later study [5], the spontaneous emission (Section B.4) was correlated with the mode proliferation. These studies show that the model describes the lateral beam increase with drive of wide sawed lasers, and the close relation between coherent properties and the spontaneous power.

A significant observation of Sommers and North [3] was that P^* in (B.3.2) was a material constant—i.e., independent of cavity geometry—and had essentially the same value for all types of heterojunction lasers. A value of P^* of order of 10 mW was reported in homojunction and single-heterojunction lasers [4], in double-heterojunction lasers radiating only the fundamental or only a high-order transverse mode [4], in broad-area lasers with box modes [6], and in narrow stripe-contact lasers supporting modes of Hermite–Gaussian character [7]. Thus, the critical parameter producing the multimoding has been reported to be independent of facet area over a range of nearly two orders of magnitude, in contrast to the model of Section B.2 where the optical field intensity is the key parameter expressed in units of watts per square centimeter.

North [3] attributes the nonlinearity to saturation of the transition probability, which he believes should occur in a strongly coupled system such as a semiconductor at a critical level

$$P^* = \hbar\omega(\Delta\omega_h)^2/\Delta\omega_s. \tag{B.3.6}$$

$(\hbar\omega)$ is the quantum energy, $\Delta\omega_h$ is the homogeneous linewidth in radians/s, and $\Delta\omega_s$ is the natural linewidth. This is of different dimensions than the constant usually associated with saturation of transition probabilities based on analysis of a collection of weakly interacting molecules [8]. The predicted level of P^* is in the milliwatt range using reasonable values of 10^{13} s^{-1} for the homogeneous line width due to electron or phonon scattering and 10^9 s^{-1} for the natural line width. However, because of lack of tests by other types of experiments, the interpretation of P^* is still tentative.

B.4   Spontaneous Power in the Lasing Region

The model of Section B.3 for the semiconductor laser predicts a quantitative connection between the coherent power and the spontaneous power at wavelengths shorter than the lasing wavelength [5]. Figure B.4.1 shows curves of the spontaneous emission from a GaAs laser measured at specific wavelengths ($\lambda_L \cong 8925$ Å). The spontaneous emission for $\lambda < \lambda_L$ continues to increase through threshold, while the longer wavelength radiation saturates because the states are filled and the spontaneous recombination rate is therefore independent of drive [9].

Other studies showed a similar growth of spontaneous emission above threshold [10], but differences have also been reported [11, 12], in particular, the behavior of a narrow stripe-contact laser [11] in which the spontaneous emission saturates at threshold, or even decreases over some current range

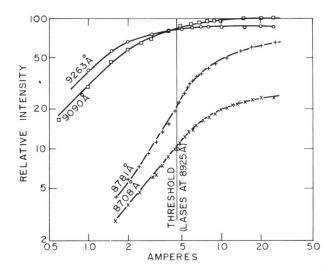

FIG. B.4.1 The relative intensity of the spontaneous radiation below and above threshold from a GaAs laser (broad-area). The radiation is measured at various wavelengths with a spectrometer resolution of 25 Å. The long wavelength emission saturates whereas the short wavelength emission increases through threshold [9].

[12]. More examples of similar behavior, with quantitative data on model powering and modeling of the gain and loss coefficients of the cavity modes, are needed to show if there is a discrepancy with the theory of North.

B.5 Summary

The small signal approximation that neglects the effect of the stimulating field on the gain coefficient is inadequate in a strong field. Two viewpoints exist regarding the relation of the gain to the optical power level in the lasing regime. These affect the explanation for lateral multimoding in laser diodes, although no consistent model exists to explain stripe-contact and wide lasers.

(1) Spatial modulation of the gain is produced by the modal standing wave pattern. The inversion is assumed reduced in the high field region with a corresponding reduction in the *local* gain coefficient. Consider a stripe-contact laser. With increasing drive above threshold, a redistribution of carriers by diffusion is assumed to occur that decreases the coupling of the gain profile to the fundamental lateral mode while producing a distribution that increases the coupling to the next order mode. Thus, the threshold of the higher-order mode is eventually reached. In this model, the prorated modal gain in a single mode laser remains fixed at its threshold value. Therefore, the *average* spontaneous emission rate is constant above threshold although local variations can

occur. This simple model is not helpful in explaining lateral mode proliferation in devices where lateral mode loss increases with order—the sawed-side laser, for example. However, note that in stripe-contact lasers, the inversion (gain) can increase above threshold if the current spread away from the contact is changing. Therefore, lateral multimoding involving the threshold of higher-order, lossier modes is consistent with the idea that local gain reduction can occur when the field intensity becomes sufficiently high.

(2)   A nonlinearity is proposed resulting from a saturation of the transition probability. Modes with increasing loss reach threshold as the drive is increased, because the prorated gain does not saturate at threshold. Therefore, the growth of the spontaneous emission above threshold is quantitatively tied to the mode proliferation. The ability to sustain operation exclusively in one lateral mode with drive will depend on the difference in threshold between modes.

There are insufficient experimental data and cavity modeling to show that either model describes all types of injection lasers. Furthermore, we have neglected index changes with drive, which perturb the cavity and thus affect modal fields. Moreover, analysis of the data from stripe-contact lasers can be hindered by the lack of precision in defining the extent of the active region. Because the current can spread as the drive is increased in the absence of strong lateral "walls," the nature of the optical cavity changes, making it difficult to attribute phenomena such as junction voltage or spontaneous emission changes above threshold to a unique origin.

REFERENCES

1. A. Yariv, "Quantum Electronics," 2nd Ed. p. 165. Wiley, New York, 1975, p. 165. (An introductory treatment.)
2. B. W. Hakki, *J. Appl. Phys.* **46**, 292 (1975).
3. H. S. Sommers and D. O. North, *Solid-State Electron.* **8**, 675 (1976).
4. H. S. Sommers, Jr., *J. Appl. Phys.* **44**, 1263 (1973).
5. H. S. Sommers, Jr., and D. O. North, *J. Appl. Phys.* **45**, 1787 (1974).
6. H. S. Sommers, Jr., *J. Appl. Phys.* **45**, 237 (1974).
7. H. S. Sommers, Jr., *J. Appl. Phys.* **46**, 1844 (1975).
8. R. Karpus and J. Schwinger, *Phys. Rev.* **73**, 2020 (1948).
9. H. S. Sommers, Jr., *Appl. Phys. Lett.* **19**, 424 (1971).
10. P. Brosson, J. E. Ripper and N. B. Patel, *IEEE J. Quantum Electron.* **9**, 273 (1973).
11. T. L. Paoli, *IEEE J. Quantum Electron.* **9**, 267 (1973).
12. P. Brosson, N. Patel, and J. E. Ripper, *Appl. Phys. Lett.* **23**, 94 (1973).

Appendix C

Pressure Effects on Heterojunction Laser Diodes

C.1 Uniaxial Stress

Double-heterojunction $Al_xGa_{1-x}As/Al_yGa_{1-y}As$ lasers were subjected to stress levels up to about 7×10^8 dynes/cm^2 and the effect on the threshold current density and spontaneous emission efficiency (i.e., below lasing threshold) was studied [1]. (It is important to note that uniaxial stress can produce crystal damage, the diode material being relatively soft. Therefore, it is important to recheck the properties of the diodes *after* the test to establish that the effects observed are indeed reversible.) In these experiments, the major conclusions were that the diode threshold current density *increased* with stress *only* if the Al concentration in the recombination region was in excess of 10%, and the greater the Al concentration (to 18%) the greater was the J_{th} increase with pressure. Diodes with GaAs in the recombination region exhibited a small *reduction* in J_{th} with pressure. The maximum J_{th} increase observed, with diodes where the Al concentration was 18%, was between 5 and 20% with a stress of 7×10^8 dynes/cm^2.

The increase in J_{th} with pressure and with increasing Al in the recombination region was correlated with a decrease in the carrier lifetime with pressure, and it was suggested that the J_{th} change resulted from a changing capture cross section of nonradiative centers. The density of such centers could be a function of the Al concentration. (The changes observed are too large to be explained by a change in the electron population in the conduction band minimum with pressure as a result of the reduced energy separation to the higher lying indirect valleys with pressure.)

Studies of DH lasers with GaAs in the recombination region have shown that the application of $\langle 100 \rangle$ uniaxial stress can result in a change in the polarization of the emitted radiation [2]. Most DH lasers operate in the TE mode, and for these Patel *et al.* [2] find that a shift to TM mode operation occurs when the stress reaches about $\sim 10^7$ dynes/cm^2. Whereas up to that value J_{th} *increases* slightly with pressure, J_{th} *decreases* with pressure after the switching to TM mode operation occurs. However, the magnitude of the effect varies from diode to diode. As explained in Chapter 6, the preferred TE mode operation is believed to be primarily the result of facet reflectivity effects which favor TE over TM modes. The stress-induced change from TE to TM operation was explained by an early model [3] based on the stress-induced splitting of the valence band valley into two doubly degenerate bands, the light hole band and the heavy hole band. This splitting may affect the relative gain coefficient of TE and TM modes by favoring TM modes.

C.2   Hydrostatic Stress

Because of the isotropic nature of the applied stress, there is considerably less danger of diode damage in hydrostatic pressure experiments than in uniaxial ones and much higher pressure levels can be safely applied. Hydrostatic stress is mainly expected to change the lasing photon energy (via the change in the bandgap energy with pressure); effects associated with changes in the crystal symmetry of the type possible under uniaxial stress are not expected. However, because the Γ conduction band minimum is raised with hydrostatic stress by 10.7 meV/kbar [4] while the X minima are lowered by ~ 1 meV/kbar, interband carrier transfer can occur since the separation between the X and Γ minima will decrease with stress by ~ 11.8 meV/kbar. Significant interband carrier transfer GaAs requires large stresses. Starting with an energy separation of ~ 0.4 eV, ~ 33 kbar will be needed to bring the X and Γ valleys into coincidence. Therefore, experiments to test these effects are best performed using alloys in which the energy separation of the valleys can be adjusted and the study of (AlGa)As lasers offers such an opportunity.

Hydrostatic pressure experiments have been conducted [5] using double-heterojunction and LOC laser diodes where the $Al_xGa_{1-x}As$ composition in the recombination region was increased from $x = 0$ to $x = 0.23$. Figure C.2.1 shows the normalized increase with pressure p in the room temperature threshold current density $[1/J_{th}(0)] (\partial J_{th}/\partial p)$ as a function of the Al fraction x in the recombination region of the diode. Considering the simplest model for the change in internal quantum efficiency in a p-type recombination region with decreasing separation between Γ and X, we expect that

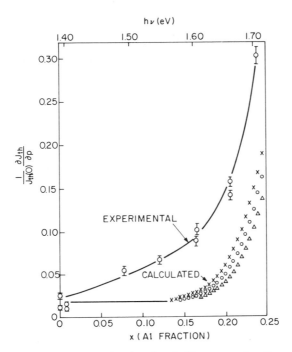

FIG. C.2.1 Normalized change in the threshold current density with hydrostatic pressure (at 300 K) of $Al_xGa_{1-x}As$ laser diodes as a function of x in the recombination region. The experimental data are compared to calculated curves assuming varying values of the electron population $(\Delta N)_\Gamma$ in the direct conduction band valley: $\times = 2.5 \times 10^{18}$ cm^{-3} $\bigcirc = 2 \times 10^{18}$ cm^{-3}, $\triangle = 1.5 \times 10^{18}$ cm^{-3} [5].

$$\frac{1}{J_{th}(0)}\frac{\partial J_{th}}{\partial p} = \frac{1}{J_{th}(0)}\frac{\partial}{\partial p}\left(\frac{1}{1+(\Delta N)_X/(\Delta N)_\Gamma}\right) \qquad \text{(C.2.1)}$$

where $J_{th}(0)$ is the threshold current density at atmospheric pressure and $(\Delta N)_X$ and $(\Delta N)_\Gamma$ are the electron concentrations in the X and Γ conduction band minima, respectively. This analysis neglects the presence of the L conduction band minima, which also increase in energy with pressure.

Various values of $(\Delta N)_\Gamma$ in the p-type recombination region at threshold are assumed in Fig. C.2.1 because of the need to take into account the electron quasi-Fermi level position (Section 12.2.3). The agreement between the simple theory and experiment is reasonable, except for the unexplained observation that the J_{th} sensitivity to pressure is excessive for $x \lesssim 0.1$. This is believed unrelated to the carrier distribution change among the bands with pressure but rather associated with changes in the nonradiative recombination processes with pressure.

With regard to the change in the lasing *photon energy* with pressure, the observed value is dependent on the dominant longitudinal mode lines. From spontaneous emission experiments, the increase in the GaAs bandgap energy is estimated to be 1.14×10^{-2} eV/kbar (as measured up to ~ 5 kbar). In fact, the GaAs bandgap pressure dependence is not quite linear, being found to be (up to 180 kbar) given by [6]

$$E_g(p) - E_g(0) = 1.26 \times 10^{-2}p - 3.77 \times 10^{-5}p^2 \qquad \text{(C.2.2)}$$

where $E_g(p)$ and $E_g(0)$ are bandgap values at pressure p (in kilobars) and at atmospheric pressure, respectively.

Figure C.2.2 shows that the individual longitudinal mode lines of the laser diode emission change at a slower rate with pressure than the spontaneous emission peak energy, although the *center* of the mode line distribution does follow the spontaneous peak energy shift. The slow *individual* longitudinal line shift with pressure is the result of a change in the refractive index with pressure,

$$\frac{1}{\lambda}\frac{d\lambda_q}{dp} = -\frac{1}{h\nu}\frac{d(h\nu)}{dp} = \frac{(1/L)(dL/dp) + (1/n)(dn/dp)}{[1 - (\lambda/n)(dn_q/d\lambda_q)_p]} \qquad \text{(C.2.3)}$$

where L is the laser length and n_q is the refractive index at the wavelength λ_q.

In Eq, (C.2.3), the length change with pressure is small whereas the term in the denominator is ~ 1.5, leaving the change of n_q with pressure the dominant effect. From Fig. C.2.2 for the shift in the mode energy with pressure $(0.27 \times 10^{-2}$ eV/kbar), we obtain in the vicinity of the lasing wavelength the index dependence on pressure,

$$\frac{1}{n}\frac{dn}{dp} = -0.33 \times 10^{-2} \, \text{kbar}^{-1} \qquad \text{(C.2.4)}$$

This value, measured at room temperature, falls within the range of measured quantities, below room temperature, or $-0.4 \pm 0.1 \times 10^{-2}$ kbar^{-1} [4, 7].

REFERENCES

1. T. Kobayashi and K. Sugiyama, *Jpn. J. Appl. Phys.* **12**, 1388 (1973).
2. N. Patel, J. E. Ripper, and P. Brosson, *IEEE J. Quantum Electron.* **9**, 338 (1973).
3. R. C. Miller, F. M. Ryan, and P. R. Emtage, *Proc. Int. Conf. Phys. Semicond. Paris* (1964).
4. J. Feinleib, S. Groves, W. Paul, and R. Zallen, *Phys. Rev.* **131**, 2070 (1963).
5. Y. Juravel, Thesis, Yeshiva Univ. (1976).
6. B. Welber, J. Cardona, C. K. Kim, and S. Rodriguez, *Phys. Rev. B* **12**, 5729 (1975).
7. M. J. Stevenson, J. D. Axe, and J. R. Lankard, *IBM J. Res. Develop.* **7**, 155 (1963).

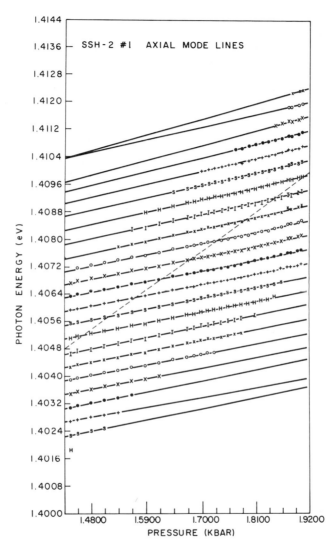

FIG. C.2.2 Shift of the axial mode lines with hydrostatic pressure compared with that of the spontaneous emission peak. As the pressure increases, some of the mode lines disappear and new ones appear. Note that the spontaneous peak shift (dashed line) follows the center of the mode line energy distribution [5].

Appendix D

Atmospheric Attenuation of GaAs Laser Emission

Line of sight communication systems offer interesting possibilities over limited distances. The atmospheric attenuation of GaAs laser radiation intensity is characterized by an equation of the form $\exp(-\alpha_a l)$ where l is the distance and α_a the attenuation coefficient. At a wavelength of ~ 9000 Å the major source of attenuation is scattering. Table D.1 shows α_a for various meteorological conditions [1]. Figure D.1 shows how the atmospheric transmission varies under various weather conditions. Design aspects of a voice communication using laser diodes are given by Hannan *et al.* [1].

TABLE D.1
Attenuation Coefficient for Various
Meteorological Conditions at 9020 Å [1]

Attenuation coefficient, α_a (km^{-1})	Meteorological description
8	Moderate fog
4	Light fog
2	Thin fog
1	Haze
0.4	Light haze
0.2	Clear
0.08	Very clear
0.014	Exceptionally clear (pure air)

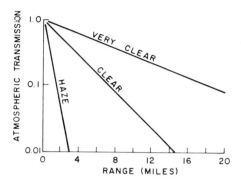

FIG. D.1 Atmospheric transmission under various weather conditions [1].

REFERENCE

1   W. Hannan, D. Karlsons, J. Bordogna, T. Penn, and W. Dravneek, *RCA Rev.* **28**, 609
     (1967).

Single Mode Emission Line Width

An approximation to the line width of the emission due to a single laser mode was given by Schawlow and Townes [1, 2], and modifications for the semiconductor laser have been discussed by several authors [3, 4]. These consider the degree of inversion of the carrier population and operating conditions, but do not change the basic form of the expression discussed here, which provides an order of magnitude theoretical estimate for the line width.

The basic reason for broadening of the emission due to a single mode in stimulated emission is the continuing spontaneous emission rate above threshold (as discussed for the simple model in Section 17.2.2). Although normally negligible compared to the number of photons in the mode due to stimulated emission, the photons emitted into the mode from spontaneous recombination do introduce random phase oscillations. However, since the number of stimulated photons in the mode increases with pump rate above threshold while in the simple theory the spontaneous emission rate is constant, the emission line width $\Delta\nu$ (full width at half-power) increases with increasing photon *number* N_{ph},*

$$\Delta\nu \approx 2(\delta\nu_c)/N_{ph} \qquad \text{(E.1)}$$

where $\delta\nu_c$, the line width of the mode, is deduced as follows. Consider the resonant modes of the cavity as independent oscillators with frequency ν. The quality factor of the cavity Q for the mode (oscillator) with frequency ν_0 is defined by

---

*N_{ph} here denotes the number of photons in the mode; in Chapter 17 this symbol was used to denote the density of photons (number in the mode per cubic centimeter).

$$Q = (2\pi\nu_0)\tau_{ph} = \nu_0/\delta\nu_c, \qquad \delta\nu_c = (2\pi\tau_{ph})^{-1} \qquad (E.2)$$

where τ_{ph} is the photon lifetime, equal to $[(c/n)(\bar{\alpha} + L^{-1}\ln(1/R))]^{-1}$ (where c is the velocity of light, n the refractive index at λ_0, $\bar{\alpha}$ the internal absorption coefficient, L the laser length, and R the facet reflectivity).

Since the power in the laser mode P_m is

$$P_m = N_{ph}(h\nu_0)/\tau_{ph} \qquad (E.3)$$

from (E.1), (E.2), and (E.3), we obtain [1]

$$\Delta\nu \approx A_0 \frac{4\pi(h\nu_0)(\delta\nu_c)^2}{P_m} \qquad (E.4)$$

The term A_0 in (E.4) is perhaps ~ 2 for operation not far above threshold. In the following illustration we assume that $A_0 = 1$ to obtain an order of magnitude estimate for the line width.

For illustration, consider a laser diode where $\bar{\alpha} = 10 \text{ cm}^{-1}$ and the cavity end loss is 30 cm^{-1}; the photon lifetime is

$$\tau_{ph}^{-1} = [(3 \times 10^{10}/3.6)](10 + 30) = 3.3 \times 10^{11} \text{ s}^{-1}$$

Therefore,

$$\delta\nu_c = (3.3 \times 10^{11})/2\pi = 5.3 \times 10^{10} \text{ s}^{-1}$$

If the laser energy $h\nu_0 = 1.5 \text{ eV} = (1.5)(1.6 \times 10^{-12}) = 2.4 \times 10^{-12} \text{ erg}$ and the power in the mode is $P_m = 10 \text{ mW} = 10^5 \text{ ergs/s}$, then from (E.4)

$$\Delta\nu \cong \frac{(4\pi)(2.4 \times 10^{-12})(5.3 \times 10^{10})^2}{10^5} = 0.85 \text{ MHz}$$

This corresponds to a spectral width

$$\Delta\lambda \cong (8.5 \times 10^5)/(4.39 \times 10^{10}) = 1.9 \times 10^{-5} \text{ Å}$$

The values routinely measured in CW laser diodes operating at room temperature are generally much larger. This is possibly because of fluctuations in the temperature of the device which introduce variations in the cavity dimensions, and unresolved broadening from lateral modes. As noted in Section 14.3, $\Delta\lambda \cong 0.16$ Å has been measured using a high resolution spectrometer for a laser operating in the fundamental lateral mode. However, at low temperatures careful interferometric measurements of the single mode emission from CW GaAs laser diodes have produced line widths of 0.15 MHz [5], which are much closer to the expected numbers from simple theory.

Measurements [6] have also been made of the single mode emission from a $Pb_{0.88}Sn_{0.12}Te$ laser diode emitting at $\lambda = 10.6 \mu m$ at very low temperatures. The modal emission intensity was found to fit a Lorentzian shape $\{1 + [2(\nu - \nu_0)/\Delta\nu]^2\}^{-1}$, with the line width $\Delta\nu = 54$ kHz in reasonable agreement with Eq. (E.4) for the specific device. This work also showed the expected reduction in the line width with increasing power in the mode.

REFERENCES

1. A. L. Schawlow and C. H. Townes, *Phys. Rev.* **112**, 1940 (1958).
2. W. P. Smith and P. P. Sorokin, "The Laser," p. 115. McGraw-Hill, New York, 1966 (an introductory treatment of the problem is presented).
3. V. F. Elesin and V. V. Rusakov, *Sov. J. Quantum Electron.* **5**, 1239 (1976).
4. Y. U. Mironov, V. I. Molochev, V. V. Nikitin, and A. S. Semenov, *Sov. J. Quantum Electron.* **6**, 123 (1976).
5. W. E. Ahearn and J. W. Crowe, *IEEE J. Quantum Electron.* **2**, 597 (1966).
6. E. D. Hinkley and C. Freed, *Phys. Rev. Lett.* **23**, 277 (1969).

Index

A

Absorption coefficient
  through atmosphere, 597–598
  in laser, 77–102, 162–165, 261–280
  in LED, 402
AlGaAsSb, 438
AlInP, 361, 388, 418
Al_2O_3, 537
AlP, liquid phase epitaxy, 353
Arrays (laser diodes), 456, 461
Atomic bonding, 11
Atmospheric transmission (GaAs laser), 597–598
Auger recombination, 29, 46–47

B

Band bending of heterojunctions, 63
Band filling, 59, 115
Bandgap energy
  of alloys, 357–363
  direct and indirect, 15
  shift with pressure, 594
  shift with temperature, 107, 433
  shrinkage, 91, 105–107
  III–V compounds, 305
  III–V compound ternaries (table), 358

Band structure
  of heterojunctions, 62–67
  IV–VI compounds, 439–440
  III–V compounds, 11–16
Bandtail states, 19–21, 25–26
Beam width, *see* Radiation pattern
Bimolecular recombination, 30, 257, 489
Blackbody radiation, 81
Bloch wave functions, 13
Bohr radius, 17
Bragg scattering, 523
Breakdown voltage (p n junction), 55
Brewster angle, 135
Brillouin zone, 14
Broad-area devices, 535

C

Capacitance–voltage relation, 51–61, 64, 66
Carrier confinement, 249–253
  effect of loss, 280–285
  interfacial recombination, 254–255
  temperature dependence, 253
Carrier diffusion length
  in (AlGa)As, 373
  in GaAs, 344–345
Carrier injection, 32

Carrier lifetime
  basic limit, 29
  effect on lasing threshold, 259–261
  below lasing threshold, 257
Carrier mobility in (AlGa)As, 372–374
Catastrophic degradation, 533–537
Cathodoluminescence apparatus, 413
Close-confinement (single-heterojunction) laser,
    2, 139, 228–230, 406–407
Coherence, 143
Collection angle, 459
Confinement factor Γ, 159, 216, 217
Continuous-wave laser
  conditions for, 428–432
  emission at 1–1.2 μm, 446–453
  IV–VI compounds, 439–446
  practical structures for room temperature
      operation, 473–485
  visible emission, 502–510
Coupled waves, 523
Coupling light into fibers, 472–473, 494–498
Covalent radii, 12
Critical angle, 188
Cross section, capture, 56
Current–gain characteristics, 92, 96
Current–voltage curve (heterojunction), 68–70

D

Dark regions, 540
Debye screening length, 18, 39
Degradation (internal) of diodes
  accelerated testing, 552–553
  causes, 546–548
  effect of materials, 542–546
  general observations, 538–542
  reliability data, 549–553
Delay (in lasing), 256–257
  relation to current, 257
Density of states, 21–26
Depletion region, *see* Space charge region
Detector (optical communications), 499
Dielectric coatings, 537
Dielectric constant
  complex, 120–122
  free space, 121
Diffusion
  coefficient, 34
  current, 53
  length, 34

  of minority carriers, 33–34
  selective (Zn), 474
Diode equation, 56
Dislocation
  description, 298–300
  etch, 400
  nonradiative recombination, 313–314
  reduction in vapor phase epitaxy, 315–318
Dispersion (in fibers)
  material, 465–472
  modal, 468–472
  relation, 242
Distributed feedback coefficient, 524
Distributed feedback laser, 523–531
  (AlGa)As/GaAs, 527–531
  theory, 523–527
Donor–acceptor pair radiation, 42–44
Dopants, 16–21
  acceptor, 16
  donor, 16
Driver circuits, *see* Pulsers

E

Edge-emitting LED, 485–500
Effective mass (carriers in semiconductors), 13,
    15–16
  (AlGa)As, 419
Eigenmodes, 150
Einstein coefficients (of induced emission), 77–84
Electric field
  related to facet damage, 536
  related to radiation power, 213
Electron affinity, 62–66
Electronegativity, 12, 39–40
Emission
  multiphonon, 44
  stimulated, 77
  wavelength dependence on doping, 109–115
Excitons, 38–42, 103–109

F

Fabry–Perot cavity, 1, 45
Facet, 191
  field distribution at, 196
Facet coatings (laser), 409
Facet damage
  catastrophic degradation, 533–537
  erosion, 537–538

Fermi–Dirac distribution, 22
Fermi level temperature dependence, 23–24
Fibers (optical)
  diode radiation coupling, 472–473
  properties, 465–473
Filaments, 402, 476
Forward mode, 524
Fourier transform of waveguide modes, 176
Free-carrier absorption, 263–264
Frequency response of diode, *see* Modulation

G

Gain coefficient
  in semiconductor, 84–102
  spatial variation, 585–586, 589–590
  at threshold, 262–275
  two-level atomic system, 82–84
GaAs, 327–345
  carrier mobility, 332
  dopant ionization energy, 329–331
  lattice, 10
GaP, 346–351
GaSb, 351–352
Gradual degradation, *see* Degradation
Grated structures, 523

H

Hermite–Gaussian modes, 168–172, 201–202
Hermite polynomials, 170
Heterojunction, 61–70
  anisotype, 61
  band diagram of, 62
  capacitance of, 64, 66
  carrier confinement, 249–253
  double, 206–222
  effect on refractive index, 413–415
  electron affinity of, 62
  isotype, 61
  laser with four heterojunctions, 222–229
  radiation confinement, 206–230
Heterojunction lasers (general), 137–143
High power (peak) lasers, 455
Hole burning, 585–590
Huygens obliquity factor, 187

I

Illumination, 455
InAs, 352, 391

InGaAs, 438
InP, 352–353, 391
InGaAsP, 390
Injection efficiency
  at heterojunctions, 68
  homojunction, 54
Infrared emission lasers
  AlGaAsSb/GaAsSb, 392, 448–453
  InGaAs, 448–452
  InGaAsP, 390–392, 448–453, 498
  InGaAsSb/InAs, 391
  IV–VI materials, 439–446
Interstitial atom, 17
Intrusion alarm, 455
Isoelectronic centers, 39–42

J

Junction delineation, 400

K

Kinks (laser power curve), 476–479, 571–573
Kirchhoff–Huygens, 187

L

Large optical cavity (LOC), 230–234
Laser diode types, description, 137–141
Laser topology, 137–143
  double heterojunction, 140
  five-layer device, 139
  four-heterojunction (FH) device, 141
  index steps, origin of, 142–143
  large optical cavity (LOC), 141
  single-heterojunction, 139
Laser transitions
  effect of dopants, 109–115
  pure materials, 103–109
Lattice parameter, 9–10
  effect on epitaxial growth, 298–318
  effect of mismatch on junction, 72
  IV–VI compounds, 439, 390–391
  III–V compounds (table), 305
Lead–salt (IV–VI) lasers, 439–446
  use in spectroscopy, 446–447
Lifetime
  minority carrier, 260
  photon, 102
  radiative carrier, 489

Light–current characteristics, spontaneous
    emission, 70
Light–voltage curve (heterojunction), 70–73
Linearity, light versus current
    laser diode, 100–101, 476–479, 571–573
    LED, 70–72, 99, 497
Lineshape (homogeneous and inhomogeneous),
    83, 558
Line width of emission spectrum, 599–601
Liquid phase epitaxy
    basic techniques, 287–294
    growth kinetics, 291–294
    multiple-bin boat, 290, 400
    ''Peltier cooling'' growth, 291
Lobe separation (emitted laser beam), 219–
    221
Luminescence
    injection, 27
    photo, 27
Luminescent efficiency, *see* Radiative
    efficiency

M

Maxwell's equations, 119–120
Microplasma, 55
Misfit dislocations
    asymmetry, 312–313
    due to doping, 303–304
    effect on heterojunction interface, 255
    effect on radiative efficiency, 313–314
    in heteroepitaxy, 304–318
    relation to strain, 298–303
    in substrate, 320–323
Mode density, 81
Mode line width, 599–601
Modes
    box modes of rectangular waveguide, 167–
        168
    conversion, 176, 189
    cutoff conditions, 156–158
    Hermite–Gaussian, 168–172
    lateral (s), 142, 238
    longitudinal (q), 96, 142
    propagation in a lossy medium, 162
    radiation of, 146, 150
    three-dimensional, 165–172
    transverse (m), 142
    transverse selection, 180–183
    trapped, bounded, 146, 148

Modulation
    laser diode, 484, 575–579
    LED, 73–75, 488–494
    types, 575–576
Molecular beam epitaxy, 296–298

N

Nd:YAG laser (LED pumped), 518
Nitrogen doping, 39–42
Noise
    degradation-induced, 542
    in laser output, 555, 556–575, 578–579
Nominal threshold current, density, 90–99
Nonradiative recombination, 44–47
Numerical aperture (fiber), 472

O

Ohmic contacts
    IV–VI lasers, 442
    III–V compounds, 400–402
Optical anomalies, 280
Optical cavity (description), 95–98
Optical flux density, 533
Optical power density, 535
Oscillations
    of laser output, 555
    resonant of lasers, 561, 566
    self-sustaining, 566

P

Package (diode), 397–399
    arrays, 398
    CW lasers, 474–476
    for fiber bundle coupling, 489
PbSnTe lasers, 439
PbSSe lasers, 439
Phase diagrams
    application to liquid phase epitaxy, 369–390
    basic principles, 363–369
Phonon kick, 547
Photoluminescence, 35–37, 410–412, 516–517
Photon lifetime, 102
    effect on laser transient properties, 556–579
    effect on mode line width, 599–600
Plane waves, 127–130
    reflection at plane boundaries, 131–135

Plasma frequency, 142
p–n junction
    capacitance, 60
    frequency response, 75
    ideal, 51–55
    nonideal, 56–60
    refractive index step, 285, 407
Polarization, electric field, 131, 174
Population inversion, 77–79, 573–575
Power efficiency, 459, 494
Power emission (LED), 494–498
Poynting's theorem, 123–125
Precipitates in GaAs, 319–320, 334
Pressure
    effect on bandgap, 594
    effect on degradation, 542–543
    effect on refractive index, 594
    hydrostatic on (AlGa)As lasers, 592–595
    hydrostatic on IV–VI lasers, 446
    uniaxial stress of lasers, 591–592
Prism coupler, 153
Propagation constant, 121
Pulsed operation (laser), 455
Pulsers, 461–464

Q

Quantum efficiency
    in direct and indirect bandgap materials, 26–28
    external, 262–275
    internal, 28
    laser differential, 101, 261–275, 403, 459, 505
    of LED, 28–29, 39–44, 405, 486–489,
        510–518
    in ternary alloys, 417–421
Quasi-Fermi level, 78–80, 250
Quaternary alloys, 390–392
    bandgap energy, 391
    diodes, 446–453, 498–500
    lattice parameter, 391

R

Radar (optical), 455
Radiance (LED), 473
Radiation confinement, loss of, 280
Radiation fields, 191–194
Radiation pattern
    box modes, 201
    comparisons of experimental and theoretical,
        234

half-power beam width of, 185, 214, 218
    Hermite–Gaussian modes, 201–202
    intensity profile, 190
    laser, 99–100, 185–247, 459, 477–483
    of LED, 494–498
    TE and TM modes, 198
Radiation zone, 190
Radiative efficiency
    in GaAs, 342–344
    ternary alloys, 417–421
Rate equations, 555–556, 576–579
Rayleigh scattering, 465
Reciprocal lattice, 13–14
Recombination
    via impurity centers, 31
    interfacial, 255
    nonradiative, 28, 44–47
    processes, 35
    radiative, 28
    region, 139–271
Recombination coefficient, 29–31, 84–85, 257–261
Reflection coefficient, 133, 188
Reflection matrix, 177
Reflectivity, 174–180
Reflectivity of facet
    effect on facet damage, 536
    measurement, 271
    role in mode selection, 177–179
Refractive index, 121
    (AlGa)As, 413–414
    effect of doping, 142, 414–417
    effect of gain, 142–143
    effective, 161
    parabolic variation, 169
Relaxation oscillations, 559–562
Resonance frequency (laser noise spectrum),
    566–573
Restricted-edge-emitting diode (REED), 497

S

Saturable absorbers, 283, 574
Saturation effects, 585–590
Sawed-sidewall lasers, 241
Scattering losses
    at laser facet, 175
    at sidewalls, 587
Segregation coefficients
    in GaAs, 334–342
    table of, 338

Schottky barrier, 442
Selfoc fibers, 467
Signal-to-noise (optical communication system), 499
Slab waveguides, 146–162
Snell's law, 132
Solubility of (AlGa)As in HF, 375–376
Space charge region (depletion region), 51–55, 64
Spatial harmonics, 525
Spectral width
    of laser diode, 99–100, 481–484
    of LED, 485–500
    of single mode, 599–600
Spectroscopy, use of IV–VI lasers, 439, 447
Spontaneous power, in the lasing region, 588
Stacks (lasers), 456
Step index fiber, 470
Stoichiometry
    effect on reliability, 543–545
    in IV–VI materials, 442
    in GaAs, 327–329
Stripe-contact laser
    current distribution, 423–428, 589–590
    definition, 138
    technologies, 421–428
    thermal resistance, 428–430
Substrate preparation, polishing of GaAs, 318
Surface-emission LED, 485–500, 510–518

T

Temperature stabilization (circuit), 480
Thermal equilibrium, spontaneous recombination
    rate at, 89

Thermal expansion coefficient, effect on epitaxy, 306, 311, 437
Thermal radiation, 83
Thermal resistance (diode), 428–434
Thin-film characterization
    techniques, 403–404
    using capacitance–voltage measurements, 412
    using photoluminescence, 409–412
Threshold condition, 165
Threshold current, 95–102, 249–280
    temperature dependence, 275–280
Transfer function, 577–578
Transitions
    interband, 98
    intraband, 98
Tunneling at junctions, 59–60

V

Vapor phase epitaxy, basic techniques, 294–295
Visible emission lasers, 500–510
    (AlGa)As, 502–505
    AlGaAsP, 438, 448–449
    Ga(AsP), 501, 506–510
    InGaAsP, 390–392, 448–449
    nitrogen doping, 510

X

x-ray topography, 313–314, 320–322

Y

Yttrium aluminum garnet laser, see Nd:YAG laser